Neuraltherapeutic Medicine

Laura Bibiana Pinilla Bonilla
Eduardo Humberto Beltrán Dussán
Agustín Ricardo Angarita Lezama
Editors

Neuraltherapeutic Medicine

An Evolution of Neural Therapy

Springer

Editors
Laura Bibiana Pinilla Bonilla
Faculty of Medicine, Master in Alternative Medicine, Neural therapy Area
Universidad Nacional de Colombia
Bogotá, Colombia

Agustín Ricardo Angarita Lezama
Faculty of Medicine, Master in Alternative Medicine, Neural Therapy Area
Universidad Nacional de Colombia
Bogotá, Colombia

Eduardo Humberto Beltrán Dussán
Faculty of Medicine
Universidad Nacional de Colombia
Bogotá, Colombia

ISBN 978-3-032-03256-0 ISBN 978-3-032-03257-7 (eBook)
https://doi.org/10.1007/978-3-032-03257-7

This Springer imprint is published by the registered company Springer Nature Switzerland AG
The registered company address is: Gewerbestrasse 11, 6330 Cham, Switzerland

In memory of Dr. Julio Cesar Payán de la Roche, who was a vortex of wisdom and tenderness where giving without expecting was his way of life. He was the joy that poured forth in hugs, smiles, and teachings. Happy and libertarian, he abandoned the security and certainties of the way of understanding life to go conquer the unknown. Training in health with human warmth was a vocation he never renounced. Reading, learning, reflecting, retracing steps, and walking again was his life's journey. His intellectual sharpness laid the new foundations of neuraltherapeutic medicine in Latin America, always listening to the message of ancestral cultures, popular wisdom, and various academic contributions. This book is an offering and a debt for his fruitful dedication.

For the doctor Ricardo Véjar Vacas, a worldly human being who lived in Ecuador with a heart full of sensitivity, love, generosity, responsibility, and an unparalleled commitment to service. From his fertile soul and enlightened intelligence, he contributed with his example, work, and teaching to the flourishing of neuraltherapeutic medicine in Latin America.

In memory of Luís Fernando Córdoba Llanos, who was a human being in love with life, with people, and with knowledge. As a sensitive and responsible man, he was an exemplary father, son, husband, and friend. He made neuraltherapeutic medicine his banner and purpose in life, and he sowed it with love and wisdom in fields and cities, without distinction of race, ethnicity, economic condition, or sexual orientation, in people who, from pain and suffering, sought his knowledgeable, gentle, and firm hand. His teachings will always be with us.

In memory of Marcela Bobbato, who, like a true "force of nature," dedicated many years to advancing the health and well-being of communities in Argentina and beyond. She emphasized the importance of fostering a matristic culture within Neuraltherapeutic medicine, building networks of collaboration, and opening new pathways at the Universidad Nacional de Mar del Plata. She was a sower of paths and a weaver of networks for life and health.

Prologue

I had just completed my first 66 laps around the Sun (and the Covid-19 pandemic had just been declared) when I accepted the recommendation that is made, especially through the so-called algorithm, to those of us who are in the "third age" (a euphemism to refer to old age). This recommendation was that to avoid or at least postpone the arrival of senile dementia, we must do crossword puzzles, put together puzzles, learn to play a musical instrument, or practice a craft.

I chose to sew patchwork quilts, the first of which I wrote an article for a Truth Commission publication entitled "Diversity" that I was commissioned to write.[1] My article was entitled "Biodiversity and self-regulation of ecosystems," which shares the focus of the different chapters of this book on Neuraltherapeutic Medicine that I have generously been invited to prologue.

With this approach, I have continued to make patchwork quilts with excerpts from articles and books that I have written over several decades. Some of these texts describe my personal experiences in "The Art of Healing,"[2] especially after two schools of life—and of what I later learned is called "resilience"—that for me have been of essential importance: the Popayán Earthquake (1983)[3] and the Tierradentro Earthquake (1994).[4]

This prologue will not be the exception because, I repeat, in the writings from which I extract several of the fragments that I share below, and in the aforementioned experiences, as well as in others not mentioned, I have applied teachings

[1] Wilches-Chaux G. Biodiversity: a patchwork quilt on the topic and the importance of its valuation. 2024. [Internet]. Available at: https://enosaquiwilches.blogspot.com/2024/08/biodiversidad-colcha-de-retazos-sobre.html

[2] Title of my conference in permanent construction on the application of the principles of Alternative Medicines in the Continuum Environmental Management-Disaster Risk Management-Climate Management, which I have been conducting in various virtual and in-person spaces since 2019.

[3] Wilches-Chaux G. Tools for the crisis. Disasters, Environmentalism, and Vocational Training. Popayán: SENA. 1989. Available at: https://repositorio.sena.edu.co/handle/11404/1034?show=full

[4] Wilches-Chaux G. On the edge of chaos. Colección Instituto Pensar. Bogotá: Pontificia Universidad Javeriana—Fundación para la comunicación Popular FUNCOP CAUCA. 2000. 138pp.

from teachers. And without medicine being my field of action, I obtained from alternative doctors and theoreticians-practitioners of Neuraltherapeutic Medicine and, particularly and directly, from Dr. Julio César Payán.[5]

My article for the above-mentioned publication "Diversity" begins with this "In Praise of Patchwork Quilts":

> For various reasons, I describe this article as a patchwork quilt. This is not only because the dictionary defines a patchwork as "a fragment of a speech or a piece of writing" (which you will find in this article), but also because, despite being stigmatized (like bottlenecks or black sheep), patchwork quilts often serve as tangible and colorfully beautiful expressions of a culture that cannot afford to waste what is still useful. This is a culture that strives to meet daily needs without unnecessary waste, driven not by greed but by a sense of responsibility. Of a culture that greatly values the imagination and manual work of those who—women in general—are dedicated to collecting pieces of fabric that remained unsold in the warehouse or who survived the loss of a garment, a covering, or a tablecloth that for some reason ceased to exist. These fragments contain textiles that were once part of family memories and identity, and they continue to hold significance.
>
> Memory, even if it is in fragments, is as important for territories, for communities, and for families as it is for each person individually. Memory loss is one of the main causes of vulnerability.

Precisely, this memory loss forced us to understand that we must change the way we conceive, plan, practice, and evaluate what we call "development" on a daily basis

> which is based on compulsive consumption, on the excessive production of waste, on the destruction of ecosystems, and on the overexploitation of soils. But above all on the disregard of the rights of all living beings, often including the rights of human beings themselves: one of them is the right to diversity over the imposition of uniformity.
>
> When we say "biodiversity," we are referring to the multiplicity of ways in which life on Earth is expressed, and that includes the enormous diversity of human beings and the cultures to which we belong, whether we realize it or not.

This book that you have in your hands will not only contribute to consolidate the conviction of its authors about the fact that the principles on which Neuraltherapeutic Medicine is based and applied are valid not only in the field of health but also in general in everything that refers to the relationship of human beings with our own bodies and spirits, two inseparable and complementary dimensions. This relationship does not end with the human being but involves ecosystems, of which that essential ingredient of life that is water is part.

This approach, inherited from the Dr. Julio César Payán de la Roche (1942–2020), one of the pioneers and masters of biological medicines in Colombia and particularly of what is now called Neuraltherapeutic Medicine, allowed me to understand

---

[5] With Dr. Payán in 1990, we produced the video titled "Health: An Alternative Vision," with the support of FUNCOP, which can be viewed here: https://www.youtube.com/watch?v=-pbjzaXZ6qU. In the video, among other topics, the two community health centers existing at that time in Barrio Colombia II in Popayán and in the Municipality of Puerto Tejada in northern Cauca are highlighted, where FUNCOP (the Foundation for Popular Communication, of which Dr. Esperanza Cerón, author of one of the chapters of this book, was director) offers the communities health and education programs based on the approach of alternative medicines.

much better our relationship with that great Living Being that is planet Earth of which we are fractals and that we know from different cultures by names such as Gaia or Pacha Mama.

It is the same vision that I express and apply in my text "Let's heal with wetlands"[6] in which I summarize the concept of fractality:

> In simple terms, fractality is the property that complex systems possess of "repeating" themselves in terms of functional and structural logic as they change scale. In its current conception, we owe it to the mathematician Benoit Mandelbrot, who was the first to speak of the "Fractal Geometry of Nature".[7] The word "fractality" links the concept of fraction with that of totality. This notion implies that, in different ways, for each fraction we can find the totality to which it belongs.

Today we also know—and this is hopeful—that by acting effectively on the part we can impact the whole.

Let Dr. Payán himself explain what the "Approaches to the concept of health from an alternative vision" consist of.[8]

He applies it to the health field. As his disciple, friend, companion, and user (not "patient"), I have applied his teachings when facing challenges in my field: the so-called Disaster Risk Management. For example, after the aforementioned earthquake in Tierradentro (June 6, 1994). That experience is narrated in the book "On the Edge of Chaos", published by the Casa Pensar of the Javeriana University of Colombia in 2000.

One of the guiding principles of human communities and their ecosystems reads as follows:

> All living beings, including human communities and their ecosystems, possess "coping mechanisms" that allow them to transform themselves creatively as a result of crises. (…) (All) different external actors that intervene or will intervene in the disaster zone (…) (should give) energy stimuli, represented in this case by the economic, methodological, or technical contributions (…) recognizing that the different expressions of the culture of the local communities are the backbone of their immune system and their creative possibilities.[9]

Now, let's listen to Payán. As you follow Payán's teachings, you will confirm that they are applicable to both human health and the living beings—thus complex systems—that constitute the territories formed by interactions among ecosystems, communities, and the institutions that comprise them:

---

[6] Result of my work in 2021 with the Wetlands Mission established by the Bogotá Environment Secretary. Available at: https://enosaquiwilches.blogspot.com/2022/01/vamos-sanar-con-los-humedales.html

[7] Mandelbrot B. The fractal geometry of Nature. New York: Henry Holt and Company, 1983.

[8] Payán JC. Approaches to the concept of health from an alternative perspective. [Internet]. Available from: https://www.terapianeural.com/articulos/14-del-concepto/103-aproximaciones-al-concepto-de-salud-desde-una-mirada-alternativa

[9] Wilches-Chaux G. Rights of individuals and communities affected or susceptible to being affected by disasters. [Internet]. Available from: https://enosaquiwilches.blogspot.com/2018/06/derechos-de-personas-y-comunidades.html

> We need to begin viewing health not merely as a state but as a process that embodies movement and change. In a human being, there are trillions of cells, each with billions of enzymatic molecules at thousands of reactions per second, in a thermodynamically open system. That is, it exchanges matter, energy, and information with its environment, with genetic memory and social, cultural, and human history. Therefore, it cannot be viewed as a static state; rather, it represents the dynamics of a process that is far from equilibrium, complex, chaotic, and deterministic, involving adaptive processes of self-eco-organization.

Precisely the territories, which are the field in which I work, cannot be understood from a static vision but must be approached and experienced as processes far from balance. In the following excerpt, Payán continues to tell us:

> In the vital process far from equilibrium (a system in equilibrium does not accept any other state outside its own and is not in a position to generate work), quantum-gravitational paradoxes arise, posed since ancient Taoism, with contradictions between its different gradients of information and energy. So the process is dialectical and biological since it is gravitational, quantum, thermodynamically open, and teleological. The process is also social since it is necessary to recognize being not only as the isolated individual but also as an entity that forms, transforms, and is transformed by the social environment. So, from being an individuality, it becomes a singularity in the biological and social with a normality and order of its own that does not have to adapt to statistical massifying normativities, so we have to accept its processes of self-eco-organization.

Ecosystems, like singular social processes, must be understood as systems that have built their own order that does not resist external regulations or impositions. This significant look at the individual singularity of complex systems is also applicable to human beings and is clarified by Payán as follows:

> The blood pressure values of blacks are higher than those of whites. The Indian works with less concentrated hemoglobin levels than the other breeds. In malaria areas, the sickle cell gene can defend the population from Plasmodium. The inflamed testicle produces substances that sometimes help the heart to function better. As examples of special behaviors.
>
> (Each human being) is a social singularity that makes him interdependent with his entire environment, something that is in accordance with his characteristic of being thermodynamically open. All this allows him to be an active part of life and behave as an emergency of it.
>
> In nature there is a true cosmic dance of photons and electrons that are primary components of our entire being. Thus, the relationship of the interdependent singularity extends to encompass the entire cosmos, consistently referencing its economic, social, political, and historical environments. This approach is how we understand the holistic.

For Julio César Payán, the health of everything that is alive, such as the nature of which the human being is a part, is not a state but a singular and emergent vital process that does not admit external restrictions…

> (…) that vital process that is health arises as a result of the events named and is expressed as the feeling of well-being in life that, being singular and interdependent, does not allow it to be reduced to predetermined norms or models.
>
> The "normal" and "normative" values that support the orthodox health model can be used as references or approximations, but only as part of the dialectical process that is health, and only if they are evaluated within the broad referent that is the holistic human being.

From Payán's biocentric-ecocentric vision, I learned that disease is the result of a unique life process interconnected with its environment, where the essence is the sick subject (such as a human being or a territory) and not the simple isolated declaration of a disease.

> From this perspective, disease is not the opposite of health; rather, it is part of a vital process and is viewed as an aggressive self-organizing mechanism within an individual (the sick person). It is not that a person simply contracts a disease; instead, they engage with it as part of their vital and teleological journey.
>
> (…) the approach to the PATIENT, not to the disease, from Neural Therapy, consists of placing impulses on the organism so that it seeks its path of self-eco-organization according to its becoming, its possibilities and its social and cosmic relationships. (…) In the end one could synthesize health as the vital process by which one accepts oneself.

So much for Dr. Julio César Payán's contribution to the weaving of my patchwork quilt. Regarding the same topic, and drawing from my environmental expertise, I contribute this piece of my own harvest to the quilt:

> I must state very expressly that I do not understand the concept of chaos as a synonym for "disorder" (with all the negative implications that this word raises) but as the non-linear order of the complex systems of nature. Likewise, I am convinced that one of the problems that currently affects some of our wetlands is that they have tried to impose on them the force of engineering and economic and bureaucratic power, our entropy-generating order.[10]

Trying to combine what has been taught from Neuraltherapeutic Medicine by Payán and others, I take this excerpt entitled Bets on Resonance, published in the text "Let's Heal with the Wetlands," which constitutes my modest personal contribution of love and hope for this significant book that you are reading:

> Resonance is the physical phenomenon that, for example, when a guitar string vibrates with a certain frequency (or natural period of vibration), without there being physical contact between them, it makes the strings of other instruments that are tuned to the same frequency vibrate.
>
> For the effects that interest us, we can define resonance as contagion through vibration.
>
> If district institutions manage to vibrate at the same frequency, which in this case is a shared vision of the territory and the function that the hydrological network plays in it (what we have called playing the same score), they will most likely resonate more easily with the communities and their organizations linked to wetland management, which in turn have the challenge of tuning into a common frequency.
>
> To make this possible and to prevent this resonance from becoming a destructive phenomenon, it is necessary to recover (if they have been lost) and strengthen (if they still exist) the socio-ecosystem controls (fundamentally the so-called negative feedback) on which the dynamic stability of the corresponding territory depends.
>
> This contagion by vibration is at the base of the so-called *Emergent Behavior*, which fundamentally consists of a series of individuals (cells, neurons, birds, fish, ants, people, social experiences, etc.) managing to couple from simple rules that they share to make the qualitative leap towards a highly complex behavior.

---

[10] Wilches-Chaux G. Downpours and leaks: Our entropy-generating order. [Internet]. Available from: https://enosaquiwilches.blogspot.com/2013/05/nuestro-orden-generador-de-entropia.html

Conclusions

It is not usual for the prologue of a book to consist of a *patchwork quilt*, nor is it typical for it to propose conclusions. But since we ventured into the former, let's venture into the latter.

1. This first one was already enunciated from the beginning of the prologue. According to its authors, the teachings, knowledge, ignorance, and principles on which Neuraltherapeutic Medicine is based, applied, and developed are valid not only in the field of health but also in general in everything that refers to the relationship of human beings with our own bodies and spirits, two inseparable and complementary dimensions. This relationship does not end with the human being but involves ecosystems, of which that essential ingredient of life, that is, water, is part.
2. It is important to highlight that the authors of the articles of this treatise on Neuraltherapeutic Medicine have—sometimes expressly, sometimes not so much—different opinions about the so-called biological or alternative medicines, which is valid and healthy because in the field of health also, the biodiversity of worldviews constitutes a primordial value.[11]

   I do not go into any specific "school" because, as I have repeated several times, that is not my field. But I am sure that the effectiveness of each and every one of them—and of Neuraltherapeutic Medicine itself, as well as of "orthodox" medicine—depends on the wisdom possessed by those who practice them to stimulate and strengthen the capacity of the sick organism. In the words of Payán, previously quoted, "the organism seeks its path of self-eco-organization according to its becoming, its possibilities, and its social and cosmic relations." That wisdom, which is not theoretical but integrally vital, undoubtedly refers to the longed-for Gift of Healing.
3. Those who are providing us with their knowledge and experiences in the chapters that follow are, for the most part, health professionals who have received orthodox academic training in their different fields and who have made the decision to guide and complement this initial training with all these concepts-tools that are part of perspectives different from the predominant "Western."

   Some of these perspectives resonate with the worldviews of the ancestral cultures of the communities that populated the territories that were now "Latin American" before the arrival of Spanish ancestors, and most of the communities descended from those cultures have managed to maintain them to this day. And thanks to them, they have managed to survive despite the multiple colonial and neocolonial threats that have put them on the verge of extinction.

   I think it's vital to emphasize this as a prime example of the dialogues of worldviews on which the survival of our human species on this planet depends.

[11] Personally, I have no hesitation in highlighting in capital letters the concepts-tools of Worldviews and Biodiversity.

And also because those of us who consider ourselves disciples of Julio Cesar Payán—whose presence emerges in each of these pages—consider that Neuraltherapeutic Medicine is a virus of life of which our teacher was its first manager (in his office in Popayán and in the Community Health Centers promoted by the Foundation for Popular Communication FUNCOP). From there arose many of the vectors of this approach that we do not hesitate to consider a Latin American contribution to the rest of the planet.

4. Several co-authors of this book, also quoting Professor Payán, expressly mention what is implicit in the other chapters: "Neuraltherapeutic medicine, as an alternative medicine, is not a mere technique, a tool, or a method, but it is a conception that must be daring and free. This is a conception impregnated with another rationality, another logic, which, in its solidarity, not vertical, recognizing knowledge and wisdom, is respectful, responsible, ethical, and deeply loving."

   This is also valid not only for those who make their contributions to society and the planet from the field of health but also for those of us who are committed to a life project around the purpose of contributing to achieving "health of the soul, health of the body, and peace."[12]

I invite you to read and commit ourselves as actors and vectors to what we learn here!

2025

Faculty of Social and Human Sciences
Universidad Externado de Colombia
Bogotá, Colombia

Gustavo Wilches-Chaux

[12] Wilches-Chaux G. The health of the soul, the health of the body, and peace. [Internet]. Available from: https://witches-chaos.blogspot.com/2014/09/la-salud-del-alma-la-salud-del-cuerpo-y.html

Preface

This text is the beautiful materialization of a long-awaited desire. It took years of combining intelligence, knowledge, and wills to make it a reality. It was a demanding educational journey that transcended geographical barriers. We had to overcome many obstacles. One very important aspect was to make it clear that our fundamental intention is and will continue to be academic and not political: to bring together the best and most current neuraltherapeutic thought from various latitudes, with a biocentric, environmental, transdisciplinary, inclusive, generous, respectful, responsible, and warm projection, to navigate the always turbulent waters of knowledge generation in medicine.

Another hurdle to overcome was the divided and separate view of those who assume that neuraltherapeutic medicine is essentially a technique versus those who think it is merely an alternative approach or perspective. To dissolve this dichotomy of the heirs in the cognitive activity of the "object-subject relationship" canonized by moderns as a classical epistemological figure, contributions have been made from the sciences of complexity, systemic, complex, feminine, and Latin American thinking to offer a comprehensive perspective that enhances our knowledge and practices.

But it is by no means a total and definitive perspective. There are many angles that will continue to be explored and several viewpoints that are still under healthy discussion. However, we seek to bring together the best in this book.

The unwavering support from the Springer publishing house and the institutional backing of the National University of Colombia in Bogotá, as well as from Colombian associations of Neural Therapy (ACOLTEN/MNT, CONETSO) and the International Federation of Medical Associations of Neural Therapy (IFMANT), is invaluable. These organizations of health professionals in neuraltherapeutic medicine contributed knowledge, feelings, intelligence, attitudes, life experiences, solidarity, and hope. Thank you very much.

The academic work carried out was a fine goldsmithing of teamwork, weaving together and interlacing the sharp texts of various authors and perspectives to offer a beautiful, thoughtful, weighed, and well-considered collective piece, refined with knowledge, meaning, and experience. A contribution to the daily construction of a just world where people are happy, free, healthy, supportive, loving, and creative. A work in the service of the community. It is the one you now hold in your hands, ready to be read, studied, and put into action.

Bogotá, Colombia

Laura Bibiana Pinilla Bonilla
Eduardo Humberto Beltrán Dussán
Agustín Ricardo Angarita Lezama

Introduction

This book arises from the desire to tell a story: the evolution of a medical practice that, by opening up to dialogue with culture, history, and life itself, underwent profound transformation. Neural therapy, originally conceived in a European context, found fertile ground in Colombia for its conceptual and practical expansion. Over time, and especially after significant events like the Popayán Earthquake in 1983, this practice began to embrace new ways of seeing life, health, illness, the body, and human suffering.

The dialogue with other forms of knowledge, such as those from communities, complexity sciences, Russian nervism, and Participatory Action Research, opened the door to a profound transformation: a paradigm shift. Thus, Neuraltherapeutic Medicine was born, a proposal that recognizes life as the central axis, and understands medical practice not only as a technical act but as a deeply human, situated, social, and relational experience.

This book is aimed at physicians and other health professionals, researchers, students, and anyone interested in understanding the epistemological stance, as well as the scientific and practical foundations that were interwoven to give birth to Neuraltherapeutic Medicine. It is, therefore, a textbook with extensive theoretical, philosophical, practical, and technical scope.

As our editor and author Eduardo Beltrán mentions in Chap. 6, this transformation led to neuraltherapeutic medicine being identified as a complex medical system, a new category proposed by Brazilian sociologist Madel Luz and her research group. Luz and her team suggest that a complex medical system is based on its own cosmology or worldview and at least five dimensions (morphological, physiological, doctrinal, diagnostic, and therapeutic dimensions).

The structure of this book follows the path of the dimensions of complex medical systems. In the first part of this book, the aim is to tell the story of a medical practice whose axis of understanding and distinguishing feature was the emphasis on the nervous system and its trophic and modulatory role in the physiological and pathological states of complex organisms. This history traces its global antecedents, moving from its structuring as a school of physiology in Russia, as a medical practice in Germany, to its transformation into a complex medical system in Colombia.

In the second part, the reader will find an introduction to the concept of complex medical systems with their dimensions, while basic and fundamental notions of complexity sciences are developed, including quantum logic, chaos theory, and fractal geometry, among others. Here, various arguments are presented that demonstrate the foundation of neural therapy/neuraltherapeutic medicine in the sciences of complexity, while also highlighting the importance of focusing on the study of health and life.

The third part discusses the morphological foundation of neuraltherapeutic medicine. It covers embryology, the anatomy of the nervous system, and highlights the role of the extracellular matrix, also known as Pischinger's basic system.

The fourth part focuses on the physiological or vital dynamic dimension of neuraltherapeutic medicine, delving into the synthetic version of physiology with two currents originating from Russia and Great Britain. This new approach includes innovative ideas and is related to the concepts of complexity sciences. It highlights the main role of the nervous system in segmental physiology and in the regulation of inflammation and the immune response at a global level. The importance of electromagnetic aspects is also highlighted, as they are part of the physiology of organisms. Specific cases of exposure and interference within organisms are reviewed.

The fifth part encompasses a comprehensive review of the philosophical aspects that integrate the doctrinal dimension of Neuraltherapeutic Medicine with epistemological and ontological implications. Likewise, its paradigmatic stance on the conception of the process of falling ill is presented, aligned with the proposals of complexity sciences, and distancing itself from reductionist, analytical, and dualistic positions.

The sixth part deals with the diagnostic approach in Neuraltherapeutic Medicine, including the life history, physical examination, evaluation of mental and emotional aspects, and paraclinical strategies. The part concludes with a proposal of synthetic diagnostic categories called pathophysiological dynamics, classified according to their location, temporality, and dominant expression.

In the seventh part, the elements that make up the therapeutic approach of this medical system are presented. It starts with therapeutic guidelines aligned with each pathophysiological dynamic, and includes aspects of lifestyle and environmental health. Likewise, general pharmacological aspects of local anesthetics are reviewed along with some recommendations to prevent adverse reactions and reduce risks in clinical practice.

The eighth part, although it focuses on the exposition of neural therapy techniques or neuraltherapeutic medicine, does not intend to be exhaustive, given that there are already numerous technique atlases that are referenced and can be consulted. However, this part prioritizes the presentation of new techniques arising from research processes, as well as those resulting from synthesis with other areas of medicine, such as manual medicine. The part also includes a chapter on the systemic approach to procaine and the focus on mental and emotional conditions.

The ninth and final part outlines the wide range of applications of neural therapy medicine in the human and animal clinical fields, including dentistry, community health, and public health.

The editors recommend reading the first seven parts in consecutive order. This is because, unless the reader already has knowledge or prior experience in Neuraltherapeutic Medicine, there are concepts that follow a clear thread in the development of each dimension of the complex medical system. In contrast, Parts VIII and IX, along with their respective chapters, can be read in any order without affecting the overall understanding of neuraltherapeutic medicine practice.

The editors of this book have written this part with the intention of providing an initial compass for the journey that begins here. Beyond being a useful guide, we hope that this text serves as an invitation for each reader to open the horizons of understanding. We hope that its pages illuminate questions, awaken curiosity, and expand the horizons of Neuraltherapeutic Medicine toward new ways of seeing and inhabiting knowledge. May this book foster a fruitful synthesis of knowledge and encourage a transdisciplinary dialogue that enriches not only professional practice but also the relationship with life itself.

Faculty of Medicine, Master in Alternative Medicine, Neural Therapy Area
Universidad Nacional de Colombia
Bogotá, Colombia

Laura Bibiana Pinilla Bonilla

Integrated Health Services Subnetwork, Research and Innovation Center
Bogotá, Colombia

Faculty of Medicine
Universidad Nacional de Colombia
Bogotá, Colombia

Eduardo Humberto Beltrán Dussán

Faculty of Medicine, Master in Alternative Medicine, Neural Therapy Area
Universidad Nacional de Colombia
Bogotá, Colombia

Agustín Ricardo Angarita Lezama

Contents

Part I
Origins and Expansion of Neural Therapy

Chapter 1
A Timeline for Milestones in the Development of Neural Therapy/Neuraltherapeutic Medicine

Jorge Kaczewer

1 Local Anesthetics, Painless Surgery

1868—TOMÁS MORENO Y MAÍZ (1766–1850): The Peruvian physician published his pioneering scientific report on cocaine, which he used in subsequent research, and performed the first peripheral nerve blockade using cocaine infiltration via hypodermic syringe [1].

1884—CARL KÖLLER (1857–1944): The Austrian ophthalmologist initiated the development of surgical local anesthesia (LA) with his article on the use of cocaine in ophthalmic surgery [2].

1884—WILLIAM HALSTEAD (1852–1922): The American surgeon performed an injection near the infraorbital nerve foramen. By demonstrating that cocaine could stop transmission in nerve trunks, he laid the foundation for nerve block anesthesia in surgery [3, 4].

1884—RICHARD JOHN HALL (1850–1897): Halsted's colleague published one of the earliest successful nerve block reports. His dentist achieved infraorbital plexus anesthesia with 0.5 ml of 4% cocaine hydrochloride, being able to obturate Hall's upper incisor [5].

1884—VASSILI VON ANREP (1852–1927): Russian physiologist published findings in *Врач* (*Physician*) on the medical applications of cocaine. He reported ophthalmic effects, including reduced photophobia in iritis and keratitis, mydriasis, and decreased lacrimation, as well as cessation of intercostal pain following the injection of 0.025 g of cocaine solution into the intercostal spaces in cases of neuralgia and acute pleuritis [6].

J. Kaczewer (✉)
School of Medical Sciences, Universidad Nacional de Rosario, Santa Fe, Argentina

Argentine Institute of Neural Therapy, Buenos Aires, Argentina
e-mail: posgradomnt@terapianeural.ar

L. B. Pinilla Bonilla et al. (eds.), *Neuraltherapeutic Medicine*,
https://doi.org/10.1007/978-3-032-03257-7_1

1886—CHARLES FRANÇOIS-FRANCK (1849–1921): French physiologist reported on the possibility of temporarily paralyzing autonomic ganglia with cocaine. In 1892, he conceived the term "nerve block" [7].

1892—CARL SCHLEICH (1859–1922): German surgeon in Berlin introduced his "infiltration anesthesia" with 0.1 and 0.2% cocaine solutions [8].

1894—CARL SCHLEICH (1859–1922): Published his monograph *Painless Operations* [9].

1895—JEAN JAQUES PAUL RECLUS (1847–1914): French surgeon in Paris published *Local anesthesia with cocaine* after 7000 surgeries without accidents using 1% cocaine concentrations [10].

2 Therapeutic Local Anesthesia

1884—SIGISMUND FREUD (1856–1939): Austrian neurologist, true pioneer in "therapeutic" local anesthesia, proposed the use of cocaine to treat patients with nervous exhaustion, depression, trigeminal neuralgia, and morphine addiction [11].

1894—J. LEONARD CORNING (1855–1923): American neurologist published a pioneering book on LA techniques for the treatment of pain [12].

1898—CARL SCHLEICH (1859–1922): He was the first to report the persistence of analgesic and anti-inflammatory effects lasting much longer than the anesthetic effects, with definitive remission or reduced recurrence following repeated "infiltrations" [13].

1898—AUGUST BIER (1861–1949): German surgeon was the first to successfully perform spinal anesthesia. He injected cocaine (3 ml of 0.5% cocaine hydrochloride) into the spinal cord of a patient [14].

1900—OSKAR KREIS (1872–1958): Swiss obstetrician used spinal anesthesia with cocaine to relieve labor pain for the first time in the world [15].

1901—THÉODORE TUFFIER (1857–1929): French surgeon used spinal cocaine to treat lower limb sarcoma pain [16].

1901—JEAN ATHANASE SICARD (1872–1929): French neurologist and radiologist described the first therapeutic use of sacral canal cocaine injection for various diseases (lumbar pain, sciatica, Tabes dorsalis, etc.) [17].

1902—GUSTAV SPIESS (1862–1934): German otolaryngologist reported that wounds and inflammatory processes resolved more quickly and with fewer complications after LA with cocaine [18].

1902—CARL LUDWIG SCHLEICH (1859–1922): First described the technique of intracutaneous injection in the form of a papule or "quaddle" [19].

1904—ALFRED EINHORN (1857–1917): The German chemist patented 18 para-aminobenzoic derivatives which he developed in the Meister Lucius and Brüning plants of the Höchst laboratory in Hesse. He named the second one Novocain (from novus, new cocaine) [20, 21].

1905—HEINRICH BRAUN (1862–1934): German surgeon was the first to use procaine on patients. The name, novocaine, first appeared in his article. Braun reported excellent results in a comparison of compounds with different concentrations of novocaine and adrenaline [22].

1906—GUSTAV SPIESS (1862–1934): Published *The importance of anesthesia in inflammation therapy*, a pioneering exploration of their influence on pathological processes such as acute inflammation, chronic inflammation, and neoplasms. He reported on its usefulness in the treatment of laryngeal tuberculosis [23].

1906—ALEKSANDR VASILYEVICH VISHNEVSKY (1874–1948): Russian surgeon perceived the anti-inflammatory effect of LA with novocaine, applying it in "zemstvo" (rural) surgery and clinic and then in military surgery during World War I [24].

1908—AUGUST BIER (1861–1949): first described intravenous regional anesthesia with Esmarch cuff. He named it "direct venous anesthesia" [25].

1910—ALBERT LEMAIRE (1875–1933): Belgian physician developed a treatment of visceral pain by means of dermal LA with novocaine [26].

1911—DIEDRICH KULENKAMPFF (1880–1963): German surgeon performed the first percutaneous supraclavicular brachial plexus block [27].

1911—GEORG HIRSCHEL (1875–1963): German surgeon invented the axillary approach for brachial plexus anesthesia. He also published a manual of local anesthesia that was translated into English, Spanish, French, and Russian, popularizing local anesthesia techniques outside Germany [28].

1911—GUIDO FISCHER (1877–1959): The therapeutic use of LA was incorporated into dentistry thanks to his major work, *Local Anesthesia in Dentistry*. The book was reprinted 10 times in Germany, 4 times in England, as well as in Russia and Spain [29].

1912—FRITZ HÄRTEL (1877–1937): German surgeon from Berlin created Gasser's ganglion and sciatic nerve injection techniques [30].

1913—KARL EWALD HERING (1834–1918): German physician, director of the Leipzig Institute of Physiology, early intuited the possible diagnostic/therapeutic value of the ANS: "The rational use of the autonomic system will one day constitute the majority of the medical arts" [31].

1913—RENE LERICHE (1870–1955): French surgeon developed periarterial sympathectomy to harness the beneficial effects of persistent vasodilation on the affected tissues [32].

1917—JAMES MACKENZIE (1853–1925): Scottish cardiologist and surgeon reported hypertonus and hyperalgesia in the subcutaneous cellular tissue and musculature when visceral diseases are present [33].

1919—HEINRICH HIGIER (1866–1942): Polish neurologist and psychiatrist published his treatise *Vegetative Neurology* [34].

1919—ANTON ELSCHNIG (1863–1939): Austrian ophthalmologist reported the first successful treatments for glaucoma with procaine [35].

1922—FARBWERKE HOECHST: In Frankfurt, the German laboratory publishes the first "textbook" of Neural Therapy *Novocaine for Anesthesia and Therapy* [36].

1923—JAKOB PÁL (1863–1936): Hungarian Austrian physician and internist used dorsal-level "Paravertebral Anästhesie" to treat bronchial asthma. He also proposed its use as a diagnostic tool in thoracic and abdominal surgeries [37, 38].

1924—MAXIME LAIGNEL-LAVASTINE (1875–1953): The French psychiatrist published *Pathology of the Sympathetic: essay of clinical anatomic physiopathology* [39].

1924—GUSTAV WILLIAM AUGUST JOSEF RICKER (1870–1948): German pathologist from Magdeburg published *Pathology as a natural science—Relational Pathology*. He argued that neural regulation of body fluids and vascular permeability is a key process in physiology. He postulated that there is no independent activity in cells; the network of relationships between the nervous system, blood, tissue fluids, and tissue itself must be seen as a single system [40].

1925—RENE LERICHE (1870–1955): During a "stelectomy" with Fontaine, he observed that infiltrating procaine into the exposed stellate ganglion induced paralysis of vasoconstriction over a wide area and alleviated pain crisis. In subsequent years, he discovered that transcutaneous novocaine injections into vegetative nerves or ganglia could avoid the need for surgical intervention [41].

3 "Heilanästhesie"[1]

1925—FERDINAND HUNEKE (1891–1966) and WALTER HUNEKE (1897–1974): The German brothers, physicians from Düsseldorf, began investigating the curative effect of local anesthetics when Ferdinand obtained immediate disappearance of his sister's migraine by intravenously applying an intramuscular drug containing procaine as a painless solvent. During the following 3 years, Walter achieved similar results with intramuscular and subcutaneous procaine in various conditions [42].

1925—FELIX MANDL (1892–1957): Austrian surgeon first used the posterior approach to the stellate ganglion to treat angina pectoris [43].

1926—ERICH SCHILF (1892–1962): Berlin physiologist translated Langley's book into German and highlighted the lack of experimental evidence supporting the antagonism between the sympathetic and parasympathetic systems [44].

1926—FELIX MANDL (1892–1957): Austrian surgeon introduced sympathetic paravertebral blockade with novocaine for therapeutic purposes. His monograph on paravertebral injection was translated into English in 1947 [45].

1927—RENÉ FONTAINE (1899–1979): French surgeon described the effects of procaine on blood vessels after trauma [46].

1928—FERDINAND HUNEKE (1891–1966) and WALTER HUNEKE (1897–1974): Published their findings on *Unknown remote effects of local anesthesia*, detailing therapeutic impacts that extended beyond the anesthetic duration and

[1] German word which means Therapeutic anesthesia.

injection site. Observing rapid onset after perivenous injections, they concluded that healing occurred through the sympathetic system and segmental cutaneous-visceral reflex connections, as described by neurologist **Henry Head (1861–1940)** [42].

1929—WALTER BRADFORD CANNON (1871–1945): American physiologist introduced the concept of "homeostasis," then adopted as guiding principle of Western medicine [47].

1929—MAX KIBLER (1900–1973): German physician developed the concept of segment therapy: visceral diseases treatment with local anesthetic injections of hyperalgesic subcutaneous zones [48].

1930—ALEKSANDR VASILYEVICH VISHNEVSKY (1874–1948): Russian surgeon published his report *Local Anesthesia using the method of the Crawling Infiltrate* in the Kazan medical journal, proving the safe use of two liters of a 0.25% novocaine solution [49].

1930—GASTON LABAT (1876–1934): French surgeon based in the United States published *Regional Anesthesia: Its Technique and Clinical Application* (1922). In 1930, he described his posterior to the stellate ganglion injection approach [50].

1932—DANIEL DANIELOPOLU (1884–1955): Romanian physiologist, clinician, and pharmacologist issued *Schema anatomo-physiologique du système nerveux de la vie végétative*. He rejected absolute antagonism in ANS function, favoring cross-stimulation as a regulatory mechanism that preserves opposing forces, a "circular system" forerunning biocybernetics [51].

1933—MIGUEL LÓPEZ ESNAURRIZAR (1901–1994): The Mexican surgeon defined the concept of "Functional Pathology" (of the ANS): a local, partial, or general imbalance of the Sympathetic System. His Sympathology was considered a nosological branch of Neurology focused on the study of the Sympathetic NS (SNS) [52].

1933—CARLOS STAJANO (1891–1976): Uruguayan surgeon published his monograph on neurodystrophies [53].

1934—ALEXEI DMITRIEVICH SPERANSKY (1888–1961): Russian neurosurgeon, a disciple of Ivan Pavlov, published *Nervous Trophism in Medical Theory and Practice*, a compilation of reports demonstrating the significant efficacy of novocaine blocks in treating various refractory diseases [54].

1934—RENE LERICHE (1879–1955): He observed the immediate disappearance of pain following surgical scar infiltration, describing the effect as occurring *"dans un clin d'œil"* (in the blink of an eye), 6 years before Ferdinand Huneke's "instantaneous phenomenon." Using procaine alone, he successfully treated migraines, gangrene, and pulmonary and cerebral embolism through sympathetic ganglia infiltration [41, 55, 56].

1934—HENRY SWARTLEY RUTH (1899–1956): American anesthesiologist published a manual of diagnostic, prognostic, and therapeutic nerve blocks [57].

1934—JAMES REILLY (1887–1974): French experimental pathologist proposed the ANS irritation syndrome, asserting a stronger link between the ANS and infectious diseases than previously recognized. Using techniques such as bacterial toxins, chemical irritants, and faradization to stimulate peripheral SNS segments across species, he confirmed Speransky's findings [58].

1934—ALEKSANDR ALEKSANDROVICH VISHNEVSKY (1906–1975): Russian surgeon published his method of injection into the sympathetic trunk at the level of the upper renal pole [59].

1935—PYOTR KUZMICH ANOKHIN (1898–1974): Russian biologist and physiologist developed the concept of Functional System. He suggested the idea of an "action outcome acceptor" and thus discovered the existence of feedback in physiological processes (but did not use this term) [60].

1935—MIKHAIL IVANOVICH ASTVATSATUROV (1877–1936): Soviet neuropathologist disciple of Vvedensky developed and disseminated the technique of intradermal novocaine blockade for various peripheral pain syndromes [61].

1936—FERDINAND HUNEKE (1891–1966): Published his book *Disease and cure: another view* [62].

1936—ALEXEI DMITRIEVICH SPERANSKY (1888–1961): He published *Bases for a New Theory of Medicine*, proposing the NS's integrative role in pathology and laying the foundation for Neural Therapy. He argued that the NS ensures internal unity and coordinates all systems. NS dysfunction induces trophic cell alterations, storing pathological information over time. He termed this process "neurodystrophy," viewing disease as a response to stimuli at any level of the NS [63].

1937—DIEDRICH KULENKAMPFF (1880–1963): German surgeon reported "miraculous results" in the treatment of epididymitis with local anesthetics [64].

1937—GINO PIERI (1881–1952): The Italian surgeon and cutaneous circulation researcher published his treatise on the neurovegetative system [65].

1937—JULES TINEL (1879–1952): French neurologist published his treatise on the neurovegetative system based on his experience with wounded soldiers during WWI [66, 67].

1938—WILHELM FALTA (1875–1950) and EGON FENZ (1907–1972): Czechoslovak physician, psychologist, poet, and essayist and his Austrian assistant published *On the Therapeutic Value of Novocaine in Internal Medicine*. Fenz reported "remarkable effects obtained with novocaine in 143 cases of sciatica" [68].

1938—KARL HANSEN (1893–1962): German physician published his book *Reflex and Algetic Signs of Internal Organs* [69].

1938—KURT RÜDIGER VON ROQUES (1890–1966): The German physician started translating the English edition of Speransky's book *Bases for a New Theory of Medicine*, which was published in Germany only in 1950 [70].

1938—ALFONSO ROQUE ALBANESE (1906–2005): The Argentine surgeon published *Manual of anesthetic blocks of the neurovegetative system; sympathetic anesthesia*, a generational bedside book in Spanish-speaking countries [71].

1939—WALTER BRADFORD CANNON (1871–1945): The American physiologist from Boston experimentally studied how the sympathetic system and adrenal medulla regulate visceral responses to stress. He introduced the term *homeostasis*, which later became a fundamental principle of Western medicine [72].

1939—OSCAR LAMBRET (1872–1943): The French neurosurgeon published his work *Technique of Sympathetic Surgery and Its Infiltrations* [73].

4 Neural Therapy According to HUNEKE

1940—FERDINAND HUNEKE (1891–1966): He observed the first phenomenon within seconds, deducing the existence of a "distortion field" that rendered local and segmental therapy unsuccessful. The remote irritative effects of the dysfunctional tissue were the real cause of medically unexplained symptoms and various chronic diseases, or aggravated incipient or preexisting pathologies, preventing their resolution. He conceived Heilanästhesie as a way of "inactivating" these "fields" that provided successful treatment of hitherto incurable diseases [74].

1940—KURT RÜDIGER VON ROQUES (1890–1966): After becoming acquainted with the lightning phenomenon, he named this approach "Neural Therapy according to Huneke" (Speransky) [75].

1940—HUBERT SIEGEN (1895–1972): The German physician conducted animal experiments on allergic phenomena, demonstrating that allergic reactions depend not only on antibodies but also on tissue memory. He showed that anesthetizing the tissue containing this memory prevents antibodies in the bloodstream from overreacting to repeated allergen exposure [76].

1940—BÉLA MEZÖ (1883–1954): Hungarian physician developed cyclic paravertebral anesthesia for the treatment of various diseases (stomach and duodenal ulcers, prostate, etc.). He used 2% pantocaine without adrenaline and repeated the injection at 5–6 day intervals [77].

1941—EGON FENZ (1907–1972): Austrian physician described the treatment of rheumatic diseases with local anesthesia based on experiences with 4116 patients [78].

1942—CURT SCHEIDT (1901–1964): The Hamburg-based dentist introduced the term "disturbance field"(interference field). According to Scheidt, a neurally interfering field refers to any tissue that is either primary or secondarily vegetatively irritated, being able to both receive and emit neural interference signals [79].

1942—WOLFGANG VEIL (1884–1946) and ALEXANDER STURM (1901–1973): The German neurologists published *Pathology of the Brainstem*, identifying the diencephalon as the central site for all pathological processes [80].

1942—NILS LÖFGREN (1913–1967) AND BENGT LUNDQVIST (1923–2001): Swedish chemists synthesized the compound we know today as "lidocaine" [81].

1943—RENE LERICHE (1870–1955): Successfully treated a migraine headache for the first time with a novocaine lavage of the temporal artery [82].

1944—BORIS VLADIMIROVICH OGNEV (1901–1978): Russian vascular surgeon injected procaine into the internal carotid artery for the first time [83].

1944—RICARDO FINOCHIETTO (1888–1962) and ENRIQUE FINOCHIETTO (1881–1948): Argentine surgeons published a comprehensive manual on local anesthesia, providing a detailed description of injection techniques and their nonsurgical therapeutic applications. Additionally, they implemented peripheral neurovegetative therapy through perifocal and intrafocal infiltrations of novocaine for the management of contusions and paratraumatic bone pain [84].

1944—KONSTANTIN BYKOV (1886–1959): Russian neurophysiologist published *The cerebral cortex and the internal organs*, proposing the concept of corticovisceral pathology [85].

1945—RENE HAZARD (1886–1974): French physician and pharmacologist specified a biological explanation for the therapeutic applications of procaine, publishing in Progrés Médical [86, 87].

1946—MAURICE LUZUY (1901–1980): The French physician published his textbook *Sympathetic infiltrations* [88].

1946—PHILIPP STÖHR Jr. (1891–1979): The German medical anatomist discovered the terminal reticulum as the final formation of the ANS, which branches into an increasingly extensive and narrow network. The final lattice consists of fibrils that cover each individual cell with a thin neuroplasmic veil [89].

1947—AUGUSTO PI SUÑER (1874–1965): The Spanish physiologist published his treatise *Neurovegetative System,* advocating for afferent sympathetic conduction and a sensory function essential for interorgan coordination and the genesis of vegetative feelings, challenging the prevailing view of the system as purely efferent [90].

1947—WALTER SCHEIDT (1895–1976): German anthropologist published *The Vegetative System*. He conceived neurofibrils as a mobile system of molecules in which new conductive pathways can arise, which he called rings [91].

1947—EGIDIO TOSATTI (1913–1990): Italian lymphangiologist published his treatise on sympathetic ganglionic LA injection techniques [92].

1948—ESTANISLAO LLUESMA URANGA (1909–1968): Spanish physician exiled in Argentina published his treatise *Neurovegetative System* [93].

1948—ALEKSANDR VASILYEVICH VISHNEVSKY (1874–1948) AND ALEKSANDR ALEKSANDROVICH VISHNEVSKY (1906–1975): Russian surgeons published *Novocaine Blockade as a Method of Acting on Tissue Trophism*, advancing local anesthesia through a gradual plane-by-plane injection approach in inflammatory processes. They viewed organic and systemic diseases as processes "under the unique orienting action of the nervous system." [94].

1948—ALEXANDER STURM (1901–1973): Published *Clinical pathology of the lung in relation to the vegetative nervous system* [95].

1948—GEORGES ARNULF (1904–1990): French vascular surgeon from Nancy developed the techniques of therapeutic local anesthesia upon the sympathetic system [96].

1948—OSWALD MARCHESANI (1900–1952): The German ophthalmologist, born in Tyrol, Austria, investigated sympathetic ophthalmia and the neurogenic basis of endogenous eye inflammation. Influenced by the ideas of Ricker and Speransky, he identified a segmental neural structure of the eye [97].

1948—PLUTARCO NARANJO VARGAS (1921–2012): Ecuadorian physician, journalist, historian, and scientific researcher published his treatise *The Neurovegetative System* [98].

1949—ALBRECHT FLECKENSTEIN (1917–1992): The German pharmacologist and physiologist, discoverer of calcium channel blockers, published *The Mechanism of Action of Local Anesthesia.* He conceptualized local anesthetics as lytic substances, describing their action as "general membrane stabilization" [99].

1949—FRITZ EICHHOLTZ (1889–1967): German pharmacologist, Fleckenstein's teacher, found that procaine exerts a vascular permeability-reducing effect [100].

1949—WILHELM NONNENBRUCH (1887–1955): The German clinician from Frankfurt published *Bilateral Renal Disease: Neuropathological Considerations*, proposing the term "irritation center" to describe the interference field more accurately [101].

1949—FRIEDRICH DITTMAR (1906–1995): The German physician, a disciple of Huneke and Karl Hansen, developed treatment for hyperalgesic zones in internal organ diseases. In *Examination of Reflex and Algesic Signs* proposed that the "neuro-angio-myosclero-dermatome" as a segmental entity responds to stimuli in any part of the segment [102].

1949—GUY LAZORTHES (1910–1982): French neurosurgeon published his treatise *The Neurovascular System*, describing in detail the autonomic regulation of cerebral blood vessels [103].

1949—KARL ANSELMINO (1900–1978): The German gynecologist published his papers, *On the prospects of cure of severe fecal obstruction by novocaine infiltration of the lumbar sympathetic trunk ganglia* and *On a new method of prolonged conduction anesthesia of labor pain: segmental epidural injection* [104, 105].

1949—JANET G. TRAVELL (1901–1997): American physician and researcher introduced the terms "myofascial pain" and "myofascial trigger point." Her pioneering work showed that each muscle possesses its own specific myofascial pain reference pattern [106].

1950—MAX KIBLER (1900–1973): German physician published his book *Segment Therapy for joint disorders and internal diseases—Experiences and considerations* [48].

1951—MAX RATSCHOW (1904–1963): The German internist, known as the "founder of angiology", tested Neural Therapy at the Medical Clinic of the University of Halle in 1950–1951. He treated 1011 patients, observing 441 complete remissions, 427 significant improvements, and 143 failures. Over 12 months, he recorded 72 flash phenomena, stating, "This is a sufficient number to underline the enormous importance of F. Huneke's observations" [107].

1951—HANS SELYE (1907–1982): The Austro-Hungarian physiologist and physician, later naturalized as Canadian, demonstrated the "general adaptation syndrome," showing that the body reacts similarly to a wide range of impulses, damages, and mental stresses. This response occurs in a nonspecific way through adaptation (alarm reaction, resistance, and exhaustion). He attributed this reaction to the pituitary-adrenal axis [108].

1951—HUBERT SIEGEN (1895–1972): German clinician from Dusseldorf published *Theory and Practice of Neural Therapy with Impletol*. With the "neural" suppression of the Sanarelli-Schwartzmann phenomenon, the greater relevance of the ANS over the humoral system was reaffirmed [109].

1951—GUIDO KRAUCHER (1886–1969): The Austrian physician published *The Intravenous Application of Local Anesthetics in Internal Medicine* [110].

1952—HERBERT SIEGMUND (1892–1954): German pathologist confirmed that both bacterial focal disorders and abacterial disturbance fields (e.g., scars) can initiate focal phenomena. And he established the focal neurovegetative theory, based on Ricker's relational pathology and Speransky's neural pathology [111].

1952—WALTER HUNEKE (1897–1974): He published *Impletoltherapy and Other Neuraltherapeutic Procedures: Fundamentals and Technique*, coining the term "interference field" to describe the *Stoerfeld*—an altered tissue region that can exert a nerve-mediated disruptive effect on distant tissues beyond its segment [112].

1953—HANS SCHMELZER (1897–1986): German ophthalmologist published his book *Neural Therapy in Ophthalmology*, describing his experience [113].

1953—PAUL VOGLER (1899–1969): Physiatrist from Berlin published, together with Herbert Krauss, the book "Treatment of Periosteum" [114].

1953—REINHOLD VOLL (1909–1989): German physician established the electroacupuncture measurements by the relationships between teeth, organs, and body structures. He listed the connections between specific acupuncture points and the ANS. His method was named Electroacupuncture according to Voll (EAV) [115].

1953—FRITZ REISCHAUER (1896–1963): German surgeon developed spinal injection techniques for lumbar nerve root blocks, as well as metameric thoracic paravertebral and sacral anesthesia [116].

1953—HANS FRIEDRICH ZIPF (1911–1969): The Director of the Institute of Pharmacology at the University of Cologne published research on the endoanesthetic effect of procaine, highlighting its beneficial modulation of pulmonary expansion, carotid body, vascular, visceral, and muscle receptors [117].

1953—ERICH STIEFVATER (1915–1994): German physician and acupuncturist developed his own acupuncture system and integrated it into Neural Therapy through his book *Acupuncture as Neural Therapy* [118].

1953—ERICH LETTERER (1895–1982): The pathologist from Tübingen argued that Ricker's "histion"—comprising the functional unit of cells, basic substance, connective tissue fibers, vessels, and nerves—should be recognized as the "primitive synergistic unit of tissue" rather than the cell [119].

1953—ERNST SCHWAMM (1913–1978): German country doctor and neural therapy (NT) expert introduced medical thermography to objectively demonstrate the link between interference fields and circulatory disorders [120].

1953—VASILY MOSIN (1917–1998): Soviet veterinarian conducted research on paravertebral sympathetic blockades in equines, sheep, and swine, demonstrating that sympathetic pathways serve as primary paths for pain sensation originating from organ receptors within the abdominal cavity. Based on these findings, he proposed that sympathetic surgery in horses could be avoided using sympathetic blockades to manage inflammatory processes affecting the peritoneum and abdominal organs [121].

1954—WALTER RUDOLF HESS (1881–1973): The Swiss physiologist published *Diencephalon, Autonomic and Extrapyramidal Functions*, including a chapter on the "Functional Organization of the Autonomic Nervous System." He argued that the ANS functions more as a visceral sensory network than a purely vegetative or automatic system [122].

1954—HERBERT JUNGHANNS (1902–1986): German surgeon first described the motion segment (MS), spine's smallest functional unit reflecting its overall biomechanics. Each MS consists of two adjacent vertebrae halves, dorsally connected by zygapophyseal joints and anteriorly by the intervertebral disc, along with spinal ligaments, joint capsules, and segmental muscles. It also includes spinal nerves with posterior horn ganglia, sympathetic paravertebral ganglia, fascial structures, the spinal dura, and the corresponding dermatome [123].

1954—HEINZ SCHOELER (1905–1973): The German homeopath published his book *The Weihe pressure points, their relations to acupuncture, neural therapy and homeopathy* [124].

1955—MELCHIOR WESTHUES (1896–1971): German veterinarian published a detailed article *On therapeutic anesthesia in veterinary medicine* [125].

1955—JOHANNES BISCHKO (1922–2004): Viennese surgeon, founder of the Austrian Acupuncture Society reported that "acupuncture treatment failures are usually due to an interference field that must first be disconnected" [126].

1956—OLOF DIETZ (1927–2007): The German veterinarian applied stellate ganglion and lumbar sympathetic block injection techniques and indications to dogs, cattle, and horses. Experiments further revealed that thoracic blockade in the sheep's splanchnic branch region enhances gastrointestinal peristalsis [127].

1958—ERNEST ADLER (1906–1996): German dentist based in Spain demonstrated that pathological interferences from dentition and tonsils affect the neurovegetative system, disrupting normal physiological function. In 1958, he coined the term *Neurofocal Dentistry* and is regarded as its founder [128, 129].

1958—INTERNATIONAL MEDICAL SOCIETY FOR NEURAL THERAPY ACCORDING TO HUNEKE (IGNH) was founded in Germany with the purpose of researching, teaching, and promoting Neural Therapy. IGNH serves as an umbrella organization for various foreign branches, maintains regular contacts, and organizes congresses both in Germany and internationally, or participates in international congresses [130].

1958—FERDINAND HOFF (1896–1988): German physician, eminent clinician who investigated the areas of vegetative regulation, internal secretion, and blood diseases, described NT according to Huneke in his textbook *Treatment of Internal Diseases*. He acknowledged not being capable of explaining but positively witnessing the Huneke phenomenon [131].

1960—JOSEF SCHMID (1919–1960): Austrian internist published his book *Neural Therapy* in Vienna [132].

1961—FRITZ REISCHAUER (1896–1963): German surgeon used a statistical report to demonstrate that effective NT is low risk. He reported 79,000 incident-free paravertebral neural anesthetic block treatments (using an average of 30 ml. of 1% procaine) over 8 years [133].

1961—FERDINAND HUNEKE (1891–1966): Published his book *The Seconds Phenomenon—Testament of a Doctor* [134].

1961—OSWALD KOTHBAUER (1926–2022): The Austrian veterinary surgeon and acupuncturist published *Novocaine therapy in horses, focusing on lumbar (perirenal) and intravenous administration*, as well as *On diagnostic pressure points and Neural Therapy in animals*. In his 1978 habilitation thesis, *Acupuncture and Neural Therapy for the Treatment of Sterility in Cattle*, he introduced the *paracervical block* (uterovaginal plexus) in cattle. Kothbauer posited that if an affected organ could generate hyperalgesic points in the segment corresponding to cutaneovisceral pathways, these could also be induced through artificial visceral irritation. By introducing irritant solutions into the ovaries or uterus of healthy cows without cutaneous hyperalgesia, hyperemic, and hyperalgesic points were observed within seconds [135].

1962—HERMANN GOECKE (1900–1994): German physician and professor of gynecology in Münster, Westphalia, applied NT on a large scale in his outpatient practice, refining with his group the technique of paracervical injection [136].

1962—HANS JOHANN SCHLIACK (1919–2008): German neurologist published *Segmental innervation. Its relevance to the clinic and practice,* together with Karl Hansen [137].

1962—ALBERT VON RICCABONA (1907–1980): The Austrian otorhinolaryngologist objectively demonstrated the Huneke phenomenon using comparative hematological analysis and iodometry, illustrating stimulus and information transport in the environment-cell system [138].

1962/1963—ALEXEY KIRILLOVICH KUZNETSOV (1915–2005): Russian veterinarian championed the use of novocaine therapy in veterinary practice. He conducted experimental studies to assess the efficacy of intravascular novocaine infusions. Additionally, he developed intravenous applications of low-concentration novocaine solutions for various noninfectious diseases in animals and proposed the blockade of skin receptors to address functional ailments [139, 140].

1963—PETER DOSCH (1914–2005): The German physician and primary disciple of the Hunekes published the *Manual of Neural Therapy According to Huneke (Regulating Therapy with Local Anesthetics)*, detailing NT's theoretical foundations, scientific principles, techniques, and key indications [141].

1963—MARCEL MONNIER (1907–1996): The Swiss neurophysiologist published *Physiologie und Pathophysiologie des Vegetativen Nervensystems*, analyzing autonomic regulation of visceral functions. For the Zurich school, the ANS extended beyond sympathetic and parasympathetic divisions, incorporating homeostatic roles of the reticular formation, diencephalon, and rhinencephalon [142].

1963—VICTOR LÉGER (1898–1968): French otolaryngologist trained with the Hunekes, published a paper on *Neural Therapy according to Huneke* in his language, introducing the Huneke line of thought in the French-speaking European area [143].

1965—ALFRED PISCHINGER (1899–1983): The Austrian physician, histologist, and embryologist—founder of histochemistry and the ground regulatory system concept—objectively demonstrated the instantaneous Huneke phenomenon using comparative hematological analysis and serum iodometry [144].

1965—GOTTFRIED KELLNER (1924–1983): The Viennese histologist defined the interference field histologically as a subchronic inflammation surrounding nondegradable foreign bodies or denatured endogenous substances, characterized by lymphoplasmacytic infiltrates and basal substance disintegration [145].

1965—HANNS FLEISCHHACKER (1910–1992): Austrian physician, head of internal medicine at the Hanusch Hospital in Vienna, proposed the clinical definition of interference field: It is an occult inflammation, which locally is oligosymptomatic to asymptomatic, but is capable of triggering symptoms in distant areas of the body [146].

1965—RONALD MELZACK (1929–2019) and PATRICK D. WALL (1925–2001): Canadian psychologist and British neuroscientist published in London their new theory of "Gate Control" to explain pain mechanisms [147].

1966—ALOIS STACHER (1925–2013): Austrian clinician and hematologist clinically defined an interference field as an occult inflammation that is locally oligosymptomatic but capable of triggering symptoms in distant areas of the body [148].

1967—EUGEN VAN DER ZYPEN (1933–2019): German ophthalmologist and anatomist discovered by electron microscopy a peripheral distribution of the ANS in a network-like and endless shape. At any point of the intertwined vegetative network, stimuli are transmitted rapidly. Crucial contribution to the understanding of the Huneke phenomenon [149].

1967—JAIME ABEL WIKINSKI (1926–2015): Argentine anesthesiologist, originally from Poland, discovered that procaine crosses the blood–brain barrier instantly. He also determined that procaine levels in cerebrospinal fluid can be detected within minutes [150].

1968—JOSÉ E. USUBIAGA (1931–1970): The Argentine anesthesiologist reported that procaine also traverses the placental barrier and has been used in obstetric anesthesia safely for the fetus with total doses of up to 4000 mg intravenously [151].

1970—FRANZ HOPFER (1917–1996): Viennese dentist, a disciple of Dosch during the 1960s, promoted the "Austrian group" together with Pischinger, G. Kellner, F. Perger, G. Kaiser, G. Feucht, O. Maresch, W. Krause, M. Eder, A. Stacher, and H. Fleischhacker. The *Austrian Medical Society for Neural Therapy according to Huneke,* was founded in 1972 [152].

1970—RONALD MELZACK (1929–2019): The Canadian psychologist published his classic work *Pain Manual* [147].

1971—GERMÁN DUQUE MEJÍA (1933–1991): Colombian surgeon, internist, and obstetrician came upon NT in Germany through Peter Dosch. In 1973, from Finca Los Robles, his family estate near Popayán, he began promoting NT throughout Latin America [153].

1971—JORGE ALBERTO DUQUE MEJÍA (1943): Together with his brother, translated multiple texts from German into Spanish [154].

1972—DIETER GROSS (1914–1986): German internist and neuropsychiatrist from Frankfurt published *Therapeutic local anesthesia*. He proposed the term irritation center to refer to the interference field [155].

1972—HEINZ RAAB (1909–1987): Austrian dentist from the Vienna University Dental Clinic elucidated the concept of focal sanitation. He emphasized that root canal treatment does not equate to "focal sanitation." The misconception lies in identifying the "focus" as the radiographically visible periapical alteration (granuloma). In his view, the "focus" encompasses any tooth with dead pulp, regardless of whether its periapical osteitis has been resolved [156].

1973—ERNEST ADLER (1906–1996): He published *General diseases caused by irritation fields of the neurovegetative system produced by dental and tonsillar problems (trigeminal area). Diagnosis and therapy*. Hundreds of detailed clinical cases descriptions before and after dental treatment [128].

1973—JULIO CÉSAR PAYÁN (1942–2020): Colombian obstetrician-gynecologist from Popayán, beginning his career at Los Robles with Dr. Duque, and after a decade transitioning to his CIMA (Centro de Investigación en Medicina Alternativa), played a key role in establishing a knowledgeable community of NT practitioners in Latin America. His "systemic and complex" approach gave NT a distinct identity, linking health and disease to social and political contexts. The "Colombian School of Neural Therapy" expanded to Argentina, Peru, Ecuador, Mexico, Venezuela, and Spain, integrating Huneke's principles, Russian Nervism, and Payan's ethical-philosophical framework. In 2016, he was recognized as the "World Philosopher of Neural Therapy" [157].

1975—ERICH MINK (1918–2009): German OB/GYN and pupil of Goecke documented his experience in gynecological NT in two textbooks. He first described in NT the vertebral facet joints injection technique, which Dosch referred to since 1984 as the "indirect sympathetic trunk injection according to Mink" [158].

1977—HANS LANGER (1936–2024): German ophthalmologist reviewed and supplemented Adler's findings on cervical projection zones of interference fields corresponding to paranasal sinuses, teeth, mandible, and tonsils (Adler-Langer points) [159].

1978—OTTO BERGSMANN (1922–2004): The Viennese pneumonologist, NT pioneer in Austria, conceived a cybernetic definition of the interference field: strong external stimuli are either processed or lead to death, while the time factor influences weak, subliminal stimuli. These stimuli cause minor external phenomena but remain latent in the NS. A second strike at a distant location triggers their emergence there [160].

1978—FRITZ KRAMER (1920–2001): German dentist described associations of teeth groups with acupuncture functional circuits together with Voll. Contributed decades of EAV research on findings of odontogenic foci and IFs [161, 162].

1979—MATHIAS DOSCH (1945): German physician based in Munich, son and disciple of Peter Dosch, published his book *Atlas of Neural Therapy with Local Anesthetics*, now translated into English, French, and Spanish and already in its third edition [163].

1980—HOLGER HUNEKE (1941–2025): German physician, son of Ferdinand Huneke, published his book "Dictionary of Neural Therapy" [164].

1981—JANET G. TRAVELL (1901–1997) AND DAVID G. SIMONS (1922–2010): John F. Kennedy's personal physician and the American physician and former astronaut published their theory of "Trigger Points" [165].

1984—MANFRED ZIMMERMANN (1933–2024): German physician and physicist specializing in pain neurobiology hypothesized that the "general response" to nociceptive signals from any segment structure can be attributed to the convergence of nociceptive afferents from the skin, musculature, or corresponding internal organs within the same dorsal horn neuron of the spinal cord [166].

1985—ESPERANZA CERÓN VILLAQUIRAN (1955): Colombian Neuraltherapist, a disciple of Payán led the *Fundación para la Comunicación Popular* (FUNCOP Cauca), a nongovernmental organization dedicated to advancing alternative approaches in fields such as democracy, gender, agrarian development, habitat, ecology, and health. The organization's initiatives were conceptualized and implemented following the principles of Participatory Action Research, as developed by the Colombian sociologist **Orlando Fals Borda (1925–2008)**. Her engagement with women's groups and her gender related contributions have been instrumental in the progressive development of the epistemic foundation of NTM [167].

1986—ANDREAS BECK (1936–2012): Swiss orthopedic surgeon and disciple of Dosch and Hopfer founded the Swiss Medical Association for Neural Therapy according to Huneke [168].

1986—WALTER ZIEGLGÄNSBERGER (1940–2024): German pharmacologist, toxicologist, and neuropsychiatrist contributed to a better understanding of the neurobiological mechanisms of nociception, chronic pain, and neuropathic pain, including a thorough analysis of interference field effects. [169].

1987—HANS TILSCHER (1935) and MANFRED EDER (1927–): Austrian orthopedic physicians published extremely low side effect rates (0.03%) in segmental and segmental-reflex complex treatment in approximately 264,000 patients [170].

1987—HARTMUT HEINE (1941–2016): German biologist, anatomist, and writer conceived the matrix research model of the interference field, describing it as a locally limited subclinical inflammation that takes place around nondegradable foreign or endogenous material, remaining below the pain threshold [171, 172].

1987—MIKHAIL VASILIEVICH PLAKHOTIN (1906–1988): The Russian veterinarian published his *Manual of Veterinary Surgery* with an extensive chapter describing the injection techniques and clinical indications of novocaine, as well as a thorough neurophysiological exploration of its action. [173].

1990—FRITZ ALBERT POPP (1938–2018): German experimental physicist specializing in biophysics and medicine, conducted extensive research on ultraweak photon emission (biophotons) from cells and tissues. His work demonstrated that biophotons serve as a mechanism for biological intercommunication and self-organization [174].

1991—HORST BECKE (1930–2019): East German gynecologist, author in 1975 of the first NT textbook in the GDR, *Brief Introduction to Neural Therapy*, was the first president of the German Society for Acupuncture and Neural Therapy, DGfAN, founded in 1990 [175].

1992—JERRY BOUQUOT (1945): American dentist and oral pathologist promoted in the English-speaking world the rediscovery of the interference field under the figure of NICO (Neuralgia-Inducing Cavitation Osteonecrosis) [176].

1993—JOHANN DIEDERICH HAHN-GODEFFROY (1939): German pharmacologist from Hamburg reviewed the potential risks of procaine therapy concluding that the rate of side effects in the literature is considerably lower than that of many comparable pharmacologic therapies [177].

1993—FELIX PERGER (1921–1993): Austrian clinician at the University of Vienna demonstrated significant cost savings by modulating the ground regulation system in chemically triggered chronic diseases—including multiple sclerosis, ulcerative colitis, rheumatic diseases, autonomic dysfunction, and select cancers [178].

1994—ANDREAS ZOHMANN (1957) and MARKUS KASPER (1958): Austrian veterinarians from Salzburg published their book *Neural Therapy in Veterinary Medicine: Fundamentals—Diagnosis—Therapy* [179].

1994—GERNOT BADTKE (1939–): German sports physician and one of the pioneers of NT in the former GDR showed how using subtle manual examination techniques can increase the success rate of neuraltherapeutic interventions [180].

1994—YOSETTE OSORIO (1958): Colombian dentist, forerunner in Neurofocal Dentistry (NFD) and promoter of its development throughout the Americas, founded the Colombian Association of Neurofocal Dentistry and Biological Medicine. She sided Dr. Julio César Payán in directing NT and NFD courses for two decades and in organizing World Congresses since 2003 [181].

1996—HANS BAROP (1949): German Neuraltherapist and trauma surgeon from Hamburg published the first edition of his textbook *Lehrbuch und Atlas der Neuraltherapic nach Huneke*. He defined the interference field as a tissue segment with sympathetic innervation, present in any part of the body, where afferent fibers exhibit chronic pathological irritation [182].

1997—LORENZ FISCHER (1953): Swiss physician published *Neural Therapy according to Huneke*. In 2002, he became a full professor of Neural Therapy at the University of Bern. In 2005 and 2010, he authored the *Health Technology Assessment (HTA) of Neural Therapy*, which was presented to the Swiss Federal Department of Health. This report led to Neural Therapy being covered by basic health care insurance in Switzerland [183].

1998—ANDREAS BECK (1936–2012): In 1998, he established the interdisciplinary chair of complementary medicine KIKOM (Kollegiale Instanz für Komplementärmedizin) in Bern, with a chair of Neural Therapy under his direction [168].

2000—RICARDO MACHIAVELLI (1950–2017): Argentine traumatologist introduced Neural Therapy in a public hospital in the province of Buenos Aires [184].

2002—SANDRA PAYÁN (1980): Colombian neural therapist and physician founded the Community Health Program of the Ministry of Health of the Province of Formosa, Argentina. The program was created to value local knowledge for integral health, promoting the collaborative sharing of knowledge, skills, and values for a better world. Its core principles are "Community is all of us," "Integral Health," and "Sum of Knowledges and Actions" [185].

2002—DAVID VINYES (1968): Catalan physician from Sabadell, Barcelona. He created terapianeural.com, a recognized reference in the field in Spanish-speaking countries. In 2003, he launched a Master in Neural Therapy at the University of Barcelona, which has trained over 700 professionals from 20 countries. He founded the Spanish Society of NT in 2014 and established the NT Research Foundation in 2019. In 2025, he edited a Spanish-language textbook on Neural Therapy, published by Editorial Médica Panamericana [186].

2002—KEVIN J. TRACEY (1957): The American neurosurgeon demonstrated that the ANS reflexively controls the immune response and that there is communication between the IS and the NS. LAs reduce neurogenically induced inflammation through their influence on neurotransmitters [187].

2003—EDUARDO HUMBERTO BELTRÁN DUSSÁN (1949): Colombian pediatrician and oncohematologist created at the National University of Bogotá, the first theoretical–practical extension course of Neural Therapy. Since 2007, a master's degree in alternative medicine was developed, including the area of Neural Therapy [188].

2003—SUSANNE HERRÖDER (1976) AND MARKUS HOLLMANN: Molecular and biological detection of the G-protein-mediated anti-inflammatory effect of local anesthetics [189].

2004—HÜSEYIN NAZLIKUL (1963): Istanbul physician founded the Turkish Society of Neural Therapy. He promoted NT through Turkey and Iran and edited a textbook in 2010 [190].

2005—ROBERT KIDD (1945–2019): Canadian physician and osteopath published his first English-language textbook on NT [191].

2006—WILFRID JÄNIG (1938): German physician and neurobiologist published his treatise on the ANS, *The Integrative Action of the Autonomic Nervous System—Neurobiology of Homeostasis*. For him various forms of coupling between sympathetic postganglionic neurons and primary afferent neurons are possible, which have been developed experimentally in animal models with controlled nerve injury, demonstrating that intimate relationships between sympathetic and afferent neurons can develop under pathophysiological conditions [192].

2010—STEFAN WEINSCHENK (1954): German gynecologist from Heidelberg authored the *Handbook of Neural Therapy: Diagnosis and Therapy with Local Anesthetics*. In 2011, he established the HUNTER Group (Heidelberg University Neural Therapy Education and Research Group), an organization committed to undergraduate and postgraduate NT training, as well as NT research advancement and scholarly publication in collaboration with the University of Heidelberg [193].

2011—ROBERTO CASTRO (1956): The Argentinian veterinarian published the first Manual of Veterinary Neural Therapy in Spanish [194].

2012—INTERNATIONAL FEDERATION OF MEDICAL ASSOCIATIONS OF NEURAL THERAPY (IFMANT): With headquarters in Meiringen,

Switzerland, the organization was founded, grouping world NT societies with the purpose of observing integration status in their respective national health systems, unifying educational standards, and easing mutual contact and cooperation [195].

2013—JORGE IVÁN SALAZAR (1959): Colombian Neuraltherapist proposed giving Neural Therapy the new name Neuraltherapeutic Medicine (NTM) as a means of acknowledging its different medical rationality and the new status of complex medical system [196].

References

1. Moreno y Maiz T. Chemical and physiological research on the Erythroxylum coca of Peru and cocaine. Paris: Louis Leclerc; 1868.
2. Koller C. On the use of cocaine for producing anaesthesia on the eye. Lancet. 1884;2:990–2.
3. Imber G. Genius on the edge: the bizarre double life of Dr. William Stewart Halsted. New York: Kaplan Publishing; 2010.
4. Osborne MP. William Stewart Halsted – his life and contributions to surgery. Lancet Oncol. 2007;8(3):256.
5. Hall RJ. Hydrochlorate of cocaine. N Y Med J. 1884;40:643–4.
6. Yentis SM, Vlassakov KV. Vassily von Anrep, forgotten pioneer of regional anesthesia. Anesthesiology. 1999;90:890–5.
7. François-Franck C. Paralytic action of cocaine on nerves and nerve centers. Applications to experimental technique. A. de P. 1892;562.
8. Schleich C. Infiltration anaesthesia (local anaesthesia) and its relation to general narcosis (inhalation anaesthesia). Verh Dtsch Ges Chiropractic. 1892;21:121–7.
9. Schleich CL. Painless operations. Berlin: Julius Springer Verlag; 1894.
10. Reclus P. Cocaine in surgery. Paris: G Masson Editeurs and Gauthier-Villars et Fils Imprimeurs-Editeurs; 1895.
11. Freud S. On coca. Centralblatt für die gesammte Therapie. 1884;11(7):289–314.
12. Corning JL. Pain in its neuro-pathological, diagnostic, medico-legal, and neuro-therapeutic relations. Philadelphia: J. B. Lippincott; 1894.
13. Schleich CL. New methods of wound healing. In: Their conditions and simplification for practice. Berlin: Verlag von Julius Springer; 1899.
14. Bier A. Experiments on the Cocaineization of the spinal cord. Langenbeck's. Arch Surg. 1899;51(3–4)
15. Kreis O. On medullary anesthesia in Parturients. Zentralbl Gynaekol. 1900;28:724–9.
16. Tuffier T. Surgical analgesia via the spinal route (subarachnoid injections of cocaine): technique, results, indications. Paris: Masson Eds; 1901.
17. Sicard JA. Medicinal drug injections via the sacrococcygeal route. C R Soc Biol. 1901;53:396–8.
18. Spiess G. The healing effect of anesthesia. Med Welt Zbl Inn Med. 1902;23:222–3.
19. Schleich C. Infiltration of anaesthesia (local anaesthesia) and its relationship to general narcosis (inhalation anaesthesia). Verh Dtsch Ges Chiropractic. 1892;21:121–7.
20. Farbwerke vorm: Meister Lucius und Brüning in Höchst AM. Method for the preparation of p-aminobenzoic acid alkyl esters. Patent. 1904;179:627. (Class 12q, Group 6)
21. Link WJ. Alfred Einhorn, Sc. D: inventor of novocaine. Dent Radiog Photog. 1959;32(1):20.
22. Braun H. On some new local anesthetics (Stovain, Alypin, Novocain). Dtsch Med Wochenschr. 1905;31:1667–71.
23. Spiess G. The importance of anesthesia in inflammation therapy. Münchn Med Wschr. 1906;53:345.

24. Wischnewski AW. The Novocaine block as a method of influencing tissue trophism. Zentrbl Chir. 1935;62(13):435–346.
25. Atanassoff PG, Lobato A, Aguilar JL. Intravenous regional anesthesia with long-acting local anesthetics. Rev Esp Anestesiol Reanim. 2014;61(2):87–93.
26. Lemaire A. The problem of visceral sensitivity and the anesthesia of Splanchnalgias. Louvain: Secretariat of the Scientific Society; 1928.
27. Kulenkampff D. Anesthesia of the brachial plexus. Beitr Klin Chir. 1912;79:550–2.
28. Hirschel G. Anesthesia of the brachial plexus in operations on the upper extremity. Münch Med Wochenschr. 1911;29:1555–6.
29. Fischer G. Local anesthesia in dentistry, with special reference to the mucous and conductive methods: a concise guide for dentists, surgeons, and students. Philadelphia: Lea and Febiger; 1912.
30. Härtel F. Conduction anesthesia and injection treatment of the Gasseri ganglion and the trigeminal trunks. Arch Klin Chir. 1912;100(1):13–292.
31. Hering E. Memory; lectures on the specific energies of the nervous system. Chicago, London: The Open Court Publishing Company; 1913.
32. Leriche R. On the elongation and sectioning of perivascular nerves in certain pain syndromes of arterial origin and in some trophic disorders. Lyon Chir. 1913;10:378–82.
33. Mackenzie J. Symptoms and their interpretation. New York: Paul B. Hoeber; 1918.
34. Higier H. Vegetative neurology – the anatomy, physiology, pharmacodynamics, and pathology of the sympathetic and autonomic nervous systems. New York: Nervous and Mental Disease Publishing Co.; 1919.
35. Graefe AK, Saemisch T, von Hess C, Elschnig A. Handbook of complete ophthalmology. Berlin/Heidelberg: Springer; 1922.
36. Farbwerke H. Clinical reports and scientific treatises on Novocain. Hoechst a. M.: Farbwerke vorm. Meister Lucius & Brüning; 1922.
37. Pal J. On the discussion of the Clinic of Angina Pectoris. Wien Klin Wchnschr. 1924;37:351.
38. Pal J. Clinical and therapeutic aspects of angina pectoris. Wien Arch Inn Med. 1923;6:153–66.
39. Laignel-Lavastine M. Pathology of the sympathetic nervous system: an attempt at anatomical-physiological-pathological clinical pathology. Paris: F. Alcan; 1924.
40. Ricker G. Pathology as natural science – relational pathology – for pathologists, physiologists, medical doctors, and biologists. Berlin/Heidelberg: Springer; 1924.
41. Leriche R, Fontaine R. Isolated anesthesia of the stellate ganglion. Its technique, indications, and results. Presse Med. 1934;42:849–50.
42. Huneke F, Huneke W. Unknown remote effects of local anesthesia. Med Welt. 1928;27:1013–4.
43. Mandl F. The effect of paravertebral injections in angina pectoris. Arch Klin Chir. 1925;136:495.
44. Schilf E. The autonomic nervous system. Leipzig: G. Thieme; 1926.
45. Mandl F. The paravertebral injection. Vienna: Springer-Verlag; 1926.
46. Fontaine R. Neurophysiology and peripheral neurosurgery of visceral pain. J Neural Transm. 1966;28:470–84.
47. Cannon WB. Organization for physiological homeostasis. Physiol Rev. 1929;9(3):399–431.
48. Kibler M. Segment therapy in joint diseases and internal diseases. Stuttgart: Hippokrates; 1955.
49. Vishnevsky AV. Local anesthesia by the method of creeping infiltrate. Moscow: Medgiz; 1956. p. 352.
50. Labat G. Regional anesthesia: its technique and clinical application. Philadelphia: W. B. Saunders Company; 1922.
51. Danielopolu D. The nervous system of the vegetative life. Paris: Masson ed; 1932.
52. López EM. Origin of functional pathology in Mexico; general principles. Cirugía y Cirujanos. 1951;19(9):494–9.
53. Stajano C. Vegetative system and trophic neurosis. Montevideo: Talleres gráficos Buenos Aires Herald; 1933.

54. Speransky AD. Nervous Trophism in the theory and practice of medicine. Moscow: Institute of Experimental Medicine of the Union; 1934.
55. Leriche R. The effect in the blink of an eye. Lyon Chir. 1932;27:62–83.
56. Leriche R. Pathophysiology of scars and the underlying sclerotic tissue studied with the aid of sympathetic Novocainization. Presse Med (Paris). 1934;42:1577–8.
57. Ruth HS. Diagnostic, prognostic, and therapeutic nerve blocks. JAMA J Am Med Assoc. 1934;102(6):419–25.
58. Reilly J, Rivalier E, Compagnon A. Hemorrhage, vascular and lymphatic lesions of the digestive tract induced by Perisplanchnic injection of various substances. Compt Rend Soc Biol. 1934;116:24–7.
59. Vishnevsky AA. Technique of Novocaine block of the sympathetic nervous system of the lumbar region. Arkhiv Biologicheskikh Nauk. 1933;34(4):519–21.
60. Anokhin PK. Biology and neurophysiology of the conditioned reflex and its role in adaptive behavior. Oxford: Pergamon Press; 1974.
61. Astvatsaturov MI. Overview of the current status of the pain problem. Sovr Psixonevrol. 1935;6:141.
62. Huneke F. Disease and healing seen differently. 7th ed. Cologne: Staufen; 1947.
63. Speransky AD. Basis for a new theory of medicine. Buenos Aires: Editorial Psique; 1954.
64. Kulenkampff D. On local anesthesia for treatment purposes, especially for acute epididymitis. Münch Med Wochenschr. 1937;84:1175–6.
65. Pieri G. Pathophysiology of the sympathetic nervous system in humans. Rome: Pozzi; 1937.
66. Tinel J. The autonomic nervous system. Paris: Masson; 1937.
67. Tinel J. Sympathetic pains. Presse Med. 1921;29:263–5.
68. Falta W, Fenz E. Remarks on the problem of thyroid-hypothalamus. J Mol Med. 1938;17(5):148.
69. Hansen K, von Staa H. Reflexive and painful disease signs of the internal organs. Leipzig: G. Thieme; 1938.
70. Speransky AD. Foundations of a theory of medicine. Berlin: Sänger; 1950.
71. Albanese A. Manual of anesthetic blockades of the Neurovegetative system; anesthesia of the sympathetic nervous system. Buenos Aires: El Ateneo; 1938.
72. Cannon WB. The wisdom of the body. New York: Norton; 1939.
73. Lambret O, Rozemon L, Decoulx P. Technique of sympathetic surgery and its infiltrations. Paris: G. Doin et Cie; 1939.
74. Huneke F. Unknown remote effects in local anesthesia. Fortschr Med. 1934;52:213–23.
75. Roques KR. The role of healing anesthesia in pathology and therapy. Münch Med Wochenschr. 1940;87:34–7.
76. Siegen H. Theory and practice of neural therapy with Impletol. Cologne: Staufen; 1951.
77. Mező BV. The origin of trophic disorders and their treatment with cyclical anesthesia. Zbl Neurochir. 1940;5:192–8.
78. Fenz E. Treatment of rheumatic diseases through anesthesia. Dresden and Leipzig: Th. Steinkopff; 1941.
79. Scheidt C. Problems and questions in cases of suspected diseases of odontogenic foci. Berlin: Lehmanns Verlag; 1942.
80. Veil WH, Sturm A. The pathology of the brainstem. 2nd ed. Jena: Fischer; 1946.
81. Löfgren N, Lundquist B. Studies on local anesthetics: II. Svenks Kem Tidskr. 1946;58:206–17.
82. Leriche R. Fronto-orbital migraines. Their treatment by novocaine injection around the superficial temporal artery. Progrès Médical. 1943.
83. Ognev BV. Intracerebral circulation, symposium of scientific investigations at the 20th anniversary of the kremlin therapeutic sanitary clinic. Moscow: State Medical Press; 1946. p. 24–8.
84. Finochietto E, Finochietto R. Surgical technique: operations and apparatus; part one: general technique; local anesthesia, vol. 2. Buenos Aires: Ediar; 1944.

85. Bykov KM. The cerebral cortex and the internal organs. 3rd ed. New York: Chemical Publishing Co. Inc.; 1957.
86. Hazard R, Chemol J, Levy J, et al. Manual of pharmacology. Paris: Masson et Cie; 1945.
87. Hazard R. A new functional proof – evaluation of blood procaine esterase. Presse Med. 1948;56:529.
88. Luzuy M. Infiltrations of the sympathetic: physiology – indications – techniques. Paris: Masson; 1946.
89. Stohr P. Nervous system nervous tissue the peripheral nervous system the central nervous system. Berlin: Julius Springer; 1928.
90. Pi Suñer A. Neurovegetative system. Mexico: Uteha; 1947.
91. Scheidt W. The vegetative system. In: Fundamentals of nerve physiology. Hamburg: Richard Hermes-Verlag; 1947.
92. Tosatti E. Infiltrations of the sympathetic. Rome: Edizioni Italiane; 1947.
93. Lluesma UE. Neurovegetative. Buenos Aires: El Ateneo; 1948.
94. Vischñevsky AV, Vischñevsky AA. Novocaine block and balsamic oil antiseptics as a form of pathogenic therapy. Ed. Cartago: Buenos Aires; 1958.
95. Sturm A. The clinical pathology of the lung in relation to the vegetative nervous system – attempt at a new general pathological order based on the example of the lung. Stuttgart: Wissenschaftliche Verlagsgesellschaft M. B.H; 1948.
96. Arnulf G. Stellate infiltration. Technique, indications, results. Paris: Masson et Cie; 1947.
97. Marchesani O. Contributions to the problem of endogenous eye inflammations. v. Graefes. Arch Ophthalmol. 1948:148.
98. Naranjo VP. The Neurovegetative system – phylogeny – embryology – anatomy – physiology – harmacology. Quito: Imprenta Universidad Central; 1948.
99. Fleckenstein A. The mechanism of excitation and inhibition with special consideration of Novocain. Anästhesist. 1954;3(1):15–9.
100. Eichholtz F, Staab A. The application of Novocain in internal medicine. In: Part II: toxicology of local anesthetic substances; 1952. p. 516.
101. Nonnenbruch W. Bilateral kidney diseases. Stuttgart: Ferdinand Enke; 1949.
102. Dittmar F. The study of reflexive and painful disease signs. Berlin and Tübingen: Haug; 1949.
103. Lazorthes G. The neurovascular system. Paris: Masson; 1949.
104. Anselmino KJ. On the prospects for curing severe constipation through Novocain infiltration of the lumbar sympathetic ganglia. Dtsch Med Wochenschr. 1947;72(43/44):641–3.
105. Anselmino KJ, Plaskuda G, Stewens R. On a new method for prolonged conduction anesthesia of labor pain: the segmental, epidural Plomb. Klin Wochenschr. 1949;27:104–5.
106. Travell J. Basis for the multiple uses of local block of somatic trigger areas (procaine infiltration and ethyl chloride spray). Miss Valley Med J. 1949;77:13–22.
107. Ratschow M. Critical review of the scope of neural therapy (healing anesthesia). Dtsch Med Wochenschr. 1951;76(1):308–11.
108. Selye H. The stress of life. New York: McGraw-Hill Book Co.; 1956.
109. Siegen H. Theory and practice of neural therapy with Impletol. Staufen: Kamp-Lintfort; 1951.
110. Kraucher GK. Intravenous use of local anesthetics in internal medicine. Berlin Heidelberg: Springer-Verlag; 1951.
111. Siegmund H. Diagnosis of focus diseases. Munich: Hanser; 1953.
112. Huneke W. Impletol therapy and other neural therapeutic methods. Stuttgart: Hippokrates; 1952.
113. Schmelzer H. Neural therapy in ophthalmology. Halle: Marhold; 1953.
114. Vogler P, Krauss H. Periostbehandlung: klinische und experimentelle Beiträge. Leipzig: VEB Georg Thieme Verlag; 1953.
115. Voll R. Topographic positions of the measurement points in electro-acupuncture, vol. 3. Kulmbach: Medizinisch-Literarische Verl.-Ges; 1977.
116. Reischauer F. On the technique of local Novocain treatment in lumbago-sciatica. Dtsch Med Wochenschr. 1953;78(40):1375–6.

117. Zipf H. Endo-anesthesia, a pharmacological way to eliminate internal sensory receptors. Dtsch Med Wochenschr. 1953;78(46):1587–9.
118. Stiefvater EW. Acupuncture as neural therapy. Stuttgart: Haug; 1953.
119. Letterer E. Interpretation of Masugi/nephritis as an allergic-hyperergic phenomenon. Dtsch Med Wochenschr. 1953;78(15):512–5. https://doi.org/10.1055/S-0028-1131312.
120. Schwamm E, Reeh J. The ultraviolet radiation of humans and its molecular spectroscopy. Hippokrates. 1953;24:737–42.
121. Mosin VV. Novocaine blockade of primary nerves as a method of protective effect on the nervous system in surgical trauma, inflammation of the peritoneum, abdominal and pelvic cavity organs in animals. Scientific Notes of. Kazan: KVI, 1954.
122. Hess WR. Diencephalon, autonomic and extrapyramidal functions, vol. 229. New York: Grune and Stratton; 1954.
123. Junghanns SA. The human spine in health and disease. New York, London: Grune and Stratton; 1971.
124. Schoeler H. The Weihe points: their relationship to acupuncture, neural therapy, and homeopathy. Ulm-Donau: Karl F. Haug; 1954.
125. Westhues M. On healing anesthesia in veterinary medicine. Berk Münch Tierärztl Wschr. 1955;24:422–5.
126. Bischko J, Kitzinger E, Nissel H. Acupuncture for advanced practitioners. Heidelberg: Karl F. Haug; 1985.
127. Dietz O. On the Ganglion blockade in animals. Habilitation Thesis, University of Leipzig; 1956.
128. Adler E. General diseases caused by irritation fields of the neurovegetative system due to dental and tonsillar problems (Area of the Trigeminal Nerve). Diagnosis and Therapy; Quito: Fundación Omniversidad de América, 2002.
129. Adler E. Focus areas and foci in the trigeminal region. 4th ed. Heidelberg: E. Fischer; 1990.
130. International Medical Society for Neural Therapy According to Huneke Regulation Therapy e.V. Neural Therapy – IGNH [Internet]. IGNH. 2024. Available from: https://ignh.de/
131. Hoff F, Janini P, María J. Treatment of internal diseases. Barcelona: Ed. Labor; 1958.
132. Schmid J. Neural therapy. Vienna: Springer-Verlag; 1960.
133. Reischauer F. Novocain therapy in surgery with contribution to the improvement of stellate ganglion block. Langenbeck's Arch Surg. 1961;298(1):391–404.
134. Huneke F. The lightning reaction. A physician's testament. Stuttgart: Haug; 1961.
135. Kothbauer O. On the pressure point diagnosis and neural therapy in animals. Wien Tierärztl Monat Vet Med Austria. 1961;48:282–94.
136. Goecke H. On experiences with neural therapy in gynecology and obstetrics. Hippokrates. 1962;33:153–6.
137. Schliack H, Hansen K. Segmental Innervation. In: Its importance for clinic and practice. Thieme; 1962.
138. Riccabona A. The Dentogenic maxillary sinus affection. Dent Pract. 1966;13:225.
139. Kuznetsov AK. Subcutaneous application of Novocain for therapeutic purposes in animals. Collection of Scientific Articles of the Leningrad Veterinary Institute. 1962;24:161–174.
140. Kuznetsov AK. Influence of Novocain on the autonomic nervous system. Collection of Papers of the Leningrad Veterinary Institute. 1963;25:215–228.
141. Dosch P, Dosch M. Manual of neural therapy according to Huneke. 2nd ed. Stuttgart: Georg Thieme Verlag; 2007.
142. Monnier M. Physiologie und Pathophysiologie des vegetativen Nervensystems. Berlin: Springer; 1963.
143. Leger V. Neural therapy in particular, according to Huneke (the phenomenon in seconds). Metz: Imprimerie Ch. Merfeld; 1963.
144. Pischinger A. The extracellular matrix and ground regulation. In: Basis for a holistic biological medicine. Berkeley: North Atlantic Books; 2006.

145. Kellner G. Basic system and regulatory disorders: (regulatory pathological conditions for diagnosis, therapy). Stuttgart: Haug; 1984.
146. Fleischhacker H. Klinik der Herderkrankungen. Therapiewoche. 1965;15:1274–8.
147. Melzack R, Wall PD. Pain mechanisms: a new theory. Science. 1965;150:971–9.
148. Stacher H. On the Huneke- phenomenon in seconds and its objectification. In: Writings of the central Association of physicians for natural medicine. Uelzen: Dr. Blume-Verlag; 1968. p. 139–49.
149. Van der Zypen E. Electron microscopic findings on the terminal spread of the vegetative nervous system and their interpretation. Acta Anat. 1967;67:431–515.
150. Usubiaga JE, Moya F, Wikinski JA, Wikinski R, Usubiaga LE. Relationship between the passage of local Anaesthetics across the blood-brain barrier and their effects on the central nervous system. Br J Anaesth. 1967;39(12):943–7. https://doi.org/10.1093/bja/39.12.943.
151. Usubiaga JE, La Iuppa M, Moya F, Wikinski JA, Velazco R. Passage of procaine hydrochloride and Para-Aminobenzoic acid across the human placenta. Am J Obstet Gynecol. 1968;100(7):918–23.
152. Hopfer F. Phenomena in neural therapeutic practice. Ärzte Naturheilverfahren. 1991;32:684–92.
153. Payán JC. Biological medicine: a commitment to life. Colombia: Fondo Editorial – Fundación Homeopática Alemana. Salve Ediciones: Buenos Aires; 2005.
154. Sarmiento Rodríguez LD. History and institutionalization of neural therapy in Colombia. Univ. Nac. de Colombia, Faculty of Medicine, Master's in Alternative Medicine, Neural Therapy area. Bogotá, Colombia; 2014.
155. Gross D. Therapeutic local Anesthesia. Volume I. basics – clinic – technique – a neurotherapeutic practicum. Stuttgart: Hippokrates; 1972. Volume II: Application in clinic and practice. Stuttgart: Hippokrates; 1988.
156. Raab H. The vegetative foundations of odontogenic focal diseases. Vienna: Maudrich; 1972.
157. Payán de la Roche JC, César J. Leap into the void, your wings will spread. Bogotá: McGraw-Hill Interamericana; 2000.
158. Mink E. Novocain therapy according to Huneke in gynecology. Heidelberg: Karl F. Haug Verlag; 1975.
159. Langer H. The Adler pressure points, causes and issues. Lecture at the 1st working conference of the neural therapy working group, Holzhau; 1977.
160. Bergsmann O. Bioelectrical phenomena and regulation in complementary medicine. Vienna: Facultas; 1994.
161. Kramer F. Textbook of Electroacupuncture, vol. 1-4. Heidelberg: Karl F. Haug Verlag; 1981.
162. Kramer F. The diagnosis of residual osteitis – another form of odontogenic focus infection. In: Biological medicine bulletin. Translated by Germán Duque Mejía; 1992.
163. Dosch M. Atlas of neural therapy techniques with local anesthetics. Heidelberg: Karl F. Haug Verlag GmbH & Co; 1979.
164. Huneke H. Dictionary of neural therapy. Heidelberg: Haug; 1980.
165. Simons DG, Travell J. Myofascial trigger points, a possible explanation. Pain. 1981;10(1):106–9.
166. Zimmermann M. Neural therapy in light of recent findings in neurobiological research. In: Seithel R, editor. Neural therapy 2. Stuttgart: Hippokrates; 1984. p. 9–27.
167. Garzón Fuentes EC. Neural therapeutic medicine in Colombia. Master's Thesis in alternative medicine, neural therapy area. National University of Colombia. 2024. Available from: https://repositorio.unal.edu.co/handle/unal/87341
168. Stettbacher MA. In memoriam Andreas Emilio Beck. Swiss Medical Bulletin. 2013;94:13–4.
169. Zieglgänsberger W. Central control of nociception. In: Mountcastle VB, Bloom FE, Geiger SR, editors. Handbook of physiology – the nervous system IV. Baltimore: Williams & Wilkins; 1986.
170. Tilscher H, Eder M. Infiltration therapy, therapeutic local anesthesia. Stuttgart: Hippokrates; 1996.

171. Heine H. Basic regulation from a new perspective. Ärzte Naturheilverfahren. 1987;28:909.
172. Heine H. Fundamentals of neural therapy theory. Ärzte Naturheilverfahren. 1988;29:851–5.
173. Plajotin M. Manual of veterinary surgery. Moscow: MIR Publishing; 1987.
174. Popp FA, Warnke U. Electromagnetic bio-information. Baltimore: Urban & Schwarzenberg; 1989.
175. Becke H. Neural therapy in lower back pain and migraine. Stuttgart: Hippokrates; 1991.
176. Bouquot JE. Neuralgia-inducing Cavitational osteonecrosis (NICO) osteomyelitis in 224 jawbone samples from patients with facial neuralgia. Oral Surg Oral Med Oral Pathol. 1992;73(3):307.
177. Hahn-Godeffroy JD. Novocain in neural therapy according to Huneke. Literature review and summary evaluation. Der Allgemeinarzt. 1993;14:876–83.
178. Perger F. Compendium of regulatory pathology and therapy – the realm of individual defense power. Berlin: Sonntag Verlag; 1990.
179. Zohmann A, Kasper M. Neural therapy in veterinary medicine: basics – diagnosis – therapy. Hannover: Schlütersche; 1994.
180. Badtke G, Mudra J. Neural therapy – textbook and atlas. Berlin: Ullstein-Mosby; 1994.
181. Osorio Y, Fajardo F. Dental foci in bone. An alternative to the electrical disturbance generated by the presence of metallic materials in the oral cavity. Oral Dia. 1994;17:10–2.
182. Barop H. Textbook and atlas of neural therapy according to Huneke. Stuttgart: Hippokrates; 1996.
183. Fischer L. Neural therapy according to Huneke – basics, technique, practical application. Stuttgart: Hippokrates-Verlag; 1997.
184. Machiavelli R. Neural therapy in a public referral hospital. 2000. Available at: https://www.terapianeural.com/articulos/22-memorias-de-los-encuentros/101-terapia-neural-en-un-hospital-publico-de-referencia
185. Morgan L, Payán SI, Pineda C. Health in the hands of the community: systematization of reflections on integral health care in Formosa. Community Health Program – Ministry of the Community – Formosa; 2002.
186. Vinyes D. Neural therapy – treatment with local anesthetics. Barcelona: Médica Panamericana Publishing; 2025.
187. Tracey KJ. Reflex control of immunity. Nat Rev Immunol. 2009;9(6):418–28.
188. Beltrán EH, Vega JA. Neural therapeutic medicine: an approach from complex medical systems. Bogotá: Editorial Universidad Nacional de Colombia; 2013.
189. Hollmann MW, Herroeder S, Kurz KS, Hoenemann CW, Struemper D, Hahnenkamp K, Durieux ME. Time-dependent inhibition of G protein–coupled receptor signaling by local anesthetics. Anesthesiology. 2004;100(4):852–60.
190. Nazlikul H. Neural therapy: another treatment is possible. Istanbul: Destek Yayinlari; 2020.
191. Kidd RF. Neural therapy: applied neurophysiology and other topics. Refrew: Custom Distribution; 2005.
192. Jänig W. The integrative action of the autonomic nervous system – neurobiology of homeostasis. Cambridge: Cambridge University Press; 2006.
193. Weinschenk S. Handbook of neural therapy. Diagnosis and therapy with local anesthetics. Munich: Elsevier; 2010.
194. Castro R. Foundations for neural therapy in canines and felines. Ed. Dunken: Buenos Aires; 2011.
195. Home. International Federation of Medical Associations of Neural Therapy. Home [Internet]. 2024. Available at: https://www.ifmant.at
196. Salazar JI. Neural therapy: from "orthodox" therapy to neural therapeutic medicine. In: Beltrán EH, Vega JA, editors. Neural therapeutic medicine: an approach from complex medical systems. Bogotá: Editorial Universidad Nacional de Colombia; 2013.

Chapter 2
The History of Neural Therapy in Germany

Hans Barop

It all began with a coincidence in F. Huneke's practice in 1925: following a recommendation from a colleague, the general practitioner F. Huneke (1891–1966) treated his sister's migraine attack with an intravenous injection of the rheumatism drug "Atophanyl," which was actually intended for intramuscular administration with the addition of procaine 2%. To his surprise, the migraine stopped. When she had another migraine attack, he injected the "correct" Atophanyl without the addition of procaine, which was intended for intravenous administration, but without success.

It is thanks to F. Huneke's precise powers of observation that he noticed the difference in the lack of procaine. When he injected pure procaine 2% intravenously, the migraine quickly subsided again. This was the first step toward neural therapy: procaine could also be used for therapeutic purposes and not just as a local anesthetic for surgical purposes. F. Huneke was not aware of the existing observations by G. A. Spiess (1862–1955) on the "healing effect of anaesthetics" in tonsillectomized patients [1–3].

Together with his brother Walter (1897–1974), also a general practitioner, F. Huneke subsequently used procaine for various diseases, initially as an intravenous injection and later also by local infiltration into painful pressure points, nerves, vessels, and joints. For this, he used procaine 2% with added caffeine (Impletol), which was produced from 1928 by Bayer AG on F. Huneke's recommendation.

Over the following years, the Huneke brothers treated illnesses such as migraines, headaches, insomnia, hearing loss, chronic kidney inflammation, neuralgia, ischialgia, chronic joint inflammation, organic and functional heart disease, Graves' disease, and various skin diseases and described this method as "medicinal anaesthesia" and "Impletol therapy."

In 1928, the first publication by F. Huneke with the title: "Unknown remote effects of local anesthesia" [4] was followed in 1936 by his book "Krankheit und

H. Barop (✉)
Specialist in Surgery, Specialising in Neural Therapy, Friedrich-Legahn-Straße 2, Hamburg, Germany
e-mail: h.barop@gmx.de

L. B. Pinilla Bonilla et al. (eds.), *Neuraltherapeutic Medicine*,
https://doi.org/10.1007/978-3-032-03257-7_2

Heilung anders gesehen," in which F. Huneke assumed that the therapeutic effect was due to the involvement of the autonomic nervous system [5].

The use of a single short-acting local anesthetic to treat different diseases was new. This was in stark contrast to the differentiated drug therapy of common medicine and led to the rapid spread of this therapy, but also to criticism and doubts about the credibility of the Huneke brothers. Today's advanced evidence-based knowledge of the neuroanatomy and neurophysiology of the autonomic nervous system in disease processes and the comprehensive effects of procaine on cell membranes, among other things, did not yet exist at the time.

Ferdinand and Walter Huneke disseminated their treatment method through numerous national and international lectures at medical events and in medical journals [6–16]. The number of doctors who successfully applied "healing anesthesia" grew steadily as doctors from medical practices, clinics, and medical schools visited Huneke's practice. On the recommendation of Prof. Max Kibler (1900–1973), a student of Huneke and familiar with the autonomic nervous system, termed the developing therapeutic use of local anesthetics as "segmental therapy."

The assumption that the therapeutic successes had to occur via the autonomic nervous system was confirmed in 1940, the time of the first "phenomenon in seconds or lightning reaction." After procaine infiltration of a patient's recurrent right-sided lower leg osteomyelitis, a painful left-sided shoulder disease that had previously been treated unsuccessfully in the segment, stopped within a few seconds.

The speed of this unexpected reaction alone led to the conclusion that it had to be a reaction via the nervous system. Obviously, osteomyelitis was the cause of the shoulder disease.

F. Huneke described the process as a "phenomenon in seconds" and the osteomyelitis of the lower leg as the "cause" of the shoulder disease, as a "interference field." This second observation was something completely new in medicine, as it was the key to the repeated failures of local application. This first observation and the many analogous therapeutic successes of F. Huneke and his students were the basis for the term "interference field therapy."

In honor of the "inventor" and in order to define the dual content of the new therapy (segmental/interference field therapy), in 1940, K. R. V. Roques (1890–1966), also a student of Huneke, called the method "neural therapy according to Huneke." This term has remained to this day, as it describes the basics of therapy via the (autonomic) nervous system in one word.

Since the first reproducible therapeutic successes of neural therapy, the desire to understand the mechanisms of action of this new treatment method had arisen at the same time. This required detailed knowledge of the neuroanatomy and neurophysiology of the autonomic nervous system.

Even before F. Huneke, the pathologist G. Ricker (1870–1948) had demonstrated the etiology of various diseases via the stimulation of the autonomic nervous system in comprehensive animal experiments. Disturbances of the microcirculation caused by different degrees of stimulation of the autonomic nervous system of the vessels turned out to be the common cause of various diseases caused by neuroplastic changes in the peripheral and central autonomic nervous system. He summarized these findings in his textbook "Pathologie als Naturwissenschaft—Relationspathologie" in1924 [17].

After F. and W. Huneke's first publication in 1928, numerous other publications appeared in the following years, both by F. and W. Huneke [6–16] and by many of his students, which dealt with the basics of neural therapy and the numerous indications. Among the authors, Siegen H., for example, demonstrated the influence of neural therapy on the immune system using the example of anaphylaxis [18–21], and Pischinger A. showed the importance of interstitial metabolism in the causal effectiveness of neural therapy [22, 23]. The French surgeon Leriche A. (1879–1955) showed in his work the therapeutic advantages of neural therapy in comparison to sympathetic surgery and described neural therapy as "the surgeon's bloodless knife" [24–27].

In 1963, the first comprehensive textbook on neural therapy was published by Dosch P. (1915–2005) with a total of 14 editions up to 1996 [28]. In their textbooks, Barop H. 1996 [29] and Fischer L. 1997 [30] presented the current scientific principles of neural therapy, which defined this treatment method as a regulatory medical procedure within overall medicine. Neural therapy is defined as an "Injection treatment method with local anaesthetics using the functions and properties of the autonomic nervous system." In the last 30–40 years, the number of scientific publications on the therapeutic use of local anesthetics has risen sharply internationally.

Due to the growing number of Huneke students, the founding of a neural therapy society was called for within the German group in order to promote the representation and dissemination of neural therapy. On March 20, 1957, the International Society for Neural Therapy according to Hunke (IGNH) was founded in Bad Pyrmont at the 12th Advanced Training Congress of Doctors of Naturopathy. It was entered in the register of associations in Munich the following year in 1958. As the number of IGNH members increased, particularly foreign doctors, further national neural therapy societies were founded, initially in Austria (ÖNR,1971) and in Switzerland (SANTH,1986). There are now national medical neural therapy societies in over 15 countries, 14 of which have been brought together in an umbrella organization (IFMANT). The aim of this medical umbrella organization is to monitor and promote standardized, scientifically oriented training, coordinate international congresses, and support the societies in their national health policy concerns.

The two-year certified training program follows an internationally valid curriculum in the respective national associations. The prerequisite is a licence to practice medicine and completed specialist training. Neural therapy has found a permanent place in university medicine in Germany at the Medical School in Heidelberg, in order to integrate the basics of this treatment method into the medical training of students.

References

1. Spiess G. The healing effect of Anesthetics. Ärztebl Inn Med. 1902;23:22.

2. Spiess G. The significance of Anesthesia in inflammation theory. Münch Med Wochenschr. 1906;53:345–51.
3. Spiess G. The significance of Anesthesia in inflammation therapy and its application, especially in the treatment of laryngeal tuberculosis. Arch Laryngol. 1912;21:120–5.
4. Huneke F. Unknown remote effects of local Anesthesia. Med Welt. 1928;27:1013–4.
5. Huneke F. Illness and healing seen differently. Bonn: Stauffen Verlag; 1936.
6. Huneke F. Focus problem and the phenomenon in seconds in its treatment for dentists. Dtsch Zahnärztl Z. 1950;23:1269–78.
7. Huneke F. Gynecology and the focus problem. Ärztl Wochenschr. 1952;7(41):967–96.
8. Huneke F. The focus problem from a neural therapeutic perspective. Hippokrates. 1952;23:625–33.
9. Huneke F. Dentists and the phenomenon in seconds. Zahnärztl Referate. 1955;56(13–14):256–9.
10. Huneke F. Neural therapy, phenomenon in seconds, and surgery. Allg Ther. 1956;27(21):675–82.
11. Huneke F. The treatment of various forms of rheumatism with Impletol. Med Klin. 1957;31(32):1127–8.
12. Huneke F. 35 years of neural therapy. Physikalisch-diätetische. Therapie. 1961:75–80.
13. Huneke F. On the frequency of the phenomenon in seconds in my practice. Hippokrates. 1969;31(3):74–7.
14. Huneke F. The phenomenon in seconds. 6th ed. Heidelberg: Haug; 1989.
15. Huneke W. Impletol therapy. Hippokrates. 1952;
16. Huneke W. Neural medicine – an overview using the example of joint diseases. Hippokrates. 1965;36:465–71.
17. Ricker G. Pathology as a natural science – relational pathology. Berlin: Springer; 1924.
18. Siegen H. Theory and practice of neural therapy with Impletol. Cologne: Staufen; 1951.
19. Siegen H. Fundamentals of neural therapy with Impletol. Hippokrates. 1961;32:348–57.
20. Siegen H. The nervous interference field. In: Voss HF, editor. That's why neural therapy. Uelzen: ML-Verlag; 1968.
21. Siegen H. The immunological balance between donor and recipient organism: a classical neuro-regulative task. In: Dosch P, editor. Neural therapy according to Huneke – Freudenstadt lectures 1974, vol. 2. Heidelberg: Haug; 1975.
22. Pischinger A. The vegetative basis of focus processes. Österr Z Stomatol. 1963;60:294–311.
23. Pischinger A. The System of Basic Regulation. Revised and edited by H. Heine. 11th ed. Stuttgart: Haug; 2009.
24. Leriche A. On stellate ganglion Anesthesia in cerebral embolism, vascular spasms, post-brain surgery, and hemiplegia. Rev Chir. 1936;55:755.
25. Leriche A. Peri- and intra-arterial novocaine injections in neural medicine. Neuralmed. 1955;3:2–5.
26. Leriche A. The treatment of post-traumatic vasomotor disorders. Neuralmed. 1955;3:15–7.
27. Leriche A. The surgery of pain. Leipzig: Barth; 1958.
28. Dosch P. Textbook of neural therapy according to Huneke. 14th ed. Haug; 1996.
29. Barop H. Textbook and atlas of neural therapy. 2nd ed. Haug; 2014.
30. Fischer L. Neural therapy, neurophysiology, injection techniques, therapy proposals. 5th ed. Thieme; 2019.

Chapter 3
The History of Neuraltherapeutic Medicine in Colombia

Edna Cecilia Garzón-Fuentes and Eduardo Humberto Beltrán Dussán

1 From Germany to Colombia

Neural Therapy arrived in Colombia in the 1970s in the southwest of the country, having been influenced by strength and recognition achieved by the Huneke brothers in Germany. With great difficulty, they positioned this new art, consolidating a robust experience and a rich casuistry (see Chap. 2). In Colombia, there is a socially, culturally and politically effervescent context, which nuanced the exercise and the gradual consolidation of Neural Therapy in this region of the world, transforming and reconfiguring its theoretical and philosophical body, as well as its practice, from a different understanding of the health-disease process and its implications for the human being and its environment. This process allows Neural Therapy to be valued by the Colombian school as a medicine with its own identity and to be recognized as a complex medical system, called Neuraltherapeutic Medicine, according to the parameters established in the literature, a process that will be described and characterized in detail in Chap. 6 [1–10].

Within the antecedents to the emergence of Neural Therapy in Germany, with the Huneke brothers around 1925, it is essential to mention the school of Russian Nervism of the nineteenth and early twentieth centuries, where Neural Therapy finds part of its roots. This school of physiology focused its research and experiments on the understanding of the functioning of the organism, recognizing the nervous system as the coordinator and integrator of all organic processes in both

E. C. Garzón-Fuentes (✉)
Master in Alternative Medicine, Neural Therapy Area, Faculty of Medicine, Universidad Nacional de Colombia, Bogotá, Colombia
e-mail: ecgarzonf@unal.edu.co

E. H. Beltrán Dussán
Faculty of Medicine, Universidad Nacional de Colombia, Bogotá, Colombia
e-mail: ehbeltrand@unal.edu.co

L. B. Pinilla Bonilla et al. (eds.), *Neuraltherapeutic Medicine*,
https://doi.org/10.1007/978-3-032-03257-7_3

health and disease conditions [6–9, 11–15]. Also preceding the appearance of Neural Therapy are the experiments with anesthetics that took place both in Russia within this same physiological current, and, in Germany, other regions of Europe and the United States [11, 12, 16]. This historical background will be discussed in depth in Chaps. 26 and 40. In Germany, there has been a great expansion and consolidation of Neural Therapy since 1925, where, in addition to its initiators, the Huneke brothers, figures such as Dr. Peter Dosch, Drs. Francel Hopfer, Scheidt, Lorenz Fischer, and Hans Barop stand out (see Chap. 2) [9, 11, 12, 17].

Around 1972, Neural Therapy arrived in Colombia through the Colombian doctor, Dr. Germán Duque Mejía. Years after completing his medical studies in Germany, Dr. Duque discovered Neural Therapy by chance while traveling with a patient to the Germanic nation to receive treatment for a medical condition for which he had not been able to find relief from the medical care he had received in Colombia. The stories tell that perhaps with disappointment, when they were already preparing to return to Colombia without having found a solution for their condition, someone told them about the existence of Dr. Peter Dosch, who performed an unconventional treatment with needles and who had reported many successes [6, 9, 10].

Dr. Duque and his patient decided to go to Dr. Peter Dosch's office, and after obtaining an unexpected and evident amelioration in the patient's ailment, Dr. Germán Duque was amazed at the results and expressed to Dr. Dosch his desire to deepen that knowledge and his desire to learn. He became a disciple of Dr. Peter Dosch's by initiating a series of learning and training trips, initially alone, and later with other Spanish-speaking doctors, and his brother Jorge Alberto Duque. On these trips, they structured their knowledge of Neural Therapy and other medical conceptions and different alternative therapies under development in Germany at that time [6, 9, 10].

2 "Los Robles" School

As Dr. Germán Duque continued his learning process, it was becoming increasingly evident that all of the new information he was gaining ought to be shared and expanded. Together with his brother, Dr. Jorge Alberto Duque, he summoned many other doctors to his trips to Germany and later to other countries, starting a training school in Colombia at the *Los Robles hacienda,* owned by his family. This hacienda, located south of the city of Popayán, department of Valle del Cauca in the southwest of the country, became emblematic in the history of alternative medicine and Neural Therapy, especially for the Spanish-speaking world.

In the gradual consolidation of *Los Robles* as a school, seedbed and center for the dissemination of alternative medicine in Colombia, the translation of a large number of publications from German to Spanish began. In this initiative, the role of Dr. Jorge Alberto Duque Mejía, a lawyer who had had his professional training in Germany, was decisive. The Duque Mejía brothers, with the support of the work team they were forming, manage to consolidate a large library of alternative medicine, both with translations of texts from German and with their own publications derived from the academic meetings that they were organizing around the dissemination and teaching of this new knowledge [6, 9, 10].

Los Robles was attended by several characters who had something to learn and something to teach in relation to health from various worldviews. According to Dr. Jorge Alberto Duque, about 1517 doctors passed, some only to be informed, others to be trained, and others, who contributed significantly to the process of consolidation of alternative medicine, as is the case of Dr. Julio César Payán de la Roche [9]. Dr. Payán arrived at *Los Robles* around 1973, invited by Dr. Augusto Leyva Samper, a renowned Colombian cardiologist and university professor, who had already had the opportunity to be in contact with alternative medicine and the experience of *Los Robles* [6, 9, 10, 18]. Dr. Julio César Payán, Colombian medical doctor, specialist in gynecology and obstetrics, who was a professor and dean of the Faculty of Medicine of the University of Cauca, marked a decisive turning point in the history and consolidation of Neural Therapy in Colombia and in the Spanish-speaking world [9].

3 Colombia, Fertile Ground

Colombia's historical and political dynamics are complex. The country has great cultural and geographical diversity and has sustained important internal conflicts over time. These conditions have generated different, unique expressions and adaptive processes in the different territories. From this perspective, the characteristics of the geographical and political context of Cauca, a department in southwestern Colombia where Los *Robles hacienda* is located, the cradle of alternative medicine in the Spanish-speaking world, mark fundamental imprints in the development and transformation of Neural Therapy in Colombia.

The conditions of manifest adversity often imply the generation and strengthening of organizational processes within the affected communities as a way of facing them and seeking possibilities of management or solution [9, 19]. In Cauca, in particular, the ethnic and cultural richness is especially diverse and has maintained the validity of ancestral knowledge and wisdom, which is expressed in a very lively way in its music, its gastronomy, and the customs of its inhabitants. Practices that have managed to remain over the centuries despite the adverse actions of cultural and social annihilation that took place between the years 1500 and 1810 during the process of conquest and colonization of these territories, and that had a strong impact on this region [9, 18, 20, 21]. Historically, in the department of Cauca, there have been multiple structured and organized social movements that have emerged in the midst of the need to manage the various crises of the territory, which have been generated and sustained over time. There, at the time of the arrival of Neural Therapy in Colombia, peasant populations, different indigenous ancestral peoples, and descendants of African settlers brought to these lands in times of slavery coexist with agreements and tensions. The capital of Cauca, Popayán, also has a strong European heritage bequeathed from the colonial era. These conditions influenced the dynamics and spaces of maturation of the thought and praxis of Neural Therapy in Colombia.

In the context described, the figure of Dr. Julio César Payán de la Roche is fundamental in the consolidation of Neural Therapy in Colombia and in the Spanish-speaking world. Dr. Payán, who had already gone through a path of social sensitivity and work with communities in the region, is one of the first doctors with a teaching career to be part of the *Los Robles* team. Dr. Payán's arrival at *Los Robles* was prompted by both skepticism and curiosity. He eventually became an undisputed leader in the consolidation of Neural Therapy as a medical system by assiduously studying and attempting to comprehend it after being astounded by the outcomes it produced in patients. From his structure and academic experience, he felt the need to seek a rational explanation for those inexplicable improvements that he observed in patients, and for which he found few or no explanations from conventional medicine. He then decisively delved into the explanations and authors behind the advances and development of Neural Therapy in Germany, gradually expanding epistemological horizons, weaving and innovating from different logics, explanatory frameworks, and fields of knowledge. Although he also knew other approaches to medicine and many other alternative practices and treatment methods that came to *Los Robles*, Dr. Payán decided on Neural Therapy and made it his partner.

In *Los Robles,* there was an effervescence of practices and knowledge, which were encompassed within the broad concept of medicine and alternative therapies. [9, 10]

> *...on the one hand, and headed by Dr. Germán Duque, a school influenced by the spiritual thought of India and that adopted, in addition to Neural Therapy, diagnostic techniques such as dowsing and other therapies that had arrived in Los Robles. On the other hand, Dr. Julio Cesar Payán de la Roche formed a school that gradually and exclusively opted for Neural Therapy* [21].

Between 1972 and 1982, the process of greatest effervescence in the development of the *Los Robles* school took place. This place for alternative medicine training and patient care center operated from the early 1970s until 1986, when Dr. German Duque made the decision to move to the country's central region, to the municipality of Arbeláez, in the department of Cundinamarca. There, he continued his work in patient care, teaching, and dissemination while developing his own alternative medicine vision. Dr. Germán Duque died on February 16, 1991, in the city of Bogotá, leaving an invaluable contribution to alternative medicine in the Spanish-speaking world [6, 9, 10, 21, 22].

4 "Payanese" School

Around 1981, Dr. Julio César Payán retired from *Los Robles,* concentrating his work in his private office in the center of the city of Popayán, opening there the possibility of receiving students to learn Neural Therapy. Thus, he continued his rigorous process of study, inquiry, and reflection, within which he founded and put into operation the *CIMA, Centro de Investigación en Medicinas Alternativas (Alternative Medicine Research Center)* that would have legal status around 1991 [6, 9, 21, 23].

A school of thought emerged that was later recognized as a complex-systemic current and, over time, was taken as a structural basis for the recognition of Neural Therapy as a medical system with its own rationality and in its designation as Neuraltherapeutic Medicine. This process developed within the framework of its institutionalization at the National University of Colombia since the end of the twentieth century. This will be covered in detail in Chap. 4. This reality became possible thanks to the path Dr. Payán continued and consolidated, as well as fortunate encounters like the one that occurs around 1985 with Dr. Esperanza Cerón Villaquirán, another character of great importance in this story [3, 5, 6, 9, 10, 21].

Dr. Esperanza Cerón, who had arrived as a patient in *Los Robles* around 1977 while still an undergraduate student of the medical career, also began her learning process there, playing a fundamental role in the social projection that Neural Therapy has in Colombia, as well as in the configuration of the scenarios that were consolidated as spaces for reflection and school of thought. Due to her social sensitivity, since her school days, she accompanied popular education processes with various communities in the department of Cauca. This work was developed from the approaches of the *Participatory Action Research (PAR) methodology*, created by Orlando Fals Borda, father of sociology in Colombia and cofounder of the Faculty of Sociology of the National University of Colombia [9]. This methodology refers to a type of non-imposing research that encourages communities to actively participate in their social transformation by facilitating the critical recovery of their history, allowing for the identification of both their reality and their potential to change it. As will be seen in Chap. 20, this methodology also contributed to the way in which both the medical consultation and the elaboration and use of clinical history were reconfigured within the exercise of Neural Therapy in this school [9].

Many factors contributed to the development of Neural Therapy in Colombia, including the robust Neural Therapy according to Huneke that came from Germany, the training and dissemination space in *Los Robles*, the tenacious efforts of the Duque Mejía brothers, the leadership of Drs. Julio César Payán and Esperanza Cerón, and the ethnic and cultural diversity of Cauca, with its long history of social and community movements. It is then described how these aspects were interwoven and generated a unique paradigmatic and identity vision for Neural Therapy in Colombia, which had a moment of unusual strengthening after an earthquake that shook the city of Popayán in 1983.

On March 31, 1983, an earthquake destroyed the city of Popayán, plunging the population into chaos, in the midst of a gloomy panorama of death, hunger, significant deterioration of the sanitary and urban infrastructure, persistent heavy rains, aftershocks that persisted, and a governmental structure incapable of attending to the magnitude of the catastrophe. During this terrible chaos, the community organized itself to face the various problems caused by the catastrophe, including the need for housing, generating different informal settlements. Within these groups, women's organizations stand out in the settlements that tried to solve the constant problems of security, provision of food and drinking water [9, 24].

Around these organized groups of women supported by students of the Faculty of Medicine of the University of Cauca, health committees were organized in tents where people were attended, dialogue was held with the community, how to heal wounds was taught, breastfeeding was educated, support was given in the search for solutions to the problems of drinking water supply, of garbage management, and other needs that the particular context was generating. In these spaces, Dr. Esperanza Cerón Villaquirán, who at the time was in the last year of her medical career and had already been attending *Los Robles* for about 6 years, had a special leadership. In addition to the accompaniment of the activities described and in view of the impossibility of a sufficient response from the health system, the lack of resources, medicines and supplies, together with a group of advanced students in the career, she supported the management and coverage of basic health needs, providing care with Neural Therapy and auriculotherapy for the populations in the settlements. At that time and specific context, a special and novel path was opened for Neural Therapy in Colombia, from the clarity that was being made in the process, of its potentialities in the care, management, and resolution of health problems; a characteristic that became more visible and useful in the framework of a public health problem of the dimensions described. Neural therapy as a therapeutic tool and *Participatory Action Research (PAR)* methodology naturally blended in these settings, accompanied by community processes and, concurrently, dialogue with a wide range of non-hegemonic knowledge and practices [6, 9, 21, 24–29].

Organized women's groups had a fundamental relevance in the reconstruction of Popayán and from there in the strengthening of Neural Therapy as well. In this process of recovery from the devastation generated by the earthquake, the *FUNCOP* collective *Fundación para la Comunicación Popular (Foundation for Popular Communication)*, of which Dr. Esperanza Cerón was cofounder, was reorganized and established its residence in the city of Popayán. This organization, which, later, given its philosophical and social orientation, was constituted as a nongovernmental organization (NGO), had been born in the city of Cali in 1981 as an education and communication project for the community. *FUNCOP* had the objective of promoting and accompanying collective and social transformations based on autonomy, freedom, sustainability, democracy, and humanism, developing its work around alternative health, the construction of democracy, the gender perspective, participatory urban planning, and food sovereignty [9, 20, 21, 30–32]. It linked popular leaders within its processes, including many of the women who had championed the processes of management and attention to basic needs in the settlements after the earthquake.

Around 1985, the women's organization of one of the nascent neighborhoods derived from post-earthquake urban settlements, the *"Colombia segunda etapa"*neighborhood, with the support of *FUNCOP*, led the implementation of the *La Nueva Esperanza* Health Center, the first in Latin America to provide care to patients with Neural Therapy. Since its affiliation with *FUNCOP*, this health center was influenced by the participatory methodologies and philosophical logic of the organization. As it was developed, it has enabled the social and community expression of Neural Therapy to flourish and mature, which had been consolidated around Drs. Julio César Payán de la Roche and Esperanza Cerón [9, 10, 21, 24, 30, 33].

Although Dr. Esperanza Cerón and Dr. Julio César Payán had already coincided and knew each other from *Los Robles*, it was around 1985, at this juncture of reorganization of the city and the community derived from the earthquake, where they began a joint work. She accepted his invitation to join him in his office for training on Neural Therapy. There, they discussed current research, issues, and realities, the city's recovery and community reorganization processes, and the settlements with the health committees and Neural Therapy with *FUNCOP* and the *Nueva Esperanza* Health Center [9, 21, 24, 31].

Over time, Dr. Payán became linked to *FUNCOP* and to the management of the *La Nueva Esperanza* Health Center, making *FUNCOP* a fundamental actor in this history as a school of thought in the epistemological maturation of Neural Therapy in this territory. The gradual consolidation of one's own thinking was more clearly structured as a result of this meeting between Dr. Julio César Payán and Dr. Esperanza Cerón, as well as the *FUNCOP* process. This was due to the spaces of collective reflection that were created, where community work, academic reflection, and the profound traces of the *Participative Research Action* methodology converge, always within a framework of respectful dialogue among different forms of knowledge. These spaces for dialogue and reflection were gradually strengthened, giving rise to the organization, from 1987 onward to a decade of meetings that were called *"Coloquios de Medicina Alternativa y Sociedad" (Colloquiums of Alternative Medicine and Society.)* In these meetings, the most diverse actors, academics, popular and ancestral knowledge, worldviews from other regions, and diverse expressions of what is known today as alternative medicine and therapeutics, find a voice creating spaces for reflection on health in a broad sense, beyond welfare or the intervention of potential risk factors. In this space, the social and political dimension of alternative medicine in general and Neural Therapy in particular began to take shape [9, 34–37].

This own way of thinking, which will be discussed in more detail in Chap. 18, which Dr. Esperanza Cerón called the "*Payanese School*" of Neural Therapy [21], was being developed in these spaces and contexts and was the basis for the structuring of the philosophical and paradigmatic vision of Neural Therapy that Dr. Payán lead [9]. Among its characteristics can be stated:

- The understanding that conventional Western medicine and alternative medicine obey different paradigmatic and conceptual structures. In other words, Neural Therapy from this perspective implies a different way of thinking, which implies that there are different rationalities or ways of thinking about health, which are not necessarily antagonistic or contradictory, but different, and from that difference we can enter into respectful dialogue [9]
- A constant search for novel explanations to the processes of health and disease, from the explanatory insufficiency of the epistemological frameworks offered by biomedicine, to the findings that were observed day by day in patients [9]

- The questioning of the concept of health as a state and of the health/disease polarity, with a rethinking and resignification of disease and diagnosis as the fundamental axis of medical practice, focusing on the processes, associations, and subjects that embody these processes and relationships, considering disease as an adaptive phenomenon [6, 9, 38, 39]
- The conviction of the need to promote and recover the autonomy of subjects and communities, as well as their capacity for action and active participation in their individual and collective health processes, recognizing them as critical actors in the possibility of transforming their own reality. It is an exercise that implies, among other variables, the critical reconstruction of the *Life History* (which will be developed in Chap. 20), the recovery of individual and collective consciousness, the strengthening of dynamics of mutual care, and the visibility and strengthening of the capacities of self-management and self-eco-organization [9].
- A critical stance against the passive role of the patient in the understanding and management of their health processes, the hierarchies implicit in the medical act, as well as the unilateral nature from which decisions are made [9]
- The rethinking of the doctor–patient relationship or community health system, tending toward non-imposing, respectful, dialogic, and participatory relationships [6, 9, 40]
- An ethical and philosophical stance that Dr. Payán calls *"Desobediencia Vital" (Vital Disobedience),* which encompasses these postulates and implies uncertainty and non-determinism in the vital and the impossibility of life "obeying" preestablished models or norms [6, 9]

With these twists and breakups to the canonical ways of understanding health and disease, a specific way of thinking was consolidated and the birth of Neural Therapy takes place as a medical system with its own rationality. [9].

5 Institutionalization of Neural Therapy

Dr. Payán met Dr. Yosette Osorio, a dentist by profession, who led the consolidation of Neurofocal Dentistry in Colombia, and with whom, around 1996, they decided to structure, in modular courses, the training that Dr. Julio César Payán had been offering both in a disciplic way in his office and in the *"Colloquiums of Alternative Medicines and Society"* [9, 10]. The courses of Neural Therapy and Neurofocal Dentistry, which were initially carried out in the city of Bogotá with the leadership of Dr. Osorio and then in the city of Cali with the accompaniment of Dr. Jorge Humberto Petta, Dr. Sandra Isabel Payán, and Dr. Edna Garzón, were formalized [9, 10, 41].

Around 1998, Dr. Eduardo Beltrán Dussán, pediatric oncohematologist and professor at the National University of Colombia, led and began the process of institutionalization of alternative medicine at that university. Dr. Beltrán initially achieved the approval of a new subject called "line of deepening in alternative medicine".

Later, extension courses for graduate doctors were approved and, finally by 2006, the master's degree in Alternative Medicine (a postgraduate official program) was consolidated with four areas of deepening: Neural Therapy (Neuraltherapeutic Medicine), Homeopathy, Traditional Chinese Medicine, and Osteopathy [9, 10, 42, 43]. This is how the National University of Colombia has been leading the teaching of Neural Therapy, taking for the design of the curricular program, the philosophical and epistemological framework developed by Dr. Julio César Payan de la Roche [44].

At the time of this publication, there are two medical associations of Neural Therapy in Colombia: The Colombian Association of Neural Therapy Julio César Payán de la Roche, CONETSO JCP [45] and the Colombian Association of Neural Therapy/Neuraltherapeutic Medicine, ACOLTEN/MNT [46] members of the International Federation of Medical Associations of Neural Therapy, IFMANT (see Chap. 2) [47], and one for neurofocal dentistry: the Association of Neurofocal Dentists of Colombia (ODNF). These three associations, in their individual projects or jointly, also work for the strengthening and recognition of Neural Therapy in Colombia, from the path bequeathed by Dr. Julio César Payán de la Roche.

References

1. Luz MT. Contemporary culture and alternative medicines: new health paradigms at the end of the 20th century. Phys Rev Saúde Coletiva. 1997;7:13–43.
2. Tesser CD, Luz MT. Medical rationalities and integrality. Ciênc Saúde Colet. 2008;13(1):195–206.
3. Beltrán EH, Vega JA. Neuraltherapeutic Medicine: an approach from complex medical systems. Bogotá: Editorial Universidad Nacional de Colombia; 2013. p. 159.
4. Salazar Marín JI. Neural Therapy: from "Orthodox" therapy to complex medical system. Master's thesis. Bogotá: Universidad Nacional de Colombia; 2010.
5. Urrego Mendoza DZ, Martiletti A, Casas del Rio GH, Ruiz Díaz P, Vega Oviedo A, editors. Alternative medicine: a view from complex medical systems. 1st ed. Bogotá: Universidad Nacional de Colombia; 2011.
6. Payán de la Roche JC. Vital Disobedience, vol. 1. 3rd ed. Sabadell: Instituto de Terapia Neural; 2016.
7. Huneke F. The phenomenon in seconds or the testament of a doctor. 1st, 2nd, 3rd vols. Translated by Dr. Germán Duque Mejía, editor. Popayán: Editorial Los Robles; 1961.
8. Asociación Colombiana de Terapia Neural – ACOLTEN/MNT, CONETSO (JCP). Neural Therapy/Neuraltherapeutic Medicine (NTM) in the Context of the Pandemic [Internet]. 2020. p. 84. Available from: https://acolten.com.co/wp-content/uploads/2020/07/LA-TERAPIA-NEURAL-MEDICINA-NEURALTERAPEUTICA-MNT-EN-CONTEXTO-DE-PANDEMIA_compressed.pdf
9. Garzón Fuentes EC. Neuraltherapeutic Medicine in Colombia. Master's thesis in Alternative Medicine. Bogotá: Universidad Nacional de Colombia; 2024. Available from: https://repositorio.unal.edu.co/handle/unal/87341
10. Sarmiento LD. History and institutionalization of Neural Therapy in Colombia. Bogotá: Universidad Nacional de Colombia; 2014. Available from: http://www.bdigital.unal.edu.co/43119/1/52145193.2014.pdf

11. Dosch P. Textbook of Neural Therapy according to Huneke (therapy with local anesthetics). 8th ed. Heidelberg: Haug Verlag; 1978.
12. Dosch P. Teaching book of Neural Therapy according to Huneke. In: (Procaine therapy). Volume one: theory and practice. Popayán: Los Robles; 1973.
13. Toscano de La Torre F, Pinilla Bonilla LB. The principles of Neural Therapy from the foundations of nervism to current neuroscience. Rev Salud UIS. 2012;44(2):57–65.
14. Bermúdez Cruz AF. The concept of reflex in Russian Nervism from a historical perspective and its impact on Neural Therapy and medicine. Master's thesis in Alternative Medicine. Bogotá: Universidad Nacional de Colombia; 2017. Available from: https://acolten.com.co/wp-content/uploads/2017/04/Tesis-Andres-Berm%C3%BAdez.pdf
15. Speransky AD. Foundations for a new theory of medicine, vol. 1. Buenos Aires: Editorial Psique; 1954. p. 7–507.
16. Vischñevsky AV, Vischñevsky AD. Novocain block and balsamic oleoresin antiseptics as a form of pathogenic therapy. Buenos Aires: Cartago; 1958.
17. Fisher Lorenz. Neural Therapy according to Huneke; neurophysiology, therapeutic injection techniques. 3rd ed. Niño Ibarra, MC, editor. Vol. 1. Mexico: [unknown editorial]; 2012. p. 1–261.
18. Garzón Fuentes EC. Tribute to Dr. Julio César Payán De la Roche [Internet]. Terapianeural.com; 2017. Available from: http://www.terapianeural.com/articulos/20-y-mas/383-homenaje-al-dr-julio-cesar-payan-de-la-roche
19. Martínez Márquez WA, Bravo AM. Fragments of the history of armed conflict in Colombia (1920-2010). Debates Univ Antioquia. 2015;72:51–6.
20. Garzón Fuentes EC. Neuraltherapeutic Medicine. Contributions from alternative medicines in the perspective of decolonial knowledge. In: Pachamama, wisdom, and territories: holding the Pluriverse with the Llauto of Our Ancestors. Cali: 2022. Available from: https://terapianeuralcolombia.com/publicaciones-articulos/articulos
21. Cerón Villaquirán E. Neuraltherapeutic Medicine, or the incessant metamorphosis of an incomplete school. Essay between the critical recovery of history and reflection on a corner of the Payan School of thought, origins of a new current. Popayán: 2023. Available from: https://terapianeuralcolombia.com/images/articulos_ensayos/Medicina_Neuralterapeutica_HISTORIA.pdf
22. Prieto C. Eastern wisdom and western technology; 2024. Available from: https://www.eltiempo.com/archivo/documento/MAM-38647
23. Payán de la Roche JC. History and current status of Neural Therapy in Colombia; 2004. Available from: https://www.terapianeural.com/articulos/13-informacion-basica/95-breve-historia-y-estado-actual-de-la-terapia-neural-en-colombia
24. Echandía Bocanegra FJ. Analysis of the articulation of Neuraltherapeutic Medicine with primary health care at the La Nueva Esperanza Alternative Health Center in Popayán, Cauca, from 1987 to 2005. Case Study. Master's thesis. Bogotá: Universidad Nacional de Colombia; 2024. Available from: https://repositorio.unal.edu.co/handle/unal/85949
25. Cerón Villaquirán E. Participatory action research and Neuraltherapeutic Medicine; 2023. Available from: https://www.terapianeuralcolombia.com/images/articulos_ensayos/investigacion-accion-participante-y-medicina-neuralterapeutica.pdf
26. Eljach M, Corredor CE, Jaramillo Salgado D, Rosero Morales JR. Fals Borda and the persistence of utopias. Popayán: Editorial Universidad del Cauca; 2009. p. 9–141.
27. Fals Borda O. Universal origins and current challenges of PAR (participatory action research). Análisis Político. 1999;38:73–90.
28. de Figueiredo GO. Participatory action research: an alternative for social epistemology in Latin America. Rev Investig. 2015;39:1–20.
29. Balcázar FE. Participatory action research (PAR): conceptual aspects and implementation difficulties. Fund Hum. 2003;7(8):59–77.
30. Ussa Calambás IC, Palacios Alomía JA, Pérez Arroyave LY. Socio-political strengthening of community organizations on human rights (HR) and international humanitarian law (IHL) for

the reconstruction of the social fabric in the central zone of the Cauca State. Thesis. Popayán: Universidad del Cauca; 2010. Available from: http://repositorio.unicauca.edu.co:8080/xmlui/handle/123456789/2252
31. Fundación para la Comunicación Popular – FUNCOP. Popayán. A social process for sustainability. Popayán: FUNCOP; 2004. p. 1–166.
32. González N. Inclusive health: a contribution from neural therapy for public health. Popayán, Cauca; 2016. Available from: https://www.terapianeural.com/articulos/14-del-concepto/359-nancy-gonzalez-bermudez
33. Payán de la Roche JC. Popayán, an Educator City. El Liberal; 1999.
34. Fundación para la Comunicación Popular FUNCOP, Centro de Información e Investigación sobre Medicinas Alternativas CIMA. Medicine, ecology, and society: critical foundations for alternative thinking. In: II National Colloquium on Alternative Medicines and Society; 1990; Popayán: Ediciones FUNCOP; 1991.
35. Cárdenas JJ. Public Health or Health for All. In: FUNCOP, CIMA, editors. Colloquiums; 2004. p. 389.
36. Caponi S. Georges Canguilhem and the epistemological status of the concept of health. Hist Cienc Saude Manguinhos. 1997;4(2):287–307.
37. Canguilhem G. Health, a common concept and a philosophical problem. Sociol Rev Fac Sociol Unaula. 1998;21:151–8.
38. Payán de la Roche JC. Diagnosis, critiques, and possibilities; 2024. Available from: https://terapianeural.com/articulos/14-del-concepto/41-el-diagnostico-criticas-y-posibilidades
39. Cardozo Pabón AM. Illness as an emerging evolutionary process. Master's thesis. Bogotá: Universidad Nacional de Colombia; 2011. Available from: https://repositorio.unal.edu.co/handle/unal/20508
40. Cerón VE. From vital disobedience to epistemic disobedience – essay on theoretical biology and health. Popayán: Ediciones Popayán Positiva; 2018. p. 7–89.
41. Payán de la Roche J. Memories. Course on Neural Therapy, Neurofocal dentistry, and complex thinking. Cali: Centro Médico Amporá; 2008.
42. Universidad Nacional de Colombia. National graduate program directorate – program. Master's in Alternative Medicine; 2024. Available from: https://posgrados.unal.edu.co/programa/?id=503
43. Cuellar LL. Towards a characterization of postgraduate programs in alternative medicine in Colombia. Master's thesis. Bogotá: Universidad Nacional de Colombia; 2011. Available from: https://repositorio.unal.edu.co/handle/unal/7685
44. Salazar Marín JI. Neural Therapy: from "orthodox" therapy to neuraltherapeutic medicine. In: Beltrán EH, Vega JA, editors. Neural therapeutic medicine: an approach from complex medical systems. 1st ed. Bogotá: Universidad Nacional de Colombia; 2013. p. 15–28.
45. Asociación Colombiana de Terapia Neural Julio César Payán de la Roche CONETSO JCP; 2024. Available from: https://terapianeuralcolombia.com/
46. Asociación Colombiana de Terapia Neural ACOLTEN/MNT. Neural Therapy for Doctors. Available from: https://acolten.com.co/la-terapia-neural-medicos/
47. International Federation of Medical Associations of Neural Therapy. 2025. Available from: https://www.ifmant.at/es/

Chapter 4
Alternative Medicine and Neuraltherapeutic Medicine in the Postgraduate Programs of the National University of Colombia

Manuel Esteban Mercado-Pedroza and Eduardo Humberto Beltrán Dussán

1 Introduction

The National University of Colombia, by initiative arising from the Faculty of Medicine, was the first public institution to incorporate into its postgraduate academic programs a master's degree in Alternative Medicine with four emphases, for graduate doctors. It was not a process without inconveniences. It was extensive and laborious, which recalls the expression of F. Engels "theoretical thought of an entire epoch, including the present, is a historical product that takes very different forms and therefore assumes a very different content also according to the different epochs" [1].

2 Determinants

The creation of the master's degree responded to the sum of a series of social, political, economic, and academic circumstances that were articulated, among which the following stand out:

The academic commitment of a public university, based on the mission of the Faculty of Medicine of the National University of Colombia, which considers "society as a complex structure that conditions us and hopes to influence it in a positive way to contribute to its social and economic, political, cultural, scientific and technological development, aiming at a participatory and equitable society. In these institutions and, researchers, graduates, students and administrators, contribute knowledge, administer, advise or provide their professional services in public and

M. E. Mercado-Pedroza · E. H. Beltrán Dussán (✉)
Faculty of Medicine, Universidad Nacional de Colombia, Bogotá, Colombia
e-mail: memercadop@unal.edu.co; ehbeltrand@unal.edu.co

L. B. Pinilla Bonilla et al. (eds.), *Neuraltherapeutic Medicine*,
https://doi.org/10.1007/978-3-032-03257-7_4

private institutions, and contribute to local and national development." [2] In this way, the Faculty of Medicine contributes to the State and the health system new knowledge, guidance, orientation, characterization of problems, solutions, and advice in the construction of science and national culture.

The paradigmatic changes in the health-disease process over time that were generated by the new models of health care in the world and the publication in Geneva of the first strategy of the World Health Organization on Traditional Medicine 2002–2005 where it is recommended that member states provide consumers and health care providers with the best information on traditional treatments, and complementary and the need to have structures and processes that would promote education in this field, research and the provision of truthful and adequate information on traditional and complementary treatments was raised in the context of health systems [3].

The interest in Alternative Medicine and Alternative and Complementary Therapies as health care systems and their expansion in different countries of the world, as a proposal for integrative health care is documented in the literature [4]. The creation in the United States of the "National Center for Complementary and Integrative Health" (NIH) in the 1990s, as a system of integration of Medicine [5].

In Colombia, since the end of the nineteenth century, there has been a growing interest in the knowledge and dissemination of this new knowledge in groups of studious doctors interested in learning initially homeopathy and later other systems of medicine practice that were called Alternative Medicine. Different training modalities were given, initially through the personal transmission of knowledge in the offices of physicians familiar with these systems and later through informal and nonformal courses. In the second half of the twentieth century, several Associations of Medical Researchers and Practitioners of Alternative Medicine emerged, some of which assumed training processes through Diplomas and other educational activities. In the 1990s and at the beginning of the twenty-first century, some university institutions offered programs such as courses and diplomas in the field of Alternative Medicine and Alternative and Complementary Therapies in the nonformal education modality [6].

During all this time, the government entities of Colombia and especially the Ministries of Health and Social Protection and Education have been legislating on the provision of health services, professional practice, and the processes of training human talent in the field of Alternative Medicine and Alternative and Complementary Therapies [7].

In 1999, under the management of Dr. Eduardo Beltrán Dussán, professor and director of the Division of Pediatric Oncohematology of the Department of Pediatrics of the National University of Colombia, the Faculty of Medicine began the training of knowledge of Alternative Medicine within the flexible component of the Medicine career for undergraduate students. On August 30, 2001, also under the management of Professor Eduardo Beltrán, the Academic Group of Alternative Medicine of the Faculty of Medicine was created, made up of different professors eager to research in this new area. In that year, the First Extension Course on Medicine and Alternative Therapeutics for Physicians at the National University began. In the following years, other Extension Courses on Homeopathy, Neural Therapy, Traditional Chinese Medicine and Acupuncture, Osteopathy, and Chiropractic were developed successfully and with great demand until 2006, when the Formal Programs of Professional Master's Degree for Doctors in Alternative Medicine began at the Faculty of Medicine [8].

3 Structuring of the Postgraduate Program: Clinical Master in Alternative Medicine

The academic success achieved in the Extension Courses, the open-minded policy of the Faculty of Medicine and its Dean, Dr. Jaime Gallego, the support of the academic group of alternative medicine, and the availability of physical and financial resources provided by the extension courses previously carried out were conjunctural to give solidity to the idea of creating the first postgraduate degree in Alternative Medicine of the National University of Colombia.

The graduate program for physicians was called the Clinical Master's in Alternative Medicine with four areas of emphasis to be chosen by applicants in: Homeopathy, Traditional Chinese Medicine and Acupuncture, Neural Therapy, or Osteopathy and Chiropractic. The program, which has a structure of 75 credits equivalent to 3800 h of academic activities, was endorsed by the Council of the Faculty of Medicine of the National University of Colombia on November 11, 2005, the curriculum was approved by the Academic Council through agreement 050 of 2006, Minute 06 of May 17, 2006, and finally it was approved and created by the Superior Council of the University National through Agreement 055 of 2006, minute 20 of September 19. In this way, the first model of postgraduate training for medical care in the field of Alternative Medicine for graduate doctors contributed to society, an innovative and revolutionary design for the country and the health system [9].

3.1 Program Objectives

3.1.1 General Objective

To train the physician to perform with the best competencies in diagnosis, paraclinical study, and comprehensive therapeutic management of the patient, considering the possibilities of Homeopathy, Traditional Chinese Medicine and Acupuncture, Neural Therapy, and Osteopathy and Chiropractic, taking into account the concepts of Classical Medicine, and thus allowing him to establish priorities.

3.1.2 Specific Objectives

1. To deepen and base the epistemological aspects of homeopathy, traditional Chinese medicine and acupuncture, neural therapy, or osteopathy and chiropractic, depending on each area of the master's degree.
2. To inform the physician to diagnose, address, and solve health problems from Alternative Medicine and alternative therapies.
3. To integrate the concepts of the therapeutic modalities of alternative medicine with those of classical medicine, under the conception of a single medicine.
4. Develop research skills in each area.
5. To generate new knowledge in the specific area of alternative medicine.
6. To define criteria and principles that guide the use of the different therapeutic modalities in health programs in the country.

The program, with a duration of 2 years, has a common core in the first semester on the concept of alternative and complementary medicine, analyzing the different medical systems that compose it, the conception of the human being and its structure, the historical and philosophical foundations, the diagnostic approach, and therapeutic strategies of each of them, highlighting the schools of integration of thought toward the conception of a single Medicine. This first semester completes a thematic seminar on Molecular Biology applied to alternative medicine, a seminar on collective health, and another on research methodology. In the following semesters, transversal academic activities are carried out in Phytotherapy, Food, and Toxicology, among others. It is from the second semester that the academic training in the specific area is oriented according to the emphasis chosen by the master's student.

From the second semester, the teaching and care practices are carried out in the university's teaching and healthcare institutions of national and international public or private institutions, in agreement with the National University and with the Postgraduate Program in Alternative Medicine. All students must carry out a degree project based on the various options of scientific research in the field of Alternative Medicine that is supported by tutors and research seminars and has a progressive development in the second and third semesters, to finish in the fourth semester with its respective socialization [10].

The program, in addition to the competency-based training of knowledge, know-how, and doing, deepens the formation of competencies of being. To this end, multiple spaces have been created where there is room for the dialogue of knowledge between students, teachers, graduates, and guests, which have allowed a continuous construction of knowledge, changes in the monitoring and evaluation system by replacing the classic methods of rote assessment with processes of reflection, synthesis, and understanding by each student, taking into account individuality in their learning processes. The know-how has been strengthened with the transdisciplinarity facilitated by the university environment, with Dentistry, Morphology, Public Health, Epidemiology, and the various models of research orientations. Competencies in doing are acquired with supervised practices in various teaching and care sites and in institutions in agreement [11].

The structuring of postgraduate training in the various areas of the master's degree has generated the initiative to create Scientific Associations in each of these areas, recognized by government institutions and validated through the Colombian Association of Scientific Societies [12].

4 From Neural Therapy to Neuraltherapeutic Medicine

The specific program of the area of neural therapy emphasizes Synthetic Physiology and the Russian School of Nervism, whose main representatives, Pavlov, Speransky, Sechenov, and Bykov, constitute the theoretical basis in the Master's Degree in Neural Therapy. It delves into other fields of knowledge, such as that of the British nervism (Chap. 12), an authority on the foundation for Segment Therapy, complemented by an extensive review of the regional anatomy and the central and peripheral nervous system to strengthen and develop various Neuraltherapeutic techniques, Speransky's contributions with neurodystrophic concepts, Vishnevsky's novocaine blocks, Pischinger's contributions on ubiquity synapses, seminars on anesthetics routinely used in neural therapy, neural semiology, colloquiums on complexity sciences and systemic thinking, seminars on methodologies for research in Alternative Medicine, seminars on special emphasis on emotions with professors of Psychology and Psychiatry that provide students with tools to treat the patient in a comprehensive mind-body way, seminars about the social and community approach of Neuraltherapeutic medicine [8].

The master's degree, with its open thinking and methodology, harmonizes the doctrine of the Russian School and its different contributions, with the German School of Neural Therapy of the Huneke brothers, segment therapy, Neurofocal dentistry, new scientific knowledge and research, with the foundation of the principles of the Complex Systemic School of Dr. Julio César Payán [8].

The Master's Degree has been structured in its academic training process, taking into account the five fundamental dimensions of any medical system: morphology, vital dynamics, philosophical foundations, diagnostic systems, and therapeutic systems, as described in the literature [13]. In the academic development, research work has been carried out by the master's degree students under the direction of the program's professors, which has served as a fundamental contribution to the structuring of Neural Therapy as a true Complex Medical System [14–16].

5 Projections

The Master's Degree has been projected due to its participation in world congresses that have been held in Colombia in cooperation with the Colombian Association of Neural Therapy Neural Medicine ACOLTEN/MNT and in other international congresses held in several countries in Europe, Asia, North America, Central, and South America. The publications derived from this academic process have also had good dissemination.

A well-deserved academic, medical, and social recognition has been generated for Neuraltherapeutic Medicine, which has played a prominent and leading role in the development of this medical rationality at an international level.

In this way, the National University of Colombia within its academic structure continues to seek the dialogue of knowledge within the various complex medical systems, in the conception of a single medicine, trying to integrate the different medical rationalities that have given rise to it, where Neuraltherapeutic Medicine occupies a preponderant place.

References

1. Engels F. Dialectic of nature. Mexico City: Editorial Grijalbo; 1961. 377p.
2. Universidad Nacional de Colombia, Faculty of Medicine. Mission. [Internet] [Cited Feb 24, 2025]. Available at: https://medicina.bogota.unal.edu.co/facultad/mision
3. WHO. WHO strategy on traditional medicine 2002–2005. [Internet]. World Health Organization 2002. [Cited Feb 24, 2025]. Available at: http://apps.who.int/iris/bitstream/10665/67314/1/WHO_EDM_TRM_2002.1_spa.pdf
4. Barnes J, Abbot NC, Harkness EF, Ernst E. Articles on complementary medicine in the mainstream medical literature: an investigation of MEDLINE, 1966 through 1996. Arch Intern Med. 1999;159(15):1721–5. https://doi.org/10.1001/archinte.159.15.1721.
5. National Center for Complementary and Integrative Health. Complementary, Alternative, or Integrative Health: What's In a Name. [Internet] [Cited Feb 24, 2025]. Available at: https://www.nccih.nih.gov/health/complementary-alternative-or-integrative-health-whats-in-a-name
6. Ministerio de la Protección Social de Colombia. National Learning Service (SENA). Occupational characterization alternative medicine and complementary therapies 2006. [Internet] [Cited Feb 26, 2025]. Available at: https://www.minsalud.gov.co/salud/Documents/Observatorio%20Talento%20Humano%20en%20Salud/CARACTERIZACI%C3%93N%20MEDICINA%20ALTERNATIVA%20Y%20TERAPIAS%20COMPLEMENTARIAS.pdf
7. Vega JA, Urrego DZ. Public policies for training, practice, and service provision in alternative medicine and complementary therapies in Colombia. In: Vega JA, Urrego DZ, editors. Alternative medicine: a view from complex medical systems. Bogotá: Editorial Universidad Nacional de Colombia; 2011.
8. Sarmiento LD. History and institutionalization of neural therapy in Colombia [Internet]. Master's thesis. Master's in Alternative Medicine, neural therapy area, Faculty of Medicine, Universidad Nacional de Colombia; 2014. Available at: http://www.bdigital.unal.edu.co/43119/1/52145193.2014.pdf
9. Universidad Nacional de Colombia, Faculty of Medicine. General information: Master's in Alternative Medicine. [Internet] [Cited Feb 26, 2025]. Available at: https://medicina.bogota.unal.edu.co/formacion/maestrias/medicina-alternativa/descripcion-al

10. Universidad Nacional de Colombia, Faculty of Medicine. Postgraduate programs: Master's in Alternative Medicine. General Information on Postgraduate Programs. [Internet] [Cited Feb 26, 2025]. Available at: https://medicina.bogota.unal.edu.co/formacion/maestrias/medicina-alternativa#enlaces-2
11. Beltrán EH. Neuraltherapeutic medicine: academic formation based on competencies. [Internet]. Master's thesis. Master's in Alternative Medicine, Neural Therapy Area. Faculty of Medicine, Universidad Nacional de Colombia. Available at: https://repositorio.unal.edu.co/bitstream/handle/unal/21635/5599037.2013.pdf?sequence=1
12. Asociación Colombiana de Sociedades Científicas. Member Societies. [Internet] [Cited Mar 3, 2025]. Available at: https://sociedadescientificas.com/sociedades-miembros/
13. Tesser CD, Luz MT. Medical rationalities and Integrality. Ciênc Saúde Colet. 2008;13(1):195–206.
14. Salazar JI. Neural therapy: from orthodox therapy to neural therapeutic medicine. In: Beltrán EH, Vega JA, editors. Neural therapeutic medicine: an approach from complex medical systems. Bogotá D.C.: Universidad Nacional de Colombia; 2013. p. 15–28.
15. Beltrán EH, Urrego DZ. A medical system called neural therapeutic medicine. In: Beltrán EH, Vega JA, editors. Neural therapeutic medicine: an approach from complex medical systems. Bogotá D.C.: Universidad Nacional de Colombia; 2013. p. 29–49.
16. Toscano F, Pinilla LB. The principles of neural therapy from the foundations of nervism to current neuroscience. Salud UIS. 2012;44(2):57–65.

Chapter 5
Origins of Neurofocal Dentistry

Sandra Lucia Patiño Niño

1 How Did the Concept of Neurofocal Dentistry Arise?

At the beginning of the twentieth century, dentistry was understood as a health practice that sought to control pain and "clean" the mouth of infections that affected people by extracting teeth, disinfecting with substances, or repairing with generally metallic materials. With the development of the concepts of Russian physiology, English physiology, and the discoveries of Huneke in Germany, a different epistemological path begins that allows us to recognize the relationship between oral structures and systemic diseases. The main elements that contributed to consolidate the concept of neurofocal dentistry are identified below.

The first conceptual element to consider is that neurofocal dentistry is born from the close relationship with neural therapy developed by the Huneke brothers; it is a term that was born in Germany in 1958, described by the Nomenclature Commission of the German scientific group for the investigation of foci, their prevention, and treatment.[1] It was the German dentist Ernest Adler (1906–1996) of Czech origin, influenced by the concepts of focal pathology and interference field developed by the Huneke brothers and the forbidden writings of Speransky [1], who described for the first time the possible irritative foci to the nervous system from the oral cavity (considering the tonsils in a relevant place) and their close relationship with the

[1] Ministry of Health and Social Protection of Colombia. Profile and competencies of the Dentist specialized in Neurofocal Dentistry in the context of the Colombian health system. 2019. [Unpublished] Document written by a team of experts: Yosette Osorio, Marcela Díaz and Sandra Lucia Patiño N. on behalf of the Ministry of Health and Social Protection of Colombia under the technical advice of Yenny Barajas.

S. L. Patiño Niño (✉)
Faculty of Dentistry, Universidad Nacional de Colombia, Bogotá, Colombia
e-mail: slpatinon@unal.edu.co

L. B. Pinilla Bonilla et al. (eds.), *Neuraltherapeutic Medicine*,
https://doi.org/10.1007/978-3-032-03257-7_5

appearance of systemic diseases [2]. From his extensive clinical observations and through the concept of interfering field, recognized by the German Huneke School, Adler identifies infectious and traumatic oral pathologies and dental interventions that generate high levels of toxicity as sources of irritation to the nervous system [2].

A second conceptual element is related to the knowledge in neuroanatomy and physiology at that time. Authors like R. Voll and F. Kramer from the concepts of electroacupuncture managed to introduce the concept of *Odonton* as a functional unit [3] that includes alveolar bone tissue, periodontal ligament, gingiva, tooth (enamel, dentin, pulp, and cementum), and alveolar bone connected to the body through nerve fibers, arterial and venous capillaries, and the lymphatic system. Based on a cartography developed by these authors, the different functions of the organs of the body are correlated with odontons [3, 4].

A third conceptual element was contributed by Pischinger a few years later with the concept of Pischinger's Basic System (see Chap. 12), who recognized the importance of the extracellular space as an ubiquitous system of the tissues in the activities of nutrition, excretion, and tissue defense, among others. The adequate fulfillment of the specific functions of the tissues within the organs and the system in general depends on the regulation generated from this extracellular space with the intervention of the autonomic nervous system [5].

From these three concepts and others from different authors, but at the same time (mid-twentieth century), we can say that the first explanation of the relationships between oral tissues with the organs and body systems, the initial foundations of Neurofocal Dentistry, were consolidated for the Western world.

2 Decision Criteria in the Development of Neurofocal Dentistry

One of the most relevant challenges of neurofocal dentists is to make therapeutic decisions that adequately support their performance. As neurofocal dentistry has developed, the therapeutic criteria have marked the following historical stages:

1. Exodontism as a way of removing interfering fields (1980–1990). Derived from the concepts of Neural therapy according to Huneke and the observations of Adler [2]. During this stage, a question was generated from the dental guild, because it was considered invasive and with a weak argumentation from the conventional paradigm.[2]
2. Stage of the biological biocompatibility of dental materials (1990–2005 approx.) This stage was born in response to the need to identify materials that did not generate irritations to oral tissues and to avoid electrogalvanism. In view of the rejection of metallic materials in the mouth, the development of alternative materials such as resins, ionomers, and ceramics for the filling of cavities and coronal

[2] Ibid.

rehabilitation is contemplated and incorporated. This coincides with the emergence of the International Academy of Biological Dentistry and Medicine (IABDM) [6] and the International Academy of Biological Dentistry and Toxicology (IAOMT) [7].

3. Stage of Integrative Dentistry (2005 onward). Integrative dentistry is understood as the search for complementarity with conventional dentistry and alternative medicine based on respect and the best interest of the patient. It recognizes the need for high-precision and biocompatible dentistry that avoids the possibility of generating irritative or inflammatory conditions in the oral cavity. It agrees with the strong development of esthetic dentistry and implant dentistry, in view of which neurofocal dentistry identifies the possible irritations that can be generated to the nervous system but recognizes that this process can occur depending on the unique characteristics of the individual and the magnitudes of the stimulus.[3] In this regard, authors Fajardo F. and Osorio Y. identify bioelectronic measurements as a diagnostic resource in Neurofocal Dentistry [8].
4. The minimally invasive dentistry stage (2018 onward) coincides with the emergence of neuraltherapeutic medicine as a complex medical system (See Chap. 3) and its epistemological stakes. When the postulates of nervism (See Chap. 13) are understood, it becomes necessary to identify the zones of irritation and inhibition, as well as the reflex adaptive processes (generated by the body understood as a whole), once the stomatognathic system is therapeutically intervened.

From conventional dentistry, under a new understanding of the pathophysiological processes in the most prevalent diseases, such as caries and periodontal disease, and their impact on systemic health, the trend in dentistry is to make micro and mini interventions, trying to prevent the disease, stop carious processes, maintain pulp vitality [9], preserve occlusal stability and periodontal health [10]. Conservative dentistry that reduces irritation and trauma to the tissues, with as few invasive procedures as possible, the use of biocompatible and regenerative materials, as well as an acceptable reduction in the use of metals in orthodontics, surgery, and rehabilitation, without impairing the efficiency and effectiveness of therapeutic results.

With the incorporation of soft technologies, strategies such as motivational interviewing are designed to maintain oral health and adherence to self-care habits over time [11]. On the other hand, it is understood that the need to take into account dental fear and anxiety in the therapeutic processes in dentistry, incorporating psychological tools such as cognitive behavior therapy [12] and acceptance and commitment therapy for pain management and stress states [13].

Therefore, it can be concluded that neurofocal dentistry at this stage makes explicit the need to generate conservative and minimally invasive therapeutic criteria in the stomatognathic system. In addition, it contemplates the approach to the biological, cognitive, and emotional spheres of people by understanding the sociocultural context, their life history, and dental history, using different paradigms and in a transdisciplinary manner.

---

[3] Ibid

These last two stages in transition in this second decade of the twenty-first century show us the future trends of dentistry with greater use of hard and soft technology and the development of options more in line with our understanding of complex systems, neurophysiology, and the stomatognathic system.

3 Neurofocal Dentistry in Colombia

Neurofocal dentistry was born from the hand of neural therapy in Colombia. At the Hacienda Los Robles in Popayán, dentists such as Dr. Luis Eduardo Alba and Lucia Barrera Girón learned the basics of neural therapy and were impregnated with the contributions of Huneke, Adler, Ricker, Voll, Kramer, Pischinger, among others, in addition to the knowledge in alternative and complementary medicine that was recreated.

In the 1980s, Dr. Luis Eduardo Alba had his office in the capital city to treat the many patients seeking solutions to their oral and systemic conditions under this look, and it is for the 1990s that Dr. Yosette Osorio ventures significantly in the development, consolidation, and dissemination of neurofocal dentistry from their personal and professional experiences. Through her active participation in the processes of medical and dental training in neural therapy in the company of doctors Julio Cesar Payan, Augusto Leyva, Hugo Castro, among others, she achieves an understanding of the morbid phenomena in the oral cavity under the paradigm of alternative and complementary medicines developed so far in Colombia and Europe. Osorio proposes a concept of neurofocal dentistry closely related to complex thinking and the integral or holistic view of the patient, "oriented to assist the natural healing processes of the individual" [14, 15].

With the development of the Colombian Association of Neurofocal Dentistry and Biological Medicine (ACONMB) and the Center for Information and Research in Alternative Medicine (CIMA), it was initiated, together with Dr. Julio César Payán, a process of formalization of education for physicians and dentists through diploma courses[4] taught in different cities of the country with the participation of local professionals from Latin America and Europe. This process of nonformal education is consolidated with the Association of Neurofocal Dentists of Colombia (ODNF) led by Osorio Y.[5]

From there, other dentists such as Jorge Petta in Cali [16] and Fernando Vanegas in Bogotá [17] made their own conceptual appropriations and developments that have been reported in academic events or publications. This process of conceptual rethinking of dentistry with a view from complex medical systems has expanded in Latin America and the development generated in countries such as Argentina, Chile, Brazil, Ecuador, and others has been especially relevant.

[4] Ibid.

[5] Ibid.

In 2019, after a long management of academic proposals, the development of the elective course of Neurofocal and Integrative Dentistry in the Faculty of Dentistry and the Master of Alternative Medicine of the National University of Colombia begins formally. This was conceived as an academic and research proposal that seeks to consolidate its development in the formal educational environment with solid bases in research processes that consider various methodologies and practices from the Alternative and Complementary Medicine, adjusted to the continuous development of dentistry. Therefore, this subject includes concepts of complexity, nervism, neuraltherapeutic medicine, osteopathy, traditional Chinese medicine, physiopathology of occlusion, and new developments in dental materials, among others. By the year 2024, other public [18] and private [19] universities throughout the country have replicated this exercise from their own understanding of neurofocal dentistry.

In conclusion, the knowledge developed in Russia, Germany, England, and Latin America from Colombia, Brazil, Argentina, Chile, among others, has been developed and continues to advance in the understanding of neurofocal and integrative dentistry, taking into account the knowledge and postulates of other complex medical systems and therapies of various origins, as well as technical and technological developments in devices, materials, and procedures from dentistry.

References

1. Marin JM. Ernest Adler: the visionary stomatologist. Available from: https://terapianeural.life/ernest-adler-el-estomatologo-visionario. Accessed 20 Dec 2024.
2. Adler E. Allgemein-Erkrankungen durch Störfelder (Trigeminusbereich): Diagnose und Therapie. In: J.A. Duque Mejía, translator. 3rd ed. Heidelberg: Edit. Heidelberg; 1983. Available from: https://n9.cl/m0eh. Accessed 20 Dec 2024.
3. Voll R. Interrelations of Odontons and tonsils to organs, fields of disturbance and tissue systems. 4th ed. Uelzen: Edit M.L.V; 1978. p. 9–173.
4. Voll R. Teeth and their relationships with the entire organism. In: Los Robles, translator. 1975. p. 167–85.
5. Perger F. Das Grundsystem nach Pischinger. In: J.A. Duque Mejía, translator. Phys Med Reh. 1979;20(6). Available from: https://n9.cl/81zy0. Accessed 20 Dec 2024.
6. International Academy of Biological Dentistry and Medicine. Sobre la IABDM. Available from: https://iabdm.org/es/sobre-iabdm/. 20 Dec 2024.
7. International Academy of Oral Medicine and Toxicology. About IAOMT. Available from: https://es.iaomt.org/about-iaomt/. (n.d.)
8. Osorio Y, Fajardo F. Bioelectronic measurements, a new diagnostic resource in dentistry. Rev Fed Odontol Colomb. 1997;54(191):36–41. Available from: https://n9.cl/dl25. Accessed 27 Nov 2024
9. González-Gil D, Flores-Fraile J, Vera-Rodríguez V, Martín-Vacas A, López-Marcos J. Comparative meta-analysis of minimally invasive and conventional approaches for caries removal in permanent dentition. Medicina (Kaunas). 2024;60(3):402. https://doi.org/10.3390/medicina60030402.
10. Sultan N, Jafri Z, Sawai M, Bhardwaj A. Minimally invasive periodontal therapy. J Oral Biol Craniofac Res. 2020;10(2):161–5. https://doi.org/10.1016/j.jobcr.2020.04.014.

11. Colvara BC, Faustino-Silva DD, Meyer E, Hugo FN, Celeste RK, Hilgert JB. Motivational interviewing for preventing early childhood caries: a systematic review and meta-analysis. Community Dent Oral Epidemiol. 2021;49(1):10–6.
12. Hoffmann B, Erwood K, Ncomanzi S, et al. Management strategies for adult patients with dental anxiety in the dental clinic: a systematic review. Aust Dent J. 2022;67(Suppl 1):S3–S13. https://doi.org/10.1111/adj.12926.
13. Feizi G, Binandeh ES, Goli F, Seraj-Khorrami N, Khalifehsoltani F. Comparison of the effect of acceptance and commitment therapy and cognitive behavioral therapy on pain tolerance and intensity perception in patients with dental anxiety: a randomized trial. Dent Res J (Isfahan). 2023;20:11.
14. Osorio Y. Neurofocal dentistry: another rationality. Rev Fed Odontol Colomb. 2003;65. Available from: https://acolten.com.co/wpcontent/uploads/2021/11/Odontologia_Neurofocal_Otra_Racionalidad1.pdf. Accessed 20 Dec 2024
15. Osorio Y. Neurofocal dentistry: a complementary approach. Encuentro Internacional de Terapia Neural, Patagonia, Argentina; 2006. Available from: https://terapianeural.com/articulos/29-odontologia-neurofocal/172-odontologia-neurofocal-un-enfoque-complementario. Accessed 20 Dec 2024.
16. Petta J. Neurofocal dentistry: from analysis to synthesis [Video File]. Congreso Internacional de Terapia Neural Sitges. Barcelona, Spain. 2012. Available from: https://n9.cl/6wfr. Accessed 20 Dec 2024.
17. Vanegas León F. Radio interviews on neurofocal dentistry. International Association of Neurofocal Dentistry and Related Sciences 2011. Available from: https://n9.cl/gx50. Accessed 20 Dec 2024.
18. Universidad de Antioquia. Facultad de Odontología. Continuing Education. Neurofocal Dentistry and Neural Therapy. Conference. 2 Aug 2024. Cátedra abierta. Available from: https://www.udea.edu.co/wps/portal/udea/web/inicio/unidades-academicas/odontologia. Accessed 1 Aug 2024.
19. Universidad CIEO. Neurofocal Dentistry Course. 2022. Available from: https://unicieo.edu.co/wp-content/uploads/2022/02/PROGRAMA-CURSO-ODONTOLOGIA-NEUROFOCAL.pdf. Accessed 2 Nov 2024.

Part II
Complexity and Complex Medical Systems

Chapter 6
Complex Medical Systems and Neuraltherapeutic Medicine

Eduardo Humberto Beltrán Dussán and Diana Zulima Urrego-Mendoza

1 Introduction: Complex Medical Systems

The concept of complex medical systems is proposed as a proposal to identify, validate, and recognize the diverse perspectives on the interpretation of the body, health, and disease that have emerged as ways of approaching the ailments of humanity, giving rise to the different practices described in the history of medicine [1]. In this way, it has been possible to identify medical systems, paradigms, and treatment strategies that are classified according to their conceptual structure and therapeutic scope [2].

This initiative arises in Latin American countries, supported by research and theoretical proposals such as that of Madel Luz in Brazil, which describes and conceptualizes the different medical rationalities, proposing the approach from medical systems integrating the concepts of health and disease, their management strategies, and identifying common and constant parameters in each, calling them complex medical systems [2–5].

The current ancestral medical cultures and medical rationalities that have been identified in history as hegemonic or conventional Western medicine and other forms of conceptualizations are based on rationalities, historical and cultural principles, and the evolution of knowledge [6].

E. H. Beltrán Dussán (✉)
Faculty of Medicine, Universidad Nacional de Colombia, Bogotá, Colombia
e-mail: ehbeltrand@unal.edu.co

D. Z. Urrego-Mendoza
Faculty of Medicine, Public Health Department, Universidad Nacional de Colombia, Bogotá, Colombia
e-mail: dzurregom@unal.edu.co

L. B. Pinilla Bonilla et al. (eds.), *Neuraltherapeutic Medicine*,
https://doi.org/10.1007/978-3-032-03257-7_6

According to these approaches, five dimensions are recognized within the conception of a complex medical system: A component referring to the morphology of the human being in its material aspect that determines its form and organization; A functionality of this body structure, based on dynamic systems that support the expression of its organization through the use of communication systems that define movements for the maintenance of life; A clear conception of what has been called *medical doctrine*, taking into account concepts of health and disease, their origins, and evolution in order to propose possible modifications; a diagnostic foundation, through which the existing alterations, their characteristics and states are identified and classified, trying to establish the underlying causes and a therapeutic component that proposes appropriate interventions seeking to recover the organization of the biological system [2–5].

These parameters characterize complex medical systems, validating them in practice and facilitating the approach to the health-disease process from different rationalities, allowing their inclusion in the recommendations of the World Health Organization (WHO) for legislation, education, and implementation worldwide [7].

The proposal of complex medical systems has been welcomed by recognized academic institutions in various countries, where they are part of educational practices and are recommended for the implementation of health services [8, 9].

Since its conception, the category of complex medical systems has been consolidated and developed as a foundation that facilitates the understanding and integration of the various medical practices, establishing guidelines for the training of human talent and health care [10, 11].

2 From Neural Therapy to Neuraltherapeutic Medicine as a Complex Medical System

Neural therapy arises from unexpected results identified during the research of local anesthetics as therapeutic elements in human beings. This generated great enthusiasm in medical professionals who replicated these experiences to seek answers about the possible mechanisms involved in these results and developed a theoretical support that structured the bases of neural therapy during the 100 years that have elapsed since its discovery [12–15] During this period, categories and paradigms have been identified that allow the concept of neural therapy to be developed as a complex medical system, which is why academia has proposed to call it neuraltherapeutic medicine (NTM) [16, 17].

The following are the components of NTM that have allowed it to be identified as a complex medical system:

2.1 Morphological Structure of the Human Being

From the NTM point of view, the human being is the result of a biological process of physical, emotional, and mental information that is integrated at the moment of conception, resulting in a new individual and unrepeatable being, with a life program that will allow the development of their potentiality [18]. This structure makes up the essence of the human being, and in its development, it interacts with physical, emotional, mental, cultural, and social factors with which it interrelates from conception, and which build and modify its individuality [19]. Other fundamental aspects will be developed in Part III of this book.

2.2 Life Dynamics or Physiologic Dimension

The functionality of the body structure of the human being in NTM depends firstly on the biological program acquired at the time of conception and secondly on the integrity of the different biological communication systems. The nervous system is comparable to an information center that transmits, regulates, and executes through its components, functionally interconnecting with the other communication systems that have been discovered and incorporated into the dynamics, such as the emotional, circulatory, endocrine, immunological, tetrahydorcannabinoid system, fractals, the basic system, intercellular communications, and electromagnetic communications, among others [20, 21] These biological communication systems are functionally interconnected both in health status and in pathological processes [22, 23].

For NTM, the dynamics of biological communication systems is based on the approach of Norbert Wiener, who in 1948 in his book "*Cybernetics or the control and transmission of information in living organisms and machines*" described the theory of what was later called biocybernetics, explaining the way in which living beings maintain an active and orderly communication with all their biological structures and with the environment that surrounds them through the so-called regulatory circuits that allow the functional harmony of life to be maintained [24].

According to Wiener, regulatory circuits are sensor-like structures with control mechanisms that allow variations within established ranges, and when they identify critical situations, they generate specific signals to establish the necessary corrections [24].

Taking into account these approaches, several researchers have generated important contributions on biological communication systems in accordance with the development of advances in knowledge with technologies such as artificial intelligence and quantum computers [25, 26]. According to this perspective, Part IV of this book will develop the physiologic concepts of NTM.

2.3 The Doctrine and Foundations

In NTM, the health-disease concept is interpreted dynamically, where health is considered as a state of compensation within the variations that the biological system tolerates to maintain vital functions; while the disease arises when the variations that occur prevent maintaining this state of functional compensation. In the face of decompensation, the body seeks new organizational strategies to adapt to extreme variations, but in some cases, a state of progressive imbalance may occur that leads to the death of the individual [27].

Triggers of this imbalance include factors that cause interference with the functioning of different biological communication systems, such as chronic inflammation, scarring, trauma and fibrotic zones, foreign bodies, proliferative cellular phenomena, prostheses, and emotional and mental events. The above conditions have been called interfering fields, irritative foci, and dysfunctional zones, among others [28, 29].

In the approach of NTM, the conception of the human being as an individual integrated into a social, political, economic, and cultural structure made up of family, friends, training institutions, work, and professional and work organizations, among others, allows us to analyze the interactions with these communication systems, especially in relation to the emotional and mental sphere [30].

From this perspective, the link between patient and treating physician must be based on the notion of the health-disease process in order to jointly identify the critical factors that have caused the alterations in biological functioning, intervene in the most appropriate way, and follow the course of the body's responses in relation to therapeutic interventions to guide subsequent therapeutic decisions [31]. Foundations, which include an exploration from complexity sciences, will be widely explained and developed in the following chapters of this part and also in Part V of this book.

2.4 The Diagnostic System

Diagnosis in NTM is based on the characterization of the conditions that generate alterations in biological communication systems. The purpose is to identify the presence of physical, emotional, mental, and social interferences, locating them as precisely as possible in order to intervene appropriately. This identification process is carried out through the medical history, physical examination, and complementary studies. The clinical history consists of an inquiry into the life history of the individual and must be approached from the narrative of the subject who suffers. The physician's understanding of the meanings that the patient attaches to his or her symptoms allows us to reveal the dimensions of the disease in its different areas: the anatomical-physiological aspect, the experiences, and the social-historical context [32, 33]. Likewise, applying the fundamentals of narrative medicine, initially described by Rita Charon [34], makes it easier for the physician to analyze in this discourse the events related to the disease, its temporalities, the inference of causal factors, the context, and the subject's perspectives on the disease. Regarding the physical examination, it must be meticulous, covering the entire body structure in order to establish the areas where the alterations of the information have originated [35] Complementary studies will be ordered according to the findings of the patient's life history and physical examination. A wider perspective of this dimension will be developed in Part VI of this book.

2.5 The Therapeutic System

The objective in NTM is to recover balance and promote the self-organization of the individual, for which it is key to restore the functionality of the interfered circuits using micro-doses of local anesthetics that are applied superficially or deeply, where interference from biological communication systems is considered to be or in sites that allow access according to the information obtained through history clinical examination, physical examination, and complementary studies [36–40].

The use of local anesthetics is due to their electrical action on the various channels, especially sodium, achieving their repolarization and acting as a stabilizing mechanism of cell membranes. The action of local anesthetics extends over the lipid bilayer of the membrane, occluding ion channels dependent on voltage variations and other channels such as calcium and chlorine. This action also includes the mitochondrial membrane and the endoplasmic reticulum system [41].

By achieving the repolarization process, interference from information is eliminated and the functionality of the system is recovered. The distance effect observed in the practice of NTM is defined as the result of the interaction of the various biological communication systems and their intimate relationship with the nervous system, taking into account their action as a regulator of biological processes. Clinical follow up through narrative is established with patients to assess the evolution during the therapeutic process, guiding the frequency of interventions and justifying new interventions in subsequent consultations [42].

In some cases, when patients do not respond to the therapeutic interventions that have been determined within the clinical analysis, there are possibilities of overloads that are difficult to eliminate, such as toxic, infectious, or inflammatory phenomena. Therefore, it is considered necessary to complement the approach with the perspective of neurofocal dentistry and analysis from other medical systems in order to achieve its elimination or stabilization [43].

In the treatment of the patient from NTM, integrated management with medical specialties and different medical systems is considered important, as part of an integrative conception of medicine. Social and emotional interferences require the identification of the factors that are generating them with the corresponding approaches and accompaniment [44]. In Part VII, VIII, and IX of this book, a broader perspective will be developed of therapeutic applications of NTM, some techniques, and fields of action.

3 Conclusions

The concept of complex medical systems has allowed the recognition of other rationalities, configuring different perspectives, conceptualizations, and approaches to the health-disease process.

Neural therapy, currently known as NTM, during its 100 years of evolution, has been enriched by incorporating theoretical dimensions into its structure that have allowed it to be identified as a Complex Medical System.

Its approach allows interaction with various medical rationalities and medical systems, complementing each other, which is why it is necessary, for the well-being of the patient, to incorporate it into the provision of health services.

References

1. Laín-Entralgo P. History of medicine. Barcelona: Editorial Masson S.A; 2006.
2. Tesser CD, Luz MT. Medical rationalities and Integrality. Sci Collect Health. 2008;13(1):195–206.
3. Luz MT. Natural, rational, social. Medical reasoning and modern scientific rationality. 1st ed. São Paulo: Editora Campus; 1997. [NT: Spanish version: Luz MT. Natural, rational, social: medical reasoning and modern scientific rationality. 1st ed. Buenos Aires: Lugar Editorial; 1997.]
4. Otani MA, Barros NF. Integrative medicine and the construction of a new health model. Ciênc Saúde Colet. 2011;16(3):1801–11.
5. Do Nascimento MC, de Barros NF, Nogueira MI, Luz MT. The category of medical rationality and a new epistemology in health. Ciênc Saúde Colet. 2013;18(12):3595–604.
6. Luz MT. Contemporary culture and alternative medicines: new health paradigms at the end of the 20th century. In: Luz MT, editor. Medical rationalities and institutions: theoretical and methodological contributions to research and thought in collective health. 1st ed. Porto Alegre: Editorial Rede Unida; 2023.
7. World Health Organization (WHO). WHO strategies on traditional medicine 2014–2023. Geneva: WHO; 2013. [Cited 2020 Sept, 26]. Available from: https://bit.ly/3WX8MiV
8. Urrego DZ. Approach to alternative medicine as a complex medical system at the National University of Colombia. Rev Fac Med Unal. 2010;58(2):155–6.
9. Urrego-Mendoza DZ, Beltrán-Dussán EH, Marilletti A, Casas del Rio GH, Ruiz-Díaz P, Vega-Oviedo JA. Alternative medicine: a view from complex medical systems. Bogotá D.C.: Universidad Nacional de Colombia; 2011.
10. Luz MT. Medical rationalities and institutions: theoretical and methodological contributions to research and thought in collective health. 1st ed. Porto Alegre: Editorial Rede Unida; 2023.
11. Abreu MB, Ferraz TSO, Albuquerque UP, Ferreira Júnior WS. Interactions between local medical systems and the biomedical system: a conceptual and methodological review in light of hybridization processes. J Ethnobiol Ethnomed. 2023;19(1):60. https://doi.org/10.1186/s13002-023-00637-w. PMID: 38093307; PMCID: PMC10720130.

12. Dosch P, Dosch M. Manual of neural therapy according to Huneke. 2nd ed. Stuttgart: Thieme; 2007.
13. Barop H. Textbook and atlas of neural therapy: diagnosis and therapy with local anesthetics. 1st ed. Stuttgart/New York: Thieme; 2018.
14. Fisher L. Neural therapy according to Huneke Mexico. Stuttgart: Spanish Version of the Publication by Hipocrates Verlag Publishing; 2012.
15. Kidd R. Neural therapy applied neurophysiology and other topics. Canada: Custom Printers of Renfrew Ltd., Renfrew; 2005.
16. Salazar JI. Neural therapy: from orthodox therapy to neural therapeutic medicine. In: Beltrán EH, Vega JA, editors. Neural therapeutic medicine: an approach from complex medical systems. Bogotá D.C.: Universidad Nacional de Colombia; 2013. p. 15–28.
17. Beltrán EH, Urrego DZ. A medical system called neural therapeutic medicine. In: Beltrán EH, Vega JA, editors. Neural therapeutic medicine: an approach from complex medical systems. Bogotá D.C.: Universidad Nacional de Colombia; 2013. p. 29–49.
18. Barresi M, Gilbert S. Developmental biology. 13th ed. Oxford: Sinauer Associates-Oxford University Press; 2023.
19. Jiao H, Kalsbeek A, Yi CX. Microglia, circadian rhythm, and lifestyle factors. Neuropharmacology. 2024;257:110029. https://doi.org/10.1016/j.neuropharm.2024.110029. Epub 2024 June 7.
20. Saks V, Monge C, Guzun R. Philosophical basis and some historical aspects of systems biology: from Hegel to Noble – applications for bioenergetic research. Int J Mol Sci. 2009;10(3):1161–92. https://doi.org/10.3390/ijms10031161. Epub 2009 Mar 13. PMID: 19399243; PMCID: PMC2672024.
21. Toscano F, Pinilla LB. The principles of neural therapy from the foundations of Nervism to current neuroscience. Salud UIS. 2012;44(2):57–65.
22. Wang RS, Maron BA, Loscalzo J. Systems medicine: evolution of systems biology from bench to bedside. Wiley Interdiscip Rev Syst Biol Med. 2015;7(4):141–61. https://doi.org/10.1002/wsbm.1297. Epub 2015 Apr 17. PMID: 25891169; PMCID: PMC4457580.
23. Kodkin VL, Artem'eva EV. Digital identification of the human condition is a prerequisite for the effectiveness of organizational automation (biocybernetic) systems operation. Sensors (Basel). 2022;22(10):3649. https://doi.org/10.3390/s22103649. PMID: 35632057; PMCID: PMC9147441.
24. Wiener N. Cybernetics: or control and communication in the animal and the machine. Paris: Hermann & Cie Editeurs; 1948.
25. Morasso P. The quest for cognition in purposive action: from cybernetics to quantum computing. J Integr Neurosci. 2023;22(2):39. https://doi.org/10.31083/j.jin2202039.
26. Xiong A, Proctor RW. Information processing: the language and analytical tools for cognitive psychology in the information age. Front Psychol. 2018;9:1270. https://doi.org/10.3389/fpsyg.2018.01270. PMID: 30135664; PMCID: PMC6092626.
27. Cardozo AM, Pinilla LB, Andrade LE. Rethinking the concept of illness from evolution and emergence. In: Beltrán EH, Vega JA, editors. Neural therapeutic medicine: an approach from complex medical systems. 1st ed. Bogotá: Editorial Universidad Nacional de Colombia; 2013. p. 73–102.
28. Dosch P, Dosch M. Interstitial connective tissue and interference fields. In: Dosch P, Dosch M, editors. Manual of neural therapy according to Huneke. 2nd ed. Stuttgart: Thieme; 2007. p. 36–45.
29. Barop H. The interference field. In: Barop H, editor. Atlas of neural therapy: Mexico. Stuttgart: Spanish Version of the Publication by Hipocrates Verlag Publishing; 2003. p. 14–6.
30. Payán JC. Vital disobedience. 1st ed. Barcelona: Editorial Instituto de Terapia Neural; 2004.
31. Payán JC. Launch yourself into the void. Your wings will extend. 1st ed. McGraw Hill: Bogotá; 2000.
32. Bordelois I. Listening to the body: bridges between health and words. Buenos Aires: Libros del Zorzal; 2009.

33. Sontag S. Illness and its metaphors/AIDS and its metaphors. 1st ed. Barcelona. Translated by Mario Muchnik Clemans.: Debolsillo Publishing; 2008.
34. Charon R. Narrative medicine. 1st ed. New York: Oxford University Press; 2006.
35. Segura PR, Beltrán EH. Design of a medical history model for neural therapy in accordance with current regulations in Colombia. In: Beltrán EH, Vega JA, editors. Neural therapeutic medicine: an approach from complex medical systems. 1st ed. Bogotá: Editorial Universidad Nacional de Colombia; 2013. p. 125–55.
36. Dosch P, Dosch M. The interference field and its elimination by means of lightning reaction. In: Dosch P, Dosch M, editors. Manual of neural therapy according to Huneke. 2nd ed. Stuttgart: Thieme; 2007. p. 78–120.
37. Fisher L. Interference field therapy. In: Neural therapy according to Huneke: Mexico. Stuttgart: Spanish Version of the Publication by Hipocrates Verlag Publishing; 2012. p. 59–62.
38. Kidd R. Treatment of interference fields. In: Neural therapy applied neurophysiology and other topics. Renfrew: Custom Printers of Renfrew Ltd.; 2005. p. 56–65.
39. Wancura-Kampic I. Segmental anatomy. The key to mastering acupuncture, neural therapy, and manual therapy. 1st ed. Munich: Elsevier; 2012.
40. Navarro K, Pinilla LB. Contributions of Henry Head to the neuroanatomical and physiological bases of segment therapy. Med UIS. 2013;26(2):33–44.
41. Brunton LL, Knollmann BC, Goodman G. The pharmacological basis of therapeutics. 14th ed. New York: McGraw Hill; 2022.
42. Kidd R. Response to treatment. In: Kidd R, editor. Neural therapy applied neurophysiology and other topics. Renfrew: Custom Printers of Renfrew Ltd.; 2005. p. 67–71.
43. Kidd R. Systemic factors inhibiting neural therapy. In: Kidd R, editor. Neural therapy applied neurophysiology and other topics. Renfrew: Custom Printers of Renfrew Ltd.; 2005. p. 95–148.
44. Beltrán EH, Vega JA, editors. Neural therapeutic medicine: an approach from complex medical systems. 1st ed. Bogotá: Editorial Universidad Nacional de Colombia; 2013.

Chapter 7
A Short Introduction to the Sciences of Complexity and Some Applications

Carlos Eduardo Maldonado and Laura Bibiana Pinilla Bonilla

1 Introduction

The sciences of complexity, also known generally as complexity theory, are a wide set of sciences, disciplines, methods and methodologies, approaches, semantics, and logics aimed at studying *increasingly* complex systems. These are, we would like to highlight, systems phenomena and behaviors that have and gained degrees of freedom. A nonlinear system is one that gains degrees of freedom, although it does not necessarily gain memory. Basically, complexity theory is made up of a twofold dimension; on the one hand a very robust epistemological apparatus that continues to be enlarged and enriched as science and research advance. On the other hand, at the same time, it is also compounded by very sophisticated techniques and rods.

According to one of us [1], the sciences of complexity can be safely said to be sciences of life, since by and large the most complex systems ever—whether intuitively or categorically, for instance, are the living beings. Nonetheless, the inverse cannot necessarily be assessed, namely that the sciences of life are sciences of complexity. The focus of this book is hence after life—and the interplay, so to speak, between health and disease; two sides of one and the same token. Distinctively, the study of life, thanks to complexity theory, entails a twofold dimension; thus, life as-we-know-it, as well as life-as-it-could-be-possible.

C. E. Maldonado (✉)
School of Medicine, Universidad El Bosque, Bogotá, Colombia
e-mail: maldonadocarlos@unbosque.edu.co

L. B. Pinilla Bonilla
Faculty of Medicine, Master in Alternative Medicine, Neural Therapy Area, Universidad Nacional de Colombia, Bogotá, Colombia

Integrated Health Services Subnetwork of the South, Research and Innovation Center, Bogotá, Colombia

L. B. Pinilla Bonilla et al. (eds.), *Neuraltherapeutic Medicine*,
https://doi.org/10.1007/978-3-032-03257-7_7

2 Background and Brief History

The theoretical origins and history of the sciences of complexity have been told several times [2–6]. Two main moments can be distinguished; firstly, some antecedents of the sciences of complexity, and then the origins and characterization of each one of the sciences of complexity. It would be necessary to characterize the various disciplines that compound complexity science, such as swarm intelligence, self-organization, self-organized criticality, and others. We leave this aside mainly due to space.

Among the antecedents, Newton and Leibniz, Poincaré, Gödel, and Turing are to be accounted as the main sources leading to complexity science. Initially, Newton and Leibniz literally saw nonlinear systems and nonlinear dynamics. The trouble, though, was that they lacked the appropriate tool to work on and with them, namely the computer. Consequently, calculus linearized nonlinearity. Poincaré has two merits, as follows: he understood the sensitivity of the interactions among three bodies, anticipating thus chaos theory. This is exactly what he did in relation with the three-body problem [7]. In strong relation with that, Poincaré was the first scientist—in this case, mathematician, who coined the term "model" as "scientific model" as it is used currently. Scientists work, debate, build, and criticize models—whether mathematical, physical, computational, or others, not just behaviors, objects, or phenomena.

In 1931, Gödel formulated the first incompleteness theorem, which was to be further developed together with the second incompleteness theorem in 1934. Gödel's main achievement consisted in making clear that most explanations and understandings, say, theories, because they are or pretend to be consistent, are really incomplete [8]. More exactly, most, if not all, explanations to date are complete or pretend to be complete; hence, they are inconsistent. In other words, a good explanation should not be tautological, which is what they are and have always been from the logical standpoint [9]. Plainly said, the truth of a set of statements or a theory or explanation cannot be accounted for within that set or explanation.

Among the pillars that lead to complexity science, Gödel's works are a landmark. Gödel wrote five theorems which gave rise to a brand-new field in logic or mathematics, or allowed to renew them. These are: (i) a theory of incompleteness or also a theory of proofs; (ii) theorems of incompleteness or also a theory of recursion; consistency of the axiom of choice and the theory of fields; (iv) the discovery that the universe is buildable, and a theory of models; and (v) Gödel is to be accounted as one of the founders and leaders of intuitionism.

One more fundamental antecedent for complexity science is A. Turing's Machine. Logically and mathematically, a Turing Machine is the result of Hilbert's Tenth Problem, stated in 1900 [10], known as the detention-problem (*das Haltungsproblem*). Basically, Hilbert's statement is that we must distinguish between decidable and undecidable problems or programs. A decidable program is the one, one can know if and when it will stop. Most problems are decidable. In other words, either there exists, or it can be developed, an algorithm to define if a problem or program is decidable.

An undecidable problem is the one for which there is not, and it is not feasible to develop, no algorithm to solve it, not even given any space, time, and resources. Undecidable problems give rise to unconventional computation. These kinds of problems or programs are by and large the most significant of all imaginable problems. Another way to reckon them is as intractable problems. These are the backbone, so to speak, of complexity science.

Turing understood and solved Hilbert's challenge exactly by pointing out in a twofold direction. A Turing machine allows understanding which problems are compressible and which are not. An undecidable program is definitely uncompressible, which means that the best thing one can do is watch the program running and see what happens. Life is an uncompressible program in that there is not a formula, an algorithm, or a joker that fits all and always. Life is the most complex system or phenomenon ever.

That said, the expression "the sciences of complexity" was coined firstly in 1984 when the Santa Fe Institute was founded. The sciences of complexity originally were chaos theory, catastrophe theory, nonequilibrium thermodynamics, the geometry of fractals, and artificial life. However. Further research proved that other sciences could be safely accounted as belonging to complexity theory. That is what has happened with epigenetics, biosemiotics, and nonclassical logics. Now, as it is well known, the whole scientific building is largely based on quantum mechanics, since it is by and large the most robust, tested, verified, confirmed, and falsified theory.

Negatively said, complexity science consists of four salient features: the rejection of, refusal, or distance from determinism, dualism, reductionism, and mechanicism. It is possible to gather these characteristics in one single term: thinking about increasingly complex systems consists of thinking—and more crucially, living, in nonalgorithmic terms.

Figure 7.1 depicts the entire panorama of the sciences of complexity.

First, chaos theory emerged within the study of meteorology, i.e., the prediction of the most basic dynamics on earth, namely the weather and climate. The lesson by meteorology is clear and fundamental: nonlinear systems cannot be predicted. Unpredictability is a substantial feature of the world. More exactly, predictability fails when considering middle and long span times. Prediction only works in a short time span, and the shorter the more accurate. In contrast, oddly enough, with modern science, chaos teaches that prediction is by no means the main concern in good science and research. As it is well known, chaos theory emerged thanks to the works of E. Lorenz.

The thermodynamics of nonequilibrium, historically the second science devoted to understanding and explaining nonlinear systems, brings to the fore that order and life emerge in far-from-equilibrium systems. The technical name dubbed was dissipative structures, which was proposed by Ilya Prigogine, who received the Nobel Prize in Chemistry in 1977 for his contributions. The biosphere, society, and living organisms are and exist as far-from-equilibrium, or also as nonlinear dynamic

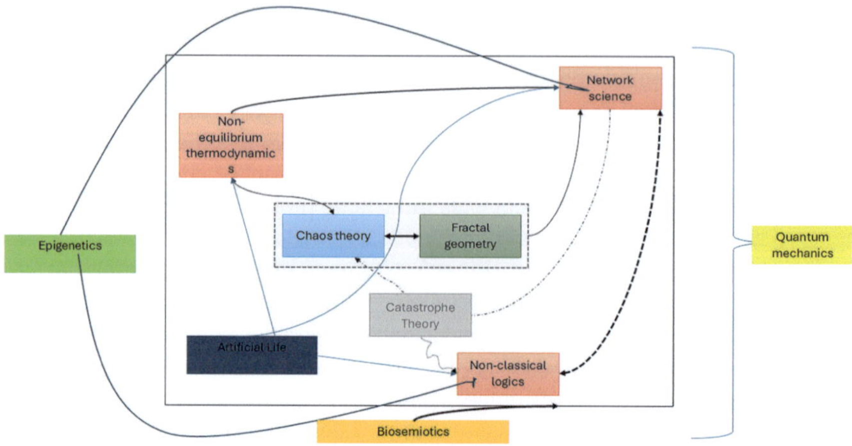

Fig. 7.1 The sciences of complexity. (Source: Own elaboration)

phenomena. Evolution can be grasped as magnificent inflections provided a number of stasis.

Furthermore, fractal geometry establishes a breakup with Euclidean geometry and makes it clear that the geometry of nature is irregular, based on ascending and descending fractals, which consists of self-similitude: the structure and behavior of the part is iteratively the same as the behavior and structure of the whole. Holism is hence impossible, or at its best, it is revealed as wishful thinking. (We will come to this immediately). The main work for the grounding of fractal geometry is B. Mandelbrot's *The Fractal Geometry of Nature*, from 1977.

Furthermore, catastrophe theory focuses on sudden, irreversible, and unforeseen changes—in nature as well as in society. A mathematical-based theory, catastrophe theory invites us to see and explain any kind of dynamics different from periodic, cyclic, or regular, in any sense of the word. It was first formulated by R. Thom working out of cobordism already from the 1960s; he received the Fields Medal in 1977.

One more science of complexity is artificial life,[1] whose origins can be traced back to 1984 and 1989, when C. Langton organized the first workshop on the field at the Santa Fe Institute. Artificial intelligence is a philosophical research program based on the best tool ever conceived—computational science aimed at understanding both the origins and the logics of the living systems. Meaningfully, artificial life proposes that the study of life is at the same time in its reality as well as in its possibilities. Indeed, the crux of the insights shed consists of making clear that the

[1]There is, as it appears, some noise here. The hype about artificial intelligence is truly—most people, lays or insiders, do not really know it- about artificial life. We have worked on this elsewhere.

concern about life is twofold: life as-we-know-it and life-as-it-could-be-possible. In other words, artificial life consists of understanding life by modeling and simulation.

The science of complex networks, firstly originated in 2001–2033 by L. Barabasi, S. Strogartz, and D. Watts shows that some things are more connected to others, and some things are also less connected to others. Consequently, it is not true that everything is connected to everything else, which is what characterizes holism. If everything was connected to everything else, nothing would be really relevant. Small-world networks, random networks, and scale-free networks are the most basic dynamic structures that help explain what complexity is and how it arises. In more general terms, systems and behaviors are context-dependent, but the contexts themselves vary and are irregular.

Nonclassical logics (NCLs) have been reckoned to be one of the sciences of complexity [11, 12]. The world in general does not consist of one single logic; instead, a wide mosaic of logics exists and is possible. Logical pluralism assesses that there is more than one singular truth-world. Moreover, different worlds exist and are possible from the logical standpoint. Technically speaking, the semantics of NCLs is the semantics of possible worlds. Thus, thinking about complexity is one and the same thing as thinking about the possible and, furthermore, even the impossible. NCLs allow for a pluralism of truth systems. Plainly said, there is not a unique or single truth and there is not and it is not a canonical form of thinking. In other words, NCLs consist in thinking non-algorithmically.

From Fig. 7.1, epigenetics can be safely said to be one of the sciences of complexity that allows overcoming dualism [13]. There are not only two things, namely, culture on the one hand and nature on the other but also nature and nurture. Epigenetics has made clear that we inherit and transmit both genes and experiences, mainly thanks to processes of methylation, phosphorylation, and acetylation. We leave the technical details aside. Thus, the distinction between the natural sciences and the social and human sciences becomes untenable.

Besides, biosemiotics can be identified as one of the sciences of complexity [14]. In biology at large, everything has to do with information. Cognition pervades biology all the way down. Already from transcription, transference, translation, and the like onto signs, signals, codes, patterns, and messages largely pervade the existence, learning, and adaptation among animals, plants, and human beings. Information becomes a more expressive concept rather than just mass (or matter) or energy. Indeed, the living beings unceasingly create, interpret, and transform signs, messages, codes, patterns, and symbols. Nature can be said to be a fantastic weave of information and communication, which furthermore brings to the fore the inconsistency of the belief that there are, on the one hand, biotic systems and, on the other, abiotic ones.

Being as it may be, the touchstone of the current knowledge building, so to speak, is based on the importance of quantum mechanics (QM). (QM) is by far the most robust of all theories currently existing. It has been verified, tested, confirmed, or falsified up to the eleventh decimal. There is no other theory with such strength. Any good understanding or explanation about the world in general or about a part of the world that either does not centrally cross or explicitly entails (QM) [15] is simply incomplete, to say the least. Oddly enough, the classical world can be safely viewed as a limited case of quantum behaviors, principles, and phenomena.

Positively said, the sciences of complexity are sciences of life [13], although the contrary cannot be assessed.

All in all, the sciences of complexity are a truly scientific revolution, for instance, in Kuhnian terms. This, we would like to argue, is one more motive for optimism.

Nonetheless, there is no definition of complexity or of a complex system. Rather, complex systems are understood by their properties or features. Various characteristics have been identified, such as emergence, nonlinearity, self-organization, swarm intelligence, turbulence, fluctuations, instabilities, learning and adaptation, evolution, first phase and second phase transitions, strange attractors, sudden, unforeseeable, and irreversible changes, irreversibility and the arrow of time, non-equilibrium dynamics, and unpredictability, among others.

3 Digging into (Some) Details

There is some confusion in the literature. It is, indeed, about the relationship and differences or commonalities between complexity theory, systems thinking, and complex thinking. The issue has to do with what the Vienna Circle dunned as some demarcation criteria, i.e., distinguishing between good science and pseudo-science, or metaphysics. The demarcation criteria can also be stated as the difference between spearhead science and normal science.

Complex thinking refers to E. Morin's work gathered around the concern of what he calls, in general, as the method. Important as it is, Morin's thinking is an ethics, i.e., it is a concern about the human being, his possibilities, and meaning. The method is a call for a change of attitude vis-à-vis the world and its complexities. More exactly, Morin does not want to change the world but to focus on how human beings can have a different attitude toward the challenges, limits, and dynamics of the world at large. In this sense, Morin's thinking coincides with religion in the amplest sense of the word as it is institutionally grasped. Presumably, religion is not about changing the world but the human beings' heart.[2] Morinians love repeating the importance of the *religare* as a salient feature of complexity as it goes. Consequently, Morinians make the difference between restricted complexity and large complexity; the former refers to the use of scientific rods whereas the latter refers to the method, as said.

Systems thinking—many time also called as systems science [16]—is a rather vast and unformed set of approaches and languages that consists of what, in the

[2] In the history of Latin America, mainly, such a conception of religions is false because it is partial. In the history of Latin America there is also liberation theology, which was and still is a commitment or an option for the poor people. Most liberation theologians were literally killed by the powers—ongoing and around—transforming thus the very experience and interpretation of religion. That is exactly what is highlighted here as "institutionalized religion."

framework of the philosophy of science, is known as coherentism (see: https://plato.stanford.edu/entries/justep-coherence/). In other words, it is the intention of grasping, taking, and understanding everything as a wonderful complex puzzle in which each piece matches perfectly with the other. Von Foerster and von Bertalanffy are usually taken as the founders of systems thinking.[3] Very frequently, it is also identified with holism, i.e., the idea that everything is connected to everything else. Systems thinking argues that there are closed, isolated, and open systems. The sciences of complexity have sufficiently shown that there are only open systems including the entire universe. There are not, and they are impossible isolated or closed systems.

In contrast, the sciences of complexity can be taken around a central issue, namely the study and concern about the degrees of freedom a system, phenomenon, or behavior has or exhibits. The higher the degrees of freedom, the more complex a system. Life can be safely understood as bearing open and unlimited degrees of freedom. Hence, the concern in this book is about health and disease, therapies, and techniques—and ultimately, about life.

Being as it may, the sciences of complexity allow us to understand, explain, and work with turbulent, nonlinear, unpredictable, fluctuating and emerging systems, phenomena, and behaviors. To be sure, the triad of life, health, and disease is such a system or phenomenon. Medicine, health, and therapies are to know, to say the least, the wide panorama of the sciences of complexity. This is the most basic invitation of this book. Some others tend to such an invitation openly and directly, while others only implicitly and derivatively.

4 Quantum Biology

Let us say it straightforwardly: biologists who work on or with quantum mechanics do see and know many more interesting things than physicists who study quantum mechanics. Moreover, life is rooted in quantum mechanics, but it is seen and largely explained as a classical system. This happens most notoriously also in medicine.

Quantum biology does not just apply quantum mechanics to living beings, but it also allows us to discover surprising quantum behaviors in nature, in general. Technically speaking, quantum biology studies quantum effects in nature, say in birds and fish, plants, fungi, and human beings, for instance. Several quantum effects observed encompass magnetoception, odor, light harvesting, photosynthesis, and the functioning of the brain, among several other behaviors [18].

The quantum principles are as follows: nonlocality, entanglement, superposition, Pauli exclusion, the wave-particle duality, uncertainty, and coherence-decoherence-recoherence. Importantly, the expression quantum mechanics does not have anything to do with any mechanic, i.e., a mechanicistic take. That was simply the way

[3] For a rather different and most solid approach cf. [17].

the founders of the theory encountered to dun it. Along the same tenure, quantum mechanics does not have any principled philosophy or state of mind.

By and large, quantum mechanics is the most robust theory ever developed, to date. It has been tested, confirmed, verified, and falsified up the eleventh decimal. There is no other theory in any field that exhibits such strength. It is indeed the best theory to explain the universe, reality, the world, nature, and life in any sense of the word. A fortiori, we would like to highlight it is the best theory to grasp health.

Quantum biology has had a clearly more solid development in biology at large, complexity theory, philosophy, and the history of science. However, in medicine it is barely been considered. This has seriously hindered applied research. Meanwhile, there has been a speculative use of the so-called quantum medicine for commercial rather than missionary health care purposes.

In the framework of an Introduction to this book, it becomes necessary to remind some of the fundamentals of quantum mechanics. Quantum mechanics is a very sophisticated, technical, and difficult mathematical apparatus aimed at explaining quantum behaviors. The quantum behaviors are expressed in the so-called quantum principles. These are teleportation, superposition, complementarity, uncertainty, the exclusion principle by Pauli, teleportation, the duality wave-particle, and nonlocality.

Quantum mechanics is articulated in a twofold mathematical expression, namely, as matrix mechanics and wave mechanics. Both are complementary. The mathematical apparatus creates even some numbers that help explain quantum phenomena. These numbers are the half-spin, the main number, the secondary number or azimuthal, and the magnetic, mainly. Quantum mechanics allows understanding quantum behaviors in physics, chemistry, current spearhead technologies, biology, and the social sciences [19, 20].

Quantum biology was born only very recently—around 2008 [21]. As it can be seen, the formation of medical doctors and, in general, health professionals has barely gone into the general domain of quantum theory. "It is time to go quantum in medicine" [22]. To date, medicine has a retardment of more than 120 years and counting. Largely, the formation and practice remain mechanistic if not reductionist. People deserve better science and practice, definitely nondualist or binary. It is indeed about the differentiation between health (physical health) and mental health (note the use of a complementation in the latter case), the strongly anatomic-physiological explanation of behaviors, diseases, and treatments, and definitely the focus on illness and disease. At its best, the medicine system has come to speak about well-being. *A petitio principii.*

Medicine in general can greatly benefit from quantum biology as follows: firstly, it consists of a rejection of mechanistic and reductionist understandings—mainly from biochemistry and the excessive focus on causality. Most notably, whereas illness or disease are clearly seen naturally or thanks to different techniques, health and life are highly counterintuitive. Quantum mechanics in general and quantum biology in particular allow for brand-new explanations and understandings that may foster new forms of intervention. It is fundamental here to highlight that usually people and medical doctors are acquainted with quantum physics. Meaningfully, quantum biologists know and see many more and quite different phenomena than quantum physicists.

To date, the clinical practice or public health -say, global health and one health, have not introduced one single element of quantum biology: not to mention quantum chemistry. The crux lies in the very conception of health/disease, i.e., life/death. This volume just wants to open a window. One of us has been systematically working along this line [18, 23, 24].

5 Some Applications from the Science of Complexity to Medicine

This section does not pretend to be exhaustive in the review of all the theories that apply to medicine from the complexity sciences. Basically, it centers on some discoveries made in the twentieth century in this field that could change the way in which we understand the physiological mechanisms in the organisms.

Firstly, the discovery of biophotons as a possible mechanism for communication within organisms would make it possible to overcome certain limitations from the biochemical field by explaining some complex physiological phenomena that occur in short intervals of time. Resorting only to neurohumoral explanations to understand all the different mechanisms of regulation of the organism could have some limitations, such as the dependence on concentration gradients and the speed of the blood distribution of these biochemical messengers, so that they can reach their site of action and be able to bind to the respective cellular receptors.

On the other hand, the history of neural therapy (neuraltherapeutic medicine) brings many challenges and questions. One of the most well-known has been reported by the Huneke brothers about the "lightning reaction" (see Chap. 2) [25], which remains unexplained by the classical theories of neurophysiology limited only to biochemical and electrophysiological descriptions. Some hypotheses have been proposed to explain this phenomenon, based on quantum principles, as will be shown below.

Another challenging aspect in the history of neural therapy has been found in the concepts of synthetic physiology, also known as the Nervism school. This school is part of the central nucleus of the physiological dimension of this medical system[4] (See Chap. 13). In 1936, Speransky, who is a prominent author of this school, proposed (with a huge experimental basis) a visionary comprehension of physiological phenomena of the organism as nonlinear, synthetic, creative, evolutionary (irreversible), and dynamic, coordinated by the nervous system according to Pinilla-Bonilla [27, 28]. At that time, there were no other explanations of Speransky's experiments. Nonetheless, with the advent of nonlinear dynamical systems and chaos theories

[4] Specifically, from the perspective of Colombian School of Neural therapy, which is a complex systemic approach according to Julio César Payán [26]

applied to physiology, their findings can be better understood. Some applications to physiology, neuroscience, and health-disease dynamics will be shown, inviting to review the classic and fundamental concepts of homeostasis in medicine.

5.1 *The Discovery of Biophotons: A New Possibility for Communication in Organisms*

Although experimental evidence for the existence of biophotons was only found from the 1950s, one of its most important antecedents is related to the discovery of the emission of ultraweak radiation from a group of cells that was undergoing a mitotic process.

In 1923, the Ukrainian biologist Alexander Gurwitsch was studying the causes of cell division. He believed that this event could be facilitated by a nonchemical external impulse that induced a collective excitation of some cellular receptors. To test this idea, he conducted an experiment involving two onion roots arranged perpendicularly and centrally aligned, with the apex of the first root (acting as the "emitter" of the impulse) directed toward the division zone of the second root (working as the "recipient"). Here, Gurwitsch could observe the induction of mitosis on the recipient through histological observations. The induction was successful with quartz tubes but failed with glass ones. He deduced that UV light was responsible for this action, which he termed "mitogenetic radiation" [29, 30].

Gurwitsch had been working on a theory that could explain the morphogenetic process in embryology since 1912. He believed that in embryological development and, also, in the mitotic process, there was a supracellular ordering factor involved. For the 1930s, he was proposing this idea under the name of "nonequilibrium molecular constellations." After that, he named this constellation the "field theory" [31].

The idea of "mitogenic radiation" was not fully accepted within the scientific community, and there were some detractors of his work [29, 30]. Nevertheless, his work influenced the development of new areas of research in biology and biophysics, especially in the exploration of nonchemical cellular communication.

From the 1950s to 1970s, biophotons of seedlings were detected by using photomultiplier tubes, and it was proposed that they were related to metabolic activities such as mitochondrial respiration and lipid oxidation, among others. After the 1980s, the hypothesis that biophotons correspond to coherent radiation that allows cell-to-cell communication has been growing (See Table 7.1) [46].

Specifically, the German physicist Fritz Albert Popp and his collaborators have found that DNA is one source of biophotons and could be the basis of cell communication. Cells emit light even when the cytoplasm is damaged, but when the nuclei are removed, there is no ultraweak photon emission anymore. Popp proposed that DNA could act as an "exciplex laser system" or "coherent light" functioning far from thermal equilibrium at threshold [30, 37].

Table 7.1 Some key publications about biophoton emission in different research fields. The information is shown chronologically

Year	Authors	Field of research
1926	Gurwitsch	Mitogenetic radiation [32]
1955	Colli et al.	Seedlings biophotons [33]
1969	Vladimirov et al.	Chemiluminescence in biological membranes [34]
1973	Zhuravlev et al.	Ultraweak luminescence in rat liver mitochondria [35]
1984	Cadenas	Biological chemiluminescence [36]
1984	Popp et al.	DNA as a source of coherent biophotons [37]
1992	Slawinski et al.	Stress-induced photon emission [38]
1994	Shen et al.	Degranulation and photon emission from granulocytes [39]
1999	Kobayashi et al.	Photon emission from rat brain with oxidative stress [40]
2000	Albrecht-Buehler	Fluorescence of live mammalian mitochondria [41]
2000	Gariaev et al.	Verifying of DNA laser emission[7]
2005	Jaffe	Luminescence in marine plants [42]
2007	Farhadi et al.	Signaling in intestinal epithelial cells [43]
2009	Fels	Cellular communication through light [44]
2011	Rastogi et al.	Photon emission from human skin [45]

Source: Own elaboration

In a similar trend, the Russian biologist Peter Gariaev began research in the field of genetics that, in 1994, he called Wave Genetics [47]. Gariaev was working to resolve the problem, in the context of the transduction of DNA into proteins, about how the third nucleotide in an encoding triplet is selected. Gariaev and his group have demonstrated what Popp previously had proposed about the laser emission from DNA. They demonstrated experimentally in Moscow this laser radiation and proposed that chromosomes had the ability to gyrate the polarization plane of the photons.[5] All these findings led them to postulate a "wave model" in which the fundamental property was the nonlocality of genetic information based on quantum principles. For this theory to work, it was necessary to admit that DNA and chromosome apparatus behave as liquid crystals, a fact that was confirmed some years later by other authors [48, 49].

Another surprising fact was the phenomenon known as the "DNA phantom effect," which was very challenging to explain for Gariaev and his collaborators. Pitkänen [50] described this phenomenon as follows: "When one removes the DNA from the chamber containing it and irradiates it by laser light, a weak pattern of scattered light is still produced as if there were a kind of phantom DNA there. The pattern can last for months."

[5] Despite the fact that Gariaev's findings were not published in any journal, this results were socialized in the Fourth International Conference on Computing Anticipatory Systems, CASYS in Belgium in 2000,available at: https://userpage.fu-berlin.de/~gerbrehm/nw/wavecomputer.pdf

Bearing in mind all these phenomena, Gariaev developed a model called "quantum holographic DNA-wave biocomputer." This model describes DNA as a "self-calibrating antenna" that can receive and send diffraction patterns representing quantum holographic information, working in a resonance phase. Based on this idea, DNA can be seen as a liquid crystal consisting of a series of conjugate mirrors, from which a laser beam carrying genetic information can be produced. These interference patterns make up the DNA holographic planes, which encode the essential data of the organism as three-dimensional representations. In conclusion, DNA molecules can be seen as a continuous network of genetic signals inside a certain biosystem. These signals can be used to create preliminary representations of biostructures, or morphogenetic information, and they link together all the organism's individual cells[7] [51].

Despite Gariaev's findings are barely known (and perhaps controversial) in the scientific community, the Nobel Prize laureate Luc Montagnier and his collaborators from Italy and Germany have also proven that DNA generates low-frequency electromagnetic waves [52]; they also confirmed that these electromagnetic signals (EMS) can be "retranscribed into DNA in living cells." They stated that these "EMS appear thus to be the carrier of the quantum coherence expressed in the DNA code" and "may play an important role in epigenetic modifications" [53].

5.2 *Brain Information Processing and Consciousness from a Quantum Perspective*

This research line has two fields of development: the first one is related to biophotonic communication on the nervous system, and the second one is related to microtubules as information processors.

In nervous systems, biophotonic emission could originate from intense metabolic and electric activity [46]. Also, these emissions have been correlated with the electroencephalographic signals [54]. There is a theoretical speculation that states that biophotons can mediate the transmission and processing of nerve signals by transmitting them along the nerve fibers, specifically through mitochondria and microtubules [46]. In the mitochondria, some processes of electrical coupling could take place [55, 56].

In the case of microtubules, Jibu and collaborators [57] have postulated that light can be transmitted on these cytoskeletal structures. It is proposed that optical signaling, as an "optic fiber," would be free from thermal and noise loss and could behave as a long-range coherent quantum phenomenon that contributes to information processing in the brain [57–59].

The conventional opinion has been held that the brain's working mechanisms should be in accordance with the laws of bioelectrical and biochemical reactions. However, this narrow view precludes us from comprehending the complex mental processes in the human brain in the formation of consciousness. In this regard, the physicist Roger Penrose and the anesthesiologist Stuart Hameroff [60] assign to microtubules the role in the emergence of consciousness. These authors claim that fundamental acts of consciousness must not be seen as algorithmic and, therefore, cannot be computed [61].

This quantum model on microtubules assumes that each dimer of tubulin is in a state that is the superposition of the α and β conformations and assumes that coherent states exist between the dimer chains. It has been suggested that states of quantum coherence could occur on microtubules that, if maintained for a long enough time, would allow signal propagation to take place without energy dissipation. This coherent and superposition state could spread over hundreds of micrometers among the other microtubules, generating a coupling dynamic, which in turn could account for the unity of consciousness. Also, it can be understood that the phenomenon of quantum wave function "self-collapse is crucial for consciousness" [57, 60, 61].

Some years later, the neuroscientist Walter Freeman and the physicist Giuseppe Vitiello proposed a model of dissipative quantum field (assuming the brain as an open system) that would explain how memories are created and updated by phase transitions. In this model, they propose that brain and mental activity cannot be separated; quite the opposite, brain and mind are "dynamically entangled" within coherent states. This model is also based on the phenomenon called Boson condensation, which facilitates the formation of neuronal correlations and behaves as a classical field not affected by quantum fluctuations, allowing memory consolidation. They additionally allege that neurons are classical objects, but the quantum variables appear when the vibrations of molecular electrical dipoles are considered. These authors also point out that the model proposed by Penrose and Hameroff does not consider the crucial aspect of the dissipation of open systems such as the brain [62].

So recently, the physicist Mikheenko [63] proposed a unified model for the processing of information in the brain based on the quantum-mechanical phenomenon of nano-superconductivity in microtubules. One hundred years ago, superconductivity was only a phenomenon evidenced at low temperatures near zero, but in the 1960s, Little [64] predicted superconductivity at very high temperatures in an organic chain of molecules of one dimension. Some years later, Kasumov et al. [65] confirmed a superconductivity phenomenon on the DNA while this was in contact with another superconductor.

Evidence of superconductivity on the brain was confirmed through electrical transport measurements on the brain slices fixed with formalin [66]. The brain slices were exposed to a water solution of graphene nano-flakes at room temperature to provide an electrical connection to microtubules before the measurement. Mikheenko claims that the measurements could give evidence of "superconductivity in the neural network of mammalian brains." Other arguments in favor of superconductivity in the brain are the observation of high conductivity within microtubules when water was put inside of them and the reported resistance near zero at certain resonance frequencies [63, 67]. More arguments have been cited by Mikheenko [63], giving a strong argument in favor of superconductivity in microtubules.

Additionally, to these mentioned facts, Mikheenko proposed that, assuming the superconductivity as a real phenomenon on the microtubules, it is also expected that the generation of coherent radiation already known as Josephson. This radiation could be estimated based on the action potential propagating on the membrane. Mikheenko suggests that its frequency could be about 33.8 THz. The model states that as each set of microtubules generates a similar radiation near the membrane, "hundreds of billions of neurons create a symphony like music in a symphony orchestra." This model explains some phenomena observed in the brain, such as memory, perception, and emotions.

5.3 Hypothesis on the Action Mechanisms of Procaine on the Nervous System from a Quantum Perspective

As mentioned before, there is a challenge in the history of discovering Neural therapy, especially when novocaine or procaine was synthesized and applied to treat several pathological conditions. Initially, researchers believed that procaine only had local anesthetic properties, but as the Huneke brothers continued to explore its therapeutic potential, they discovered unexpected effects. The Huneke brothers, and later neural therapists worldwide, observed empirically that applying procaine to a specific part of the organism sometimes resulted in a nonlocal or remote effect. These remote effects had the particularity that could occur in a very fast way, which they called "lightning reaction." They wanted to mean with this expression that the reaction happened in seconds.

Some authors have proposed a hypothesis about the action mechanism of procaine on the microtubules from a quantum perspective [68]. Understanding this hypothesis requires keeping certain elements in mind. First, it is important to remember that, despite microtubules being part of the cytoskeleton of all cells, they are especially abundant in neurons [69]. The second element is that some decades ago, Fröhlich proposed that in biological systems, there could be long-range coherence and energy storage due to dielectric properties based on the component parts that possess dipole vibrational activity, where free electrons are found [70]. This suggests the possibility of finding coherence states in the propagation of signals that travel with low energy dissipation. Precisely, the third element is based on a quantum model of electrical signaling transfer on the microtubules [71, 72]. Fourth, the National University of Colombia tested the dielectric properties of procaine in a high-tension laboratory.[6] Román et al. found that procaine has an extremely high dielectric permittivity, which means that it behaves as a condenser with enormous

[6] Roman F, Jaimes R, Osorio Y. Acercamiento al comportamiento dieléctrico de la procaína y sus soluciones: análisis de la permitividad dieléctrica con la procaina, 2003. These results were never published but were presented at the 2003 World Meeting of Neural Therapy in Bogotá. See: https://www.terapianeural.com/congresos/46-congresos/109-colombia-2003-congreso-internacional-de-terapia-neural-resumenes

capacity to store electrical charges. This is an important aspect because it is known that signal propagation in microtubules depends on the electrical properties of the medium in which they are immersed, particularly permittivity. However, there are still no systematic studies on the alteration of this property by the inclusion of local anesthetics in the medium [68].

Bearing in mind these four elements, Cruz and Fayad [68] suggest that due to the distribution of charges between the inner and outer medium in the microtubules, and given the high permittivity of procaine, it could be inferred that an ionic cloud would be created in the external medium adjacent to the microtubules that would allow the amplification of signals propagating along the microtubule axis. Consequently, this would be an important result for interpreting microtubule-to-synaptic transmission communication and could serve as a basis for explaining why low concentrations of procaine are required to achieve therapeutic effect.

Also, this hypothesis could explain the dual effect of procaine observed by Vishnevsky [73], in which there is a blockade of the nerve conductivity in the first instance, and then an active process of excitation, which implies an improvement of the trophic function of the nervous system and, in consequence, of the innervated tissues. This aspect could also be correlated with the experimental findings about the intracellular action of procaine that can induce microtubule assembly or inhibit it [74].

This proposal paves the way for a wide range of research, including the potential implications of altering signal propagation in microtubules on the development of various pathologies. According to reports, microtubules play a role in the pathogenesis of certain diseases like Alzheimer's [75] and some types of cancer [76], yet there remains a vast field to explore in this area.

5.4 A New Perspective for Physiology from Nonlinear Dynamics and Chaos Theory

For many years, the mechanistic and linear view of nature took precedence over scientific research, reducing systems into their component parts to understand them. Linear systems are characterized by the magnitude of their responses being proportional to the amplitude of the stimulus and by their predictability [77, 78].

However, the systems of nature, including human beings, lack mechanical periodicity or linear dynamics, contradicting the predictions of homeostasis of classical physiology. Physiological variables, such as the normal human heartbeat, actually have a complex behavior that fluctuates permanently under basal conditions [78, 79].

Chaos dynamics, which are associated with nonlinear and complex dynamics, have found application in various fields, particularly in the exact sciences. The application of chaos dynamics to medicine remains challenging and under development, and according to research by Boubaker [80], it accounts for only 3.8% of the scientific production in literature.

While certain publications in the field of physiology began to appear in the 1980s, a significant increase was observed in the 1990s, primarily centered on cardiovascular physiology, with "heart rate variability" serving as the pioneering application of chaos theory to this discipline [80]. Nonetheless, publications in this area expanded their scope to encompass respiratory physiology, immunology, neurology, psychiatry, epidemiology, the locomotor system, oncology, and metabolic diseases, among others [78, 80].

This section will focus on two main areas: the application of the theory of nonlinear dynamical systems and chaos theory to the concepts of health and disease; and applications to the area of neurophysiology.

5.4.1 Implications for Health-Disease Concepts

A group of researchers from the Laboratory for Computational Physiology of the Massachusetts Institute of Technology and from the Margret and H.A. Rey Institute for Nonlinear Dynamics at Beth Israel Deaconess Medical Center in the United States have been working since the 1980s to understand nonlinear dynamics in physiology. In 1999, these scientists created the Research Resource for Complex Physiologic Signals under the auspices of the National Center for Research Resources of the National Institutes of Health, and one of its objectives is to stimulate research in complex physiological variables from several methodologies, including nonlinear dynamics [81].

Based on an analysis of physiological variables such as the heart rate, this group had discovered some characteristics that could differentiate the process of health and diseases from the chaos theory and nonlinear dynamics perspective. When they analyzed dynamics from healthy subjects, they found that the cardiac interbeat intervals fluctuated in an unpredictable way. Neuroautonomic inputs, which create a nonlinear interaction between the sympathetic and parasympathetic branches of the nervous system, could explain this variable behavior [82].

On the other hand, when they observed the dynamics of some pathologies, such as the tremors of Parkinson's disease, the obstructive sleep apnea, and the epilepsy and fetal distress syndromes, they found a tendency to a periodic or regular pattern of behavior [77]. Goldberger [79] referred to these behaviors as a "decomplexification of systems," signifying a deterioration of information within them, implying a limited capacity to adjust to the demands of a constantly changing environment. When the dynamics of systems become more regular and periodic, it is easier to predict their evolution because they are much more stable than other dynamics. This is the characteristic that enables physicians to make a diagnosis and to make a prognosis of the disease's course [77].

Healthy dynamics demonstrate a capacity to adapt to unpredictable stimuli and stress situations, a phenomenon also known as functional plasticity [79] For this reason, Peng et al. [82] proposed a modification of the term "homeostasis," which refers to the pursuit of "constancy," in place of the term "homeodynamics," to better account for dynamics that deviate from equilibrium under basal conditions.

As a hypothesis, this functional plasticity could explain why healthy organisms are fully capable of generating a good immune response to microorganisms. Conversely, organisms that have an alteration of their "ground" or nervous tone, either due to irritation or dystrophy coordinated by the nervous system, according to Speransky, are much less adaptable and become easy prey for infections.

Now, speculating in the mental sphere, human beings are faced with situations that challenge them either at a social, work, family, or personal level. Depending on the way in which this information is "integrated" into the dynamic system, which in part is naturally linked to the interpretation of organisms about what happens to them, it will lead to a more adapted or less adapted self-organization. In the second case, the less well-adapted dynamics will cause organization patterns that tend to be a cyclical or periodic dynamic. This is what makes people go through manic-depressive episodes or processes where the same memories and feelings keep coming up, like a circuit that keeps going around and around, which can lead to mental illness.

Based on these postulates from nonlinear dynamical systems, there is much room to explore in the field of health and disease processes.

5.4.2 Implications for Neurophysiology

Since the 1970s, the already mentioned Walter Freeman, Professor of Neurobiology at the University of California in Berkeley,[7] integrated mathematics, biophysics, and engineering to understand neurophysiology from the new perspective of chaos theory and nonlinear dynamics. Freeman's work aimed to comprehend the brain as a self-organizing, nonequilibrium, and dissipative structure. As a philosopher, Freeman was also in line with Heidegger's and Merleau-Ponty's philosophies, as well as the idea of embodied cognition [83].

Freeman [84] suggests that "perception cannot be understood solely by examining properties of individual neurons, a microscopic approach that currently dominates neuroscience research." Therefore, he integrated the chaos theory to explain the ability of a wide range of neurons in the olfactory cortex to abruptly switch from one pattern of activity to another, which constitutes a perception activity through a "phase transition" [84, 85].

Freeman observed an auto-generated electrical activity in the olfactory bulb neurons that facilitates this aspect, even in the absence of external motivation [84]. In other words, chaos provides the system with a "ready state" where a broad band of many templates or neural cell assemblies is involved [86].

The experiments conducted by Freeman and his colleagues demonstrated that all neurons in the bulb contribute to the generation of each olfactory perception,

[7] Freeman also studied mathematics and physics at M.I.T., philosophy at Chicago University, medicine at Yale University, and neuropsychiatry at the University of California at Los Angeles. He was also the president of the Pavlovian Society in 1977 and a founding member of the Journal's Editorial Board of "Cognitive Neurodynamics." His scientific tradition traced back to Charles Sherrington and Karl Pribram.

indicating that the entire bulb is always activated, not just a small subgroup, with only the pattern of activation differing [84]. The study of the electroencephalographic signals reveals that the act of perception creates a spatial pattern of oscillations, known as amplitude modulation patterns, that constantly alter to reflect the animal's goals and expectations. The olfactory system, as well as the auditory, visual, and somatosensory cortex, demonstrated this activity [83].

Using a computational model, Freeman showed that the addition of a new odor to the olfactory cortex model's perceptual repertoire altered the activity patterns of all other maps, indicating a true associative memory system, as described by Pavlov [84]. In the 1930s, the disciple of Pavlov, Alexei Speransky, discovered that when a stimulus entered the nervous system, its information never remained confined to a specific location, but instead, it triggered a reflex response that encompassed the entire nervous system (see Chap. 13). Regardless of whether the response was adaptive or pathological, the nervous system always responded as a whole to all stimuli in a nonlinear way [26, 87].

This computational tool provided a graphic representation of the dynamics of olfactory systems, illustrating a chaotic attractor. Each attractor represents the behavior of systems established under the influence of a particular stimulus. From this perspective, an act of perception consists of an explosive leap of system dynamics from one basin of a chaotic attractor to another [84].

Furthermore, Freeman described intentionality as the process via which brains address the symbol-grounding dilemma and create the psychological "now" [61]. He firmly challenged reductionism, which perceives brains solely as information-processing entities, transforming input data into output neural representations. According to Kozma [83], he came to understand the brain as an integrated organ that is fundamental to the unity of the mind, body, and brain. Additionally, Freeman held the belief that the chaos theory approach could explain the brain's ability to adapt flexibly to the external world and generate new patterns, including "fresh ideas." In this regard, Speransky has also described the sudden integration of information from external agents with the organism, leading to the creation of a new organism [87], which explains the brain's ability to self-organize continuously.

Alexei Ukhtomsky, another author from the Nervism School or Synthetic Physiology, proposed concepts that bore a striking resemblance to those put forth by Freeman. In the 1920s, he established the concept of dominance or dominant center (refer to Chap. 13). This physiologist developed in 1940 a mathematical model of excitation for the nervous system that was based on the concept of a "nonlinear oscillatory ensemble" [88]. In this regard, Golbin and Umantsev [89] proposed a hypothesis based on Ukhtomsky's concepts and on chaos theory. They speculate that in diseases, there is an inability to self-produce chaos in a specific part of the organism, for example, the heart. They held the belief that in order to survive, a pathological organism activates a "compensatory dominant system" in a high-level chaotic pattern (for example, scratches themselves without a clear cause) to compensate for the loss of healthy chaos in the main subsystem (the heart). We can also observe this behavior in the paroxysmal outbursts of anger and tears, which relieve emotional tension and lead to a brief period of calm.

Other authors who follow this field of research have found that the inhibitory process of neuronal assemblies plays a crucial role in nonlinear neurodynamics. The inhibitory interneurons participate in the shaping of these dynamical assemblies or activation patterns that can generate chaos. Another learned lesson is that neither a neuron nor a cell assembly is designed to serve a single purpose [86]. Rather, they can implement several functions depending upon the internal states of the brain and the constraints placed upon it by environmental factors, as Piotr Anokhin said with his functional systems theory (See Chap. 13) [90].

In conclusion, the application of the theory of nonlinear dynamic systems and the theory of chaos to physiology and neurobiology enables us to understand phenomena such as creativity, spontaneity, perception, the integrity of the nervous system, and the transitions between healthy and sick dynamics. This approach finds several points of convergence with the approaches of synthetic physiology (see Chap. 13). We can outline these convergence points as a promising path for future research.

References

1. Maldonado C. Las ciencias de la complejidad son ciencias de la vida. Santiago de Chile: Trepen; 2021.
2. Scott AC. The nonlinear universe: chaos, emergence, life. Berlin: Springer; 2007.
3. Maldonado CE. Ciencias de la complejidad: ciencias de los cambios súbitos. Odeón Observ Econ Oper Numér. 2005;2:85–125. Available from: https://revistas.uexternado.edu.co/index.php/odeon/article/view/2643
4. Waldrop MM. Complexity: the emerging science at the edge of order and chaos. New York: Touchstone; 1993.
5. Lewin K. Complexity: life at the edge of chaos. Chicago: University of Chicago Press; 1992.
6. Gleick J. Chaos: making a new science. Londres: Penguin Books; 1987.
7. Barrow-Green J. Poincaré and the three-body problem. Providence: American Mathematical Society; 1996.
8. Gödel K. On formally undecidable propositions of principia Mathematica and related systems. New York: Dover; 1992.
9. Wang H. A logical journey: from Gödel to philosophy. Cambridge: The MIT Press; 1996.
10. Gray JJ. The Hilbert challenge. Oxford: Oxford University Press; 2001.
11. Maldonado CE. Pensar: lógicas no clásicas. Bogotá: Universidad El Bosque; 2016.
12. Maldonado CE. Pensar: lógicas no clásicas. Bogotá: Universidad El Bosque; 2020.
13. Maldonado CE. Epigenetics and/as complexity. In: Cómbita JL, Maldonado CE, editors. Biología teórica, explicaciones y complejidad. Bogotá: Universidad El Bosque-Bievep; 2021. p. 53–70.
14. Maldonado CE. Biosemiótica y complejidad. Bogotá: Universidad El Bosque; 2022.
15. Maldonado CE, Giraldo J. El mundo es cuántico: una teoría a partir de las múltiples interpretaciones de la mecánica cuántica. Bogotá: Desde Abajo; 2022.
16. Meyers RA, editor. Encyclopedia of complexity and systems science. New York: Springer-Verlag; 2009.
17. Midgley G, editor. Systems thinking. Vol. I: general systems theory, cybernetics and complexity. Vol. II: systems theories and modeling. Vol. III: second-order cybernetics, systemic therapy and soft systems thinking. London: Sage Publications; 2003.

18. Maldonado CE, Gómez-Cruz N. Synchronicity among biological and computational levels of an organism: quantum biology and complexity. Proc Comput Sci. 2014;36:177–84. https://doi.org/10.1016/j.procs.2014.09.076.
19. Haven E, Khrennikov A. Quantum social science. Cambridge: Cambridge University Press; 2013.
20. Maldonado CE. Quantum theory and the social sciences. Momento Rev Fis. 2019;59:34–47. https://doi.org/10.15446/mo.n59E.81645.
21. McFadden JJ, Al-Khalili J. Life on the edge: the coming age of quantum biology. New York: Crown; 2014.
22. Bisiani J, Anugu A, Pentyala S. It's time to go quantum in medicine. J Clin Med. 2023;12(13):4506. https://doi.org/10.3390/jcm12134506.
23. Maldonado C. A quantum coherence-recoherence-based model of reality. Neuroquantology. 2018;16(11):44–8. https://doi.org/10.14704/nq.2018.16.11.1858.
24. Maldonado C. The world as a quantum information processor. Praxis Filosófica. 2021;53:53–68. https://doi.org/10.25100/pfilosofica.v0i53.11448.
25. Barop H. Neural therapy. In: Textbook and atlas of neural therapy. New York: Thieme Medical Publishers Inc.; 2017.
26. Sarmiento LD. Historia e institucionalización de la terapia neural en Colombia [Master's thesis]. Bogotá: Universidad Nacional de Colombia; 2014. 72 p. Available from: https://repositorio.unal.edu.co/handle/unal/49642.
27. Pinilla-Bonilla LB. Análisis crítico de los procedimientos teórico-metodológicos de las investigaciones de A. D. Speransky que sustentan la terapia neural desde la lógica peirceana [Master's thesis]. Bogotá: Universidad Nacional de Colombia; 2010. 119 p. Available from: https://repositorio.unal.edu.co/handle/unal/6873.
28. Pinilla-Bonilla LB. Aplicación del método de investigación peirceano a la obra de Speransky. In: Oostra A, Zalamea F, editors. Cuadernos de sistemática peirceana. Bogotá: Editorial Nomos; 2012. p. 93–114. Available from: https://www.unav.es/gep/bibliopeirceana.html.
29. Volodyaev I, Beloussov LV. Revisiting the mitogenetic effect of ultra-weak photon emission. Front Physiol. 2015;6:241. https://doi.org/10.3389/fphys.2015.00241.
30. Grass F, Klima H, Kasper S. Biophotons, microtubules and CNS: is our brain a "holographic computer"? Med Hypotheses. 2004;62(2):169–72. https://doi.org/10.1016/S0306-9877(03)00308-6.
31. Beloussov LV, Opitz JM, Gilbert SF. Life of Alexander G. Gurwitsch and his relevant contribution to the theory of morphogenetic fields. Int J Dev Biol. 1997;41(6):771–7.
32. Gurwitsch A. Das Problem der Zellteilung physiologisch betrachtet. Berlin: Springer-Verlag; 1926. https://doi.org/10.1007/978-3-642-90660-2.
33. Colli L, Facchini U, Guidotti G, et al. Further measurements on the bioluminescence of the seedlings. Experientia. 1955;11:479–81. https://doi.org/10.1007/BF02166829.
34. Vladimirov IA, Suslova TB, Olenev VI. Chemiluminescence associated with the formation of lipid peroxides in biological membranes. II. The role of Fe^{2+} in the development of chain oxidation of lipids and of ultra-weak luminescence. Biofizika. 1969;14(5):836–45. Russian
35. Zhuravlev AI, Tsvylev OP, Zubkova SM. Spontaneous endogenous ultraweak luminescence of rat liver mitochondria in conditions of normal metabolism. Biofizika. 1973;18(6):1037–40. Russian
36. Cadenas E. Biological chemiluminescence. Photochem Photobiol. 1984;40(6):823–30. https://doi.org/10.1111/j.1751-1097.1984.tb04657.x.
37. Popp FA, Nagl W, Li KH, et al. Biophoton emission: new evidence for coherence and DNA as source. Cell Biophys. 1984;6(1):33–52. https://doi.org/10.1007/bf02788579.
38. Slawinski J, Ezzahir A, Godlewski M, Kwiecinska T, Rajfur Z, Sitko D, et al. Stress-induced photon emission from perturbed organisms. Experientia. 1992;48(11–12):1041–58. https://doi.org/10.1007/BF01947992.
39. Shen X, Mei W, Xu X. Activation of neutrophils by a chemically separated but optically coupled neutrophil population undergoing respiratory burst. Experientia. 1994;50(10):963–8. https://doi.org/10.1007/BF01923488.

40. Kobayashi M, Takeda M, Sato T, Yamazaki Y, Kaneko K, Ito K, et al. In vivo imaging of spontaneous ultraweak photon emission from a rat's brain correlated with cerebral energy metabolism and oxidative stress. Neurosci Res. 1999;34(2):103–13. https://doi.org/10.1016/s0168-0102(99)00040-1.
41. Albrecht-Buehler G. Reversible excitation light-induced enhancement of fluorescence of live mammalian mitochondria. FASEB J. 2000;14(13):1864–6. https://doi.org/10.1096/fj.00-0028fje.
42. Jaffe LF. Marine plants may polarize remote Fucus eggs via luminescence. Luminescence. 2005;20(6):414–8. https://doi.org/10.1002/bio.866.
43. Farhadi A, Forsyth C, Banan A, Shaikh M, Engen P, Fields JZ, Keshavarzian A. Evidence for non-chemical, non-electrical intercellular signaling in intestinal epithelial cells. Bioelectrochemistry. 2007;71(2):142–8. https://doi.org/10.1016/j.bioelechem.2007.03.001.
44. Fels D. Cellular communication through light. PLoS One. 2009;4(4):e5086. https://doi.org/10.1371/journal.pone.0005086.
45. Rastogi A, Pospíšil P. Spontaneous ultraweak photon emission imaging of oxidative metabolic processes in human skin: effect of molecular oxygen and antioxidant defense system. J Biomed Opt. 2011;16(9):096005. https://doi.org/10.1117/1.3616135.
46. Tang R, Dai J. Biophoton signal transmission and processing in the brain. J Photochem Photobiol B. 2014;139:71–5. https://doi.org/10.1016/j.jphotobiol.2013.12.008.
47. Institute of Linguistic of Wave Genetics. Dr. Peter P. Garyaev, Doctor of biological sciences, Academician of the Russian Academy of Natural Sciences and RAMTN [Internet]. Wave Genetics; 2023. Available from: https://wavegenetics.org/en/garyaev/aspectyi/
48. Zakharova SS, Jesse W, Backendorf C, van der Maarel JR. Liquid crystal formation in supercoiled DNA solutions. Biophys J. 2002;83(2):1119–29. https://doi.org/10.1016/S0006-3495(02)75235-1.
49. Chow MH, Yan KT, Bennett MJ, Wong JT. Birefringence and DNA condensation of liquid crystalline chromosomes. Eukaryot Cell. 2010;9(10):1577–87. https://doi.org/10.1128/EC.00026-10.
50. Pitkänen M. The Notion of Wave Genome and DNA as Topological Quantum Computer. SciRePrints [Internet]. 2010. Available from: https://scireprints.lu.lv/69/
51. Gariaev PP, Vasiliev AA, Berezin AA. Holographic associative memory and information transmission by solitary waves in biological systems. Proc SPIE Int Soc Opt Eng. 1993;3:249–59. https://doi.org/10.1117/12.155056.
52. Montagnier L, Aissa J, Del Giudice E, Lavallee C, Tedeschi A, Vitiello G. DNA waves and water. J Phys Conf Ser. 2011;306:012007. https://doi.org/10.1088/1742-6596/306/1/012007.
53. Montagnier L, Del Giudice E, Aïssa J, Lavallee C, Motschwiller S, Capolupo A, Polcari A, Romano P, Tedeschi A, Vitiello G. Transduction of DNA information through water and electromagnetic waves. Electromagn Biol Med. 2015;34(2):106–12. https://doi.org/10.3109/15368378.2015.1036072.
54. Persinger M, Dotta B, Saroka K. Bright light transmits through the brain: measurement of photon emissions and frequency-dependent modulation of spectral electroencephalographic power. World J Neurosci. 2013;3:10–6. https://doi.org/10.4236/wjns.2013.31002.
55. Skulachev VP. Mitochondrial filaments and clusters as intracellular power-transmitting cables. Trends Biochem Sci. 2001;26(1):23–9. https://doi.org/10.1016/s0968-0004(00)01735-7.
56. Müller M, Mironov SL, Ivannikov MV, Schmidt J, Richter DW. Mitochondrial organization and motility probed by two-photon microscopy in cultured mouse brainstem neurons. Exp Cell Res. 2005;303(1):114–27. https://doi.org/10.1016/j.yexcr.2004.09.025.
57. Jibu M, Hagan S, Hameroff SR, Pribram KH, Yasue K. Quantum optical coherence in cytoskeletal microtubules: implications for brain function. Biosystems. 1994;32(3):195–209. https://doi.org/10.1016/0303-2647(94)90043-4.
58. Hameroff SR, Watt RC. Information processing in microtubules. J Theor Biol. 1982;98(4):549–61. https://doi.org/10.1016/0022-5193(82)90137-0.

59. Thar R, Kühl Little M. Propagation of electromagnetic radiation in mitochondria. J Theor Biol. 2004;230:261–70. https://doi.org/10.1016/j.jtbi.2004.05.021.
60. Hameroff S, Penrose R. Orchestrated reduction of quantum coherence in brain microtubules: a model for consciousness. Math Comput Simulat. 1996;40(3–4):453–80. https://doi.org/10.1016/0378-4754(96)80476-9.
61. Atmanspacher H. Quantum approaches to consciousness. In: Zalta EN, editor. The Stanford encyclopedia of philosophy; 2015. Available from: https://plato.stanford.edu/entries/qt-consciousness/.
62. Freeman W, Vitiello G. Matter and mind are entangled in two streams of images guiding behavior and informing the subject through awareness. Mind Matter. 2016;14:7–24.
63. Mikheenko P. Symphony in the brain. Preprints. 2024;2024041254. Available from: https://doi.org/10.20944/preprints202404.1254.v1
64. Little WA. Possibility of synthesizing an organic superconductor. Phys Rev. 1964;134:A1416–24. https://doi.org/10.1103/PhysRev.134.A1416.
65. Kasumov AY, Kociak M, Guéron S, Reulet B, Volkov VT, Klinov DV, Bouchiat H. Proximity-induced superconductivity in DNA. Science. 2001;291(5502):280–2. https://doi.org/10.1126/science.291.5502.280.
66. Mikheenko P. Possible superconductivity in the brain. J Supercond Nov Magn. 2018;32:1121–34. https://doi.org/10.1007/s10948-018-4965-4.
67. Sahu S, Ghosh S, Hirata K, Fujita D, Bandyopadhyay A. Multi-level memory-switching properties of a single brain microtubule. Appl Phys Lett. 2013;102:123701.
68. Cruz Y, Fayad R. Microtúbulos y terapia neural. Propuesta de una investigación promisoria. Rev Med. 2011;19(1):82–92. https://doi.org/10.18359/rmed.1228.
69. Baas PW, Rao AN, Matamoros AJ, Leo L. Stability properties of neuronal microtubules. Cytoskeleton (Hoboken). 2016 Sep;73(9):442–60. https://doi.org/10.1002/cm.21286.
70. Fröhlich H. Long-range coherence and energy storage in biological systems. Int J Quantum Chem. 1968;2(5):641–9. https://doi.org/10.1002/qua.560020505.
71. Tuszyński JA, Brown JA, Hawrylak P. Dielectric polarization, electrical conduction, information processing and quantum computation in microtubules. Are they plausible? Philos Trans R Soc A. 1998;356(1743):1897–926.
72. Martínez J, Ávila C, Fayad R. Transporte de señales eléctricas en microtúbulos: una aproximación cuántica. Rev Col Fis. 2010;42(2):104–6.
73. Vishnevsky A. El bloqueo novocaínico y los antisépticos oleo balsámicos como una forma terapéutica patógena. Buenos Aires: Cartago; 1958.
74. Coffe G, Foucault G, Raymond M, Pudles J. Dual effect of procaine in sea urchin eggs. Inducer and inhibitor of microtubule assembly. Exp Cell Res. 1985;156(1):175–81. https://doi.org/10.1016/0014-4827(85)90271-X.
75. Alonso AD, Grundke-Iqbal I, Barra HS, Iqbal K. Abnormal phosphorylation of tau and the mechanism of Alzheimer neurofibrillary degeneration: sequestration of microtubule-associated proteins 1 and 2 and the disassembly of microtubules by the abnormal tau. Proc Natl Acad Sci USA. 1997;94(1):298–303.
76. Hagen NA, du Souich P, Lapointe B, Ong-Lam M, Dubuc B, Walde D, Love R, Ngoc AH. Tetrodotoxin for moderate to severe cancer pain: a randomized, double-blind, parallel design multicenter study. J Pain Symptom Manag. 2008;35(4):420–9. https://doi.org/10.1016/j.jpainsymman.2007.05.011.
77. Goldberger AL. Non-linear dynamics for clinicians: chaos theory, fractals, and complexity at the bedside. Lancet. 1996;347(9011):1312–4. https://doi.org/10.1016/s0140-6736(96)90948-4.
78. Higgins JP. Nonlinear systems in medicine. Yale J Biol Med. 2002;75(5–6):247–60.
79. Goldberger AL, Amaral LA, Hausdorff JM, Ivanov PC, Peng CK, Stanley HE. Fractal dynamics in physiology: alterations with disease and aging. Proc Natl Acad Sci USA. 2002;99(Suppl 1):2466–72. https://doi.org/10.1073/pnas.012579499.

80. Boubaker O. Chaos in physiological control systems: health or disease? Chaos Theory Appl. 2024;6(1):1–12.
81. Goldberger AL, Amaral LA, Glass L, Hausdorff JM, Ivanov PC, Mark RG, Mietus JE, Moody GB, Peng CK, Stanley HE. PhysioBank, PhysioToolkit, and PhysioNet: components of a new research resource for complex physiologic signals. Circulation. 2000;101(23):215–20. https://doi.org/10.1161/01.cir.101.23.e215.
82. Peng CK, Buldyrev SV, Hausdorff JM, Havlin S, Mietus JE, Simons M, Stanley HE, Goldberger AL. Non-equilibrium dynamics as an indispensable characteristic of a healthy biological system. Integr Physiol Behav Sci. 1994;29(3):283–93. https://doi.org/10.1007/BF02691332.
83. Kozma R. Reflections on a giant of brain science: how lucky we are having Walter J. Freeman as our beacon in cognitive neurodynamics research. Cogn Neurodyn. 2016;10(6):457–69. https://doi.org/10.1007/s11571-016-9403-3.
84. Freeman WJ. The physiology of perception. Sci Am. 1991;264(2):78–87.
85. Freeman WJ. Simulation of chaotic EEG patterns with a dynamic model of the olfactory system. Biol Cybern. 1987;56(2–3):139–50. https://doi.org/10.1007/BF00317988.
86. Korn H, Faure P. Is there chaos in the brain? II. Experimental evidence and related models. C R Biol. 2003 Sep;326(9):787–840. https://doi.org/10.1016/j.crvi.2003.09.011.
87. Speransky AD. A basis for the theory of medicine. New York: International Publishers; 1943.
88. Zueva EY, Zuev KB. The concept of dominance by A.A. Ukhtomsky and anticipation. In: Nadin M, editor. Anticipation: learning from the past. Cognitive systems monographs, vol. 25. Berlin: Springer; 2015. p. 13–35. https://doi.org/10.1007/978-3-319-19446-2_2.
89. Golbin A, Umantsev A. Adaptive chaos: mild disorder may help contain major disease. Med Hypotheses. 2006;66(1):182–7. https://doi.org/10.1016/j.mehy.2005.06.031.
90. Sudakov KV. Theory of functional systems: a keystone of integrative biology. In: Nadin M, editor. Anticipation: learning from the past. Cognitive systems monographs, vol. 25. Berlin: Springer; 2015. p. 153–74. https://doi.org/10.1007/978-3-319-19446-2_2.

Chapter 8
Complexity Science, Life and Health: Foundation for a Theory of Health

Carlos Eduardo Maldonado

1 Introduction

Ever since the term and programs about public policies arose, the whole issue has truly been about disease, not health. The word "health"[1] has been and is still largely used; however, the real concern is about illness. They speak about health, but they really mean sickness. This is a most crucial problem that gravely affects society and each individual. Public health, global health, and One Health are truly about disease. Moreover, the Quadripartite organizations—the Food and Agricultural of the United States Organization (FAO), the United States Environment Program (UNEP), the World Health Organization (WHO), and the World Organization for Animal Health (WOAH) in their collaboration for One Health incur in the same mistake. Making no odds, it appears that they are doing things with words [1]. It is indeed the performative function of language.

Classically and normally, most institutions, policies, and actions talk about health, but they really mean disease.

Knowing about illness and disease, as well as caring about suffering and sickness, is certainly important. No question about this. Such is indeed the whole history of medicine and the health sciences as currently known. Without turning our backs on disease, both a moral and epistemological imperative arises, namely knowing and caring also about health. This chapter is all about the justification of this claim. We must know about health—not just about the word "health".

[1] In the following I will use "health" between quotation marks to refer to the standard use of health, as motive for suspicion or doubt. In contrast, the word health will be used plainly to mean exactly *health* and not disease, which is exactly the core if this chapter.

C. E. Maldonado (✉)
School of Medicine, Universidad El Bosque, Bogotá, Colombia
e-mail: maldonadocarlos@unbosque.edu.co

L. B. Pinilla Bonilla et al. (eds.), *Neuraltherapeutic Medicine*,
https://doi.org/10.1007/978-3-032-03257-7_8

This chapter's main argument is that we must know about health; however, in order to know about health, we must first know about life. After all, health is most probably the most important expression of life, i.e., being alive. Thus, the sciences of life emerge as a propaedeutics for the health sciences. Yet, life is by and large the most complex phenomenon, system, or behavior existent or imaginable. If so, making clear what life is and could be is crucially the concern of the sciences of complexity. Following the argument, the sciences of complexity are the rationale for the sciences of health. Such is indeed the interplay between complexity, life, and health.

This chapter consists of, and crosses, a theoretical perspective, a methodological approach, and a heuristic challenge as follows. It is important to clear up the language of public health, global health and One Health as it has been, and is currently, largely used and implemented. This is an analytical endeavor that comprises a conceptual workout. Nothing goes without saying, and certainly language is not immaculate and obvious. On the contrary, language appears as the ground for ways of living, forms of life, and standards of life together with policies of all kinds that entail programs and actions, ends and means largely set and understood. The first section of this text is devoted to such clarification.

The aim of the first section consists of making clear that there is a grave misunderstanding about health, as it happens. Various arguments and reflections will be brought out.

The second section argues that knowing about health is a consequence of truly knowing about life [2]. Thus, life in general, and the life sciences in particular, are to be reckoned as propaedeutics for health, or the health sciences. In other words, what is really at stake in health is not just well-being, the absence of illness, or the survival of the patient, but his liveliness, his joy-for-living, his capacity for conceiving of incompleteness-as-an-horizon. The trouble, though, is that despite there being more than one hundred definitions of life, none of them really work [3].

The third section is concerned with the complexity of health. Against the standard comprehension, there are not two kinds of health, namely health (= physical health) and mental health, which is normally taken as the two main domains in medicine and the health sciences at large. Health is one and the same, from the outset.

The risk could emerge that such an understanding coincides with One Health. The latter is clearly anthropocentric, as it will be proved. Health cannot be fully grasped aside from the importance of the environment. The crux of the argument in this section is that the environment encompasses not just the ecosystems and the planetary stance, but goes far beyond a mere planetary approach. Thus, the interplay between planetary health and One Health are revealed as highly limited. The great cultures, peoples, and civilizations have had and still do have a strong connection with the cosmos or the universe. Such is the clearest divide between the standard discourses and policies and the real complexification of health, i.e., life.

The fourth section argues that life is adamantly undetermined. This is an invitation to underdetermine nature, the world, the human existence, for example. Certainly, this is a most astonishing invitation. Various arguments will be provided that support the claim. The point is that very just as life entails a mindset of indetermination, so too health requires being undetermined. Whereas within the paradigm of current biomedicine, illness or disease should be determined by any possible means, health and life demand a completely different mindset. Indetermination is the central pivot, so to speak, of any complexity approach and understanding [4]. To say the least, Heisenberg's work stands in the background, shedding very suggestive lights on the whole issue here [5].

The fifth section digs into the previous arguments and leads the entire reflection to a new level. Life cannot by any means be reduced to human experience, and certainly not to the planetary frame, either. The complexity of life consists in the fact that it is definitely not any kind of "stuff". Instead, life should be understood by what it does—it is a process [6]. The living beings do a manifold of processes. A general picture of what living beings do is depicted and explained. The conclusion is surprising and counterintuitive.

Following up the latter argument, the sixth and final section concentrates on what the complexity of being alive means—which cannot be reduced to the human expression of life. Life in general is a most complex weave made up of numerous dynamic threads and crossings, and exchanges. One of the most important contributions of the sciences of complexity consists in bringing out the fact that caring about life entails a twofold perspective, thus: life-as-we-know-it, and life-as-it-could-be--possible [7]. No other scientific, philosophical, or disciplinary take allows for such a comprehension. This section helps make clear what this means.

At the end, some general conclusions are drawn.

2 Distinguishing "Health" from Health

There are currently four main characterizations of a corresponding number of general policies about health. These are public health, global health, planetary health, and One Health. Presumably, they are different in that at each step, successively, the aim consists in being always more encompassing. They are concerned with the health of human collectives, society, people, and cultures, and ultimately mankind as a whole. The basic common minimal denominator for those four forms of caring about health for the public in general, is clinical medicine[2]; in other words, caring for each individual. There is, as it happens, an essential tension between the individual and society or also between each individual and mankind. Such is the current crux of the standard health and life sciences.

The rationale for public health at large is epidemiology. Epidemiology stands indeed as the real and final measure for health/disease in a population; in other words, it is the final ground that allows speaking about epidemics, pandemics, and outbreaks. The recent experience of COVID-19 is illustrative enough not only at the global level but also at each national and continental scale [8]. Epidemiology, so to

[2]The term "clinical medicine" or biomedicine will use to designate the medicine that is conceived from a western perspective. The western civilization has always known about death and suffering and very little about health and life, if at all.

speak, utters the final word about the conditions of health/disease of a population. Of course, epidemiologists have their own battery of tools, rods and concepts that are always more refined thanks to big data.

On the other side, regarding the health/sickness conditions of individuals, clinical analysis and diagnostics speak out the final word, generally speaking. However, the final judgment about the real condition of a patient is provided by the results of pathology, physiological, and biochemical tests. The examinations of cells, tissues, tumors, blood, and organs, and even of the corpse, bring light to the anatomical and chemical signatures of cells. This study of physiopathological state serves as the real and final ground that allows us to determine, without any doubt, the condition of a person, alive or dead.

The two following formulas state the relations:

(i) Epidemiology $\models$ Public Health.
(ii) Physiopathology $\models$ Clinical Medicine.

The logical sign $\models$ signifies here a correspondence that shows ground, reason, or fundament. Thus, formula (i) says that epidemiology serves as the ground for public health. Correspondingly, formula (ii) argues that clinical medicine is ultimately based on a physiopathological analysis or study.

The formulas (i) and (ii) can be integrated thus:

(iii) Epidemiology $\models$ Public Health $\therefore$ Physiopathology $\models$ Clinical Medicine.

The logical sign $\therefore$ allows us to identify here an analogy. It is namely, the analogy between the formula (i) and the formula (ii). The result is as follows: both clinical medicine and public medicine are about disease, not truly about health. In one case, physiopathology serves as rationale, whereas on the other side, it is epidemiology that emerges as ground. The difference pertains to the scale of human experience. Both are fundamental in determining illness or disease.

Important as they are, clinical medicine and public health do not really know about health. They are about diseases. This albeit, is not a minor issue in any sense. Biomedicine in the largest and deepest sense of the world is about sickness and pain—which are to be battled and defeated by any means. (I call *en passant* the attention on the warmonger language used recurrently in medicine and the health sciences).

We cannot and should never turn our backs on suffering and disease. That would be morally, epistemologically, and humanly perverse. Diseases are to be treated and intervened in as many means as possible. After all, what is at stake is human suffering. No practice, theory, or attitude can be sustained in any sense if it does not directly attack and overcome suffering, pain, or disease. It is not sufficient to reduce them; period.

That said, this text contends that we must *also*—and most probably *beforehand* know about health. The hurdle lies in the fact that Western civilization has never directly, i.e., by itself, known about health; only always about fears, death, suffering, pain, sickness. History, anthropology, philosophy and cultural studies can provide enough arguments about why such is indeed the case. For reasons of space, I leave aside a further explanation of the issue. The focus is health, i.e., life.

All current public, national and international, continental and local discourses, actions and policies are truly about disease, in spite of the fact that they speak about health. Society, it appears, has and is currently largely manipulated by the use of "health" when what is really meant are sickness, illness, and disease. There are crucial social, cultural, and civilization dangerous obstacles here.

They speak about "health" by they really mean disease. Moreover, they speak about "health," but they talk about disease.

The analysis of the use of words or the use of language is and has been a most fruitful, critical, and democratic philosophy. The leading thread here will be logic understood in a broad sense. I shall come back to this observation.

The main argument of this chapter affirms that in order to (truly) know about health, one must also know about life. In other words, the utterance of health must resonate as life, liveliness, and the like. Any action, speech, discourse, or policy, for instance, about health which does not openly and directly entail life is plainly a contradiction; a strategy, if you wish, which is the same. Talking, as it is the standard discourse "out there", about well-being, or the absence of disease, or the importance of primary attention in health, for instance, clearly obliterate life at large. As it will be argued below, life is not just a concern for and about human beings. The concern about life largely surpasses the human expression of life, and definitely any planetary concern.

Knowing about health encompasses a sense of inner satisfaction with existence, a sound balance of and with the environment in the largest sense of the word, which includes the social and human environment, a sensation of joy, tranquility, and peace that cannot be manipulated in any jargon possible. An authentic joy of living can overcome any fear, no matter what. Classically said, i.e., more standardized, it is all about the lack of stress—particularly chronic stress, namely knowing how to live well (*suma qamaña* or *sumak kawsay*, for the Andean cultures, for instance) and certainly a healthy or sound or livable lifestyle.

More exactly, medicine in the Western world is and has always been reactive. Its core is about curing, much more than healing—distinction that makes nervous some orthodox people who work with the clinical model. Nonetheless, medicine in the largest sense of the word, which includes the entire set of the health sciences, has given to mankind one of the best imaginable gifts that any human being can receive, namely a larger or deeper life, hope, and life expectancy. The relations between them are a highly complex matter that cannot be superseded just in terms of the distinction between subjective and objective stances.

It would be rhetorically demanding that instances such as the WHO, its corresponding continental chapters, such as the African Health Organization or the Pan American Health Organization, for instance, or any of the other members of the quadripartite—WHOA, FAO, UNEP, reckon that their whole endeavor is about disease. Ultimately, the concern is just about the global burden of disease—or just the burden of disease at a more local scale. Disease, and not properly health. There is, as it happens, a gap between decision-makers at large and the scientific community, as well as the basis of society.

The moral and epistemological demand that immediately arises here consists in tracing a clear-cut distinction between disease and health. We all should know about health, not just using a word to mean something else. To know about health requires knowing about life.

Knowing about life opens up the doors wide open to bringing into the daily light on the table, a most sensitive and complex issue, life. Complexity science has made a sensitive call, namely, knowing about life entails a twofold perspective, thus: life as we know it, very much as life-as-we-it-could-be possible [7]. No other science, discipline, or approach has such a distinctive trait.

Getting cured—or healed is definitely not a one-way action or process. Epistemologically, that implies the distinction between subject and object. And humanly and socially, that entails the affirmation of a certain power and an asymmetry of actions. There is a large literature about these aspects that includes the perils of the medicalization of society, the use of biopolitics, and the entire panoptic of powers and institutions.

Against that, the truth is that no one is truly cured if he/she does not become a curer/healer. This is what medical anthropology teaches us, among diverse other studies, approaches, and disciplines. Getting cured and/or healed is a two-way process that sensibly affects both sides. The standard discourse about One Health—with capital letters, *en passant*, global health, planetary health, and public health do not know anything about such a two-way action and process.

More exactly, getting cured entails an entire web of relations in which each self is a sensitive node that helps trigger curation and healing for the others. In other words, whereas there are some diseases that are particularly individual, health comprises a large and indeterminate weave of direct and indirect connections. Caring for one's own health is one and the same thing as caring about others' health, and life.

3 One Basic Proviso: Knowing About Life

In order to know about health, one must know firstly and continuously about life. One serious obstacle emerges immediately, namely, there are more than one hundred definitions of health, and none is valid—or (definitely right; only, in the best of cases, partially correct). This means we simply do not know what life is, what living beings are, and do. After all, life as a research program is very recent [9].

Plainly said, we do not know really what life is, as yet.

The standard understanding and explanation of life assesses that life arose in a space that made it possible. The best known of such spaces is the Earth. More exactly, the origins of life are one and the same thing as the origin of the space in which life emerges. Such space is rightly not the (planet) Earth but the biosphere, a cross-disciplinary term originally coined by E. Suess by known thanks to V. Vernadsky [10]—a living entity. In other words, the classical time-line that puts physics at the origin, then follows inorganic chemistry, then organic chemistry, after that biology, and finally culture is wrong, to say the least. The endeavor to understand life implies a total redefinition of the story of science and the relations among sciences and disciplines. Here, I do not enter into this question. I restrict here the interest to life and health.

It is almost impossible to turn one's head around and *not* find life. The most basic assumption to soundly enter into the realm of understanding and explaining what the living beings are and do is by acknowledging that life is not any "stuff" of any sort. More explicitly, life does not reduce to a singular "stuff"—in our case, carbon [11, 12]. It is already well known that there is no need whatsoever for the DNA to turn to the right; it could very well turn to the left; for instance.

Life is a physical phenomenon; however, it cannot be reduced to physics. According to Schrödinger, living beings deny physics; negentropy is the term we coined, with which, furthermore, he was not happy, after all [9]. Life entails a physics of immateriality [13]. Living beings can be characterized not ontologically, i.e., by something they are, but by what they do. There is a vast array of things living beings do that make them possible: they metabolize, they process information (non-algorithmically!), they create continuously brand-new messages, codes, signs, patterns, symbols, and signals, they evolve unceasingly, they never stop learning for stop learning entails ultimately death, they coevolve with their environment, for instance.

More fundamentally, in nature they never behave algorithmically. Life in general, from enzymes to proteins, from the cell to the tissues and organs, from each individual organism to a given ecological niche, for example—nothing, behaves algorithmically, i.e., a behavior reduced to laws, norms, commandments, and the like. Instead, there is a highly complex weave made up of creation and novelty. Such a weave is to be read and interpreted in the long run.

Largely speaking, the living beings do not live algorithmically, either. In the case of human beings, though, behaviors are highly algorithmic due to the weight of culture, taken in the largest sense of the word, which includes religion, education, politics, economy, and the legal system, mainly.

Surprisingly, there are bnot, first, conditions (for) and then life that exists, afterwards. On the contrary, living beings both create the conditions for their emergence and their sustainability. In complexity theory, this is known with two expressions, thus: autopoiesis and self-organization. Classically said that life is *causa sui*. In other words, there is not a cause, external thereafter, that originates life. Life creates itself. More radically, there is not a space, say a planet, where life appears. Life emerges in a system that behaves like a living system. In the case of our biosphere, she has a physiology [14], metabolizes, exhibits all properties of far-from-equilibrium systems, which means that she is a dissipative structure, and the like [15, 16]. Gaia is one of the names for our living Earth. Anthropology teaches that all cultures and civilizations have their own name for her. Meaningfully, in all languages, nature is female.

The story of the study and understanding of life in general is very recent. As a research problem, not without several backgrounds, it originated in 1944 thanks to

Schrödinger's book *What Is Life?* [9]. Surprisingly, it was not a philosopher, a theologian or a biologist who discovered life as a scientific research problem. It was a physicist working in quantum physics. Life is a counterintuitive phenomenon; more exactly, it is not a classical phenomenon, but a limit case of the quantum world. The living beings dig their roots in the quantum realm [17]. More broadly said, the classical world is a limit case of the quantum world.

That means that life is and has been grasped as a classical phenomenon, but it truly is quantum. To date, numerous quantum effects have been studied and observed at various scales in the web of life, even at normal environment temperatures, in the seas as well as on earth. Recurrently, the relationship between health and disease has also been explained in classical terms. It appears, therefore, that we do not truly know about health, but about disease, either.

Illness or sickness is an alarm; sometimes, a most serious and important alarm. According to Canguilhem, sometimes we get sick in order not to die [18–20]. The normal (= health, vitality) does not reside within the living being, but it passes through it. Life is literally a resonance box, if allowed. In other words, any disease is a sudden or subtle call that *means* something. Usually, it means that something is going wrong or has been going wrong. That something is basically the way existence has been lived so far, or also the relations with others and the environment. More exactly, a disease is an alarm that things must change. The trouble, though, is that such an alarm sometimes arrives too late, because the mind has not been able to pay attention to previous alarms. Cultures largely distract the mind with unnecessary or banal things—unnecessary or banal from the standpoint of biology in the deepest sense of the word.

The structure, logic, and forms of diseases are well-known. Such is the claim of biomedical and clinical medicine hand in hand with the pharmaceutical companies. There are chronic, acute, complex, rare, orphan, infectious, hereditary, congenital, acquired, and several other diseases. The map, the diagnostics, and the structures are, it seems, all too well known.

However, the understanding of what diseases are and *mean* remains obscure for a mindset that is typically classical. The question, as it clearly appears, does not just consist of objects, subjects, phenomena, dynamics, problems, or solutions, but also about their *meaning*. In the case of life and health in general, it makes absolutely no sense to deal with things apart from their meanings. As a matter of fact, in historical terms, such a distinction and opposition are very recent. It appears indeed with the distinction and sometimes the opposition between ideas and values, or facts and meanings, or also, facts and values—which emerges firstly sometime around the end of the nineteenth century and the beginnings of the twentieth century.

In other words, classically said, it is time we overcame the distinction and even the separation between facts and values.

Plants, I would like to suggest, offer a most suggestive view of the relations about life and health.

Plants are, comparatively with animals and humans, slow; very slow. They do move; however, they move too slowly to evade or escape from problems. Plants are sessile. When facing troubles, say heavy rains, earthquakes, or drought, plants must face the problems from within, so to speak. Typically, the attitude of animals and humans vis-à-vis problems is always the same: escape, running away. Human beings have a variety of escaping, such as running away, rationalizing, sublimation, negation, and many others.

Since plants cannot evade the problems, they have learned to modify their metabolism. More exactly, plants solve problems by slowing down their metabolisms [21]. Dormancy is the best response plants develop for solving problems. In other words, plants decrease their metabolic activity and recede to their core and roots, which are the real and perhaps most fundamental structures or anatomies. Dormancy can take years, decades and even centuries, according to the circumstances.[3]

A most valid and legitimate analogy emerges, hence after. No one and nothing—plant or animal, truly gets cured if he or she does not (learn to) modify his own metabolism. Straightforwardly said, curing and healing entail radically modifying the ways which living beings have been living—in the largest sense of the word; i.e., how they have been eating, living, loving, sensing, thrilling, and relating to themselves, to others, and the environment.

Anthropology sheds very suggestive light on the issue. Ancient cultures and peoples teach that no one is really cured if he or she does not also help cure others. Thus, curing or healing is not a passive or submissive attitude—which can easily be inferred from conventional medicine, i.e., clinical medicine—where the medicine doctor knows and the patient provides only his own body and, sometimes, his mind. Curing and healing are all about transforming oneself and helping others to cure and heal. Health is relational hence complex.

As it can be easily seen, the weave of life allows for learning from other dimensions, contexts, and forms of life, not just from the very human or anthropological perspective. Caring about health is thus the same thing as knowing about the weave and complexity of life in general.

En passant, it could be useful to remember that plants' anatomy or architecture is modular, that they do not have eyes, but see, they do not have brains, but think, they do not have a stomach, but eat and digest. A number of other examples could be easily provided. Furthermore, plants make up about 80% of the biomass of the earth—up to 97%.

Without any doubt, plants do solve problems and are, by and large, much better problem solvers than animals and humans. If one of the main characteristics that define intelligence is the capacity to solve problems, plants are far more intelligent than animals and humans combined. Botany was always a minor science within the landscape of sciences and disciplines. It was relevant only when botany was applied, referred to, or applied to human beings. Such is grossly said the entire history of the Nobel Prizes in Medicine and Physiology. However, botany has been radically transformed thanks to research pioneered by F. Baluska and his teams. As a result, botany exists currently as the neurophysiology or also neurobiology—of plants [22].

[3]Presumably, tardigrades are among the extremophiles some of the best organisms more capable of dormancy in extreme conditions.

Now, it has become clear that plants are highly complex living beings in that there is no clear-cut frontier among plants, fungi, and bacteria, for example. Instead, there is a wonderful interactive network among plants, viruses, fungi, and bacteria [23]. Symbiosis literally roots in the deepest dynamics of life. If so, the analytical mindset inherited from Western tradition must be radically changed, particularly when dealing with issues of health and life. A much re-intertwined, large-scope and transversal view is to be developed—whence we all must learn to know and view life. The trouble though is that rightly taken life is not a system of phenomena that rests on natural perception and the weight of the senses. Meaningfully, life is a counterintuitive phenomenon—that cannot be reduced to the classical world or stances.

4 The Complexity of Health

Whether confusing health with disease, or else intending to really talk about health somehow, the truth is that health has always been considered just as a human concern. After all, Western civilization has largely been anthropocentric, anthropomorphic, anthropological. The human being is the apex of evolution.

More recently, regarding global health, the planetary health and One Health—surprisingly with capital letters, the inclusion of animals, waters, and plants is a sort of circle whose center or radius is always the human being, whether individually or as society. The transposition of the issue into global or planetary, for instance, is just the overlapping of the human scale to the planet; nothing more. The prevailing discourses and practices about health are and remain largely and plainly anthropocentric and anthropomorphic. The truth is that such policies and discourses do not truly care about the weave of life, but only about human beings—their well-being, benefits, and survival.

Knowing about life is much more and indeed very different to knowing just about mankind. Life does not know about centers or hierarchies—in spite of some biologists' interpretations. An eco-centered or also bio-centered view of the world is an explanation of a weave without a central thread, form or expression—and certainly not a priori. Nature, the world, or life is a complex set of sets, interdependencies, co-adaptations, interrelations, intertwining and entanglement where there is literally no center and no radius, in any sense. In other words, it is a highly evolving and unceasingly adaptive process in continuous achievement with only local optimality. Darwin coined a lucky expression, namely an adaptive rugged landscape [24], a concept that has been adopted and developed by complexity theory theorists and researchers.

At the human scale, it is essential not to distinguish, and definitely not to oppose or hierarchizing between health, i.e., physical health and mental health. Such a distinction and sometimes even opposition is completely erroneous and ultimately dangerous vis-à-vis the life care. It does not truly benefit health or life, for, again, it is a parlor for talking about illness or disease. Human beings cannot be fragmented in any sense, not even epistemologically. Epigenetics has come to shed valuable light on the health sciences in general, on clinical medicine, psychology, and psychiatry in particular, by explicitly assessing that they are not two different dimensions, nature and culture, but they are one and the same thing. I leave aside here the mechanics set out that make such a process possible, namely phosphorylation, acetylation, and methylation at the chromatin and histones in the cells.

Fantastically, the organism as such does not exist. It is an abstraction. Rather, the human body is an ecosystem, an idea that can be easily grasped thanks to systems biology, network biology, the Global Bacteriome Project, as well as the Global Virome Project, e.g.—not the mention the theory of endosymbiosis, and the importance of the microbiome [25].

Moreover, the human body is the interface between a highly complex internal ecosystem and a wide-open and indeterminate external ecosystem. The most basic way to refer to each ecosystem is exteroception and interoception, being the latter complementary with proprioception. The dynamic balance between homeostasis and homeorrhesis can safely depict the idea. The organism is the outcome of the tensons and relations between homeorhesis and homeostasis [26]. In that interplay, the microbiome plays a most crucial role.

It is necessary to recall that the microbiome changes every 24 h, in accordance with lifestyles, food, relations, feelings, and emotions, co-existing with animals and pets, most notably. Rightly understood, the ancient Greek idea of an individual has become a mere empty word valid at most in the classical social and human sciences. The individual is in reality the outcome or the interface between complex internal and external networks, processes, intertwining, fields, and entanglements. One more abstraction, to say the least. In the health and life sciences, the organism is the translation of the philosophical idea of the individual.

Being as it may be, health does not concern merely human experience, but also the health of the environment largely taken, which includes, among others, air and waters, plants and animals, fungi and earth. Such, nonetheless, is by no means just a planetary concern. Gaia or the biosphere is a living organism in an immediate ecosystem, the solar system, which is an ecosystem that exists within another one, namely the Milky Way—all, at fantastically rapid and unrepeatable velocities. The biosphere moves at about 107.000 km/h around the sun (or about 30 km/sec), the solar system rotates around the Milky Way at an average speed of 230,000 km/sec, and the Milky Way moves at an average speed of 2.1 million km/h around the local cluster. The importance of the dynamics of Gaia does not depend solely on the internal processes and cycles. Subtle, cosmological influences must also be taken into account.

Indeed, the standard understanding of health in the Western world was immediate and direct. Vast, large relations, fields, and entanglements are to be considered, too.

The spectrum of the environment could be easily enlarged and enriched. The basic idea is the acknowledgement that the idea of the environment as it was originally set at the end of the nineteenth century is basically inaccurate because of limited. The entire issue is definitely not just a planetary concern. Undoubtedly, life and health entail much more complex weaves than previously thought. Western civilization, at the end of its days, reached maximum a planetary worldview. It would always be refreshing remembering that all great cultures, peoples, and civilizations had furthermore a connection with the universe. If so, the concept of environment should be enriched and enlarged till the universe—as we know, as it is and would be. After all, the concept of the environment is essentially open and indeterminate.

As a consequence, health does not only correspond to lifestyles in general, but also to the interdependencies of each singular existence with the vast array of living phenomena and their surroundings. The complexity of health corresponds with large phase spaces—i.e., spaces of possibilities that comprise fields, interplays, intertwining, entanglement of layers, contexts, sets, and networks. Without any kind of dualism, whereas disease or being sick is obvious or evident, being healthy entails a kind of subtlety, namely, health can only be grasped from within. Such an attitude entails that you care about the health of others because you have known the various alarms sent by the body and mind and can rightly read and interpret those signs from *within*. An externalist approach to health or disease does a very little favor to others. Information and professionalism, as they are often stated, are important and yet very limited. Besides and most probably the foremost significant attitude comprises compassion, empathy, feelings, and sensitivity. The trouble though is that these are usually left aside in the name of objectivity. Life cannot be fully grasped in an objectivistic manner. The arts and aesthetics, notably, can shed important light on the complexity of the attitude toward health and life in general.

5 From Health to Life

Health is most probably the most important experience of life, i.e., being alive. Truly knowing about health is crucial to affirm and make life possible. It is not battling a disease that is at stake; it is also not even the well-being of a person, animal, or plant, for instance. It is the sense of vitality, the very joy of living, the striving for dreaming, longing, wanting, desiring, sewing and building horizons, relations, actions, possibilities, what is really at stake.

Curing and healing, important as they are, are just a condition for relating with life, i.e., with oneself, the others, and the natural world in the amplest sense of the word. It is really myopic to care for human beings' well-being as a target, leaving nature in the backstage, on a lower level, or as taken for granted. More radically, there are not two things: human beings and nature. They are one and the same process, one and the same reality. Nature does not know of hierarchies or centralities.

It should always be highlighted: human beings belong to nature, they are not in any sense above it. Humans are just one expression of the manifold forms of life. It is only in and vis-à-vis nature that they can be rightly understood and their life fully achieved.

An analogy could be convenient at this level. In the American legal system, a person can be judged and probably sentenced ultimately as guilty or non-guilty, being the latter quite different from being innocent—most notably vis-à-vis the presumption of innocence. In the same tenure, a person can be simply cured without truly awakening in him/her a real joy or satisfaction with life. This is what occurs in most clinical cases, basically due to the fragmentation of and within sciences and biomedicine.

The analytical tradition is, after all, a great burden for understanding health and making life possible. Thinking about life and health requires a capacity for synthesis. To be sure, imagination is one of such forms of thinking—and living in and as synthesis.

Inversely, one can be sick and yet very much alive. Therefore, being healthy entails having, dreaming about, sowing horizons and possibilities—having still things to do, things to know, places to go to, for instance. Liveliness is the core of being healthy, hence an act of disobedience [27], of non-submission when viewed from a standard or standardized form of life. In physical terms, such a disobedience is coined as negentropy to mean that living beings exist by negating physics—physics in the classical sense of the term, i.e., classical mechanics, at large. When overlapped to the social and human sciences, negentropy acquires magnificent scopes and horizons.

Anthropology and history show that in other peoples, cultures and civilizations, no one can be truly cured or healed: (a) if he/she does not radically change the way he/she was living until they got sick; (b) if in turn, he/she does not actively make that others to get cured or healed of their own illnesses. *Voilà* a most striking discovery vis-à-vis the clinical medicine, its practices, and institutionality. In other words, getting cured or healed is much more than an individual entity—it is a relation, an essentially open relation.

In contrast, all institutions are closed or self-referential. The range of institutionalism and neo-institutionalism studies is meaningful enough.

Being healed or cured is a matter of committing with oneself and the others, of changing and helping change—the forms, styles, and standards of life. (Between brackets, anthropology and history have traditionally been politically incorrect sciences or disciplines.) In other words, getting cured or healed is a real metamorphosis in that it comprises the unity of mind and body, of the own organism and the environment, both natural and cultural. It comprises a structural modification of things as they have been till now.

Let us make clear what is already implicit here. Knowing of and making health possible entails a change of the world—as it has been, as it currently goes.

As it is clearly seen, this entails a process of lucidity and radicality. Certainly, most diseases are not serious and do not necessarily lead to the dead end of death. As mentioned, each singular illness or sickness is an alarm, and it should be taken as such. Following up on the metaphor, there are, as it happens, levels or layers of alarm. A low level does not necessarily entail or lead to a final alarm.

Nobody really gets cured or is healed if he/she does not understand nature, the place, the signs and symptoms of the sickness. Rightly reading and interpreting them is crucial and yet very difficult. It has to do with a much deeper dimension than the mere symptomatology or signs of a disease—namely, the semiotics of the disease, in the sense of conventional Western medicine. Sickness talks about sensations, feelings, stories, metabolizations, homeostasis, and relations, past and present—all of which are not necessarily direct or immediate.

This calls for a technical aspect, as follows.

Traditional and conventional thinking has focused on direct inferences, that is, inferences of the kind: A B. Anything else is just a variant of the direct or immediate inference; for example, whether A entails necessarily or hypothetically B, or also, if B follows A contingently or apodictically, for instance.

However, complexity theory in general and non-classical logics in particular teaches that direct inferences are trivial. Instead, there are also indirect inferences, inferences by analogy, by contingency, and uncertain inferences, for instance [28]. These are sorts of inferences that are never evident, to say the least, in any possible sense, tacitly or potentially, for instance.

The human body speaks at least three main languages. One is pleasure, another is pain, and the third one is most probably the most significant; it is the language of silence. Interoceptive perception as well as exteroceptive perception, manifestly illuminate the first two. Nonetheless, the most important and subtle of all three languages the body speaks is silence, in that it is normally not heard or listened to in everyday life. Certainly not in a noisy world as it currently happens.

The trouble begins when silence is superseded by pain or the feeling of uncomforting of some kind. Normally, people do not pay attention to the subtle language of the organism—whether in the physical or the mental or in the interplay between both dimensions. Rather, sometimes, when they pay attention to the mind or the body, it may be already too late. Culture overvalues and overstimulates the significance of pleasure in any sense, which tends to overshadow silence, the most beautiful and complex of all languages.

The banality of a culture of easy and immediate, engineered pleasures severely impedes the authentic language of the mind and body—of the spirit.

In order to make health possible, good science and technology, high-quality research and information, even fine arts and philosophy are necessary. However, they are insufficient. To live and have a healthy life, one also, and most probably mainly, needs wisdom. The problem lies in that wisdom cannot be taught. There are no courses, seminars, classes, or conferences on wisdom. Nonetheless, wisdom can be learned.

Wisdom appears thus as *conditio* sine qua non for living, i.e., living-well and having and caring for good health. This is, it is my contention, the real complexity of life and health.

A brief sketch of the history of medicine shows how doctors can be useful here. Indeed, in the beginning—Th. Mann used to say, “in the night of times” [29], a doctor was a shaman. He or she knew about herbs, plants, animals, the cycles of the moon, the tides of the waters, the human heart, the secrets of loneliness, the importance of music, and the speech of the stones, for instance. A shaman was and is still capable of listening to silence and interpreting it adequately. This was, roughly speaking, during the Paleolithic. In many places around the world, such is still the case.

Perhaps it could be useful to remember that human existence has taken place in about 97% of time in the Paleolithic and only about 3% from the Neolithic until now [30]. Significantly, the anatomy and the physiology of human beings were shaped by evolution for the conditions of the Paleolithic, not for the current conditions.

Later on, in ancient Greece and Rome—that is, at the dawn of Western civilization, the doctor was also a philosopher. This can be easily seen in Hippocrates' and Galen's writings and teachings [31, 32]. In contrast, for the best standards in biomedicine, a medical doctor should be a specialist and hopefully have sub-specializations and sub-sub-especializations.

Without any prevention, a sharp contrasting picture appears to a sound understanding. Currently, doctors have at their best wonderful research, strong and large databases, special studies, and information. In many cases, many of them may be even polymaths, if you wish, very educated people, indeed.

Yet, wisdom seems to be hidden—lacking.

Such is the complexity of the relationship between health and life. A spontaneous invitation to wisdom would be more than desirable. After all, it is not just the human form of life that is important, but the entire weave of life, in its vast array of processes, relations, fields, and interactions.

The rationale of wisdom does not consist in preventing, but in understanding. Yet, no one truly understands with his or head. Understanding is a matter of the heart. Many times, understanding is already a way of being healed or cured.

6 Life Largely Surpasses the Human Experience

Oddly enough, human beings are not the apex of evolution. They are just one more node in a highly complex and still not fully known network. We live—life exists and exists in and as a living and creative universe [33, 34]. Ecology has sufficiently made it clear that in nature, there are no key species. In the best cases, there are umbrella species. Neither are human beings the culmination and last word of evolution, nor are they the basic layer, from any standpoint.

There have been five major mass extinctions. We are currently witnessing the sixth extinction due to anthropogenic reasons. Surprisingly, after each mass extinction, life has emerged more diversified, robust, and resilient than before. In evolutionary terms, human beings are still infants—a most recent experiment of evolution. It might be useful to remember that Saurians dominated the earth for around 250 million years, until the catastrophe was produced by the meteorite that fell in Yucatan. Cephalopods, on the other hand, dominated the seas for over 500 million years. The species of hominids barely have some 400,000 years—less than the minimum time scale that geology uses for its measuring—1 million. Literally, human beings are far from being a geological stance or force or period. (Talking about the Anthropocene, catchy as it might appear, is bad science.)

We are just scratching the early stage of a time that is beginning to think and care about health, i.e., life—far more meaningfully than the standard jargon about public health, global health, planetary health, and One Health, as already mentioned. There are reasons for optimism when looking sensibly around [27, 35, 36].

To be sure, human health and life are absolutely untenable without, above, or aside from the essentially open and indeterminate weave of the living beings both as-we-know-them as well as they could-be-possible. More exactly, life and health are directly proportional to the relations and interactions with the environment—nature.

The environment, however, comprises both a natural and a cultural dimension. Hence, health depends also on hereditary traits, just as epigenetics has made it clear. Till 2021, it was known that the intergenerational information covered up to eight generations [37–39].

Everyone's life does not entirely depend on him/herself. Complexity theory can be partially said to be about that pitch of flavor that is inescapable and irreducible in any sense, namely, randomness. I do not intend to affirm that the world, life, or everyone's existence is random or contingent. Rather, there is, if allowed, a pitch of condiment called randomness that cannot be discounted. Whereas normal science—in the Kuhnian sense of the word—does know about randomness but wants to harness or master it by any means, complexity theory argues that we must learn to live with (a pitch of) uncertainty [40, 41].

The inheritance of genes does not depend on anyone, not explicitly or voluntarily, at least. Neither does the inheritance of experiences via methylation, for instance. Nonetheless, it is also true that there is not any kind of determinism in any sense. Increasingly complex systems are non-deterministic [42, 43]. Living beings control a few things, say their mate, their progeny, relatively, but the most important condition for their lives cannot be completely controlled, namely, the environment. Vis-à-vis the internal environment, human beings for example, have barely any control over their microbiome.

At the human scale, paradoxically as it may appear, human beings do not properly have free will [44, 45], although, as it will be shown below, they must be capable of being free, moreover, liberated from social forces and contrivances.

Rightly seen, there is not a clear-cut frontier or barrier among the various levels, forms, expressions of life; technically said, among the different domains of life. The theory of symbiogenesis and the recognition of the holobiontic character of living beings help understand the fuzziness or many-valuedness nature of life. Everything is interdependent although in degrees and modes that vary according to the niche, biome, and ecosystem.

It is indeed empty to say that everything depends on anything else, or also that everything is connected to everything else. Holism is not exactly a good science. If such was the case, then nothing would be truly relevant. Instead, there are more and less degrees of connectedness, more and less degrees of relations. Both graph theory and the science of complex networks illustrate this sufficiently [46, 47]. Knowing, to say the least, about small-world theory, random networks and free-scale networks permit understanding that some things are more connected than others. More rigorously, complex networks exhibit power law distributions, which is something that holism and systems science totally ignore.

The theory of evolution is a historical science. Astonishingly, all theories that seek to explain the origins of life are experimental—in vivo, in vitro, *in info*, most notably, according to researchers, and research centers and institutes. The core of the issue lies in the fact that evolution is chaotic, i.e., an evolving system that never repeats the same trajectory [48, 49].

From Western medicine, being sick is a state. Indeed, it does not define life or being alive even though it may happen in a variety of modes: acute, chronic, complex, orphan, and the like. It is, I would like to argue, being healthy, what defines striving, dreaming, longing for something or someone, so to speak. To be clear, health is a process [6]. Health means, entails, a process that can ultimately be grasped as a sense for living, a joy for life, a feeling of having achieved goals and targets, if one wishes. More exactly, it is in so far as health is a process, not a state, that there is perfect bridge with wisdom. After all, wisdom is much more than an acquisition or an asset, it is a process of having encountered the right way and keeping it.[4]

Against all odds, it is not the goal which is really relevant, but the process of searching and attaining it—the path.

Indeed, being healthy is not just a sense of well-being, as it is currently explained, but a sense of integration with the entire weave of life. It is exactly in this sense that enters and anchors life as-it-could-be-possible. On the other side, anthropocentrism characterized Western civilization up until now. However, nothing allows assessing that it is sound and desirable. Quite on the contrary, it was and still is that anthropocentrism which regards nature as resource and, by extension, other human beings as resources too, i.e., human resource which is sick—and sickens. Institutional economists even talk about relational capital, or human capital and the like (*horribile dicta*).

Health comprises a connection of life in general in all forms and expressions. Some of the translations for such attitude are: compassion, *Einfühlung*, putting-oneself in other's shoes, and several others. Much more than a concept, health is also and mainly an experience.

7 The Complexity of Being Alive

Life is not easy, certainly, but it would be pretentious and vain, claiming also that it is a ballast. The geography of existence can adequately be seen as a rugged adaptive landscape. Valleys and hills, abysses and high mountains, coasts and streambeds, among other characterize in general any general view of a landscape, not to mention

[4] A sense of way here recalls in the horizon some coincidence with the Tao, in the Chinese tradition. Cf. [50]. Some sort of resonance can be heard also in regard to Heidegger's philosophy [51, 52].

clouds and rains, sunny days and calm nights, storms and stillness, for instance. It does go without saying, indeed.

There is not one clue for life to be persistent. Its best capacity—definitely not skill, is learning [53]. The better and the quick living beings learn the more chances they have to adapt. Living beings must learn—at any cost! This means, against the anthropological take on education, that learning is not precisely a matter of models, programs, philosophies or policies. Many times, learning is a question of rightly reading the environment and interpreting what happens—and will or may happen. Anticipation and modelling are clues of biological intelligence.

Learning is not necessarily rational or reflective. The living body does learn, too.

Learning can be said to be a condition for being healthy. If so, knowledge, information and wisdom are far determinants for liveliness. Knowledge, however, is not exactly a rational or intellectual achievement. Cognition is far more a complex and encompassing process than mere knowledge. Cognition can be said one face of the token, whose complementary side is wisdom.

We need wisdom to live. Yet, crucially, no one and nothing is truly wise when they turn the back to nature. Only *in the midst of* nature and facing and living *along with* nature in the largest sense of the word can wisdom be achieved. As already said, nature comprises society, the world, the biosphere and the cosmic background—but also each single leaf, every single bird or cow, the passing by of a river, the stillness of a lake, the varying game of the cloud forms, for instance.

Nonetheless, for each single person, the most immediate expression of nature is his or her own body—provided, of course, that there is not a separation or a distinction between mind and body. Nature speaks to each one throughout his/her own body. In other terms, nature speaks to everyone prima facie through the body, i.e., the living ecosystem [54, 55].

One important hurdle for living a good life consists in social pressures. These are authentic physical forces—such as gravity, resistance, nuclear force, contact or tension forces, electromagnetism or spring force, for instance. The mass society with its means, social apparatuses, institutions, and social media constitute real physical forces each individual as well as society as a whole are normally subject to. It is normally extremely difficult for each single individual to overcome the social forces and pressures and be liberated from them. The thermodynamic cost is very high even though it has never been explicitly measured. The issue has not even been explicitly considered by scientists or researchers [56, 57].

The liberation from social forces—being customs, culture and history some of them, too, has been indirectly understood as revolutions, such as spiritual, religious, political or economic revolutions. Here I want to argue that health consists in the capacity of liberating oneself from those social contrivances—when needed.

Indeed, this can be illustrated by the Lyon Declaration on mental health [58]. Summarily, the mental health can be characterized by the capacity to saying: no!—no to injustices, atavisms, powers and forces of any kind. Being healthy, it appears, is one and the same thing as a process of liberation, emancipation or illumination—three different ways to point out to one and the same direction.

Inversely, those who are unable to liberate themselves and help others to be liberated can safely be said to be sick; sometimes seriously sick. Liberation simply consists in developing and keeping the capacity to say: no!—when necessary. A series of civil action emerge immediately, namely disobedience, in submission, disrespect, for instance—all of which are non-violent action.

Let's make it explicit: it is not easy to be healthy—whereas falling sick does not require any effort. Falling sick is most of time something that just happens. People do not know it, but they very often get sick out of impotence, due to limitations, because of stress and despair, just because they cannot cope with a given circumstance. Literally, the body somatizes a given circumstance, happening or process. One of the three languages—indeed the most common in the mass society utters, yields or screams. In contrast, in normal conditions, the body does not have to scream or yield.

Somatization incarnates the complexity of living. It is a name and a sign for the complex intertwining between the mind and the body, the internal ecosystem and the external one, between oneself and the others, and so forth. It is a sign or an effect. Somatization is the effect of affections of which consciousness is not always present or aware of. Clinical medicine, important as it is, is just a science of effects even though it speaks about causes. At the end of day, biomedicine doctors, in so far as practitioners, are envoys and spokesmen of a model based on external interventions, mainly pharmacological, which end up favoring the pharmaceutical industry, period.

Thinking and knowing about the complexity of health and life means reaching a complex weave of, many times, indirect, hidden or subtle causes. Many times, too, evident and direct causes can be identified. When such is the case, many times it may be already too late for getting cure or being healed.

Mind and body are just two names for one highly complex experience which is living. Let us say *en passant* that the Cartesian division between *res cogitans* and *res extensa* is a most serious mistake [59, 60] with serious and undesirable consequences. The whole history of science up until now is the follow-up of the Cartesian error. Since Descartes until now science has assumed uncritically and has systematically repeated what in another context C. P. Snow called "the two cultures." Crudely said, it is the distinction between, on the one side, biotic processes, and on the other hand, abiotic systems and phenomena.

Knowing about life and health is the safest key, I argue, to definitely overcome such division, opposition or hierarchy. *Ditto*: reality is not what it seems—nothing goes without saying.

A variety of forms have been uncovered or re-framed that shed lights on that; some examples are the *ikigai*, *shinrin-joku*, *ubuntu*, *suma qamaña* and *sumak kawsay*, *hygge*, *lagom*, *utz k'aslemal*, among others. Significantly, the background of such concepts, experiences and relations roots deep in history, anthropology, religion and spirituality, ethnic practices and wisdom—all of which are peripheral knowledge. A minimal common denominator is the importance of nature in the largest sense of the word and experience, the importance of spirituality, the non-division between the self and the others or the body and mind.

Indeed, nature is much more than a forest, a sea, or a landscape, for instance. It is rather the experience that we all are integrated, including rivers, mountains, plants and animals. Nature is not just a *thing*, but a *feeling*, an *experience*.

Other worlds are possible, other forms of living are possible far beyond the western standards and reinforcing mechanisms. There are peoples, cultures and societies that knew why, and how, to say no! to atavisms of all kinds coming from the western world as it arises from the above writ.

Being alive does not go without saying, in any sense. It demands a thermodynamic cost—some work—for all sentient beings. The most basic token is learning, as already mentioned. Yet, the most valuable coin, so to speak, is being healthy. The quality, extend, and depth of health corresponds exactly to the horizons, possibilities and richness of life. Being healthy and caring for health is, I argue, the real cost for being alive.

All sentient beings care about health, even though most do not have the concept. In fact, most living beings do not need such a concept. Experience is enough. Negatively, being healthy consists in avoiding or reducing as much as possible pain and suffering of all sorts. Positively stated, health consists in the silence of the body, and in an accountable number of capabilities, among which the most basic ones are caring for others—family members and in general all sentient beings, playing, enjoying and rejoicing with little, tiny things. The phenomenology about this is truly ample; it is caring about the environment as of oneself, and acknowledging the importance of elders, contemporary and the younger ones alike, without preferences or hierarchies.

The entire issue is much less complicated as it appears. After all, living is nothing else as rejoicing the present, period. Life happens in the present—although, as mentioned, all living beings have a clear sense of modeling and anticipation.

Being healthy is thus one and the same thing as living lucidly the present as it flows. Lucidity, though, does not entail any reflective or conscious experience in the intellectual sense of the word. Lucidity refers here to the capacity of reading the environment and interpreting it—without any a priori fear, anxiety or uncertainty. Unlike the mass society (Canetti), or of the one-dimensional man (Marcuse), or the society of spectacle (Debord), or the liquid modernity (Bauman), among many other diagnostics and pictures, nature knows much better than the human western society—about living without fears and authentically.

8 Conclusions

A theory of health must be possible, which we did not have until now. The rotatory axes so to speak of such a theory, it is claimed here are complexity theory, life and health—a threefold way for referring to one and the same thing.

Surprisingly, a theory of health is not so much an intellectual building as a living experience that can albeit be shared with others in a manifold way.

Whereas biomedicine uses algorithms for diseases—which are the battery of protocols, measurements, various kinds of committees among which one is about ethics, and the like including inter-consultancy, there are not, and indeed they are impossible, algorithms for health. It is exactly in this sense that living and being healthy entails wisdom.

For living, and being healthy we certainly need information, education, science, research, technology, arts, and philosophy. But they are not sufficient. To live one additionally needs (some) wisdom. The trouble though is that wisdom cannot be taught, although it can be learned.

There is no kind of teaching, didactics, methodology, pedagogy, plans of programs of and for wisdom. However, many of us do know, for instance because we have encountered them along our lives, (many) wise men and women. The most basic trait about them is that they do not announce themselves—they do not promote, they do not sell or publicize themselves, nor do they allow to be announced and publicized. They walk with pigeon's steps, paraphrasing Nietzsche from a different context.

Nothing about and around the institutional discourses about "health" says one single word about wisdom. And if by chance they happen to cross the word and experience, they naturally might tend to formalize wisdom—which is a *contradictio in terminis*.

Significantly, however, wisdom was always a matter of individuals. The shaman, man or woman, always has used to select a young boy or girl to be educated as a future shaman. Now, meaningfully, vis-à-vis the present and the upcoming future, a big difference arises.

Indeed, for the first time in the history of the human family, a new unprecedented challenge emerges. We need to care about wisdom, a social or collective experience. Given the learning new have reached during history together with the learning of the contemporary age, having a, or some wise men and women is not sufficient any longer. The real challenge consists in having *collectives* of wise men and women, wisdom *as a social and cultural experience*. Never before has humanity faced such a challenge and opportunity. This is the crux and fix of this text.

I argue that such a challenge is feasible, doable, or reachable. The key, it is clear from the body of this chapter, consists in caring about life and/or health.

A last remark becomes compulsory here. An ethics of care, i.e., caring, is a feminine ethics, and indeed the first moral or ethics with a feminine word and spirit—in the entire history of ethics or morals.[5] The entire history of ethics was and still largely still masculine, i.e., patriarchal. For the first a feminine ethics emerges: ethics of care.

Traditionally and universally, women care—for children, the elderly, the neighbors and the others, even if unknown. Women usually cared about the home fire, the

[5] I take here morals and ethics as equivalent, for the sake of argumentative line of this text. Any further distinction, useful in other contexts, appears here as merely academical.

heart, the crops, the cycles of the moon, the winds, rains and draughts, the passers-by and the foreigners, for instance, not to mention the sufferers, the sick.

Caring consists in and entails proximity, contiguity, skinship, holding hands, looking at the other's eyes—alas! understanding without judging.

Meaningfully, men can also learn to caring—not only women.

To be sure the most fundamental care is about health, namely, liveliness and joy. After all, caring means living-together-with-others—even if there are no troubles, problems or sorrows. Living together, voilà the most basic form of complexity, for human beings, for it is not just about other humans, but also any other sentient being, as-we-know-it, as well as-it-could-be-possible.

References

1. Searle J. How to do things with words. Cambridge: Cambridge University Press; 1961.
2. Maldonado CE. Preliminaries for a theory of health, not disease. Bogotá: Ed. Universidad El Bosque; 2021.
3. Bedau MA, Cleland CE, editors. The nature of life: classical and contemporary perspectives from philosophy and science. Cambridge: Cambridge University Press; 2010.
4. Maldonado CE. Indeterminacy as complexity. Revista de Filosofía de la Universidad de Costa Rica. 2024;63(167). (upcoming).
5. Heisenberg W. On the intuitive content of the quantum-theoretical kinematics and mechanics. Z Physik. 1927;43:172–98. https://doi.org/10.1007/BF01397280.
6. Nicholson DJ, Dupré J, editors. Everything flows: toward a processual philosophy of biology. Oxford: Oxford University Press; 2018.
7. Langton CE, editor. Artificial life: an overview. Cambridge: The MIT Press; 1998.
8. Almeida Filho ND. Modeling the Covid-19 pandemic as a complex object (Samajian notes). Estudos Avançados. 2020;34(99):97–118. https://doi.org/10.1590/s0103-4014.2020.3499.007.
9. Schrödinger E. What is life? Cambridge: University of Cambridge Press; 2012.
10. Vernadsky VI. The biosphere. Copernicus; 1998.
11. Dartnell L. Origins: how the earth made us. Random House; 2019.
12. Canfield DE. Oxygen: a four billion years history. Princeton: Princeton University Press; 2015.
13. Maldonado CE. Five arguments toward understanding life in light of a physics of the immaterial. PRO. 2022;81:19. https://doi.org/10.3390/proceedings2022081019.
14. Volk T. Gaia's body: toward a physiology of earth. Copernicus; 1998.
15. Thompson WI, ed. Gaia: a way of knowing. Political implications of the new biology. Lindisfarne Books.
16. Lovelock J. The ages of Gaia: a biography of our living earth. Oxford: Oxford University Press; 1989.
17. McFadden J, Al-Khalili J. Life on the edge: the coming of age of quantum biology. Broadway Books; 2016.
18. Canguilhem G. The knowledge of life. Paris: J. Vrin; 1993.
19. Canguilhem G. Ideology and rationality in the history of the life sciences. Paris: Vrin; 2009.
20. Canguilhem G. The normal and the pathological. Paris: PUF; 2013.
21. Baluska F, Mancuso S, Volkmann D. Communication in plants: neuronal aspects of plant life. Springer Verlag; 2006.
22. Baluska F, Mancuso S. Plant cognition and behavior: from environmental awareness to synaptic circuits navigating root apices. Biol Environ Sci. 2018; https://doi.org/10.1007/978-3-319-75596-0_4.

23. Sheldrake M. Entangled life: how fungi make our worlds, change our minds & shape our futures. New York: Random House; 2020.
24. Darwin C. The origin of species by means of natural selection. New York: The Classics of Science Library; 1995.
25. Ball P. How life works: a users' guide to the new biology. Picador; 2023.
26. Odum EP. Ecology: a bridge between science and society. Sunderland: Sinauer Associates, Inc; 1997.
27. Payan de la Roche JC. Vital disobedience. Barcelona: Instituto de Terapia Neural; 2016.
28. Kyburg HE Jr, Teng CM. Uncertain inference. Cambridge: Cambridge University Press; 2001.
29. Mann T. Joseph and his brothers: the stories of Jacob, young Joseph, Joseph in Egypt, Joseph the provider. Everyman's Library; 2005.
30. Attali J. The nomadic man. Paris: Livre de Poche; 2005.
31. Galen. On diseases and symptoms. Cambridge: Cambridge University Press; 2006.
32. Hippocrates. On air, waters, and places. Harvard University Press; 2004. https://doi.org/10.4159/DLCL.hippocrates_cos-airs_waters_places.2022.
33. Kauffman S. Humanity in a creative universe. Oxford: Oxford University Press; 2016.
34. Smolin L. The life of the cosmos, vol. 51. New York: Oxford University Press; 1998.
35. Payan de la Roche JC. Biological medicine: a commitment to life. Instituto de Terapia Neural; 2006.
36. Almeida FN. Complexity and Transdisciplinarity in the field of collective health: evaluation of concepts and applications. Salud Colectiva. 2006;2(2):123–46.
37. Burton NO, Greer EL. Multigenerational epigenetic inheritance: transmitting information across generations. Semin Cell Dev Biol. 2022;127:121–32. https://doi.org/10.1016/j.semcdb.2021.08.006.
38. Zhang Y, Sirard MA. Epigenetic inheritance of acquired traits through DNA methylation. Anim Front. 2021;11(6):19–27. https://doi.org/10.1093/af/vfab052.
39. Jablonka E, Lamb MJ. The inheritance of acquired epigenetic variations. Int J Epidemiol. 2015;44(4):1094–103. https://doi.org/10.1093/ije/dyv020.
40. Kauffman S. Investigations. Oxford: Oxford University Press; 2000.
41. Prigogine I. The end of certainty. New York: Free Press; 1997.
42. Lorenz E. The essence of chaos, vol. 48. Washington: The University of Washington Press; 1995.
43. Gleick J. Chaos: the making of a new science. New York: Viking Adult; 1987.
44. Sapolsky RM. Behave: the biology of humans at our best and worst. Penguin Books; 2017.
45. Sapolsky RM. Determined: a science of life without free will. Penguin Press; 2023.
46. Hoffman P. The man who loved only numbers: the story of Paul Erdös and the search for mathematical truth. New York: Hyperion; 1998.
47. Barrat A, Barthélemy M, Vespignani A. Dynamical processes on complex networks. Cambridge: Cambridge University Press; 2008.
48. Gould SJ. Wonderful life: the burgess shale and the history of nature. W. W. Norton & Co.; 1990.
49. Gould SJ. The structure of evolutionary theory. Belknap Press; 2002.
50. Lao-tzu. The Way and its virtue. Chinese text presented and translated by F. Houang and P. Leyris. Paris: Éditions du Seuil; 1979.
51. Heidegger M. What is thinking? Tübingen: Max Niemeyer Verlag; 1984.
52. Heidegger M. Path to speech. Paris: Gallimard; 1959.
53. Nussbaum M. Creating capabilities: the human development approach. Cambridge: Belknap Press; 2013.
54. Spinoza B. Ethics. Oxford: Oxford University Press; 2000.
55. Atlan H. Course on biological and cognitive philosophy. In: Spinoza and current biology. Paris: Odile Jacob; 2018.
56. Ball P. Critical mass: one thing leads to another. New York: Farrar, Straus and Giroux; 2006.

57. Zurek WH, ed. Complexity, entropy and the physics of information. Vol. VIII Santa Fe institute studies in the sciences of complexity. Westview Press; 1990.
58. Furtos J, Sundram S. Globalization and mental health: the Lyon declaration. Asian J Psychiatr. 2012;5(3):283–5. https://doi.org/10.1016/j.ajp.2012.07.006.
59. Damasio A. Descartes' error: emotion, reason and the human brain. Penguin Books; 2005.
60. Damasio A. The strange order of things: life, feeling, and the making of cultures. Pantheon; 2018.

Further Readings

Maldonado CE. A look at quantum biology with an interest in health. Investigaciones en Complejidad y Salud. 2021;14:1–84. https://doi.org/10.18270/wp.n3.14.
Maldonado CE. A look at tragedies, death, pandemics as a look at life. Investigaciones en Complejidad y Salud. 2023;20:1–147. https://doi.org/10.13140/RG.2.2.16985.49761.
Maldonado CE. A world made of numerous narratives establishes health. Investigaciones en Complejidad y Salud. 2022;16:1–54. https://doi.org/10.18270/wp.n4.16.
Maldonado CE. An introduction to epigenetics. Complexity and health. Investigaciones en Complejidad y Salud. 2019;1:1–35.
Maldonado CE. Biosemiotics and complexity. Bogotá: Ed. Universidad El Bosque; 2022.
Maldonado CE. Complexity and health: thinking radically. Revista Hojas del Bosque. 2020;8(4):6–15. https://doi.org/10.18270/heb.v4i8.2994.
Maldonado CE. Complexity of health and the role of homeostasis. Investigaciones en Complejidad y Salud. 2020;7:1–70. https://doi.org/10.18270/wp.n2.7.
Maldonado CE. Complexity of health, not disease. In: Valeology, game theory, narrative. Bogotá: Ed Universidad El Bosque; 2020. p. 16–51.
Maldonado CE. Critical reflections on public health theory. In: On the way to complexity sciences. Bogotá: Ed. Universidad El Bosque; 2019. p. 19–50.
Maldonado CE. Disease, health, time: revolving around vicissitudes. Investigaciones en Complejidad y Salud. 2020;6:1–62. https://doi.org/10.18270/wp.n2.6.
Maldonado CE. Epigenetics and the radical transformation of biology. Investigaciones en Complejidad y Salud. 2019;2:1–58. https://doi.org/10.18270/wp.n1.2.
Maldonado CE. Health and not disease. In: Transitions to complexity. Bogotá: Ediciones Universidad El Bosque; 2020. p. 1–25.
Maldonado CE. History of science as the game of the visible and invisible. Investigaciones en Complejidad y Salud. 2019;3:1–51. https://doi.org/10.18270/wp.n1.3.
Maldonado CE. Horizons of bioethics. In: Health and social reality. Bogotá: Academia Nacional de Medicina/Universidad El Bosque; 2004. p. 27–46.
Maldonado CE. Information theory and complexity. In: The third scientific revolution. Bogotá: Ed. Universidad El Bosque; 2020.
Maldonado CE. Introduction to the complexity of eating. Investigaciones en Complejidad y Salud. 2023;19:1–97.
Maldonado CE. One brain, two brains: complicating medicine and biology. Investigaciones en Complejidad y Salud. 2020;8:1–50. https://doi.org/10.18270/wp.n2.8.
Maldonado CE. Preliminary thoughts for a theory of health, not of disease. Health sciences and complexity sciences. Investigaciones en Complejidad y Salud. 2021;5:1–102. https://doi.org/10.18270/wp.n20.5.
Maldonado CE. Public health and complexity. In: History, concepts, and axes. Bogotá: Ed. Universidad El Bosque; 2019. p. 147–73.
Maldonado CE. Public health and quantum theory. In: A bridge for research. Bogotá: Ed. Universidad El Bosque; 2019. p. 19–28.

Maldonado CE. Quantum biology and health sciences. A possible dialogue. Investigaciones en Complejidad y Salud. 2021;13:1–62. https://doi.org/10.18270/wp.n3.13.
Maldonado CE. Quantum physics and medicine: pros and cons of a necessary dialogue. In: Maldonado CE, editor. Approaches to health from complexity, ethics, and medicine. Bogotá: Ed. Universidad El Bosque; 2023.
Maldonado CE. Science as the tension between the visible and the invisible. Investigaciones en Complejidad y Salud. 2019;4:1–49. https://doi.org/10.18270/wp.n1.4.
Maldonado CE. Six theses on health and complexity. Revista Salud Bosque. 2018;8(1):5–7. https://doi.org/10.18270/rsb.v8i1.2370.
Maldonado CE. Tensions between feelings and consciousness: understanding homeostasis. Investigaciones en Complejidad y Salud. 2021;10:1–62. https://doi.org/10.18270/wp.n3.10.
Maldonado CE. The biological roots of knowledge. Investigaciones en Complejidad y Salud. 2021;12:1–69. https://doi.org/10.18270/wp.n3.10.
Maldonado CE. The challenges of reaching a large picture of the world and life. Investigaciones en Complejidad y Salud. 2022;15:1–44. https://doi.org/10.18270/wp.n4.15.
Maldonado CE. The complexity of health. Interactions between the biological and the social. In: Morales MC, editor. Rethinking the social nature of health in contemporary societies. Perspectives, challenges, and alternatives. Bogotá: Universidad Nacional de Colombia; 2008. p. 96–108.
Maldonado CE. The role of chance in the complexity of history, existence, and health. Investigaciones en Complejidad y Salud. 2022;19:1–155. https://doi.org/10.13140/RG.2.2.13918.41289.
Maldonado CE. The strange nature of life: quantum biology, complexity, life, anad health. Investigaciones en Complejidad y Salud. 2021;9:1–65.
Maldonado CE. Time between health and disease. Physics and complexity. Investigaciones en Complejidad y Salud. 2020;5:1–60. https://doi.org/10.18270/wp.n2.5.

Chapter 9
What Is Living? A View from the South

Agustín Ricardo Angarita Lezama

1 Introduction

> We live in a capitalist, patriarchal-matriarchal, anthropocentric society, crossed by profound social inequalities, cultural and economic, in addition to multiple violences and great and serious environmental damage. The patriarchal-matriarchal anthropocentric culture is centered on distrust, control, authority, and submission in the appropriation of things and of truth and in the blindness or ignorance and invisibilization of others. (Humberto Maturana and Ximena Dávila [1])

According to Humberto Maturana, at the end of the 60s, during a biology class on the origin of living things at the University of Chile, a student asked him: "What is it that began approximately 3800 million years ago and that has remained alive, with thousands of variations, to this day?" Maturana, after thinking for a long time, did not know how to answer and offered to provide an answer much later. With this question going around in his head, he embarked on a long path of investigation in search of an answer.

Years later, and together with another Chilean researcher, Francisco Varela, they coined the term, *autopoiesis,* to try to answer the question they had been asked: "What is life? or What is a living being?" [2].

A. R. Angarita Lezama (✉)
Faculty of Human Sciences and Arts, Tolima University, Ibagué, Tolima, Colombia

Faculty of Medicine, Universidad Nacional de Colombia, Bogotá, Colombia
e-mail: agustinangarita@yahoo.es

L. B. Pinilla Bonilla et al. (eds.), *Neuraltherapeutic Medicine*,
https://doi.org/10.1007/978-3-032-03257-7_9

2 Autopoiesis

The concept of autopoiesis caused a stir and multiple comments and influences in different fields of knowledge. Its future is not the subject of this chapter. However, academic discussion and permanent reflection over the years pushed Maturana to reflect and think that he was wrong in the sense of the question he had been asked years ago. Instead of asking "What is life? or What is a living being?" He wondered: what criteria should he use as an observer to affirm that he sees a living being when he is seeing a living being? Or this other question: what does an observer have to see happening in a system to be able to affirm that this system is a living being?

This change in the question is due to a transformative change in the traditional view [3]. It is to stop asking oneself, from the dual thought of life as something external, anchored in the supposedly real, in the objective, in the being in itself of being, that is, in the transcendent, to start looking at a process that occurs in an ever-changing present, which does not happen in isolation but is very interconnected, in a network, in context, and in a systemic and complex way, that is, living in a networked process. A network is an interrelated operation of successive processes that occur in the same phenomenal domain. It is a process in which a large number of processes are systemically articulated, generating a large dynamic network of processes [4].

The expression autopoiesis, as already mentioned, was created in the 70s, describes in a single word the dynamic configuration of molecular processes that constitute a living being as a living being. The notion of autopoiesis is not a definition of life or living, nor is it an explanatory notion. What this expression, *molecular autopoiesis*, does is to synthetically describe the configuration of molecular processes that constitute a living being, as a living being [5]. Living beings exist and are living beings in the continuous production of themselves: autopoiesis is the being and realization of living. It is worth clarifying, Maturana explains, that living beings do not have autopoiesis; they do not use autopoiesis to live, as if it were something external to them, but the continuous realization of molecular autopoiesis *is the living* of what we distinguish as a living being [4].

Autopoiesis is understood from the cell as a minimal living being, because all living beings are composed of cells. But an organism is also an autopoietic being composed of cells. According to Francisco Varela, co-creator of the term and concept, first from the cell and then as an organism, autopoiesis indicates:

1. The cell, as a minimal living being, is made up of a closed network of molecular productions, in which the molecules produced with their multiple interactions generate the same network of molecular productions that produced them, generating what is called molecular *self-organization*.
2. The molecular components of a cell unit must be dynamically *related* in a continuous network of interactions. This dynamic network of chemical and physical interactions produces concrete transformations and new elements. Why are these new elements not dissolved or diluted in a dynamic medium of change? [6].

3. A characteristic of minimal living systems is that their organization includes the creation of a perimeter, a boundary, an edge, a segmentation that specifies the territory of the network's operations and defines the system as a unit. However, this edge is not isolated; rather, it is an integral part of the system's self-organization. This same self-organizing process then specifies its extension as a discrete unit by constituting its own operational edges. Therefore, this self-managed organization *from within* defines an *edge* or a limit to establish how far there is a self and where the difference from that self begins.
4. The dynamics of this closed network of molecular productions in the cell results in the continuous production of the same cell and its edge, constituting everything as an autopoietic system.
5. The cell as a molecular autopoietic system is closed in its dynamics of self-production, but open to the flow of molecules and energy through the edge that it itself created. That is, the autopoietic cell is thermodynamically open but operationally closed.
6. By creating this limit that is open and dynamic, the living system, to exist, does so in a functional or operational closure, existing as a totality in the environment in which its identity is preserved. This edge or *membrane* is a universal feature of living things, and it presents the same type of structure throughout the living world. The membranes maintain the cell as a differentiated entity, being non-rigid structures that are always active. The membrane is the condition of possibility for the operation of the network of transformations that produced it as a unit. It happens that the cell does not contain several membranes but is *a single system* of interconnected membranes that remain in constant movement [6].
7. The cell membrane, as already mentioned, defines a boundary that is open and dynamic. This edge differentiates it from the environment in which it exists. However, no living being can live in isolation. The living of the living being, by creating its limits, establishes an *internal micro world* for the organization itself to recognize itself (*identity*). And at the same time, it establishes an external world, or *macro world*, that contains it and that, as a living being, it needs. This is the *dependence* of all living beings. This macro world is the niche, the environment or context on which *the living being depends*, but this dependence is mutual; the living being and its context are interrelated in a two-way dependence. This is why the entire living organization is said to be *codependent*.
8. The living being exists in a continuous present, in a continuous now, in the flow of a changing and continuously transforming present.
9. The life of a living being occurs in its molecular autopoiesis as internal dynamics of processes and does not depend on the molecules that make it as a particular organism. To speak of an autopoietic systemic dynamic indicates and aims to make visible the rich internal interrelation of processes that make up the molecular, recursive, cyclical dynamic network, which produces itself in an operationally closed system. This *network of processes* is profusely interconnected in a *systemic* way, in such a way that acting on one of them is acting on

all. The *systemic network organization* is a pattern common to all living beings. Where there is life, there are networks.

10. The autopoietic internal dynamic network is systemic and defines the rhythm and volume of self-production. The operational self-organization of an autopoietic unit is not linear but is *recursive* or looping. The flow of components changes permanently, and autopoiesis remains without being static or predictable.
11. *Ontogeny* is the story of the structural change of a living being, seen as a unit, without losing its identity. This change or ontogeny occurs by the decision of the living being or triggered by the environment in which it lives and which is constantly changing, but this change depends on its internal dynamics and not on the external stimulus. Two or more autopoietic units can meet in their ontogeny and couple if their interactions are recurrent or very intense. This coupling of two or more ontogenies occurs in an operational closure or functional closure.
12. If two or more autopoietic units are coupled in their ontogeny, with their recurrent or permanent interactions, the result would be a history of mutually concordant and coherent structural changes, that is, a *structural coupling* between these two or more autopoietic units.
13. The couplings of several autopoiess in their ontogeny generate another unity that is also self-organized but of a higher order than the cellular ontogeny. This new self-organizing unit is an organism.
14. In an *organism* such as an autopoietic system, living is an *emergent property*, which results from an *organization*, not from the reaction of certain components. This organization is *self-created* as a *distributed property* of the interaction between the dynamic network of global processes and local reactions. Like a network of processes, *it functions without a center* and without external direction, obeying its self-created internal rules. This is its *autonomy*. An autopoietic organism is both autonomous and codependent.
15. Autopoietic systems are autonomous. For them, the most important thing is to maintain their own organization, their self-created order, no matter what transformations they have to make in the face of external stimuli to maintain their own organization. An organism generates a permanent network of reactions that make itself a pattern of self-created and autonomous basic organization.
16. A living being is an autopoietic molecular system, and an autopoietic system is a living being. In autopoiesis, the living occurs; it occurs in living itself, and it is not something that the organism or the living being does [7].

The *preservation of living* is the foundation of all that is possible in living beings, and it is the preservation of a particular way of life for the living being as an organism in the succession of generations, which constitutes and realizes the identity of that living being as a particular kind of existence [4].

3 The Organisms

Living beings, in general, are molecular autopoietic systems that operate as discrete units in a relational space in which, by existing as totalities, they exist as *organisms*. We speak of *a system* every time we distinguish a set of interconnected, interacting elements of any nature, so that if we act on one, we act on all.

In their living, living beings as organisms, whether human or not, exist in two spaces: in the space where their living takes place, existing in the continuous production of themselves in the flow of the realization of their molecular autopoiesis. And at the same time, they are realized as totalities by existing, operating as organisms, and interacting in the *relational space* that contains them. This applies to all living beings, including human beings [4].

An organism is a functionally closed dynamic system. This exists in the conservation of its organization in a process that happens through a continuous change of interactions with the environment. This environment does not pre-exist but arises and changes with the organism in the constant flow of that becoming. An organism is an existence of the autopoietic system as a totality: every living being exists as an organism in its historical becoming or flow. The preservation of its own organization in an ever-changing environment defines the course of an organism's historical evolution. The history of an organism is a becoming of change around *something that is conserved* [4].

An individual who looks at and analyzes a process from a distance is an observer, that is, outside the process and could say that he sees an organism in the realization of its life when he distinguishes a *changing molecular architectural singularity*. This architectural singularity, seen in its historical evolution, operates as a closed network of processes that make up a molecular autopoietic system.

According to Maturana, in an organism, autopoiesis is a process that occurs and happens. In this biological event, there is no purpose, there is no control, there is no better or worse, there are no adaptive advantages nor hierarchies. The different kinds of living beings live all their different lives without external or internal orientation toward a particular purpose or operational purpose. What happens is that they arise as a continuous result of the permanent change of the dynamic architecture that they are [4].

4 Operational Closure

Living beings, all of us, are the present of a history of *conservation of living* that has occurred and is occurring spontaneously without purpose or causality. There is no teleology of life.

Autopoietic systems are systems in which they operate, their operation is closed, and whose components are produced within a cyclical and systemic process that takes place in the internal microenvironment of the cell. *Operational closure* refers to the control by which the internal elements self-organize in an emergent way within the cell or the living being, achieving stability, and permanence, all under *their own* dynamics of operation. In other words, the living being constructs its own vital norms. It is their autonomy [8].

According to Margulis, from the beginning, the process of living responded to its *autopoietic* imperative in a universe that obeyed thermodynamic laws. Delimited and separated from the world by a border created by itself, life was added in the form of lipid droplets that increased its internal order and generated its membrane or edge [9].

To understand and comprehend autopoiesis is to realize that an observer sees, for example, how wound healing is not a special process from the organism to end tissue damage, but is a circumstantial aspect of the continuous production of itself, such as healing. The same happens with the regeneration of an organ, with tissue differentiation, or with the growth of the organism.

5 Structural Coupling

We have already explained that an *organism* is a closed dynamic system that exists as a temporal–spatial architectural totality that preserves its organization as an organism of a certain kind in its historical becoming (preserving its *identity*), through its continuous change in interactions with an environment or medium that arises and changes with it in the flow of that constant becoming.

It had previously been said that autopoietic systems existed in two domains. On the one hand, they exist in the flow of its internal dynamics, which allows it to operate as a molecular autopoietic system in a *dynamic and closed network of processes* in the continuous production of itself, in its autopoietic and autonomous process. This would be the body of the living being. On the other hand, it also exists as an organism in its very rich *relational dynamics*. It would be his psychic body or his soul. These two domains, the internal or biological autopoietic (the body), and the relational or social (the mind), where intersubjectivity occurs and is enriched, merge into a totality as a single existence, as a total being. The mind-body fusion. This organism, as a whole, relates to an ever-changing environment [10].

Organism and environment *arise together* in the same time and place. In other words, they coexist. They depend on each other. It is a *codependency*. They interact permanently with each other. To speak of the *medium* is not to speak of a static or abiotic space or container. On the contrary, it includes everything biotic and its circumstances. Therefore, an organism coexists with its environment and with other organisms that live there and depend on each other [4].

An organism, when coexisting in an environment and with other organisms, in their correlation, receives stimuli of various kinds. Faced with a stimulus that it receives from its environment, the organism can react by modifying its operational architecture, but always maintaining its autopoietic organization. If the stimulus is very powerful, the body does not resist it and dies. Otherwise, the organism reacts by modifying its structure according to its autopoiesis, its own norms. In other words, *the stimulus has an impact, but it does not decide* [11].

It is from this internal wisdom accumulated in the vital maintenance of its order, self-organization, and autonomy that the organism, in the face of a stimulus, modifies its operational functional structure, always maintaining its organization, its order, or its autopoiesis [12].

Let us recap, what happens if the stimulus is strong and hurts the operational architecture of the organism? The self-organizing internal dynamics will establish the necessary adjustments to modify its operational and functional architecture, reestablishing its organization and maintaining its autopoiesis. If the stimulus is too strong, the organism will lose its order, its self-organizing process, and its functional architecture will be altered, and then the organism will die.

This is why it is stated that, as molecular autopoietic systems, living beings are systems or organisms *determined* in our own structure so that nothing external to us that affects us can determine what happens to us or what can be trigger in us certain structural changes in our structure [7].

An autopoietic organism has as its priority, so to speak, to maintain its internal organization, its vital order, in the face of any change. It modifies its operational architecture to maintain its internal organization. It is important to emphasize that the central and fundamental thing about change is not the change itself, but *what is preserved in the dynamics of change*, in its permanent flow. In any dynamic relational situation, what is conserved will define what could be changed [4].

6 The Organism-Niche Ecological Unit

Every living being in existence always arises in an environment that makes it possible. In other words, both the living being and the circumstance or context that makes it possible arise, occur, happen, transform, and exist together. Living beings exist, then, in an ecological unit that has been called since conception *the ecological organism-niche unit*. This is an ecological unit because the living being and its circumstance or environment, structurally coupled, always change together.

Everything that happens to an organism, whether in its internal dimension (body) or in its relational flow (mind), happens in the realization of its autopoiesis as the dynamics of recursive changes of a spontaneous and dynamic architecture. This architecture, as a temporal or spatial entity, constitutes a closed system in a permanent flow of operational relations disjoint with its context or niche [4].

As said, the living of an organism always occurs in a dynamic and intimate coupling between the living being and its environment. This dynamic structural coupling constitutes the *ecological organism-niche unit* and is the existential space of every living being. There is no living being outside this ecological organism-niche unit, that is, without its environmental context of life.

In short, the scope of operation and relationship that makes it possible for a living being to live constitutes the *ecological organism-niche unit*. The moment a living being emerges, the niche that makes it possible arises in a close relationship of unity. Living being and niche arise together in codependence. When we talk about the origin of living beings, what we must talk about is the origin of the dynamic organism-niche ecological unit.

Therefore, the niche and living being form, when living, the *ecological niche-organism unit,* in which they change together in a congruent way. The niche of a living being would disappear as such when the living being establishes a structural coupling in another environmental space. In practice, the niche is the world of the system [6].

As already mentioned, the organism and the context of its life, or its niche, change at the same time in the conservation of a relationship of *structural coupling* so that the living being lives while this relationship is spontaneously preserved in the flow of its life. This is why every living being, every organism, functions and lives in a *structural coupling* with the environment, with its context, with its environment or niche as its condition of life and existence. Therefore, it is in the permanent conservation of its structural coupling that every living being operates and lives or disintegrates.

A living being, and the niche that contains it, change at the same time in a congruent way as the spontaneous result of their recursive interactions only if, in the flow of the changes in the structural architecture, which these interactions trigger in both, the living being retains its autopoiesis and its relationship of structural coupling to the environment in its niche. If the structural coupling is lost and the *emergent coherence* between the organism and its niche that arises with it is no longer preserved, then the organism dies [4].

7 The Niche-Culture Ecological Unit

Human beings, as living organisms, live in a flow of recursive interactions with our niche, which in turn is made up, among many others, of different human beings and culture, which we all permanently build.

Humans become human; we are not born human [13]. The evolution of the lineage of bipedal primates (hominids) to which all humans belong originated in the evolution of a way of *living together*. In other words, *living together* made possible a co-evolution of a lineage of bipedal primates that preserved a way of living together, a coexistence that arose when an ancestral family was constituted as a very close and intimate space of life together, of sensual coexistence around a female [14]. This living together around the sharing of food, shelter, care, sensuality, tenderness, sexuality, and the pleasure of the closeness of the cohabitant was preserved in learning to understand and experience that others were legitimate in the doing of living together [15].

Respect for the cohabitant and the cohabitation that is born from the biology of loving constituted an environment of closeness in the sharing of the doings of living together, in the pleasure of living together around a female, and in enjoying the company in sensuality, care, sexuality, and tenderness. In the recursion and conservation in this space of coexistence, *language* emerged as what made us human [16]. The human is the *emergence* of a recursive coexistence in respect of the biology of loving in language. Loving is the emotion that always happens before the action, which constitutes the cement, the pleasure and joy of being together, which legitimizes and makes coexistence possible [17].

Culture is everything that is preserved and maintained in the evolution of the coexistence of human lineages. Culture, being part of coexistence, constitutes a pillar of the *organism-niche ecological unity,* expanding it to the *organism-niche-culture ecological unity.* This unity possesses all the *epigenetic* power of a dynamic structural coupling that culture can generate [4].

8 Emergencies and Dissipative Structures

As already explained, humans would be an *emergency* in the future for bipedal primates. A new order that burst in, that sprouted, that emerged in a quantitative leap, but, above all, a qualitative one, in which characteristics appeared that could only be deduced once the new order appeared. They are the bifurcations of complexity that appear when living beings move away from thermodynamic equilibrium, and the creation of new structures and qualities becomes possible. Emergencies are the rise of new qualities that cannot be explained by the characteristics of the components that already existed. They are a qualitative leap that breaks linearity and that would explain the non-existence of the missing link in the history of humanity. Life then does not pre-exist; it is an emergent property.

We have already stated that living systems are open to the flows of matter and energy. However, complex systems are organizationally closed, with operational closure.

Living systems could not be explained from the linear and deterministic perspective of physics and its traditional thermodynamic equations. Therefore, the concept of *negentropy emerged* as an explanatory proposal to understand living beings that move away from thermodynamic equilibrium and would live *denying* entropy [18].

If entropy refers to the measure of the disorder of a system, and autopoiesis is the dynamic process in which an organism maintains its own order, living beings must *dissipate the entropy* generated by living in order to stay alive. An organism, then, is an *autopoietic dissipative structure*. An autopoietic structure or architecture of a living system is always a dissipative structure, but not all dissipative structures are autopoietic networks [19].

9 Cognition and Living Systems

All systems that are alive would be cognitive systems, that is, systems that know, understand, and learn, and when this *cognition* exists, the existence of an autopoietic network that dissipates energy must always be presupposed. If the simplest organisms are capable of perception, then they would be organisms capable of *cognition* [20].

In the act of living, by the very structural coupling that gives *identity* to the system, a double bond is generated at that moment that is part of the *organism-niche ecological unity*: the recognition of the self and the non-self. As living is doing, all doing is knowing. This recognition of the *self* constitutes the identity of the system.

Knowing is functioning; it is the permanent operation of the components of a system in their internal dynamics, in their microenvironment, and their respective changes in the structural architecture. The close relationship between doing and living, that is, between experience and doing, relates knowledge to the changes that occur in the structural architecture of the autopoietic system, in the context of its structural coupling with its niche, with its environment. So, we could say that in the living being, knowing, doing, and living are inseparable facts [21].

Cognition would then be the very process of living. This process is inextricably linked in an organism to autopoiesis and its dissipative structure: three different aspects of the same dynamic of living. The being and doing of living systems are united and inseparable during their specific mode of self-organization. All living systems are cognitive systems, which know and understand, and *cognition* always involves the existence of a network of autopoietic processes that dissipate entropy. The concept of cognition is greater than that of thought and includes perception, emotion, and action. That is, the entire life process [20].

The concept of cognition indicates the entire relational or mental process of knowledge construction. In general, the vital processes of systems are identified with cognition and the process of knowing, that is, with the mind. Cognition in the humans includes language, conceptual thinking, and consciousness [21].

It is worth clarifying that the mind is not a thing that exists in isolation. It is a process, the very process of life. All the self-organized activity of living systems is a mental activity. The interactions of a living organism in *The-niche-culture ecological unit* are cognitive-mental interactions. It should also be made clear that mind and matter are not separate but are two inextricable aspects of the vital phenomenon. The mental process is immanent in matter. And as such, the brain is not necessary for the mind to exist. It is worth noting that knowledge, consciousness, and mind are *embodied emergences* of the whole mind-body [20].

The brain is one of the structures through which the mental process operates, however, the CNS, the immune system, the endocrine system, the intestinal microbiome, among others, form a single cognitive network of the complete autopoietic organism.

10 Conclusions from Neuraltherapeutic Medicine

Neuraltherapeutic medicine is *biocentric, not dual.* The human being is not divided into matter and energy, mind and body, or soul and flesh. The mind is an incarnated emergent property. As Julio César Payán said, the human "is mind and body at the same time; that is, he is a *total being*" [22].

All their thinking, feeling, and action orbits around living. Living is an *emergent,* self-created, perfectly distributed property, without a center and without external control, without hierarchies to maintain its own organization and maintain its living. Living does not accept external rules or impositions, even if they are of good will. Living is against the tide. It is vital disobedience [22].

Its *self-organization* establishes its own rules and mandates, that is, its *autonomy.* The organism manages its limits from within to define itself (its internal micro world). Therefore, it is from within that human behaviors are decided, not from the outside.

The organism is thermodynamically open but operationally closed, and its functional closure determines its *identity.* The external stimuli of its environment have an impact but do not decide the life of an organism.

Human living occurs in the ever-changing, interconnected, networked, and systemically shaped present. It is a life in continuous transformation, never static or predictable. Both the organism and its environment, its context or environment, arise together, coexist, have relationships and interactions of processes in a systemic and networked way. In such a way that acting on a particular process, even if we do not realize it, is to act on everyone [5].

The human being is an autopoietic organism, a self-organized living being, which exists in an environment or environment that makes it possible. This union is a structural coupling that generates the ecological unity of the niche organism that is an emergent coherence. Humans were not born human; we became human in living together, in language, in the biology of loving, in the cooperative creation of a niche, which results in the ecological unity of organism-niche-culture. Therefore, humans are co-dependent on other organisms. They live together; they coexist.

The organism-niche-culture ecological unit accounts for codependence, and for the epigenetic transformations of the human being. From this point of view, humans live with the viruses that appeared earlier in history and with a large number of microorganisms, fungi, plants, animals, and in connection (structural coupling) between all of them. This interdependence must always be taken into account by Neuraltherapeutic medicine.

The human being realizes his living, in his biological internal space (autopoiesis) and in his relational or social space, as a unified existence. Cognition is the process of life.

The behavior of a human being is what an external observer sees in him, and on this, he proposes an explanatory proposal.

Living together is living with the cohabitant in the biology of respect, in the biology of loving, and in care [5].

Neuraltherapeutic medicine is living in an alternative, biocentric, non-patriarchal, non-hierarchical, feminist, Latin American coexistence, weaving interculturalities, and accepting and experiencing ignorance in order to be able to carry out dialogues.

Finally, Neuraltherapeutic medicine, as an alternative medicine, is not a mere technique, a tool or a method, but it is a conception that must be dared and free, a conception impregnated with another rationality, another logic, which in its solidary, non-vertical interaction, recognizing knowledge and wisdom, is respectful. Responsible, ethical, and deeply loving [22].

References

1. Maturana H, Dávila X. The tree of living. Santiago de Chile: Matriztica MVP Editores; 2015.
2. Maturana H, Varela F. The tree of knowledge. Santiago de Chile: Universitaria; 1990.
3. Maturana H, Varela F. Of machines and living beings: autopoiesis, the organization of the living. Buenos Aires: Lumen; 2004.
4. Dávila X, Maturana H. Human dwelling in six essays of biological-cultural studies. Santiago de Chile: Instituto Matriztico; 2008.
5. Maturana H. Transformation in coexistence. Santiago de Chile: Océano-Dolmen; 2004.
6. Varela F. The phenomenon of life. Santiago de Chile: Dolmen; 2002.
7. Maturana H. Reality: objective or constructed? I. Biological foundations of reality. Barcelona: Anthropos; 2009.
8. Maturana H. Reality: objective or constructed? II. Biological foundations of knowledge. Barcelona: Anthropos, Universidad Iberoamericana, ITESO; 2009.
9. Margulis L, Sagan D. What is life? Barcelona: Tusquets; 1996.
10. Harari YN. Nexus. Bogotá: Penguin Random House; 2024.
11. Maturana H. Emotions and language in education and politics. Santiago de Chile: Universidad de la Frontera; 1990.
12. Maturana H. Biology of cognition and epistemology. Temuco: Universidad de la Frontera; 1990.
13. Angarita Lezama A. We are not born human, we become human. Ibagué: Academia JUNTOS; 2021.
14. Maturana H. From biology to psychology. 4th ed. Santiago de Chile: Universitaria – Lumen; 2003.
15. Angulo Rasco JF. Affective justice: an urgent educational and political need. Hemiciclo. 2022;24:51–64.
16. Maturana H. The meaning of the human. Santiago de Chile: Ediciones Pedagógicas Chilenas; 1992.
17. Maturana H, Dávila X. The tree of living. Santiago de Chile: MVP Editores; 2015.
18. Prigogine I. Is it just an illusion? An exploration from chaos to order. Barcelona: Tusquets; 1983.
19. Prigogine I. The end of certainties. Madrid: Taurus Santillana; 1997.
20. Capra F. The web of life. Barcelona: Anagrama; 2000.
21. Maturana H, Bloch S. Biology of emotions and Alba emoting. Santiago: Dolmen Océano; 2020.
22. Payán de la Roche J. Vital disobedience. Sabadell: Instituto de Terapia Neural SL; 2016.

Part III
Morphologic Dimension in Neuraltherapeutic Medicine

Chapter 10
Basic Embryology for Neuraltherapeutic Medicine

Luz Amparo Arias-López

1 Development of the Nervous System

Very early in development, around the third week of gestation, a crucial process is generated that results in the establishment of the three germ layers; this event is known as *gastrulation*. This is how an outer layer called the ectoderm is created, an intermediate layer that is the mesoderm, and an inner layer that is the endoderm (Fig. 10.1). The cells that make up these three layers will give rise to all tissues and organs. Similarly, it is during gastrulation that the specification of the anteroposterior axis and the determination of the midline of the developing embryo take place [1].

Below the ectoderm and along the midline, a cord of mesodermal cells forms the definitive notochord, which serves as the basis for the induction of neural plaque formation and the subsequent neural groove that will give rise to the neural tube, from ectodermal cells, a stage known as *neurulation* [2]. The first induction for the development of the nervous system is the formation of the neural plate from the thickening of the dorsal ectoderm that is located above the notochord. This ectoderm receives inducing signals that block the influence of bone morphogenetic proteins 4—BMP4—causing nervous tissue to form [3].

The lateral edges of the neural plate begin to rise at the third week of development, forming the neural folds; secondary to this elevation in the central a cleft called the neural sulcus is formed (Fig. 10.2). When the neural folds rise, they approach the midline until they contact the one on one side with the other, and thus they fuse from the cervical from the fifth somita to the caudal, thus forming the *neural tube*. The neural tube will give rise to the central nervous system and a cavity

L. A. Arias-López (✉)
Faculty of Medicine, Morphology Department, Master in Human Morphology, Universidad Nacional de Colombia, Bogotá, Colombia
e-mail: luaariaslo@unal.edu.co

L. B. Pinilla Bonilla et al. (eds.), *Neuraltherapeutic Medicine*,
https://doi.org/10.1007/978-3-032-03257-7_10

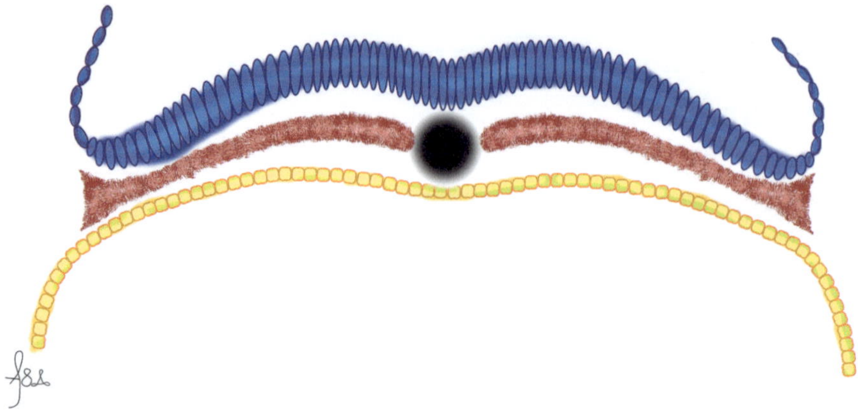

Fig. 10.1 Schematic of gastrulation that gives rise to the three germ layers in the embryo. (Source: Adapted from [1]. Illustration by Angélica Ochoa)

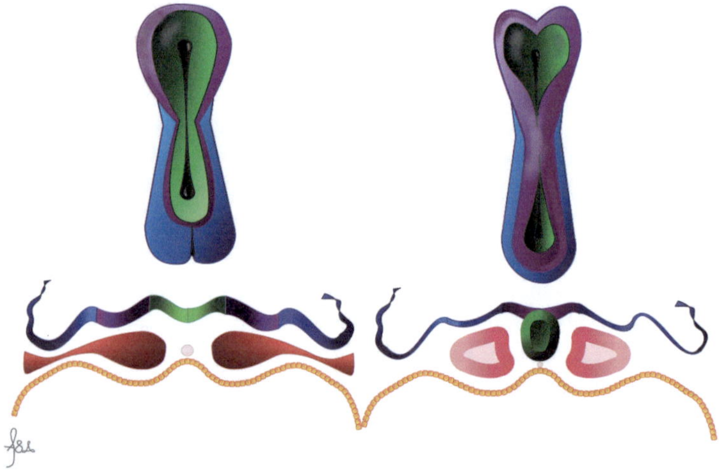

Fig. 10.2 Diagram of the neural sulcus, neural crest, and onset of neural tube formation. (Source: Adapted from [2]. Illustration by Angélica Ochoa)

will have formed inside it that will later give rise to the ventricles in the case of the brain and the ependymal duct in the case of the spinal cord [1, 2].

When neural tube fusion begins, neuropores are formed, which are the open ends of the tube; the anterior or cranial neuropore and the posterior or caudal neuropore that communicate with the amniotic cavity. These two neuropores must finally close; the cranial has its definitive closure on day 25 of development in the phase of 18–20 somites and the caudal on day 28 approximately. If neural tube closure does not occur within the scheduled developmental times, closure defects will occur with varied pathological presentations [1].

As the neural sulcus forms, there is a migration of cells from the lateral part of the neural plate to the dorsal part; these cells form the so-called neural crest and they detach once the neural folds join, thus forming a separate layer of neuroectodermal cells. These cells will undergo an epithelial-mesenchymal transition and enter the underlying mesoderm once they leave the neuroectoderm. Neural crest cells are multipotent and will transform into different populations of neurons and migrate to fulfill broad functions. Some will form sensory neurons of the cranial nerves; others will form ganglia and afferent neurons of the spinal nerves. They will also form paravertebral and prevertebral ganglion neurons and postganglionic neurons of the visceral efferent system of the autonomic nervous system. Likewise, the neural crest will give rise to neuroendocrine cells such as chromaffin cells in the medulla of the adrenal gland; they will also form glial cells in the peripheral nervous system, such as Schwann cells and skin pigment cells, which we know as melanocytes. It also originates a large part of the craniofacial skeleton, connective tissue, cartilage and dentin; in addition, it gives rise to the carotid body, the enteric nervous system, and the heart's outflow tract [4, 5].

2 Primary and Secondary Vesicles

Once the neural tube is configured, the region that constitutes the brain will undergo a series of divisions or segmentations from the already existing neural tube. The primary subdivisions divide the brain into three dilations or vesicles, the *forebrain*, the *midbrain,* and the *hindbrain*. These three vesicles, during the fourth week of development, will give rise to a more specific subdivision of five dilations, thus, the forebrain will form the *telencephalon* and the *diencephalon*. The *telencephalon* will expand and form the cerebral hemispheres developed into complex structures such as the cerebral cortex, which is responsible for higher cognitive functions, and the basal ganglia, which form inside the hemispheres and are essential for movement control. It will also give rise to the lateral ventricles. The *diencephalon* will give rise to thalamic and hypothalamic structures, the pineal gland and the pituitary gland, the latter considered to be the master gland of the endocrine system. It will also give rise to the optic vesicles and the third ventricle. The diencephalon acts as the primary center for the transmission and processing of sensory information and autonomic control. The vesicle called *the midbrain* continues without subdividing and will give rise to what we know as the midbrain, where structures such as the tectum with its upper and lower colliculi will develop with important roles in the processing of sensory information and motor control; likewise, the midbrain will give rise to the cerebral aqueduct. Finally, the *hindbrain* will give rise to fundamental segmentations for craniofacial organizations. In general, the hindbrain is subdivided into *the metencephalon* and the *myelencephalon*; the former will give rise to the cerebellum as a coordinator of movement and balance, and the *pons* that acts as a connection center between the brain and the spinal cord and contains nuclei that regulate respiratory functions. The second will form the medulla oblongata. The cavity that

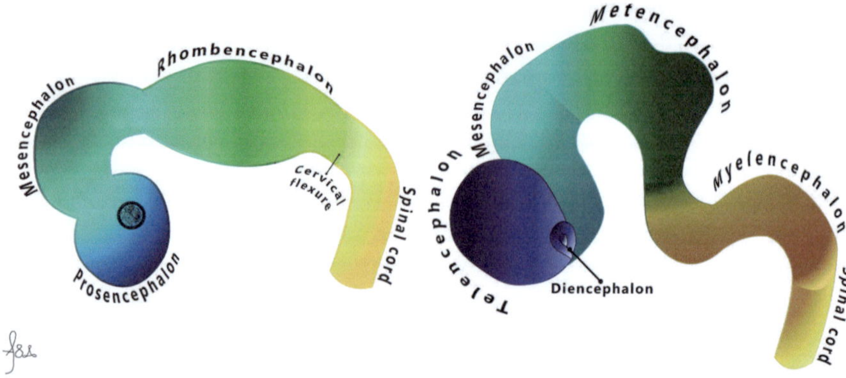

Fig. 10.3 Diagram of the stage of the three vesicles with the forebrain, midbrain, and hindbrain, and the stage of the five vesicles where the forebrain has formed the telencephalon and the diencephalon, and the hindbrain has given rise to the metencephalon and the myelencephalon. (Source: Adapted from [2]. Illustration by Angélica Ochoa)

forms in the metencephalon and myelencephalon is the fourth ventricle (Fig. 10.3) [1, 3, 6, 7].

3 Segmentation

Segmentation is one of the most transcendental critical prerequisites in development and is particularly important in the nervous system, including the neural crest, rhombomeres, as well as in the somites, pharyngeal arches, and aortes [8].

The hindbrain has a particular segmentation into seven rhombomeres as a result of the action of different types of genes. Each rhombomeric segment gives rise to different types of neuronal cells that do not mix with those of another rhombomere despite being very close. Likewise, this segmentation establishes an essential anticipatory fundamental program for the formation of functional circuits (Fig. 10.4) [9].

The rhombomeric segments give rise to the motor nuclei of the cranial nerves Trochlear (IV), Trigeminal (V), Abducens (IV), Facial (VII), Glossopharyngeal (IX), Pneumogastric or Vagus (X), Spinal (XI), and Hypoglossal (XII) that emerge from the brain stem.

The third common cranial nerve does not emerge from the rhombomeres any more than the olfactory and optic nerves. The sensory nuclei of the cranial nerves are generated from the nasal, otic, and epibranchial ectodermal placodes and neural crest cells. The epibranchial placodes also contribute to the formation of ganglia for the nerves of the pharyngeal arches V, VII, IX, and X. On the other hand, the parasympathetic ganglia (visceral efferents) come from neural crest cells and their fibers are transported by cranial nerves III, VII, IX, and X [1, 10].

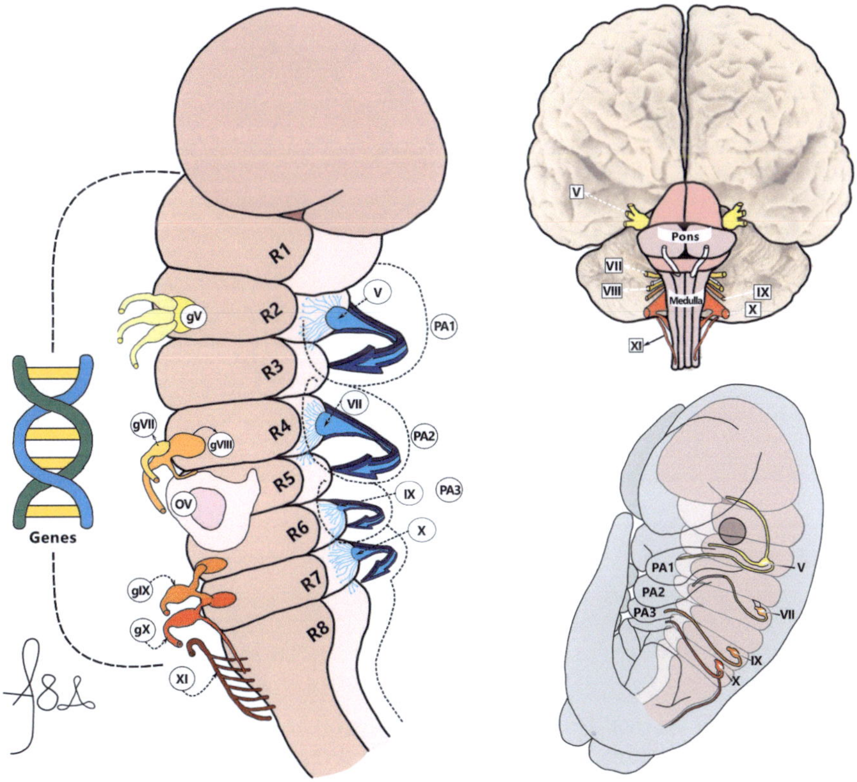

Fig. 10.4 Diagram of the rhombomeric segments giving rise to the nuclei of cranial nerves V, VII, IX, and X. (Source: Adapted from [9]. Illustration by Angélica Ochoa)

Once the neural tube is closed, neural crest cells migrate from the rhombomeres to the pharyngeal arches where they surround and fuse with the mesodermal layer to form definitive structures. Cells from the first and second rhombomere migrate to the first pharyngeal arch, cells from the fourth rhombomere migrate to the second arch, and cells from the sixth and seventh rhombomere will populate the third, fourth, and sixth arches with cells (Fig. 10.5). The cells of the third and fifth rhombomere are not mentioned because they are not part of any pharyngeal arch. The pharyngeal arches are crucial in the development of bone, muscle, vessels, and nerves in the face, neck, and oropharyngeal apparatus. In addition, four of the cranial nerves invade the pharyngeal arches and give rise to branches that will provide the innervation of the structures derived from each arch. These nerves are the trigeminal, facial, glossopharyngeal, and vagus nerves [11].

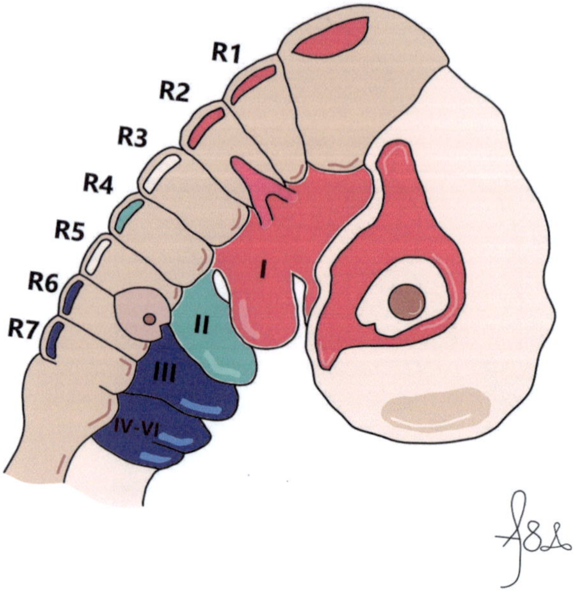

Fig. 10.5 Diagram of rhombomere segmentation and cell migration for pharyngeal arch formation. (Source: Adapted from [11]. Illustration by Angélica Ochoa)

4 Spinal Cord

Caudally to the cervical bending, what remains of the neural tube will form the spinal cord, where three zones are differentiated: *ventricular valve, mantle, and marginal*. The mantle layer contains neuronal bodies of the gray matter, while the marginal zone contains the axons that constitute the white matter [2].

As neuroblasts are added to the mantle layer, thickenings are generated at the ventral and dorsal levels of the tube. The ventral plates are the basal plates that contain motor neurons, while the dorsal thickenings are the wing plates. The former will give rise to the motor areas of the spinal cord and the latter to the sensory areas of the spinal cord (Fig. 10.6). Between the two previous areas, another group of nerve cells accumulates, giving rise to the horna intermedia, a small region that is only found at the thoracic and upper lumbar levels and contains sympathetic nerve cells of the autonomic nervous system [1].

5 Spinal Nerves

By the fourth week of development, motor nerve fibers begin to appear in the basal plates of the spinal cord, grouping together to form the ventral roots of the nerves, while the dorsal roots form fibers from dorsal root ganglia cells. The distal prolongations join the ventral and dorsal roots to form the spinal nerve [6, 10].

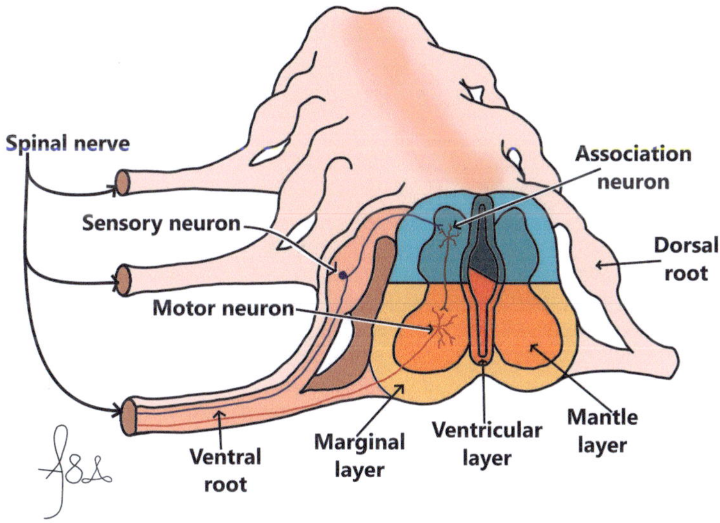

Fig. 10.6 A. Diagram of the basal plates that will give rise to the motor areas and the wing plates that will give rise to the sensory areas of the spinal cord. (Source: Adapted from [6]. Illustration by Angélica Ochoa)

6 Vegetative Nervous System

When neural crest cells migrate by the fifth week of development, they migrate from the thoracic region to the region behind the dorsal aorta on either side of the spinal cord. Once located there, they form a bilateral sympathetic chain of ganglia interconnected with each other by longitudinal nerves, thus forming the sympathetic trunks that we know from anatomy. From the thoracic position, neuroblasts migrate to the cervical and lumbosacral regions. At first the segmental division is very clear; however, later it ceases to be so, and that is because at the cervical level that arrangement changes due to the fusion of the ganglia at this level. Neuroblast migration also takes place to the anterior part of the aorta to form the celiac and mesenteric ganglia. Other neuroblasts migrate to the heart, lung, and gastrointestinal tract to give rise to sympathetic plexuses of these organs. The fibers that synapse at the same level in the sympathetic chain or pass through it are myelin-containing preganglionic fibers that stimulate the sympathetic ganglia cells. When the fibers pass from the spinal nerves to the sympathetic ganglia, they form white communicating branches that are only found from the first thoracic segment to the second lumbar segment. Postganglionic fibers do not have myelin and pass to other levels of the sympathetic chain or extend to organs. There are also gray communication branches that pass through the sympathetic chain and go to the spinal nerves and from there to blood vessels and sweat glands and are found at all levels of the spinal cord. At the parasympathetic level, the preganglionic fibers originate at the level of the brainstem and sacral region of the spinal cord. These fibers travel through the cranial nerves III, VII, IX, and X. Postganglionic fibers originate from neurons in the neural crest-derived ganglia and go to the viscera, salivary glands, and pupil sphincter muscle [1, 6, 10].

References

1. Sadler TW. Langman: medical embryology. 12th ed. Barcelona: Lippincott Williams & Wilkins; 2012. p. 384.
2. Osuna E, Caro LE, Patiño G. Neuroanatomy: fundamentals of structural, functional, and clinical neuroanatomy. 1st ed. Bogotá: Universidad Nacional de Colombia; 2016. p. 215.
3. Carlson BM. Human embryology and developmental biology. 5th ed. Barcelona: Elsevier; 2014. p. 505.
4. Theveneau E, Mayor R. Chapter 4 – neural crest cell migration: guidance, pathways, and cell–cell interactions. In: Trainor PA, editor. Neural crest cell: evolution, development, and disease. San Diego; 2024.
5. Lefcort F. Development of the autonomic nervous system: clinical implications. Semin Neurol. 2020;40(5):473–84.
6. Gilbert S, Barresi M. Developmental biology. 11th ed. Massachusetts: Sinauer Associates, Inc; 2016. p. 940.
7. Purves D. Neuroscience. 3rd ed. Buenos Aires: Editorial Médica Panamericana; 2007. p. 891.
8. Müller F, O'Rahilly R. Segmentation in staged human embryos: the occipitocervical region revisited. J Anat. 2003;203(3):297–315.
9. Krumlauf R, Wilkinson DG. Segmentation and patterning of the vertebrate hindbrain. Development. 2021;148(15)
10. Moore K, Persaud TVN. Clinical embryology. 8th ed. Barcelona: Elsevier; 2008. p. 522.
11. Toro-Tobon S, Manrique M, Paredes-Gutierrez J, Mantilla-Rivas E, et al. Pharyngeal arches, chapter 1: Normal development and derivatives. J Craniofac Surg. 2023;34(7)

Chapter 11
Anatomy of the Nervous System

Luz Amparo Arias-López

1 Head and Neck

Head and neck neuroanatomy is fundamental in the practice of neural therapy medicine, as it allows an understanding of the nerve pathways and structures essential for the modulation of physiological responses and the restoration of homeostasis in the patient's body.

From the first anatomical studies since the renaissance to modern imaging techniques, knowledge of neuroanatomy has transformed therapeutic intervention strategies in the craniocervical region, allowing safer and more effective approaches in the practice of neural therapy.

A precise anatomical approach allows the neuraltherapist to identify structures such as the upper cervical ganglion or the trigeminal nerve, in interventions aimed at improving the neural response and reducing symptoms related to certain dysfunctions.

1.1 Trigeminal Nerve Anatomy: V CP

The trigeminal nerve is the main sensory nerve of the face and has motor function for the muscles of mastication [1]. Its importance in neural therapy lies in its wide distribution and in the specific points where it can be addressed therapeutically.

L. A. Arias-López (✉)
Faculty of Medicine, Morphology Department, Master in Human Morphology, Universidad Nacional de Colombia, Bogotá, Colombia
e-mail: luaariaslo@unal.edu.co

L. B. Pinilla Bonilla et al. (eds.), *Neuraltherapeutic Medicine*,
https://doi.org/10.1007/978-3-032-03257-7_11

1.1.1 Origin and Location

The nerve emerges over the mid-lateral aspect of the pons or pons with a large sensory root and a smaller motor root. It has a large sensory ganglion called the semilunar or trigeminal ganglion, or Gasser's ganglion, which is located near the apex of the petrous portion of the temporal bone in the middle cranial fossa. The sensory axons form the three major divisions: the ophthalmic branch known as V1, the maxillary ramus as V2, and the mandibular ramus as V3. Motor root axons travel with the mandibular division (Fig. 11.1) [2].

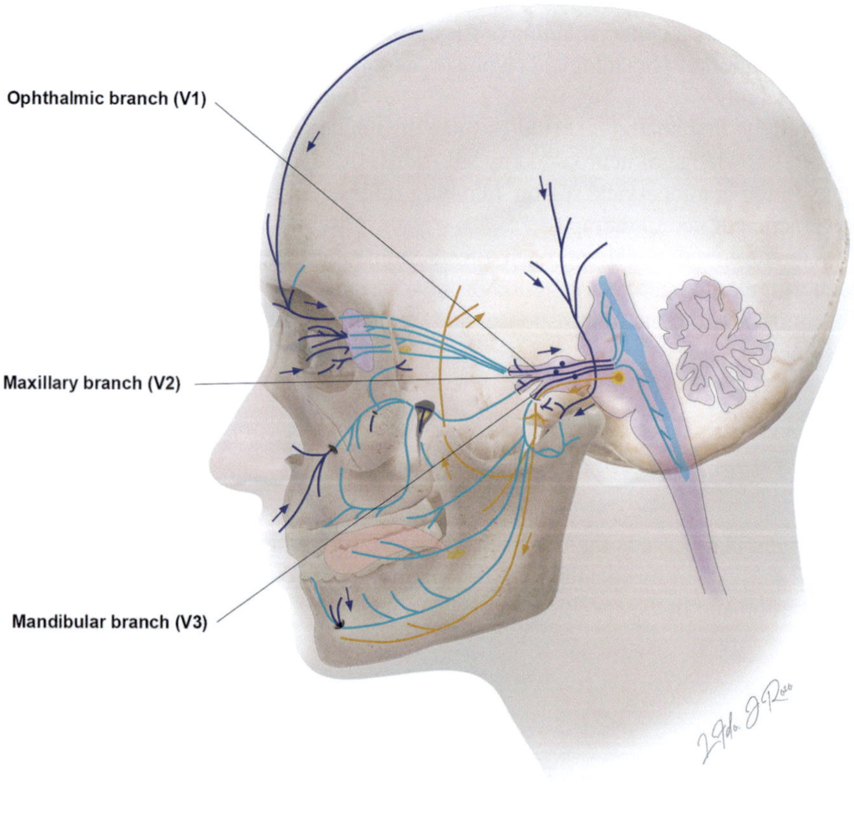

Fig. 11.1 Overview of the trigeminal nerve. (Source: Adapted from [3]. Illustration by Luis Fernando Jaimes)

1.1.2 Branches and Trajectories

The ophthalmic division of the trigeminal nerve (V1) penetrates the lateral septum of the cavernous sinus, where it divides into its three terminal branches: frontal, nasociliar, and lacrimal. These branches enter the orbit through the superior orbital fissure (Fig. 11.2) [2, 3].

The frontal nerve runs along the lateral part of the superior orbital fissure, located outside the common tendon ring or Zinn's ring. It then follows the path of the upper wall of the orbit and, when it reaches the orbital rim, divides into the supratrochlear nerve and the supraorbital nerve. The supratrochlear nerve provides sensory innervation to the forehead, nose, and upper eyelid. On the other hand, the supraorbital nerve crosses the supraorbital incision and ascends under the skin of the forehead, innervating its anterior region [4, 5].

The nasociliary or nasal nerve, upon entering the orbit, passes through the common tendon ring and bifurcates in the medial wall. Some of its collateral branches go to the ciliary ganglion, forming the sensory root of this ganglion; others project toward the eyeball as long ciliary nerves; and others are distributed to the mucosa of the ethmoid and sphenoid sinuses [5]. Finally, the nasociliary nerve gives rise to two terminal branches: the anterior ethmoidal nerve and the infratrochlear nerve. The former runs through the anterior ethmoidal canal, reaches the upper part of the cribriform plate of the ethmoid, crosses it, and enters the nasal cavity to provide sensory innervation to the mucosa of its lateral walls. The infratrochlear nerve remains in the orbit and innervates the mucosa of the tear ducts [3, 4, 6].

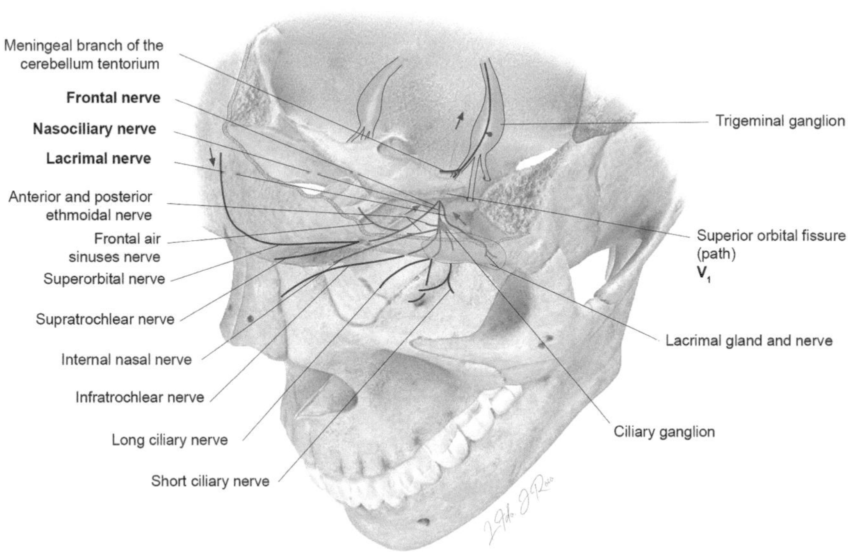

Fig. 11.2 Ophthalmic division of the trigeminal nerve. (Source: Adapted from [3]. Illustration by Luis Fernando Jaimes)

The lacrimal nerve enters the orbit and is located lateral to the common tendon ring. Along its lateral orbital path, it emits a communicating branch with the zygomatic nerve, which participates in the innervation of the lacrimal gland. However, it is essential to point out that this nerve, derived from the ophthalmic division (V1) of the trigeminal, does not have a secretomotor function. The regulation of tear secretion depends on the facial nerve (VII), through fibers that originate in the pterygopalatine ganglion [7, 8].

1.1.3 Ciliary Ganglion

The ciliary ganglion is located on the lateral aspect of the optic nerve and presents variability in its size and morphology. Its functional components include afferent fibers from the sensory root of the ciliary ganglion, which is a branch of the nasociliary nerve (V1), as well as parasympathetic fibers from the oculomotor nerve root (III) and sympathetic fibers with dilating motor function of the iris, which originate in the internal carotid plexus [6]. From this ganglion emerge the short ciliary nerves, which go directly to the eyeball (Fig. 11.3).

The maxillary nerve, the second division of the trigeminal nerve (V2), is exclusively sensory. It crosses the middle cranial fossa in an anteroinferior direction and leaves the skull through the greater foramen teres. Subsequently, it crosses the pterygopalatine fossa and projects forward, entering the orbit through the inferior orbital fissure. Its journey continues through the infraorbital canal until it emerges through

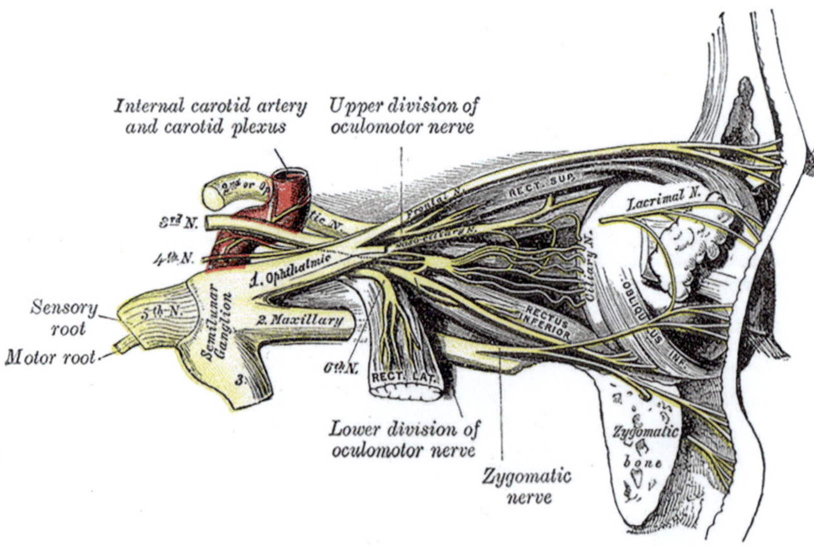

Fig. 11.3 The ciliary ganglion, its connections, and its relationship with the optic nerve are shown. (Source: Taken from [9])

the infraorbital foramen on the face, where its terminal branches are arranged in a fan-shape [8, 10].

Among its main collateral branches are the zygomatic, superior alveolar, and palatine nerves, as well as minor branches such as the meningeal and pharyngeal nerves. The zygomatic nerve arises in the pterygopalatine fossa next to the maxillary nerve and ascends to the orbit, where it runs along the lateral wall and is connected to the lacrimal nerve by a communicating branch. Subsequently, it is divided into two main branches: zygoticofacial and zygomatotemporal (Fig. 11.4) [4].

The branches of the superior alveolar nerve pierce the tuberosity of the maxilla, providing innervation to the roots of the upper molars and sending fibers to the maxillary sinus. The anterior superior alveolar branches originate in the infraorbital canal and are distributed toward the maxillary incisors and canines, leading sensory afferents related to dental pain [9].

1.1.4 Pterygopalatine Ganglion

The pterygopalatine ganglion, of cranial parasympathetic origin, is located in the pterygopalatine fossa and is associated with the maxillary nerve. Its main function is the regulation of tear and vasomotor secretion from the nasal cavities (Fig. 11.5) [10, 11]. This control is exerted by the pterygoid canal nerve, which results from the convergence of the greater petrosal nerve (derived from the facial nerve) and the deep petrosal nerve, which carries sympathetic fibers from the internal carotid plexus.

The mandibular nerve (V3) is the only mixed division of the trigeminal, as it has a wide and short sensory root and a more extensive motor root [13]. Both roots cross

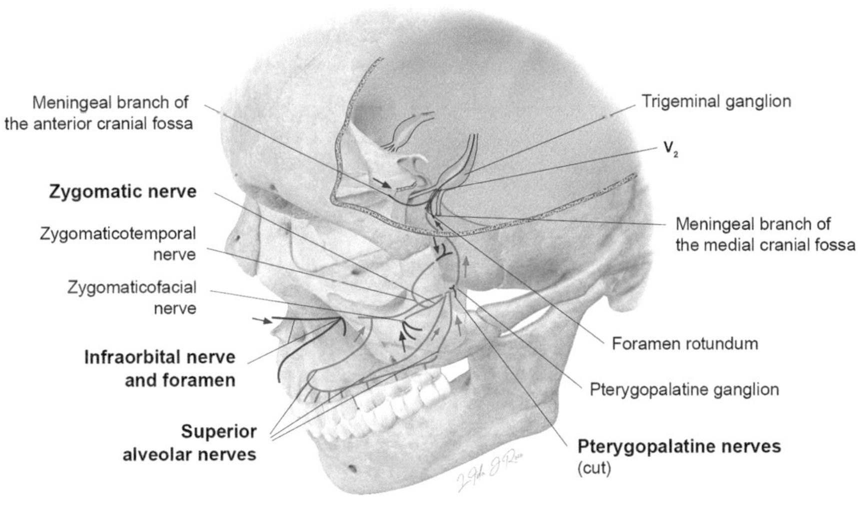

Fig. 11.4 Maxillary division of the trigeminal nerve. (Source: Adapted from [3]. Illustration by Luis Fernando Jaimes)

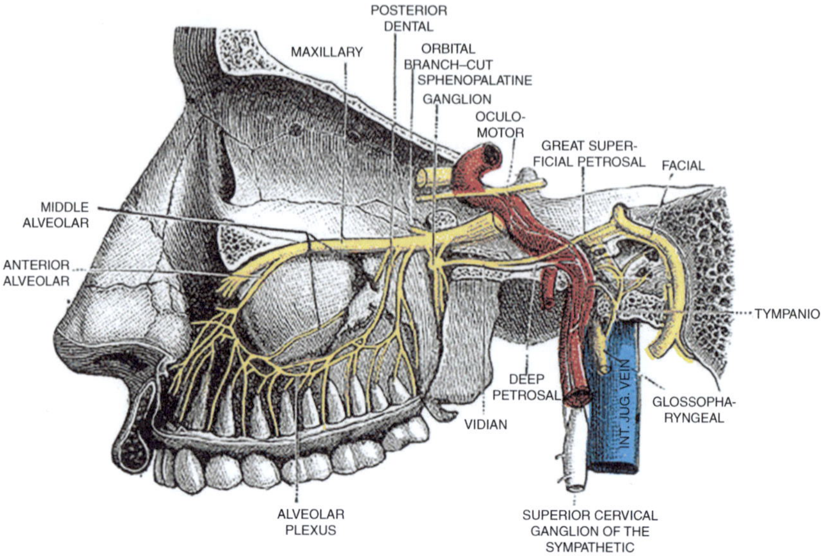

Fig. 11.5 The pterygopalatine ganglion is shown within the pterygopalatine fossa. (Source: Taken from [12])

the foramen ovale to enter the infratemporal fossa. In this region, the main nerve trunk emits meningeal branches that return to the skull through the spinous foramen along with the middle meningeal artery. It also originates a motor branch for the medial pterygoid muscle (Fig. 11.6).

Subsequently, the mandibular nerve divides into two trunks:

- *Anterior trunk*: Smaller in volume and mainly motor function. From this are detached the masseterine, deep temporal, and lateral pterygoid nerves, which innervate the homonymous muscles. It also originates a sensory branch, the buccal nerve, which carries sensory information from the gums and cheek mucosa.
- *Posterior trunk*: Larger in volume, it emits the auriculotemporal nerve, the inferior alveolar nerve, and the lingual nerve.

The auriculotemporal nerve arises from two roots surrounding the middle meningeal artery and runs toward the neck of the mandibular condyle. After penetrating the parotid gland, it ascends through the temporal region next to the superficial temporal artery, innervating the skin in this area [13, 14].

The mixed-function inferior alveolar nerve descends between the pterygoid muscles and enters the mandibular canal along with the inferior alveolar artery. It provides sensitivity to the posterior dental roots and even the canine, in addition to emitting lower gingival branches for the gums. Its terminal branch, the mental nerve, emerges from the mental foramen and is distributed in the skin of the chin and lower lip [2, 5, 6, 15, 16].

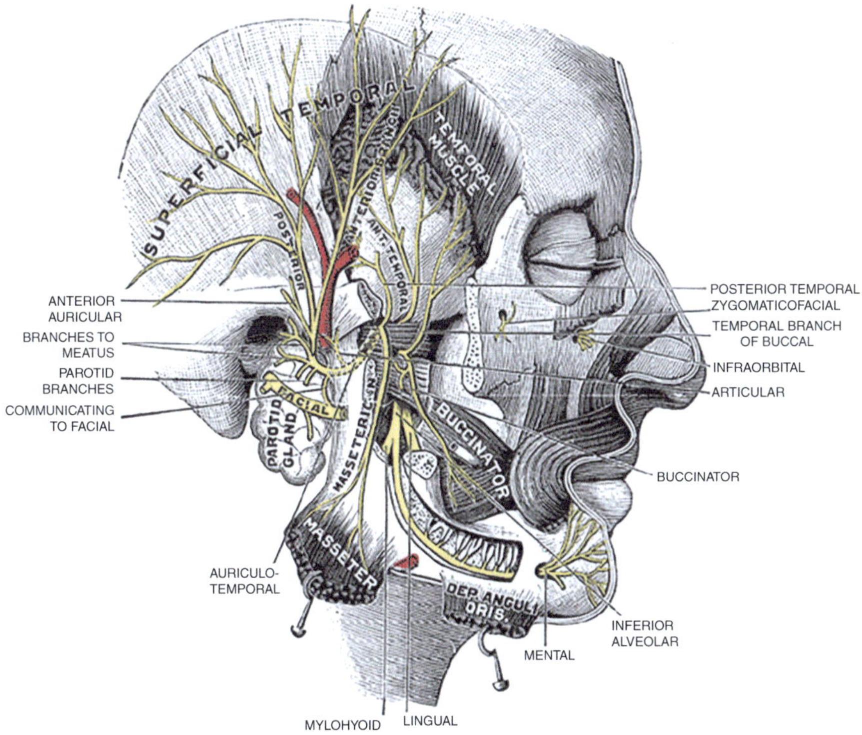

Fig. 11.6 Mandibular division of the trigeminal nerve, its trunks and branches. (Source: Taken from [17])

1.1.5 Otic Ganglion

It is a small nerve mass located below the foramen ovale and medial to the mandibular nerve. Its afferent branches come from the mandibular nerve, while its visceral efferents arrive through the lesser petrosal nerve—the glossopharyngeal nerve—and a sympathetic plexus root around the middle meningeal artery (Fig. 11.7). The efferent fibers of the ganglion are directed to the parotid gland via the auriculotemporal nerve [2, 4, 5, 8].

1.1.6 Submandibular Ganglion

This ganglion is connected to the lingual nerve by small nerve fillets. It receives sympathetic fibers from the periarterial plexus of the facial artery, as well as communicating branches with the chorda tympani nerve (the facial nerve) and with the hypoglossal nerve on the floor of the mouth (Fig. 11.7) [2, 11].

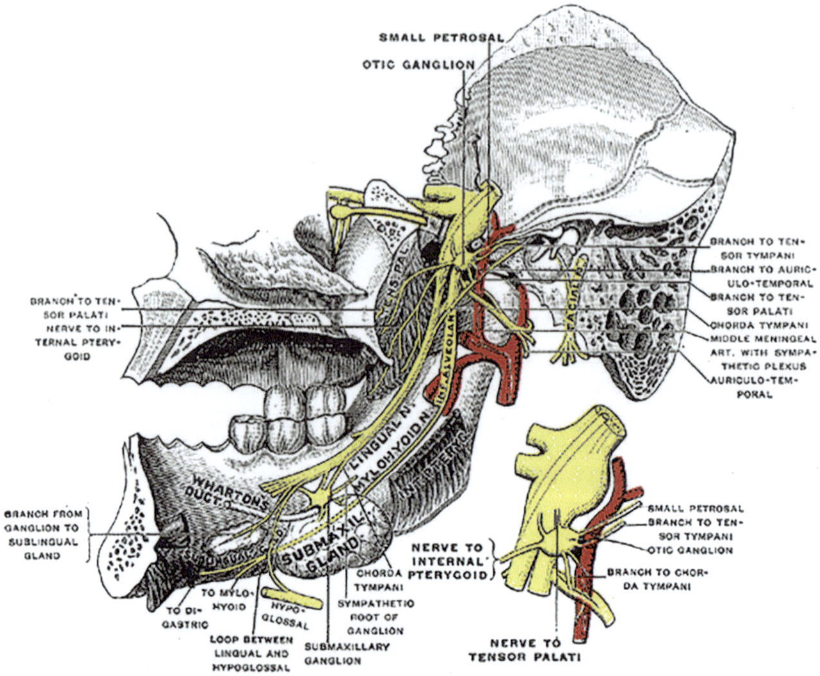

Fig. 11.7 Mandibular division of the trigeminal nerve with the otic ganglion and submandibular ganglion is observed. (Source: Taken from [18])

1.2 *Facial Nerve Anatomy: VII PC*

The facial nerve, also known as the seventh cranial nerve (VII CP), is a mixed nerve with motor, sensory, and autonomic functions.

1.2.1 Origin and Location

The facial nerve has a complex anatomical path. It originates in the brainstem, at the level of the pons, and extends through the temporal bone, crossing the duct of the facial until its exit through the stylomastoid foramen. From this point, it is widely distributed on the face, innervating muscles essential for facial expression, as well as salivary glands, the lacrimal gland, and areas of the tongue and soft palate [3, 19, 20] (Fig. 11.8).

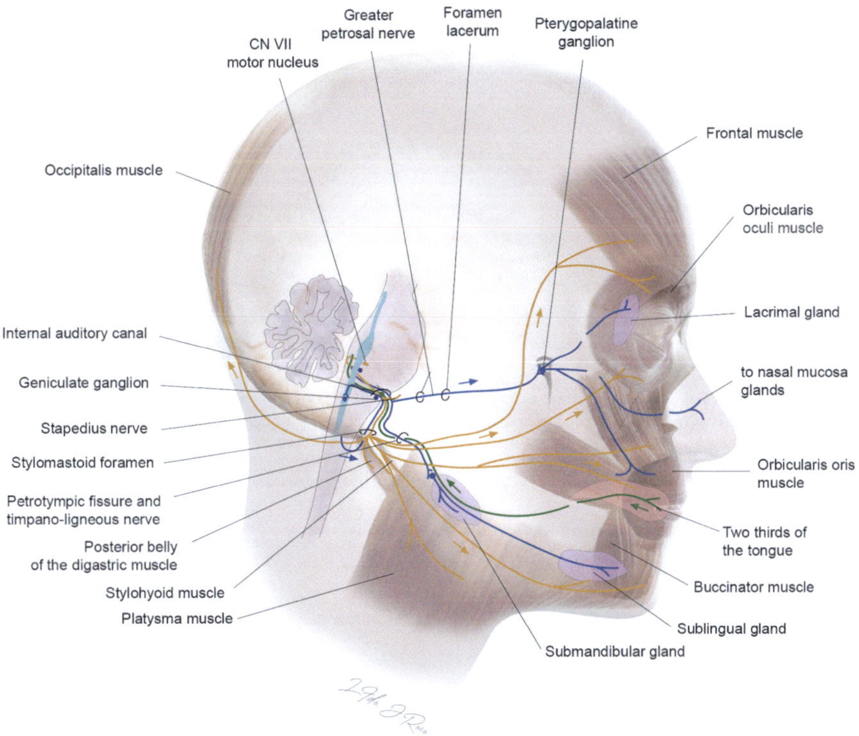

Fig. 11.8 Facial nerve and its functional components. (Source: Adapted from [3]. Illustration by Luis Fernando Jaimes)

1.2.2 Branches and Trajectory

The axons of the general, special sensory, and parasympathetic motor components form the intermediate nerve, which leaves the brainstem at the bulboprotuberance junction, lateral to the motor axons. Within the internal auditory canal, the intermediate nerve joins with the motor axons in the facial canal, where the facial nerve abruptly changes direction forming the facial knee. This site is home to the geniculate ganglion, where general and special sensory neurons reside [2, 3, 5, 7].

From the geniculate ganglion, the facial nerve gives rise to several branches (Fig. 11.9):

- *Major petrosal nerve*: It transports parasympathetic information to the lacrimal gland and the oral, pharyngeal, and nasal mucous glands, as well as sensory fibers of taste from the soft palate.
- *Nerve for the stapes muscle*: It arises in the vertical portion of the facial canal and innervates the stapes muscle in the middle ear.
- *Chordaus nerve of the eardrum*: It crosses the cavity of the middle ear and emerges in the infratemporal fossa through the petrotympanic fissure. It attaches

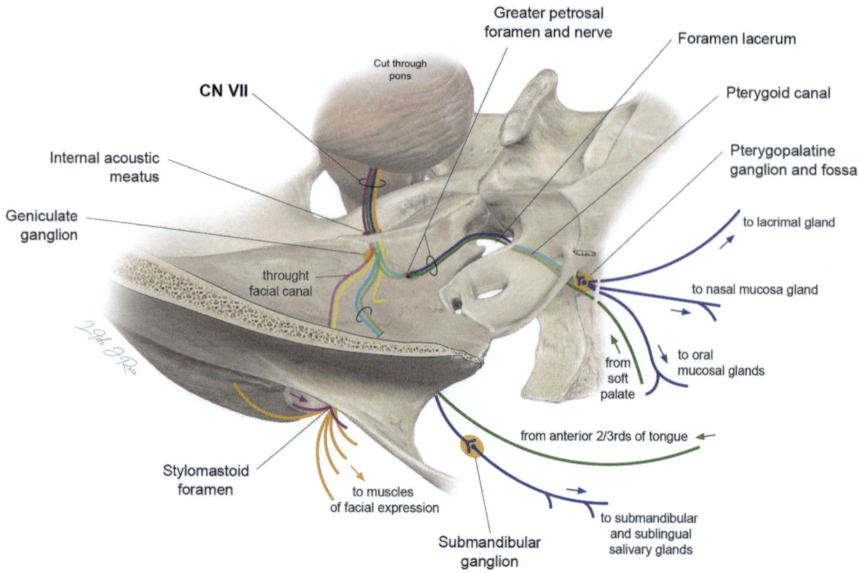

Fig. 11.9 Branches of the facial nerve from the geniculate ganglion. (Source: Adapted from [3]. Illustration by Luis Fernando Jaimes)

to the lingual nerve (branch of the V CP) to carry taste sensations from the anterior two-thirds of the tongue and parasympathetic motor fibers directed to the sublingual and submandibular salivary glands.

The rest of the general sensory and motor axons continue their journey down the posterior wall of the tympanic cavity to the stylomastoid foramen, where the facial nerve emerges and gives rise to several branches:

- *Posterior auricular nerve*: Targets the occipital muscle and carries general sensitivity of the pinna, external ear canal, and tympanic membrane.
- *Branches for the stylohyoid and posterior belly of the digastric*: they innervate these muscles.

Within the parotid gland, the facial nerve divides into two main trunks:

- *Temporofacial trunk*: originates the temporal, zygomatic branches and a branch communicating with the oral nerve of the facial.
- *Cervicofacial trunk*: gives rise to the buccal, mandibular, and cervical branches, responsible for the innervation of the facial muscles [3, 8, 20].

Once the main nerves of the head have been described, the components of the cranial nerves that reach the neck will be reviewed.

1.3 Glossopharyngeal Nerve: IX PC

1.3.1 Origin and Location

The glossopharyngeal nerve originates in the dorsolateral sulcus of the medulla oblongata, behind the olive, in association with the vagus nerve (X) and the accessory nerve (XI). Its journey begins through the jugular foramen or posterior tear, where it has two ganglia: one superior and one inferior. Subsequently, it descends adjacent to the pharyngeal wall, between the superior and middle constrictor muscles, until it reaches the oral cavity, distributing itself in the pharynx and the posterior portion of the tongue [2, 4].

1.4 Branches and Functional Components

The glossopharyngeal nerve contains motor fibers directed to the stylopharyngeal muscle, general sensory fibers for the mucosa of the nasopharynx and oropharynx, the pharyngotympanic tube (which connects the pharynx to the middle ear), the middle ear cavity, and the posterior third of the tongue. In addition, it carries taste fibers (special sensitivity) destined for the posterior portion of the tongue and parasympathetic fibers directed to the parotid gland as well as to the carotid body and sinus [2, 4, 8] (Fig. 11.10).

The branches of the IX cranial nerve reflect their different functional components. Among them, the tympanic nerve (Jacobson's) emerges at the level of the jugular foramen and enters the tympanic cage to innervate structures of the middle ear and pharyngotympanic tube. It also emits a branch to the carotid body and sinus, in relation to the bifurcation of the common carotid arteries. It also provides pharyngeal branches that innervate the nasopharynx and oropharynx, as well as branches destined for the palatal tonsil and the dorsal portion of the tongue. The only motor branch of the glossopharyngeal nerve is the one that goes to the stylopharyngeal muscle.

1.5 Vagus Nerve or Pneumogastric: X PC

The word vagus comes from vagabond that characterizes those who spend their time traveling and in the case of the vagus nerve it bears that name because it is the cranial nerve that is most widely distributed throughout the body. So much so, that the X PC goes to the neck, chest, and abdomen, and carries the sensory, parasympathetic, and motor innervation from the intestinal tract to the transverse colon. It is called pneumogastric because it will innervate the organs of the respiratory ventilatory system and a large part of the digestive system.

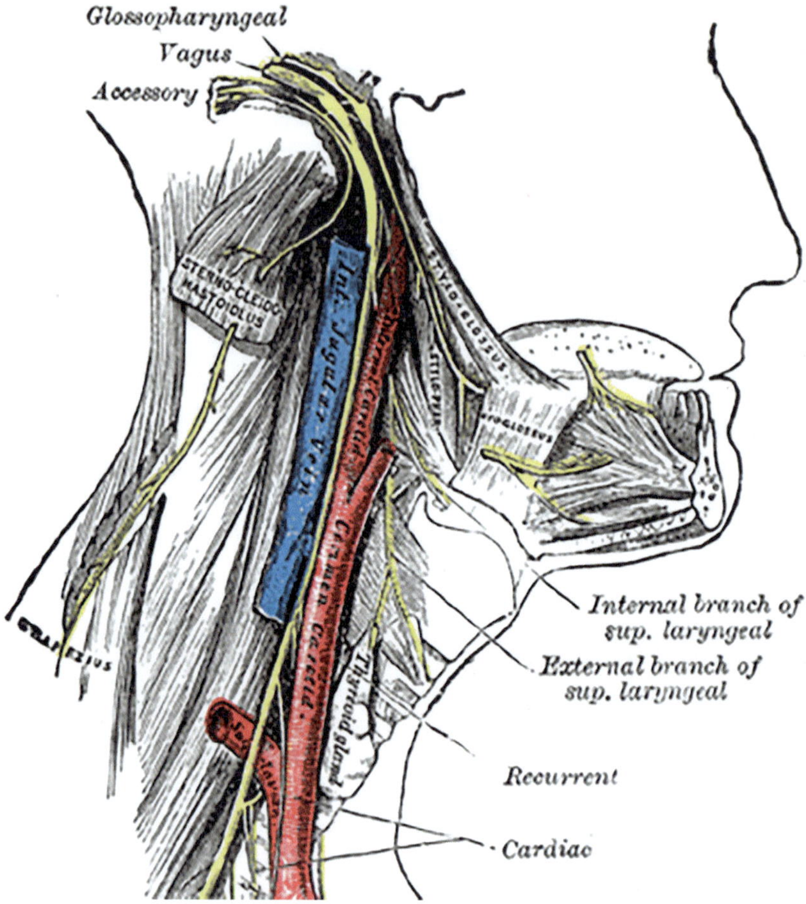

Fig. 11.10 Glossopharyngeal nerve entering the pharynx between the superior and median constrictor muscle and in its relationship with the styloglossus muscle. (Source: Adapted from [21])

1.5.1 Origin and Location

The nerve originates in the dorsolateral sulcus of the medulla oblongata, then emerges through the jugular foramen accompanied by cranial nerves IX and XI. At its exit, the vagus nerve has two sensory ganglia, superior and inferior. It enters the carotid sheath and accompanies the common carotid artery, the internal jugular vein, and the internal carotid artery, forming the vasculonervous bundle of the neck. It is located posteriorly between the internal jugular vein and carotid artery within the sheath. In the neck, it descends vertically and then passes to the chest between the vein and the subclavian artery (Fig. 11.11).

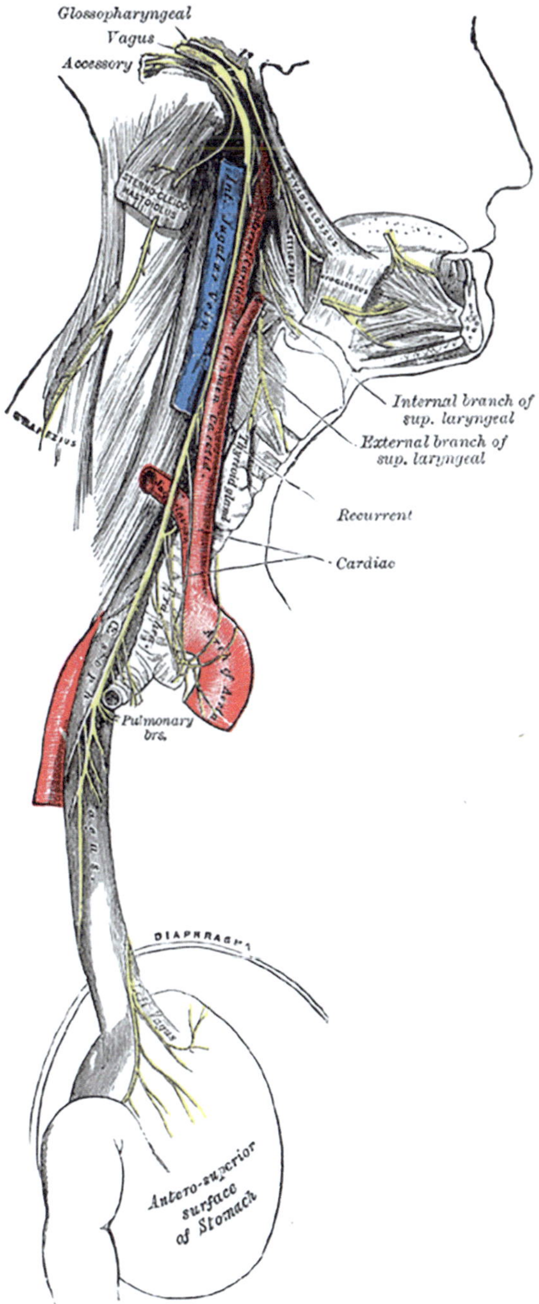

Fig. 11.11 Pneumogastric or vagus nerve, its location, and its functional components. (Source: Taken from [21])

1.5.2 Branches and Functional Components

The vagus nerve is motor for the muscles of the larynx, all the muscles of the pharynx (except the stylopharyngeal), and all the muscles of the palate (except the tensor of the soft palate). In addition, it provides motor innervation to the muscles from the esophagus to the transverse colon.

In terms of sensory distribution, the vagus nerve innervates the larynx, laryngopharynx, trachea, and esophagus to the transverse colon. Its taste function is limited and only covers the posterior region of the tongue. In young children, there may also be gustatory innervation in the palate and pharynx due to the presence of taste corpuscles, which disappear in adulthood. Its parasympathetic component is directed to the viscera up to the transverse colon.

The vagus nerve originates several branches:

- *Meningeal nerve*: Sensitively innervates the meninges of the posterior cerebral fossa.
- *Atrial branch*: Provides sensory innervation to the external ear canal.
- *Pharyngeal branches*: They contain motor fibers for the pharyngeal muscles and additional sensory fibers.
- *Carotid branches for the body and sinus*: Involved in cardiovascular regulation.

The superior laryngeal nerve is divided into two branches:

- *Internal laryngeal nerve*: It enters the larynx through a hole in the thyrohyoid membrane and provides sensory innervation to the laryngeal vestibule and ventricle.
- *External laryngeal nerve*: It innervates the cricothyroid muscle.

The inferior or recurrent laryngeal nerve is mixed and contains motor fibers for all muscles of the larynx except the cricothyroid. Its recurring branches have different origins on each side of the body:

On the left side, it descends to the aortic arch and then ascends the tracheoesophageal groove to the larynx. On the right side, it originates at the level of the subclavian artery and follows a similar path to the larynx.

Recurrent nerves cross the inferior thyroid artery before entering the larynx, where they provide sensory innervation to the glottis and infraglottic cavity [22] (Fig. 11.12).

From the vagus nerve in the neck also emerge 2 to 3 parasympathetic cardiac nerves to contribute to the formation of the cardiac plexus with contributions from the cardiac nerves of the sympathetic chain.

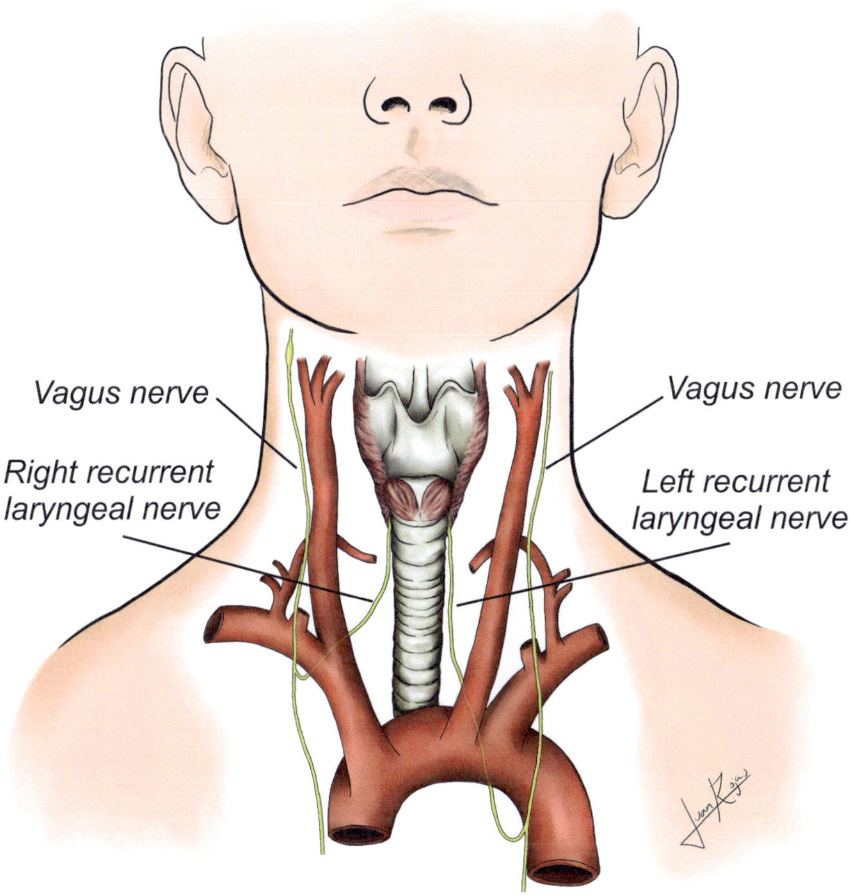

Fig. 11.12 Left and right recurrent laryngeal nerves, posterior view. (Source: Adapted from [23]. Illustrated by Juan Rojas-Arias)

1.6 Spinal or Accessory Nerve: XI PC

1.6.1 Origin and Location

The accessory nerve originates like its two predecessors in the dorsolateral sulcus of the medulla oblongata. It has two roots, the cranial root originating from the ambiguous nucleus of the vagus nerve and a spinal root originating from the medullary nucleus of the superior portion of the spinal cord from C1 to C6. The spinal root ascends to the skull through the foramen magnus and joins the cranial root, the two roots together exiting the skull through the jugular foramen (Fig. 11.13).

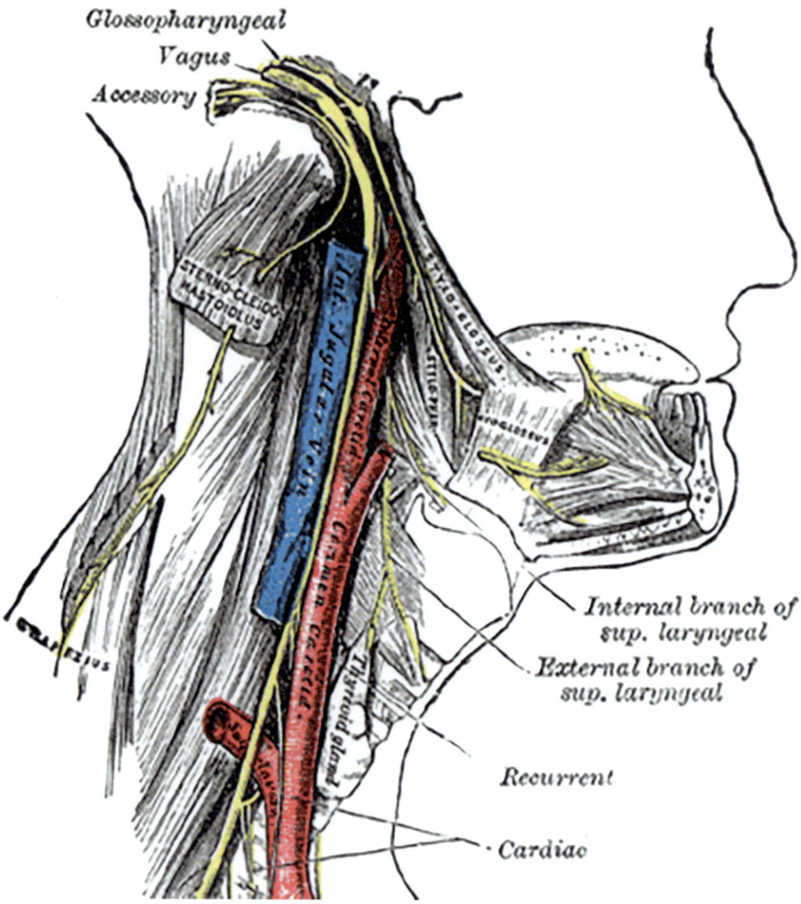

Fig. 11.13 Accessory or spinal nerve crossing the sternocleidomastoid and trapezius muscles to which it provides motor efferents. (Source: Adapted from [21])

1.6.2 Branches and Functional Components

Once the nerve comes out of the jugular foramen, the two roots separate again. The spinal root is directed toward the sternocleidomastoid muscles (ECM) and trapezius for motor innervation, while the cranial root separates and joins and distributes with the vagus nerve.

The accessory or spinal nerve exits the jugular foramen, crosses behind the vasculonervous bundle of the neck, reaches the deep aspect of the ECM, crosses the ECM, and gives a branch that crosses the occipital triangle and will innervate the trapezius muscle [2, 8, 11].

1.7 Hypoglossal Nerve: XII PC

It is a specifically motor nerve and its innervation is exclusive to the muscles of the tongue except for the palatoglossus muscle which is innervated by the vagus nerve. The hypoglossal nerve is related to the internal carotid artery, external carotid artery, and lingual artery. The hypoglossal nerve crosses into the lingual artery (Fig. 11.14).

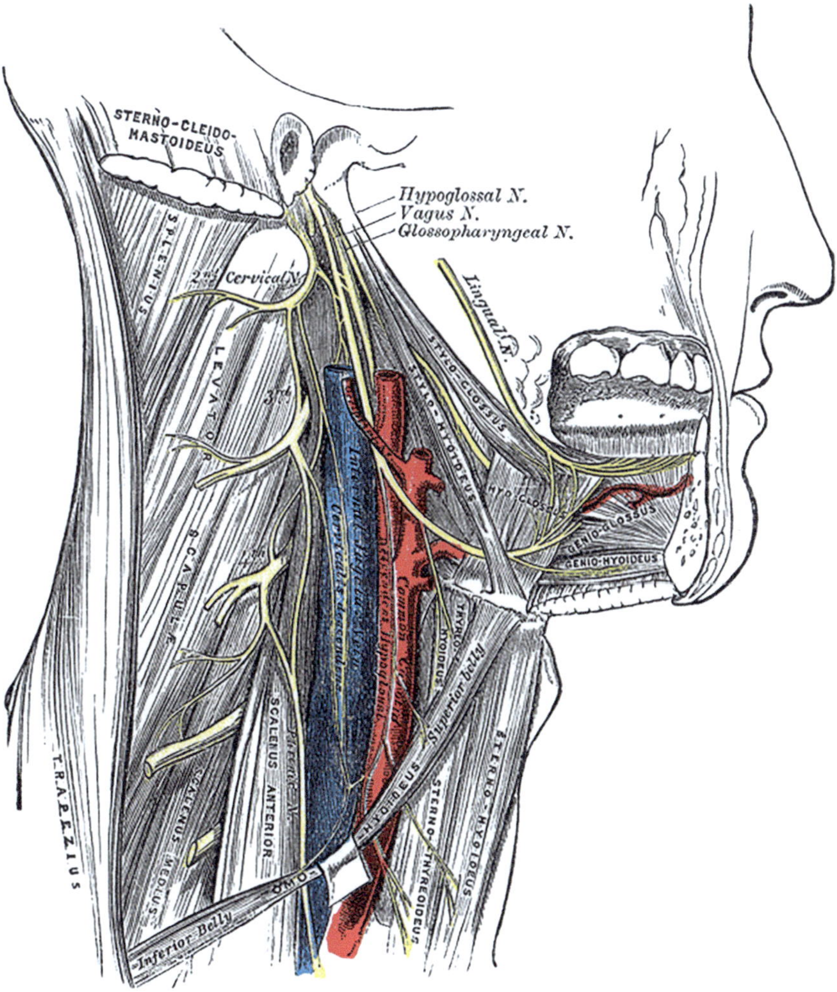

Fig. 11.14 Hypoglossal nerve crossing the lingual artery. (Source: Adapted from [24])

1.7.1 Origin and Location

The hypoglossal nerve exits through the duct of the anterior hypoglossal or foramen condylarus, between the occipital condyle and the occipital bone, exits behind all the elements, crosses behind the internal carotid artery and then is located between the internal jugular vein and the internal carotid artery, makes an arch toward the mouth and passes medially to the internal jugular vein, It is there where it crosses the carotids and the lingual artery and then heads toward the tongue. The hypoglossal nerve is accompanied by a branch of C1 that goes to the genihyoid and thyrohyoid muscles [11].

1.7.2 Cervical Plexus

The cervical plexus is made up of anterior roots of the spinal nerves from C1 to C4. These roots are in the paravertebral region in front of the middle scalene. The cervical plexus gives deep medial and lateral branches that are mixed, sensory, and motor. In addition, it gives superficial branches that are exclusively sensitive (Fig. 11.15).

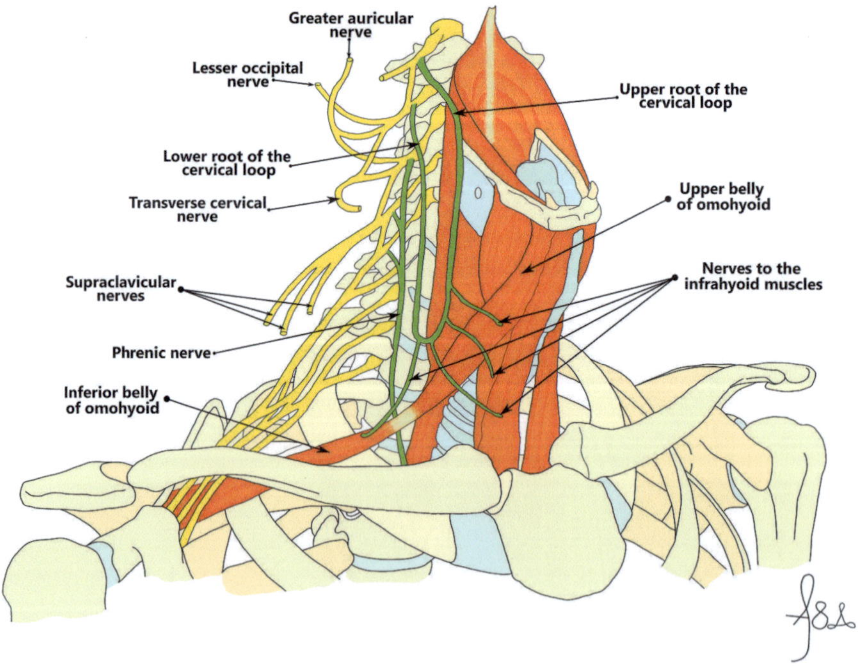

Fig. 11.15 Cervical plexus with its medial and lateral branches. Likewise, the cervical loop is shown. (Source: Adapted from [11]. Illustrated by Angélica Ochoa)

1.7.3 Deep Branches

- The deep branches of the cervical plexus are divided into lateral and medial branches. Deep lateral branches include:
- The communicating branch with the spinal nerve.
- The branch for sternocleidomastoid muscle (ECM).
- The branch for the trapezius muscle.
- The branch for the middle scalene muscle.
- The branch for the levator scapula muscle.

The branch that innervates the ECM and trapezius is a proprioceptive branch, since the motor innervation of these muscles comes from the accessory nerve (XI cranial nerve) [1, 2]. Similarly, the levator scapula muscle receives motor innervation from the brachial plexus, but proprioceptive innervation is supplied by the cervical plexus [3, 4].

Medial deep branches include:

Communicating branches for the vagus (X) and hypoglossal (XII) nerves, as well as for the cervical sympathetic chain.

Mixed branches for the prevertebral muscles, such as the long head muscle and the long neck muscle.

The lower branch of the cervical loop.

The phrenic nerve (C3–C5), the main motor nerve of the diaphragm [5].

The phrenic nerve is considered the most important nerve of the cervical plexus due to its function in ventilatory movements [6]. It descends over the anterior scalene muscle, is located between the subclavian (posterior) artery and the subclavian (anterior) vein, and enters the thorax until it reaches the diaphragm [7, 8].

- *The cervical loop* is a fundamental structure in the innervation of the infrahyoid muscles. It is also known as loop of the hypoglossus, because its upper root seems to originate from the hypoglossal nerve; however, this root comes from C1 and not from the hypoglossus [9, 10]. The cervical loop is formed from the anterior branches of C1 to C3, organized into two roots:
- *Top root*: It is formed by C1 fibers.
- *Lower root*: It is formed by C2 and C3 fibers.

Both roots join together to form a loop-like structure that innervates the omohyoid, sternothyroid, and sternohyoid muscles. The cervical loop is superficial to the carotid sheath [11].

1.7.4 Superficial Branches

The superficial branches of the cervical plexus are exclusively sensory and are located between the platysma muscle and the posterior border of the ECM [1, 2].

- *Minor occipital nerve (C2)*: It ascends laterally, passing behind the ECM from Erb's point (nerve point of the neck) to the occipital and posterolateral area of the head, located behind the ear [3]. It provides sensory innervation to the scalp skin in the lateral and posterior occipital region, as well as to a small portion of the pinna. This nerve has clinical relevance, as it may be involved in occipital neuralgia, a condition that causes severe pain in the back of the head [4, 5].

- *Transverse cervical nerve (C3):* It crosses the superficial aspect of the ECM in the anterior direction and, upon reaching the anterior border of the muscle, divides into ascending and descending branches. Its terminal branches perforate the platysma and innervate the skin of the supra- and infrahyoid regions [6, 7].
- *Greater auricular nerve (C2–C3):* It surrounds the posterior border of the ECM and ascends toward the pinna, accompanied by the external jugular vein. It gives sensitive branches for the parotid gland and the skin of the ear and angle of the jaw [8, 9].
- *Supraclavicular nerves (C4)*: They cross the supraclavicular region and sensitively innervate the skin of the shoulder, the pectoralis major muscle, and the skin over the sternum [10, 11].

1.7.5 Cervical Sympathetic System

The cervical sympathetic system is the upper portion of the sympathetic trunk and is part of the autonomic nervous system, responsible for regulating involuntary functions such as vasoconstriction, sweating, and pupillary dilation in the head and neck. The cervical sympathetic system is composed of a chain of ganglia located laterally to the spine in the neck and communicates with other sympathetic segments to facilitate the "fight or flight" response in this region. It is formed by a nerve trunk that descends in front of the cervical spine, anterior to the transverse processes or slightly lateral to them. It descends vertically to the thorax and there continues with the thoracic sympathetic chain [3, 4].

1.7.6 Cervical Sympathetic Ganglia

The sympathetic chain in turn has three cervical sympathetic ganglia, the superior cervical ganglion or magnum, is the largest, it is located at the level of C1 to C2, it is immediately inferior to the carotid duct and that ganglion gives rise to the internal carotid nerve which is the cranial branch of the sympathetic system that will penetrate with the internal carotid artery to the intracranium (Fig. 11.16).

The middle cervical ganglion, located at the level of the C5 and C6 vertebrae, is the smallest of the three nodes and may be absent in some people. It is related to the inferior thyroid artery [1, 5, 6].

The lower cervical ganglion may be fused with the first thoracic ganglion forming the so-called stellate ganglion. It is located near the neck of the first rib, anterior to the transverse process of C7. It is related to the first portion of the subclavian artery and to the vertebral artery in the triangle between the lateral border of the

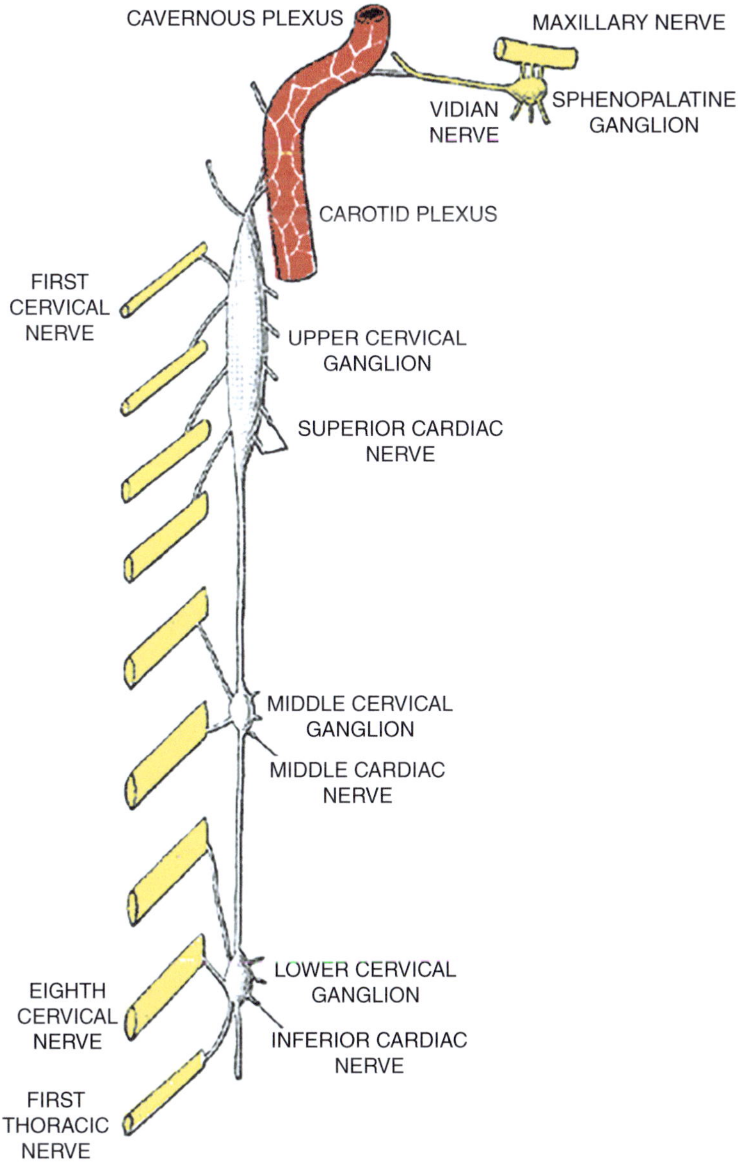

Fig. 11.16 Cervical sympathetic chain with its three sympathetic ganglia, superior or magnum, middle, and inferior. (Source: Adapted from [25])

long neck muscle, the medial border of the anterior scalene, and the first rib. A part of the chain that passes in front of the subclavian artery forms a structure called the loop of the subclavian, but it is part of the sympathetic chain [7, 8].

1.8 Branches of the Cervical Sympathetic Chain

The branches are of two types: the gray communicating branches that are sympathetic fibers that come out of the ganglia and are distributed with the peripheral nerves that come from the spinal nerves and go to the neck or upper limb, and the branches that give the ganglia to each other that are distributed together with the arteries. The medial branches that come out of the ganglia are distributed as follows: those that come out of the upper cervical ganglion go to the larynx, pharynx, cardiac branches that go to the thorax to form the cardiac plexus, branches for the common carotid, external carotid, and its branches. From the middle ganglion come postganglionic branches for the thyroid gland, cardiac branch for the cardiac plexus, and branches for the esophagus and trachea. The inferior ganglion also gives a cardiac branch and branches that are distributed with the branches of the subclavian artery. It is important to mention that there are no white communicating branches in the cervical region [9, 10].

2 Chest Neuroanatomy

The nervous system at the thoracic level is composed of the 12 pairs of thoracic spinal nerves, which are distributed without forming plexuses and mainly constitute the intercostal nerves. These nerves correspond to the anterior branches of the thoracic spinal nerves, are mixed in nature, and are numbered according to the overlying rib [2, 4, 6, 8].

From the exit of the intervertebral foramen, the spinal nerve bifurcates and the tape-shaped anterior ramus penetrates the intercostal space in front and is then located between the intimal and internal intercostal muscles. The nerve follows the thoracic concavity and ends at an anterior cutaneous branch that emerges near the lateral border of the sternum for the first six nerves. The next five nerves terminate in a branch that penetrates the abdominal wall anterolaterally between the oblique internus and transverse abdominis muscles.

The intercostal nerve is always accompanied by the arterial branches from the aorta or internal thoracic and by the venous vessels, constituting a vasculonervous axis that extends beyond the intercostal space. In the intercostal space the vein is more superior, then the artery follows and the nerve is more inferior [8].

The intercostal nerves give branches for the costovertebral joints and collateral branches which are the intercostal muscular branches, the rib levators and the transverse thorax, a cutaneous branch, the lateral perforator that emerges out of the intercostal space to innervate the skin of the corresponding region and gives pleural and mediastinal sensory branches. The intercostal nerves communicate with the thoracic sympathetic chain, with the brachial plexus and lumbar plexus, and with the medial brachial cutaneous nerve, through the second lateral cutaneous nerve to form the intercostobrachial nerve [9, 10].

The twelfth intercostal nerve does not occupy an intercostal space but is the subcostal nerve that passes in front of the quadratus lumborum muscle and behind the pleura, kidney, and adrenal gland, which is why it has been considered rather a lumbar nerve.

2.1 Thoracic Sympathetic Chain

It extends from the stellate ganglion at the top to the diaphragm, where it continues with the lumbar sympathetic trunk. It is a thin trunk located in the laterovertebral region, in relation to the costovertebral joints, and follows the thoracic curvature in a concave shape. This structure is attached to the skeleton by the endothoracic fascia, which separates it from the parietal pleura, and is connected to the intercostal nerves by communicating branches.

The sympathetic chain is interrupted in the middle of each vertebra by a ganglion of varying shape and size. From the seventh thoracic ganglion onward, the caliber of the chain decreases due to the formation of the splanchnic nerves. Often, the last thoracic node fuses with the first lumbar node.

2.2 Thoracic Sympathetic Chain Distribution

The thoracic sympathetic innervation is distributed through different branches:

- *Communicating branches* with the intercostal nerves emerge laterally from the sympathetic ganglia.
- *Visceral and vascular branches*, which innervate the lung (through the pulmonary plexus), esophagus, aorta, and heart (through the cardiac plexus).

In addition, the thoracic sympathetic chain provides abdominal branches through the splanchnic nerves:

- *Major splanchnic nerve*: It originates from the thoracic ganglia 7, 8, and 9, crosses the diaphragm, and goes to the celiac ganglion.
- *Lesser splanchnic nerve*: It comes from the thoracic ganglia 10 and 11, crosses the diaphragm, and ends at the celiac plexus.
- *Inferior splanchnic nerve or "imo":* It is inconstant, originating in the thoracic ganglion 12 and ending in the aorticorrenal ganglion, near the origin of the renal artery [2, 4, 8, 10, 11].

3 Neuroanatomy of the Back

The dorsum is an anatomical region that houses key neurological structures, such as the spinal cord, nerve roots, and associated neural networks. Its study is essential to understand neuromuscular physiology and pathologies that can affect mobility and sensitivity in different regions of the body [8].

The spinal cord is the main component of the central nervous system in the dorsum region and extends from the medulla oblongata to the medullary cone, at the level of L1–L2 in the adult. Its internal configuration is divided into gray matter and white matter. In the dorsal horns are the sensory neurons that receive afferent information from peripheral receptors. The bodies of the motor neurons responsible for controlling the skeletal muscles reside in the ventral horns. On the other hand, the lateral horns (present in the thoracic and upper lumbar segments) contain neurons of the sympathetic nervous system [9].

Spinal nerves emerge from the spinal cord through the intervertebral foramina and divide into dorsal and ventral branches. The dorsal branches innervate the intrinsic muscles of the dorsum and the skin of the posterior region of the trunk. The ventral branches innervate the anterolateral wall of the body and extremities [11].

4 Neuroanatomy of the Abdomen

The neuroanatomy of the abdomen comprises the structures of the nervous system that innervate the viscera and abdominal wall. This innervation is crucial for the regulation of autonomic functions such as gastrointestinal motility, glandular secretion, and visceral pain modulation. Neural control occurs through the somatic and autonomic nervous systems [1, 4].

Abdominal innervation is composed of afferent and efferent fibers from the central nervous system (CNS) and the enteric nervous system. The enteric nervous system is a network of intrinsic neurons that regulates intestinal motility and secretion autonomously, although it receives modulation from the sympathetic and parasympathetic systems. It is composed of the myenteric (Auerbach) and submucosal (Meissner) plexuses [2] (Fig. 11.18).

4.1 Somatic Innervation of the Abdomen

The abdominal wall is innervated by the intercostal nerves (T7–T11), the subcostal nerve (T12), and the iliohypogastric and ilioinguinal nerves (L1). These nerves provide skin sensitivity and motor control over the abdominal muscles [5, 6].

4.2 Sympathetic Nervous System of the Abdomen

The lumbar sympathetic chain is made up of two ganglion structures located on each side of the spine, extending from L1 to L5 within the retroperitoneal space. Its precise location is on the anterolateral border of the lumbar vertebral bodies, adjacent to the internal insertion of the psoas muscle. This sympathetic chain is separated from the lumbar somatic nerve roots by the psoas muscle itself and its fascia. As it descends, it is positioned in front of the vertebral bodies and, further down, it continues posterior to the primitive iliac vessels to integrate with the pelvic sympathetic trunk [26] (Fig. 11.17).

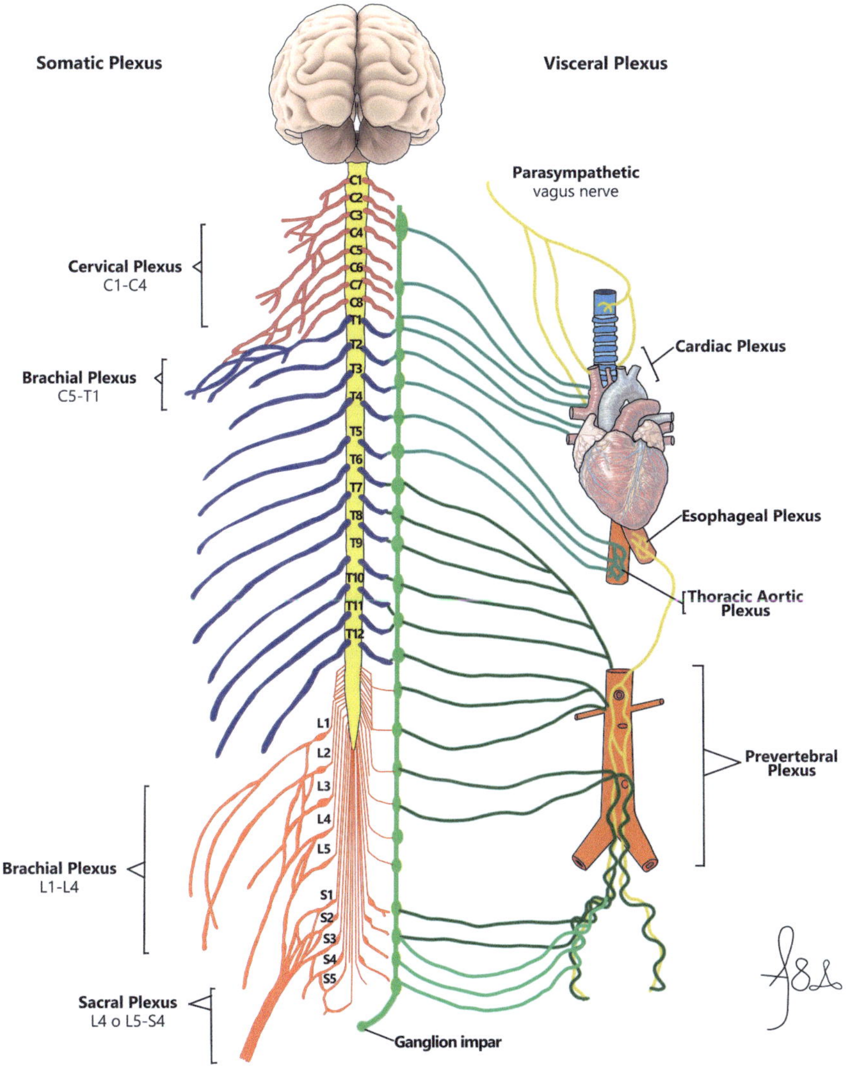

Fig. 11.17 Thoracic and abdominopelvic sympathetic chain. (Source: Adapted from [20]. Illustrated by Angélica Ochoa)

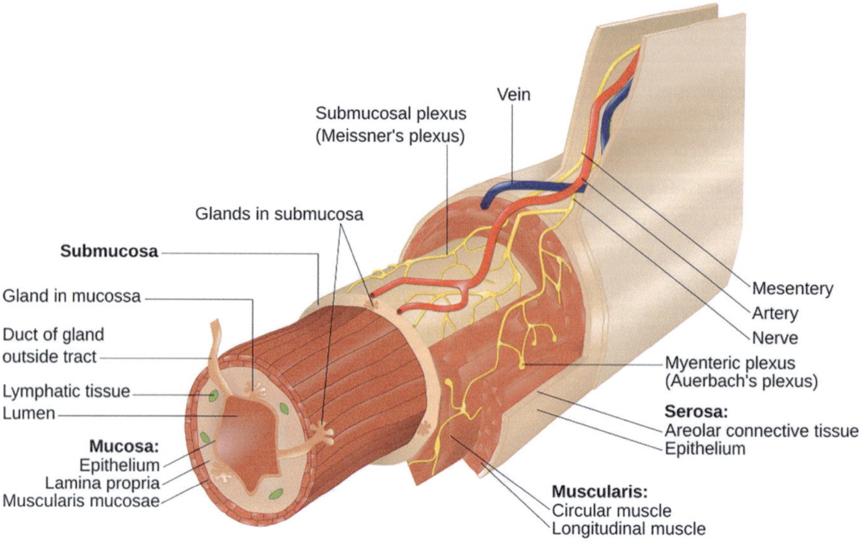

Fig. 11.18 Enteric nervous system with its myenteric and submucosal plexuses. (Source: Taken from [27])

The number of lumbar sympathetic nodes varies between four and five, depending on the fusion between the T12 and L5 ganglia. Its shape is fusiform and its size is variable. The distance between each ganglion and the transverse process of the corresponding vertebra is between 4 and 5 cm.

As for their connections, the first two lumbar sympathetic ganglia receive white communicating branches that establish contact with the corresponding spinal nerves. These branches have an oblique path and cross the fascicles of the psoas muscle. The postganglionic axons emerging from the sympathetic chain are organized in a plexus around the iliac arteries, allowing sympathetic innervation of the femoral and obturator nerves. The lumbar ganglia originate four splanchnic nerves. The first goes to the celiac plexus, the second to the intermesenteric plexus, the third crosses the primitive iliac vessels to reach the hypogastric plexus, and the fourth, coming from the inferior lumbar sympathetic ganglion, is located posterior to the primitive iliac vessels before projecting toward the pelvis. The latter also contributes fibers to the lower portion of the superior hypogastric plexus [26].

Of the four lumbar splanchnic nerves, the first two remain in the abdomen, while the last two are directed toward the pelvis. For this reason, the latter are also known as abdominal splanchnic nerves or hypogastric nerves.

4.2.1 Parasympathetic Nervous System of the Abdomen

The vagus nerve (X cranial nerve) innervates most of the gastrointestinal tract to the splenic flexure of the colon. From this point on, parasympathetic innervation comes from the sacral segments (S2–S4) via the pelvic splanchnic nerves, which regulate the function of the distal colon and pelvic viscera [4].

5 Neuroanatomy of the Pelvis and Perineum

The nerves of the pelvis are represented by the sacrococcygeal plexus, the splanchnopelvic nerves, the inferior hypogastric plexus, and the visceral plexuses. The sacrococcygeal plexus originates from the anterior branches of L4–L5, S1–S5. This plexus is responsible for providing innervation to the lower limb, pelvis, and perineum (Fig. 11.19). The pelvic branches go to the muscles that form the levator ani, coccygeus, obturator internus and piriformis and the perineal branches include the inferior rectal nerve and the pudendal nerve [5].

The **superior hypogastric plexus** (T10–L2) and the **inferior hypogastric plexus** contain sympathetic and parasympathetic fibers that regulate visceral functions such as urinary continence and intestinal motility [6].

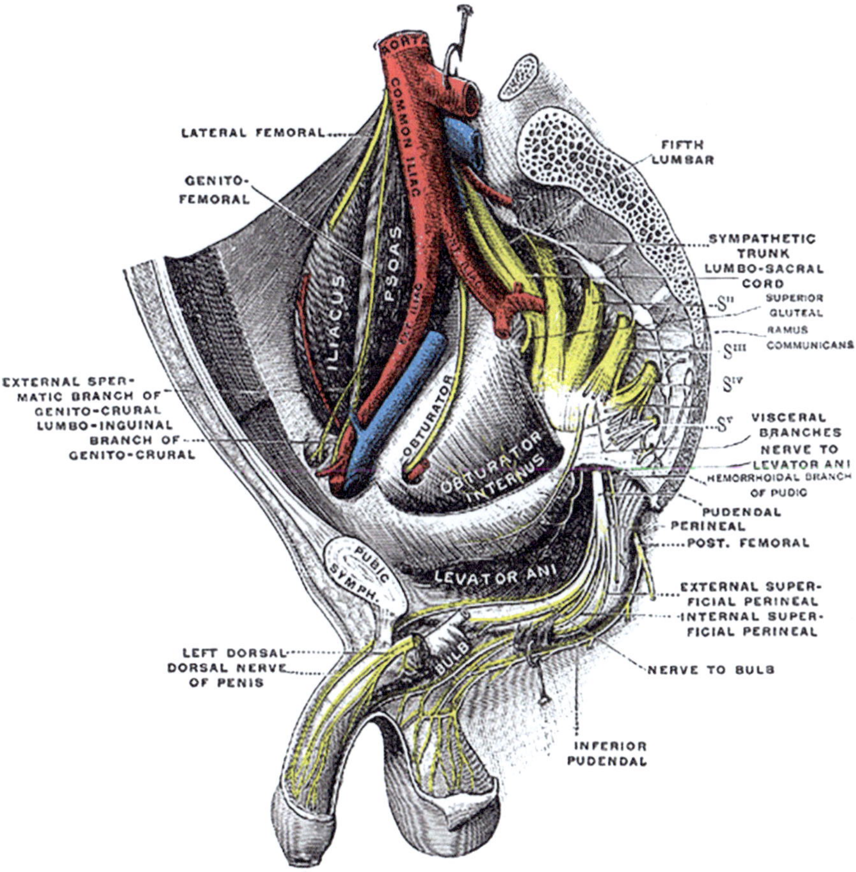

Fig. 11.19 Sacrococcygeal plexus and lumbosacral sympathetic trunk. (Source: Taken from [28])

6 Upper Limb Neuroanatomy

The upper extremity receives most of its motor and cutaneous innervation from the brachial plexus, which comes from the anterior roots of C5, C6, C7, C8, and T1. Likewise, there is a contribution of the supraclavicular nerves that are part of the superficial branches of the cervical plexus to the skin of the upper part of the shoulder and the intercostobrachial nerve from the second intercostal nerve that innervates a small area of the skin of the armpit and the medial aspect of the arm [29].

At the neck level between the anterior scalene and the middle scalene the roots of the plexus form the primary trunks, thus C5 and C6 form the upper primary trunk, C7 forms the middle primary trunk, and C8 and T1 form the lower primary trunk. Each of the primary trunks is divided into an anterior division and a posterior division, in such a way that the union of these will give rise to the secondary trunks or cords, thus, as all the posterior divisions join and form the posterior secondary trunk, the anterior division of the upper and middle trunk will form the lateral secondary trunk and the anterior division of the lower primary trunk will give rise to the medial secondary trunk [1].

The location of the brachial plexus allows us to identify two portions, the supraclavicular portion formed by the primary trunks in relation to the anterior and middle scalenes and the subclavian artery (Fig. 11.20). The infraclavicular or axillary portion is in relation to the axillary artery [29].

From the supraclavicular portion come the dorsal nerves of the scapula for the greater rhomboid, lesser rhomboid, and levator scapula muscles; the suprascapular nerve for the supraspinatus and infraspinatus muscles; the long thoracic nerve for the serratus major or anterior muscle; and the subclavian nerve for the innervation of the muscle of the same name.

The cords give preterminal branches before the inferior margin of the pectoralis minor muscle, this is how the lateral cord gives rise to the lateral pectoral nerve, the posterior cord emits the superior and inferior subscapularis nerves and the thoracodorsal nerve. The medial cord gives rise to the medial pectoral, medial brachial cutaneous, and medial antebrachial cutaneous nerves [31].

Once the cords or secondary trunks exceed the lower border of the pectoralis minor, they give rise to the terminal nerves. The lateral cord extends to form the musculocutaneous nerve that crosses the coracobrachialis muscle and reaches the anterior muscles of the arm innervating the biceps brachii, brachialis, and coracobrachialis. This nerve ends as the lateral antebrachial cutaneous nerve and carries the sensory afferents from this region of the forearm. Likewise, the lateral cord gives rise to the lateral root of the median nerve (Fig. 11.21). The posterior cord originates the axillary and radial nerves, and the medial cord extends to form the ulnar nerve (ulnar) and the medial root of the median nerve.

As for the location of the most representative nerves of the upper limb, the suprascapular nerve can be located topographically, which, once formed, goes down and back to pass through the suprascapular notch inferior to the transverse ligament and there reaches the supraspinous and infraspinous muscles [31].

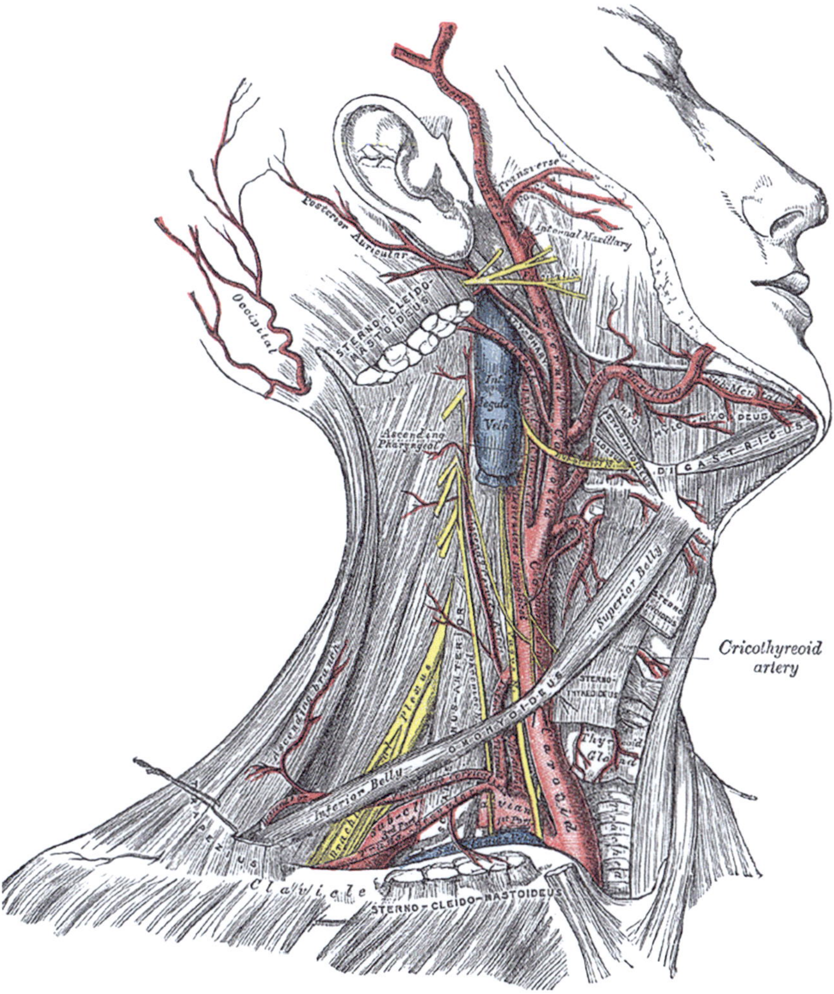

Fig. 11.20 Supraclavicular portion of the brachial plexus, note the relationship with the anterior and middle scalene muscles and the subclavian artery. (Source: Taken from [30])

The axillary nerve is initially located posterior to the axillary artery and in front of the subscapularis muscle and runs accompanied by the posterior humeral circumflex artery with which it crosses the biredondo-humerus-tricipital or lateral axillary quadrangular space and innervates the deltoid and teres minor muscles.

The radial nerve is located posterior to the axillary artery. At the level of the arm, it enters the round-humerus-tricipital triangular space accompanied by the deep brachial artery, crosses the torsion channel of the humerus, perforates the lateral intermuscular septum and passes to the anterior region of the arm between the brachial and brachioradialis muscles in the lateral bicipital sulcus, where it divides into a

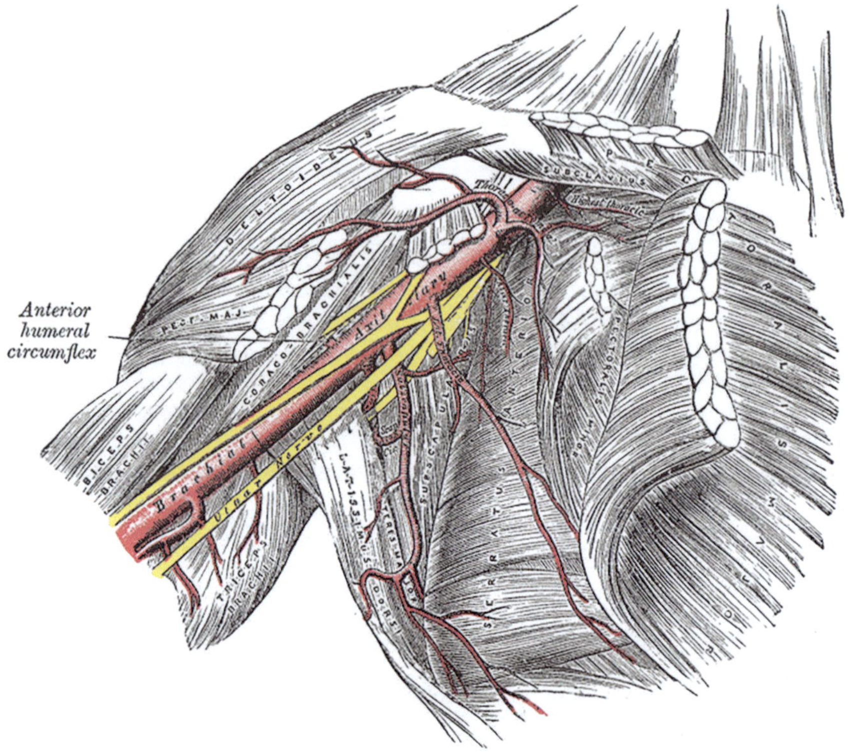

Fig. 11.21 Brachial plexus, infraclavicular portion. Note the musculocutaneous, median, and ulnar nerves. (Source: Taken from [32])

superficial sensory branch and a deep branch, engine. The deep branch passes between the heads of the supinator muscle, enters the posterior compartment to innervate the extensor muscles of the forearm, then emits its terminal branch or posterior interosseous nerve that is located in the interosseous membrane and reaches the radiocarpal joint.

The superficial branch is located in the anterior region of the forearm accompanied by the radial artery along the brachioradialis muscle, then reaches the dorsum of the hand and fingers for cutaneous innervation of this region [31].

The ulnar nerve arises in the axillary fossa and runs along the medial aspect of the arm to the medial epicondyle accompanied by the superior ulnar collateral artery. At the elbow level, it occupies the olecranial epitrochlea fossa and is covered by the epitrocleoolecranial ligament, then crosses the insertions of the flexor carpi ulnaris to reach the anteromedial region of the forearm. At the level of the forearm, in its distal third, it originates the palmar branch for the skin of the ulnar region of the palm of the hand. In the radiocarpal joint, it is located in front of the flexor retinaculum, occupying the ulnar canal and thus reaching the hand. The ulnar nerve provides motor innervation to the flexor carpi ulnaris, third and fourth flexor digitorum deep, third and fourth lumbrical, the deep portion of the flexor pollicis brevis, the adductor pollic, the interosseus palmaris and dorsal, and the flexor and abductor pinky muscles.

On the other hand, the median nerve is located in front of the axillary artery. In the arm it occupies the brachial canal, in the elbow fossa, the median nerve is located in the medial bicipital sulcus, then it runs between the two heads of the pronator teres muscle, then it is located between the superficial and deep flexor muscles of the fingers, then it is related to the deep aspect of the flexor flexaculum flexor superficialum locating between the flexor digitorum superficialis and the flexor pollicis longus and then passes to the hand and give there the recurrent branch of the median and the terminal branches in the interdigital spaces.

7 Neuroanatomy of the Lower Limb

The lower limb receives its innervation from the lumbar and sacral plexuses, which give rise to mixed nerves responsible for sensory and motor function (Fig. 11.22).

The lumbar plexus is a nerve network that originates from the anterior branches of the L1–L4 spinal nerves, with occasional contribution from T12. It is located within the psoas major muscle and its branches innervate structures of the abdominal wall, pelvis, and lower limb [1].

Anatomically, the lumbar plexus presents an arrangement in which its main branches emerge progressively from the depth of the psoas. Among its collateral branches are the iliohypogastric nerve and the ilioinguinal nerve, both derived from L1 and responsible for the innervation of the abdominal wall and the skin of the inguinal region [2]. The genitofemoral nerve (L1–L2) perforates the psoas and divides into genital and femoral branches, which innervate the cremaster muscle and the skin of the femoral triangle, respectively [3].

The terminal branches of the lumbar plexus include the lateral femoral cutaneous nerve (L2–L3), the femoral nerve (L2–L4), and the obturator nerve (L2–L4). The lateral femoral cutaneous nerve is responsible for the sensory innervation of the anterolateral aspect of the thigh. The femoral nerve is the main nerve of the anterior thigh region, providing motor innervation to the anterior compartment muscles and sensory to the anteromedial aspect of the thigh and leg [4]. For its part, the obturator nerve crosses the obturator foramen and innervates the muscles of the medial compartment of the thigh, essential in the adduction of the lower limb [5].

The nerves that emerge from the sacral plexus (L4–S4) are the sciatic nerve (L4–S3), which is the largest in the body, innervates the posterior compartment of the thigh, and is divided into:

- *Tibial nerve*: It innervates the posterior muscles of the leg and the sole of the foot.
- *Common peroneal nerve*: It is divided into deep (innervates the anterior muscles of the leg) and superficial (lateral muscles of the leg).

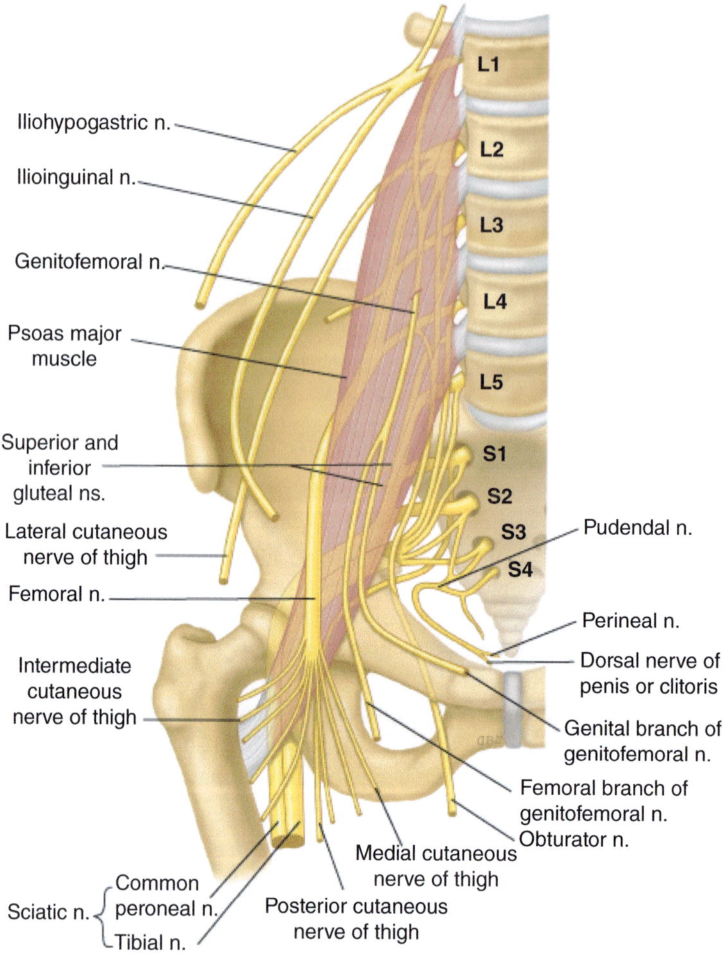

Fig. 11.22 Lumbar and sacrococcygeal plexus. (Source: Taken from [33])

- *Superior gluteal nerve (L4–S1)*: It provides motor innervation to the gluteus medius and minimus muscles and to the tensor fascia latae.
- *Inferior gluteal nerve (L5–S2)*: It innervates the gluteus maximus.

The autonomic nervous system regulates involuntary functions of the lower limb, such as vascular control and sweating. Sympathetic innervation comes from the lumbar and sacral sympathetic ganglia, while parasympathetic innervation comes from the sacral plexus through the pelvic nerve [2, 4, 6, 7].

References

1. Bustamante J. Functional and clinical neuroanatomy. 4th ed. Colombia: Celsus; 2007. p. 215.
2. Latarjet M, Ruiz A. Human Anatomy. 4th ed. Buenos Aires: Editorial Médica Panamericana; 2012. p. 304.
3. Wilson-Pawels L, Stewart P, Akesson E, Spacey S. Cranial nerves in health and disease. 3rd ed. Mexico: Editorial Médica Panamericana; 2013. p. 84.
4. Standring S. Gray's anatomy: the anatomical basis of clinical practice. 42nd ed. China: Elsevier; 2020. p. 607.
5. Moore KL, Dalley AF, Agur AMR. Clinically oriented anatomy. 7th ed. Philadelphia: Wolters Kluwer; 2013. p. 1065.
6. Snell RS. Clinical neuroanatomy. 7th ed. Philadelphia: Wolters Kluwer; 2010.
7. Netter FH. Atlas of human anatomy. 4th ed. Barcelona: Elsevier; 2007.
8. Moore KL, Dalley AF, Agur AM. Clinically oriented anatomy. 8th ed. Spain: Wolters Kluwer; 2018.
9. Gray H. Anatomy of the human body: Plate 777. Philadelphia: Lea & Febiger; 1918. Available at: https://archive.org/details/anatomyofhumanbo1918gray/page/n5/mode/2up
10. Pansky B. Human anatomy. 6th ed. Mexico: McGraw-Hill Interamericana; 1996.
11. Drake RL, Vogl W, Mitchell AWM. Gray's anatomy for students. 4th ed. Philadelphia: Elsevier; 2020.
12. Gray H. Anatomy of the human body: Plate 779. Philadelphia: Lea & Febiger; 1918. Available at: https://archive.org/details/anatomyofhumanbo1918gray/page/n5/mode/2up
13. Rhoton AL. Cranial anatomy and surgical approaches. New York: Wolters Kluwer/Lippincott Williams & Wilkins; 2023.
14. Williams PL, Warwick R. Gray's anatomy. 36th ed. Philadelphia: W.B. Saunders Company – Churchill Livingston; 1980.
15. Kierner AC, Zelenka I, Gstoettner W. The Auriculotemporal nerve. Clin Anat. 2003;16(3):192–9.
16. O'Brien MD. The trigeminal nerve. J Neurol Neurosurg Psychiatry. 2020;91(1):104–10.
17. Gray H. Anatomy of the human body. Plate 781. Philadelphia: Lea & Febiger; 1918. Available at: https://archive.org/details/anatomyofhumanbo1918gray/page/n5/mode/2up
18. Gray H. Anatomy of the human body. Plate 782. Philadelphia: Lea & Febiger; 1918. Available at: https://archive.org/details/anatomyofhumanbo1918gray/page/n5/mode/2up
19. Drake R, Vogl W, Mitchell A. Gray: anatomy for students. 3rd ed. Barcelona: Elsevier; 2015. p. 898.
20. Paulsen F, Waschke J. Sobotta atlas of human anatomy. 25th ed. Barcelona: Elsevier; 2020. p. 419.
21. Gray H. Anatomy of the human body. Plate 793. Philadelphia: Lea & Febiger; 1918. Available at: https://archive.org/details/anatomyofhumanbo1918gray/page/n5/mode/2up
22. Allen E, Minutello K, Murcek BW. Anatomy, Head and Neck, Larynx Recurrent Laryngeal Nerve. 2023 Jul 24. In: StatPearls [Internet]. Treasure Island (FL): StatPearls Publishing; 2025.
23. Drake R, Vogl W, Mitchell A. Gray: anatomy for students. 5th ed. Barcelona: Elsevier; 2024.
24. Gray H. Anatomy of the human body. Plate 794. Philadelphia: Lea & Febiger; 1918. Available at: https://archive.org/details/anatomyofhumanbo1918gray/page/n5/mode/2up
25. Gray H. Anatomy of the human body. Plate 844. Philadelphia: Lea & Febiger; 1918. Available at: https://archive.org/details/anatomyofhumanbo1918gray/page/n5/mode/2up
26. González Mesa JM, Otero Granados E, Valle Hoyos MD, Rivera M. Lumbar sympathetic blockade. Rev Soc Esp Dolor. 2013;20(6):324–31.
27. Betts G, Desaix P, Johnson E, Korol O, Kruse D, Poe B, et al. Anatomy and physiology. 2nd ed. Houston: Rice University; 2022. Available at: https://openstax.org/details/books/anatomy-and-physiology-2e

28. Gupton M, Varacallo MA. Anatomy, Abdomen and Pelvis: Genitofemoral Nerve. [Updated 2022 Oct 24]. In: StatPearls [Internet]. Treasure Island (FL): StatPearls Publishing; 2025. Available from: https://www.ncbi.nlm.nih.gov/books/NBK430733/
29. Jacob S. Human anatomy: clinically-orientated approach. 1st ed. Churchill Livingstone: Elsevier; 2007.
30. Gray H. Anatomy of the human body. Plate 507. Philadelphia: Lea & Febiger; 1918. Available at: https://archive.org/details/anatomyofhumanbo1918gray/page/n5/mode/2up
31. Pró EA. Clinical Anatomy. 1st ed. Buenos Aires: Editorial Médica Panamericana; 2012.
32. Gray H. Anatomy of the human body. Plate 523. Philadelphia: Lea & Febiger; 1918. Available at: https://archive.org/details/anatomyofhumanbo1918gray/page/n5/mode/2up
33. Foreman M, Maddy K, Patel A, Reddy A, Costello M, Lucke-Wold B. Differentiating lumbar spinal etiology from peripheral Plexopathies. Biomedicine. 2023;11(3):756. https://doi.org/10.3390/biomedicines11030756.

Chapter 12
Pischinger's Basic System

Eduardo Humberto Beltrán Dussán and Mónica Lucía Name-Guerra

In 1975, Dr. Alfred Pischinger (1899–1982), Austrian physician, professor at the University of Vienna, researcher in Embryology, Morphology, Physiology, Biochemistry, and Histochemistry, described what was called the Basic System, referring to a system of information regulation, also called the extracellular matrix, whose functions are carried out mainly in the interstitial space. In the history of medicine and his approaches to organic systems, the writings of Hippocrates (460 BC) based on the humoral theory, the organic theory and the importance of blood circulation proposed by Galen (129–201), the cell theory of Rudolf Virchow (1858) and the contributions of later researchers such as Bordeau (1767) are recognized. Reichert (1845), Rindfleisch (1869), Hertwig M (1881), Buttersack SB (1910), and Von Mollendorf (1943) who made important observations related to connective tissue, initially considered as structural support, and later recognized as a complex biological communication system [1].

In publications, Dr. Pischiger, taking into account the approaches of Ricker's (1924) "Regulatory Pathology" and Eppinger's (1949) "Pathological Permeability," he described the structure of the interstitial space made up of extracellular water, the capillary network, connective tissue cells, the proteoglycan and glycosaminoglycan system, hematological cells related to the immune response, proteins, which were later recognized as semiconductors and superconductors of signals, and the endings of the autonomic nervous system, among other fundamental elements for the processing of all information related to the maintenance of life from various regulatory centers, particularly from the brain [2].

E. H. Beltrán Dussán (✉)
Faculty of Medicine, Universidad Nacional de Colombia, Bogotá, Colombia
e-mail: ehbeltrand@unal.edu.co

M. L. Name-Guerra
Asociación Colombiana de Medicina Integrativa y Homeopática and Private practice, Bogotá, Colombia

L. B. Pinilla Bonilla et al. (eds.), *Neuraltherapeutic Medicine*,
https://doi.org/10.1007/978-3-032-03257-7_12

The regulations of this processing system were initially understood based on the theory of open systems proposed by Von Bertalanfi in 1950 [3] and on the approaches of biocybernetics developed by Wiener in 1948 [4].

In this way, the Basic System has been identified as the regulatory center of all biological processes, such as nutrition, metabolic processes, tissue oxygenation, cellular detoxification mechanisms, inflammation processes, endocrine activity, immune response, autonomic nervous system activity, psycho-neuro-endocrine-immunological interaction, genetic and epigenetic signaling, the molecular processes and biophysical processes that occur in living beings [5–7]. It is now recognized that molecular information, based on the structures of nucleic acids, receives or emits its information through interstitial water [8]. The functionality and ubiquity of the so-called Basic System in the organism has been evidenced by judicious scientific research [9].

In the advancement of knowledge about the biology of living beings and, particularly about the human being and its structure, the concept of molecular biology has now been incorporated, and research is being oriented towards the conception of subatomic particles and biophysics, based essentially on information [10–12]. These biophysical communications, which have an electromagnetic foundation, travel through this space to come into contact with the cellular information processors that are the cell membranes and generate the corresponding responses [13]. The extracellular matrix has been described as a processing mechanism of circadian cycles related to organic homeostasis and many pathological processes [14].

The evolution of knowledge about the Basic System, extracellular matrix or interstitial tissue has generated clarity about the origins, evolution, and regulation of pathological processes, and from the different complex medical systems, the mechanisms of action of the different therapeutic strategies of medicine and their rational and integrated use have been better understood [15–18].

It is for this reason that therapies aimed at eliminating signaling interferences located in the matrix, which arose in the conception of the various complex medical systems, are of capital importance in the process of integrating medicine for the solution of pathological states [19–21].

Taking into account the various biological actions that have been described in local anesthetics [22], when used in micro-doses applied in the interfering fields within the conception of neuraltherapeutic medicine, it can be considered as a valuable strategy in the processes of regulation of extracellular matrix alterations and thus contribute to the solution of pathological processes [23].

1 Reflections on the Extracellular Matrix in the Light of Current Knowledge

Could the extracellular matrix be a communication structure as fast as that of the nervous system, so that it can carry information at a distance and produce a distant regulation of other areas? In the following paragraphs, hypotheses and ideas are put forward as to how the application of local anesthetics in certain regions of the body (scars, painful areas, etc.) can have a therapeutic effect at a distance, via extracellular matrix and not only through the nervous system.

The extracellular matrix (ECM) is a ubiquitous organ with an integrative capacity for the organism, described for decades by different researchers, among whom Dr. Alfred Pischinger stands out. Recently, this tissue has been recognized as *an interstitium*, a structure that is little recognized in human tissues [24]. In this research, Benias et al. were able to observe the in vivo dynamics of this important tissue through laser confocal endomicroscopy (pCLE). This equipment provides real-time histological images of human tissues at a depth of 60–70 μm during endoscopy (in vivo microscopy). Researchers recognize that this anatomical structure may be involved in processes such as cancer metastasis, edema, fibrosis, and the mechanical functioning of many or all tissues and organs [24].

The extracellular matrix is a new communication organ responsible for carrying external information into the cell and represents 20% of the total body mass. It is the structure where the immune, nervous, and hormonal systems dialogue with the cell. So, it is much more than the "mere cement of cells"or a tissue with a support function, as it was previously believed.

Important figures mentioned in this book, such as Claude Bernard (French physiologist), may have been referring to the extracellular matrix when he spoke of the "inner environment"(*Le terrai intérieur*). On the other hand, Dr. Carl Rokitansky, published his most important histological investigations in 1854 in an article entitled "On the growth of connective tissue" showing since that time the importance of this tissue in health and disease. Likewise, other researchers such as Dr. Hartmut Heine and Dr. James Oschman conclude that the cell is influenced by its immediate environment, and this interaction is needed in the communication of the extracellular space with the interior of the cell [25].

Alexis Carrel (1873–1944), a French biologist and physician, won the Nobel Prize in Physiology and Medicine in 1912. He described the first operative techniques of vascular anastomosis and the transplantation of blood vessels and organs, carrying out an experiment in which he kept alive for several years in vitro a strain of chicken fibroblasts by constantly changing their extracellular environment until the death of the culture occurred by a laboratory accident [26]. This experiment led to the conclusion that the state of these matrix structures is very important for local and distant communication and to regulate the homeodynamics of the organism.

Name (one of the authors of this chapter) hypothesizes that the matrix network that extends across the entire body is a semiconductor electronic network. Collagen fibers are the structural component of ECM and the most abundant protein in the human body. This structure is a semiconductor with piezoelectric properties, which could transmit information from one place to another quickly and accurately. The semiconductor capacity of collagen fibers is highly dependent on the water content. It is a hydrated protein that optimizes its ability to transmit information [27].

Collagen is a complex supramolecular structure with very diverse morphologies in different tissues, which gives it a wide range of biological functions in the body [28, 29]. Collagen is a big part of both specialized and non-specialized connective tissue in vertebrates. It makes up about a quarter of the body's proteins, three quarters of dry skin, more than 90% of tendon and corneal tissue, and about 80% of bone organic matter. To date, 29 types of collagen have been identified, the difference in these types being due to the difference in triple polypeptide chains and the difference in helical length [27, 30].

As collagen fibers are hydrated, water molecules give them certain biophysical characteristics such as conductivity and electrical permittivity. In aqueous media, conductivity is mainly due to the presence of charged ions in the environment. Dielectric permittivity is defined as the material's ability to store energy (electric capacitor). Proteins are sensitive to electrical excitation and exhibit specific electrical properties under certain conditions [27].

Collagen fibers contain amino acids like glycine, proline, hydroxyproline, glutamine, arginine, aspartic acid, and hydroxylysine. These amino acids have ions that move to the negative pole of an electric field when exposed to it, making the fibers very conductive [27]. The hydroxyl groups of amino acids in collagen macromolecules form hydrogen bonds with water molecules and increase the conductivity of the collagen solution. Ring structures lead to better conductivity due to their β bonds [6]. Some amino acids in the collagen macromolecule, such as phenylalanine, tyrosine, and histidine, have a benzene ring with α bonds and, thanks to the free electrons, increase the conductivity of the collagen solution [27, 31].

This information from research carried out on aqueous collagen solutions suggests that collagen fibers could play a leading role in the transmission of information when the local anesthetic is injected in a specific place and responses are obtained at a distance. Collagen fibers carry bioelectrical signals between different parts of the body, speaking a new language of communication, of microcurrents of electron and proton fluxes that travel through the body through these dielectric protein structures capable of transmitting information throughout the system. Electrons are semi-conducted through this helical protein and protons (H^+) and hydroxyl groups (OH^-) migrate through the hydrated layer, generating a flow of information that travels throughout the matrix.

In addition, piezoelectric effects have been documented in collagen fibers [32], a fact that could facilitate the ability to store and transmit information throughout the body, generating bioelectrical signals at a distance.

References

1. Oschman HH, Pischinger A, editors. The extracellular matrix and ground regulation. Basis for a holistic biological medicine. Berkeley: North Atlantic Books; 2007.
2. Pischinger A. The system of basic regulation. Zahnarztl Mitt. 1977;67(21):1255–6. German
3. Von Bertalanffy L. The theory of open systems in physics and biology. Science. 1950;111(2872):23–9. https://doi.org/10.1126/science.111.2872.23.
4. Wiener N. Cybernetics: or control and communication in the animal and the machine. Paris: Hermann & Cie Editeurs; 1948.

5. Stewart RH. A modern view of the interstitial space in health and disease. Front Vet Sci. 2020;7:609583. https://doi.org/10.3389/fvets.2020.609583. PMID: 33251275; PMCID: PMC7674635
6. Isaac R, Reis FCG, Ying W, Olefsky JM. Exosomes as mediators of intercellular crosstalk in metabolism. Cell Metab. 2021;33(9):1744–62. https://doi.org/10.1016/j.cmet.2021.08.006. PMID: 34496230; PMCID: PMC8428804
7. Bohr T, Hjorth PG, Holst SC, Hrabětová S, Kiviniemi V, Lilius T, Lundgaard I, Mardal KA, Martens EA, Mori Y, Nägerl UV, Nicholson C, Tannenbaum A, Thomas JH, Tithof J, Benveniste H, Iliff JJ, Kelley DH, Nedergaard M. The glymphatic system: current understanding and modeling. iScience. 2022;25(9):104987. https://doi.org/10.1016/j.isci.2022.104987. PMID: 36093063; PMCID: PMC9460186
8. Tyson JJ, Novak B. A dynamical paradigm for molecular cell biology. Trends Cell Biol. 2020;30(7):504–15. https://doi.org/10.1016/j.tcb.2020.04.002. Epub 2020 Apr 30. PMID: 32362451; PMCID: PMC8665686
9. Cenaj O, Allison DHR, Imam R, Zeck B, Drohan LM, Chiriboga L, Llewellyn J, Liu CZ, Park YN, Wells RG, Theise ND. Evidence for continuity of interstitial spaces across tissue and organ boundaries in humans. Commun Biol. 2021;4(1):436. https://doi.org/10.1038/s42003-021-01962-0. PMID: 33790388; PMCID: PMC8012658
10. Schlissel G, Li P. Synthetic developmental biology: understanding through reconstitution. Annu Rev Cell Dev Biol. 2020;36:339–57. https://doi.org/10.1146/annurev-cellbio-020620-090650. PMID: 33021822; PMCID: PMC8139837
11. Beck M, Covino R, Hänelt I, Müller-McNicoll M. Understanding the cell: future views of structural biology. Cell. 2024;187(3):545–62. https://doi.org/10.1016/j.cell.2023.12.017.
12. Liberali P, Schier AF. The evolution of developmental biology through conceptual and technological revolutions. Cell. 2024;187(14):3461–95. https://doi.org/10.1016/j.cell.2024.05.053. Epub 2024 Jun 20
13. Funk RHW. Biophysical mechanisms complementing "classical" cell biology. Front Biosci (Landmark Ed). 2018;23(5):921–39. https://doi.org/10.2741/4625.
14. Dudek M, Swift J, Meng QJ. The circadian clock and extracellular matrix homeostasis in aging and age-related diseases. Am J Physiol Cell Physiol. 2023;325(1):C52–9. https://doi.org/10.1152/ajpcell.00122.2023. Epub 2023 May 29. PMID: 37246635; PMCID: PMC10281784
15. Liu WT, Cao YP, Zhou XH, Han D. Interstitial fluid behavior and diseases. Adv Sci (Weinh). 2022;9(6):e2100617. https://doi.org/10.1002/advs.202100617. Epub 2022 Jan 2. PMID: 34978164; PMCID: PMC8867152
16. Long AM, Lee G, Demonbreun AR, McNally EM. Extracellular matrix contribution to disease progression and dysfunction in myopathy. Am J Physiol Cell Physiol. 2023;325(5):C1244 51. https://doi.org/10.1152/ajpcell.00182.2023. Epub 2023 Sep 25. PMID: 37746696; PMCID: PMC10855263
17. Aman J, Margadant C. Integrin-dependent cell-matrix adhesion in endothelial health and disease. Circ Res. 2023;132(3):355–78. https://doi.org/10.1161/CIRCRESAHA.122.322332. Epub 2023 Feb 2. PMID: 36730379; PMCID: PMC9891302
18. Soles A, Selimovic A, Sbrocco K, Ghannoum F, Hamel K, Moncada EL, Gilliat S, Cvetanovic M. Extracellular matrix regulation in physiology and in brain disease. Int J Mol Sci. 2023;24(8):7049. https://doi.org/10.3390/ijms24087049. PMID: 37108212; PMCID: PMC10138624
19. Mormone E, Cisternino A, Capone L, Caradonna E, Sbarbati A. The model of interstitial cystitis for evaluating new molecular strategies of interstitial regeneration in humans. Int J Mol Sci. 2024;25(4):2326. https://doi.org/10.3390/ijms25042326. PMID: 38397003; PMCID: PMC10889234
20. Wang Y, Jiao L, Qiang C, Chen C, Shen Z, Ding F, Lv L, Zhu T, Lu Y, Cui X. The role of matrix metalloproteinase 9 in fibrosis diseases and its molecular mechanisms. Biomed Pharmacother. 2024;171:116116. https://doi.org/10.1016/j.biopha.2023.116116. Epub 2024 Jan 5

21. Ortega JA, Soares de Aguiar GP, Chandravanshi P, Levy N, Engel E, Álvarez Z. Exploring the properties and potential of the neural extracellular matrix for next-generation regenerative therapies. Wiley Interdiscip Rev Nanomed Nanobiotechnol. 2024;16(3):e1962. https://doi.org/10.1002/wnan.1962.
22. Catterall WA, Mackie K. Local anesthetics. In: Brunton LL, Knollmann BC, editors. Goodman & Gilman's the pharmacological basis of therapeutics. 14th ed. McGraw Hill; 2002. p. 489–504.
23. Vinyes D, Muñoz-Sellart M, Fischer L. Therapeutic use of low-dose local anesthetics in pain, inflammation, and other clinical conditions: a systematic scoping review. J Clin Med. 2023;12(23):7221. https://doi.org/10.3390/jcm12237221. PMID: 38068272; PMCID: PMC10707454
24. Benias PC, Wells RG, Sackey-Aboagye B, Klavan H, Reidy J, Buonocore D, Miranda M, Kornacki S, Wayne M, Carr-Locke DL, Theise ND. Structure and distribution of an unrecognized interstitium in human tissues. Sci Rep. 2018;8(1):4947. https://doi.org/10.1038/s41598-018-23062-6. Erratum in: Sci Rep. 2018 May 10;8(1):7610. doi: 10.1038/s41598-018-25732-x
25. Naranjo TA, Noguera-Salva R, Fariñas-Guerrero F. The extracellular matrix: morphology, function, and biotensegrity (part I). Rev Esp Patol. 2009;42(2):249–61.
26. Carrel A, Ebeling AH. Age and multiplication of fibroblasts. J Exp Med. 1921;34(6):599–623. https://doi.org/10.1084/jem.34.6.599. PMID: 19868581; PMCID: PMC2128071
27. Ashoorirad M, Saviz M, Fallah A. On the electrical properties of collagen macromolecule solutions: role of collagen-water interactions. J Mol Liq. 2018;300(14):112344. https://doi.org/10.1016/j.molliq.2019.112344.
28. Gopalakrishnan D, Balachandar V, Kumbharkhane AC, Sampathkumar R. Dielectric relaxation studies of collagen–surfactant complexes in aqueous buffer solution. Int J Biol Macromol. 2019;138:215–23.
29. Gendron R, Kumar MR, Paradis H, Martin D, Ho N, Gardiner D, et al. Controlled cell proliferation on an electrochemically engineered collagen scaffold. Macromol Biosci. 2012;12:360–6.
30. Sorushanova A, et al. The collagen suprafamily: from biosynthesis to advanced biomaterial development. Adv Mater. 2019;31:1801651.
31. Chen X. Theoretical electrical conductivity of hydrogen-bonded benzamide-derived molecules and single DNA bases. J Biol Phys. 2013;39:607–24.
32. Marino AA, Spadaro JA, Fukada E, Kahn LD, Becker RO. Piezoelectricity in collagen films. Calcif Tissue Int. 1980;31(3):257–9. https://doi.org/10.1007/BF02407190.

Part IV
Physiologic Dimension in Neuraltherapeutic Medicine

Chapter 13
Synthetic Physiology: A Visionary Conception

Laura Bibiana Pinilla Bonilla

1 Introduction

Despite the perception of a linear and homogeneous historical development of physiology, the nineteenth century witnessed a conceptual bifurcation of so-called modern physiology, giving rise to two distinct versions: an analytic version and a synthetic version [1]. Their differences lay in their ontological and epistemological stances, which allowed them to follow different research methodologies, describing the physiology of organisms from two perspectives that generated discrepancies in the understanding of the concept of reflex, the concepts of health and disease, the relationship between mind and body, among other concepts [2, 3].

In the first two parts of this chapter, the historical background of physiology will be reviewed, addressing its methodological approaches that led to divergences in the positions on the functional dynamics of organisms, defining two currents in the history of medicine. The third part will address the history of the creation of a new conception in physiology that was called synthetic physiology. The fourth part illustrates the fundamental concepts of this synthetic approach, which will be the basis for the subsequent development of Ukhtomsky's theory of the dominant focus or center (fifth part), Speransky's new conception of the health-disease process (sixth part), the therapeutic proposals derived from this new vision in medicine (seventh part), the cortico-visceral theory (eighth part), ending with the most recent, most visionary and conceptually advanced theory proposed by Anokhin (part nine).

L. B. Pinilla Bonilla (✉)
Faculty of Medicine, Master in Alternative Medicine, Neural Therapy Area, Universidad Nacional de Colombia, Bogotá, Colombia

Integrated Health Services Subnetwork of the South, Research and Innovation Center, Bogotá, Colombia
e-mail: lbpnillab@unal.edu.co

L. B. Pinilla Bonilla et al. (eds.), *Neuraltherapeutic Medicine*,
https://doi.org/10.1007/978-3-032-03257-7_13

At the end of this chapter, as the tenth part, the applications of the theories presented here in the clinical and practical field are outlined, as well as a reinterpretation of the concept of Interfering Field from these new approaches.

2 The Methodological Renewal and the Birth of the Analytic Current in Physiology

Physiology has been considered an independent science since Jean Fernel in 1542, who proposed that the object of its study is to understand the "nature of the healthy man, of all his forces and all his functions." But it was only towards the end of the eighteenth century and the beginning of the nineteenth century that several events occurred that were oriented towards a methodological renewal of it, thus emerging modern physiology [4].

During the eighteenth century, the contributions that the chemist and biologist Antoine-Laurent Lavoisier made to the physiology of respiration were important, introducing laws of chemistry that facilitated the discovery that it was a process of oxidation of organic compounds by oxygen in the air [1]. In addition, together with fellow mathematician and physicist at the Royal Academy of Sciences, Pierre-Simon Laplace, he built new instruments and developed new experimental methods to accurately measure heat transfer in biological and chemical processes [5, 6].

These new experimental methods served as inspiration for the methodological renewal of modern physiology that took place during the first half of the nineteenth century. This renewal was largely led by the Frenchman Francois Magendie, who had been sponsored and influenced by Laplace, importing the sense of "true science" into physiology [4, 7]. In 1821, Magendie founded the Journal of *Physiologie Expérimentale*, the year in which the Academy of Sciences had awarded him the Prize for Experimental Physiology, incited by Laplace and, in 1930, he instituted the first laboratory of experimental physiology at the *Collège de France* [4]. Among his most recognized findings are the studies on the cerebrospinal flow system and the differentiation of the sensory and motor action of the spinal nerves, which is also known as Bell-Magendie's Law [8].

Within the framework of the French school, Claude Bernard was Magendie's assistant, substitute, and successor, and although he stood out for his experimental orientation, he kept his distance as a biologist from the other sciences, which marked the difference with Magendie. Bernard considered it a mistake to completely liken the phenomena of living bodies with inert bodies. His conception of the *milieu interne* was based on an elastic condition of autonomy of the organism taken as a whole that allows it to resist with respect to changes from the external [4]. Bernard believed in the intelligence of the organism and in the vital force that animated it, which is why he opposed the physical and mathematical reductionism, tending towards more qualitative descriptions in the biological [9].

Johannes Peter Müller stood out as an important figure and leader within the German school of physiology, oriented towards a more experimental style. In the works of 1826, the law of the specific energy of the nerves was induced, based on both philosophy and physiology. He also worked on reflex actions, confirming Bell and Magendie's findings. Among Muller's disciples are Virchow, Schwann, and Haeckel in the line of cell theory; but other authors such as du Bois-Reymond, von Brucke, and Helmholtz, who founded the German Physical Society, also stood out. Du Bois-Reymond and Helmholtz excelled mainly in the area of electrophysiology. In fact, Helmholtz was the first to measure the speed of the nerve impulse. Carl Ludwig, on the other hand, was very influential in the German school, emphasizing the introduction of measurement and number as pillars in physiology [4, 9].

The arrival of positivism and materialism towards the middle of the nineteenth century ended up stripping away the vestiges of vitalism to move on to an era dedicated to the concrete, the observable, the detail and began the study of nature through empirical laws and analytical methods [9]. The analytical scientific method, precisely, tended to separate the particular from the general and the simple from the complex in order to gain access to the understanding of phenomena. Within this program of thought, isolated elements were found (and henceforth considered) as constant and participating in the organism as independent entities. That is, of the great discoveries that greatly affected the development of physiological research in this century, the discovery of the cell theory was the one that predominantly had the greatest influence on most of the schools of physiology in the West. Thanks to R. Virchow's proposals, the organism was studied from the perspective of the "cellular state,"where it was considered as a mere sum of cells and whose pathological processes were also assumed to be a sum of alterations in the function of individual cells [1].

For this reason, the predominant scientific research method was aimed at studying isolated organs in the context of "acute" experiments, excluding the investigation of the influence of the nervous system under normal conditions on all physiological processes [1]. The study of the concept of reflex as a physiological unit of the nervous system was also aimed at eliminating any psychological or teleological vestiges that had developed during the seventeenth and eighteenth centuries. This allowed it to move towards a "rectification"that was greatly facilitated when Todd proposed in 1839 the term "afferent" to replace the concept of sensation (which had been associated with the field of psychology) [4]. From this approach, the concept of reflex is confined to the lower nervous centers, assuming it as a linear phenomenon (stimulus-response) with fixed characteristics. Consequently, all higher forms of CNS activity that determine the behavior of the organism in its surrounding environment were excluded from the sphere of physiological research [1].

On the other hand, the theory of evolution was not proposed until the second half of the nineteenth century, so that physiological research methods during the first half would not take into account the relationships between the functioning of the nervous system and the surrounding environment [1].

During the second half of the nineteenth century, a new interest in physiology arose in North America. Dalton introduced Bernard's operative physiology to Buffalo in 1854. Bowditch was a student of Ludwig in 1869 and founded in 1871 the first physiology laboratory at Harvard University. Among Bowditch's students are Cushing and Walter Cannon. Other prominent researchers were Draper, Austin Flint, and Mitchell [4, 9].

During this second half, the English school of physiology, which had been left behind by the lack of suitable laboratories, began to emerge. The driving force behind the reform of physiology research and teaching was William Sharpey, who, together with his disciple Michael Foster, taught physiology at University College. Foster later founded the first physiology laboratory and took up the chair of physiology at Cambridge in 1870. One of Foster's disciples was John Newport Langley, who studied at Cambridge and proposed the names "autonomic nervous system"and "parasympathetic."Another disciple was Charles Sherrington, who dedicated his career to working on the nervous system. In 1897, he coined the word "synapse" and decided to work intensively on the study of spinal cord reflexes and on the differentiation between proprioceptors and superficial receptors of the skin [9]. On the other hand, Henry Head, who had studied with Hering in Prague [10] and with Julius Bernstein in Germany, was later invited by Michael Foster to Trinity College, Cambridge, as an assistant professor. Head had very close academic relations with William Rivers and Charles Sherrington [11]. As will be seen later in Chap. 15, Henry Head constructed one of the first dermatome maps in the history of medicine, and today, it serves as the basis for segmental physiology. Additionally, Chap. 14 illustrates Head's contributions to a current of thought in medicine centered on the nervous system, also called British Nervism.

Although the Russian school of physiology also had its heyday from the beginning of the nineteenth century, its development and methodological approach deserve a greater depth that will be addressed in the next section.

2.1 The Foundation of Physiology in Russia

Within the framework of the teaching-learning system of physiology from the eighteenth century, with the reign of Peter the Great in Russia, the European system of teaching medicine for the training of doctors in Russia was introduced. Especially Dutch and English doctors were taken to Russian medical schools to extend their knowledge in these universities [12].

One of the most relevant authors in the history of Russian thought was the Russian physician, surgeon, and physiologist Efrem Osipovich Mukhin (1766–1850) [13]. In 1800 he defended his thesis, "On the stimuli acting on the human body," thanks to which he received the degree of doctor of medicine from the University of Göttingen in 1804. In his thesis, for the first time, the elements for a reflex theory were presented, which made him one of the founders of the theory of nervism [14, 15].

Another of the most relevant Russian physicians in the history of Russian physiology was Ivan Timofeevich Glebov, whose mentors were E. O. Mukhin and I. E. Dyadkovsky [16]. Glevob graduated from Moscow University and was later trained in several laboratories, such as Claude Bernard's and Johannes Peters Muller's in Berlin. On his return to Russia, Glebov taught human physiology and general and comparative anatomy and histology, as well as carrying out the important task of translating Magendie's works into Russian, among others [9, 12].

Glebov was not only the first person in Russia to teach comparative or evolutionary physiology, but he also reformed the teaching of this branch of knowledge through the introduction of an extensive course of practical training in physiology of the nervous system (NS) and physiology based on physics, chemistry, and natural history. His doctoral thesis was entitled "Mental phenomena from physiological, therapeutic and pharmacological points of view." Since he was appointed vice-president of the St. Petersburg Medical-Surgical Academy, he took care to bring teaching and research to a very high level and, therefore, founded an institute of anatomy and physiology, as well as several well-equipped clinics for mental and nervous diseases and many other research laboratories. His new way of teaching was responsible for the training of many outstanding medical professors. Among his Russian disciples were Ivan Mikhailovich Sechenov (1829–1905), as well as the clinician Sergei Botkin (1832–1889). Both were very close and shared his ideas in science, particularly on the central role of NS in physiological and pathological processes in animals and humans [12].

In particular, Sechenov is of enormous importance in Russian history since he is considered the founder of a school of physiology to which Pavlov belonged, the school of *Nervism*. During his studies in Russia, he was widely influenced by materialistic currents and, around 1850, he graduated as a Doctor of Medicine at the University of Moscow, where, under the guidance of Glebov and Orlovsky, he learned the principles of experimental and theoretical physiology [1, 9]. Around 1856 he went abroad and worked with Ludwig, Helmholtz, and Du Bois-Reymond in Berlin, as well as with Bernard in Paris. Together with Bernard, he incorporated the idea of determinism and that of the *milieu interne*. In 1863 he published his book "The reflexes of the Brain" in which he gave a materialist interpretation of the mental phenomenon, a book that would later be confiscated for its strong criticism for being a propagator of immorality and nihilistic philosophy. However, some authors claim that Sechenov managed to develop an intermediate position between the idealistic and materialist aspects of reality through a neutral monist proposal rather than a merely materialist one [17].

Sechenov also described the summation of subthreshold stimuli and the phenomenon of inhibition in the central nervous system (CNS). And one of his relevant disciples was Nikolai Yevgenyevich Wedensky (1852–1922), who worked on the phenomena of stimulation and inhibition and on the important concept of internal unity. Wedensky replaced Sechenov in St. Petersburg and then studied with Du Bois in Berlin and with Bowman in London. Wedensky relied on the study of electrical potentials that originated as a result of the stimulation of a nerve or muscle to create the important concept of "excitation wave or nerve impulse." One of Wedensky's disciples was Alexei Ukhtomsky, who, as will be seen later, was the one who developed the principle of dominance or the nerve centers in persistent stimulation and who was also in charge of developing and extending the ideas of his mentor [1, 9].

Sergei Botkin, who worked in St. Petersburg, was noted for his interest in the clinic but also for his interest in physiology, which encouraged him to establish a comparative physiology laboratory in his own clinic. Among his main proposals is the statement that the learning and teaching of physiology should be based on knowledge of experimental physiology [9, 12].

Both Sechenov and Botkin were invited by their mentor Glebov to be professors at the Medical-Surgical Academy in St. Petersburg and are considered to be pioneers of the school of Nervism, which considers the nervous system to play a central role in the organism and emphasizes the importance of reflexes in physiology and pathology. Precisely, the idea of the central role of the nervous system in the organism, characteristic of the Russian school of physiology, originating in Glebov, was developed in Botkin and Sechenov and provided the experimental and theoretical basis for the future research of Ivan Petrovich Pavlov (1849–1936) and his disciples in Russia (see Fig. 13.1) [12].

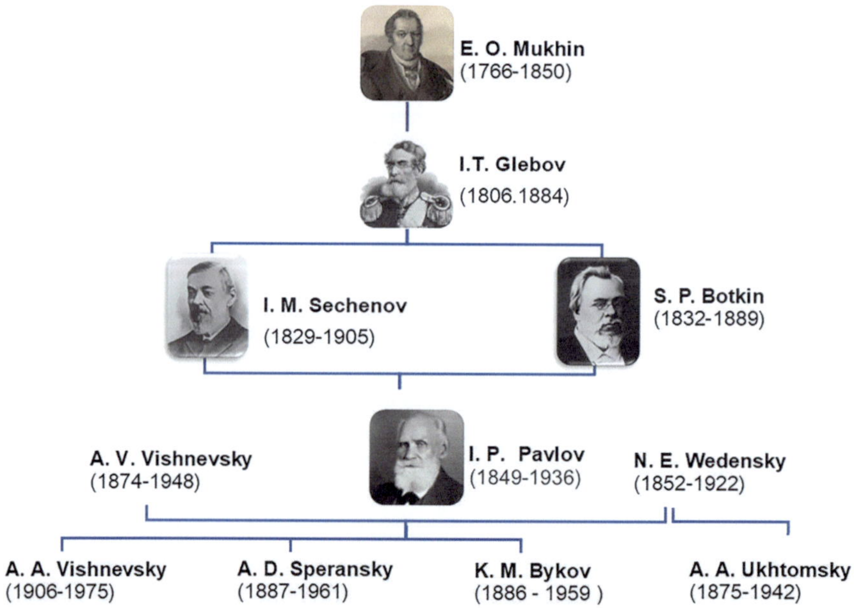

Fig. 13.1 Scientific tree with the main authors of the synthetic physiology school. (Source: Own elaboration. Photographs of Mukhin and Glevob were taken from Analytical Service of Lomonosov Moscow State University, 1993–2025 (Available at: https://letopis.msu.ru/peoples/). Photographs of Sechenov, Botkin, and Pavlov are courtesy of the National Library of Medicine)

2.2 *The Foundation of Synthetic Physiology with Ivan Petrovich Pavlov*

Ivan Pavlov was born in Ryazan in 1849. In 1879, he obtained his medical degree from the Medical-Surgical Academy in St. Petersburg. During 1879–1890 he was the director of research in Botkin's laboratory, although during the years 1885 and 1886 he was studying with Carl Ludwig in Leipzig and with Heidenhain in Breslau. During the 1890s, he was appointed as professor of pharmacology and physiology at the Academy of Military Medicine and, simultaneously, he was asked to organize the Department of Physiology of the Institute of Experimental Medicine in St. Petersburg. Pavlov received the Nobel Prize for his work on the digestive process, where he used the surgical method of creating fistulas in dogs to study them. During the 1890s, Pavlov identified the pathways by which bowel movement reflexes and gastric secretions are modified through the nervous system. He also highlighted the importance of "psychic" factors where, for example, the sensation of hunger could activate the secretion of gastric juice [18, 19].

Pavlov's school marked a fairly clear methodological-theoretical difference in physiology. In fact, Pavlov himself called his line of thought the school of "synthetic physiology," in which the physiological phenomenon is considered as an integral whole in the various conditions of its development (see Table 13.1). In the same way, in this new scientific-methodological line, the fundamental principle is to combine analysis with synthesis within the framework of physiological research. Pavlov

Table 13.1 Characteristics of the school of analytical and synthetic physiology

Characteristics	Analytic	Synthetic
Types of reasoning	It is mainly based on analysis (fragmentation of the object of study, abstracting from the relationships with other parties).	Union of analysis and synthesis. The synthesis phase focuses on identifying correlations and patterns emerging from the whole.
Biological theory of influence	Cell theory	Theory of evolution
Research methods	Organs and functions isolated from the whole	The whole organism and the relationships between its parts.
Duration of experiments	Acute (short duration)	Chronic (until the death of the animal)
Characterization of the body's reflexes	Constant and fixed. Limited to lower nerve centers	Dynamic and changing in relation to higher nerve centers.
Concept of disease	Sum of alterations of individual cells	Initial alteration of the NS with subsequent alteration of organs and functions. The process is not restricted to one area, since it can be reflected to other parts of the nervous system until generalization.

(continued)

Table 13.1 (continued)

Characteristics	Analytic	Synthetic
Conception of higher nervous functions	Not easily knowable	Knowable
Consideration of the interrelationship with the environment	Scanty	High; from there derived the branch of Russian "ecological" physiology.

Source: Taken and modified from Pinilla-Bonilla et al. (2024)

did not agree with studying the physiological phenomenon in mutilated animals or in acute experiments; on the contrary, his method was characterized by thoroughly investigating physiological processes in healthy animals and in the context of a chronic experiment. Another relevant difference of the Pavlovian school consists in the consideration that theory cannot be separated from praxis. Indeed, in 1900 Pavlov affirmed that the "physiological synthesis agrees with medicine and is identified with it" [1].

Unlike the Virchowian view, which had its greatest influence on the development of the other schools of physiology, the legacy of Sechenov and Pavlov in Russian physiology is characterized by their adherence to the principles of the theory of evolution. This theory is represented in the consideration that the properties of organisms and their cells take shape during evolutionary development, where continuous modifications are experimented within the framework of an interaction with the surrounding environment. The organism can exist in a continuously changing external environment only if it is able to respond to such changes by adapting to them. In higher animals, connections with this surrounding world, as well as the interconnections of internal functions, are made possible by the action of the NS, especially the cerebral cortex in vertebrates, which determines the organism to behave as a whole [1].

Since Sechenov, there has been the idea that all forms of nervous activity could be considered as reflex activity, and this conception was fundamental to understanding the causal dependence of the behavior of animals and humans on the past and present conditions of existence. In other words, every physiological process in the organism is dependent on the reflex activity of the NS, but not the reflexes understood as fixed and invariable like the other schools of physiology. Pavlov, in the course of his research, was able to demonstrate that the notion of reflex should be applied even to the phenomenon of mental activity, which supported the idea of his mentor Sechenov that "every act of conscious and unconscious life is a reflex in its original sense" [1].

Pavlov considered Nervism as a physiological orientation "that aims to extend the influence of the nervous system to the greatest possible number of activities of the organism" [20].

2.3 Fundamental Concepts of Synthetic Physiology According to the Pavlovian School

Within the concepts developed by the school of synthetic physiology, prior to understanding the theory of conditioned and unconditioned reflexes, it is essential to review the notions of irritability, excitation, and inhibition. The next step involves reviewing the concepts of reflexes and their different variations according to the school of Nervism. Likewise, the concepts of corticalization and generalization of reflexes will be addressed, to end by addressing the Pavlovian proposal on the first and second signal systems.

Irritability It is a fundamental concept that refers to the ability of organisms to respond to changes in the environment, which also generates a modification in their internal physiological dynamics. In this conceptual framework, the "agents" are those that generate the "stimuli" that trigger changes in organisms. This irritability also depends on the "stimulation threshold" of each organism. There is an inverse relationship between "irritability" and "stimulation threshold" so that more irritable organisms are those with a lower stimulation threshold [1].

One might think that stimulation thresholds are predetermined or fixed in organisms; however, Speransky showed that these thresholds are dynamic and vary according to the history of previous irritations, which modify what would be called "(base) tone of the nervous system" [21].

The Excitation Process In the NS, an excitatory process refers to the activation response to certain electrical, chemical, or mechanical stimuli. In a fiber, a simple stimulus produces an excitatory impulse. But in the centers, to produce a reflex, several successive stimuli are required in the afferent fibers that reach a minimum range so that it then extends to the axons and synapses. In the nerve centers, excitation often persists for some time after stimulation of the receptors.

Excitation can also radiate or spread through the CNS, leading to generalized reflexes. A certain generalization of reflexes is observed under the increase of stimulation of the receptors (until the strength of the stimulation reaches a point beyond which it becomes an inhibition) [22].

The Inhibition Process In the nerve fiber, inhibition manifests itself in the suppression of excitation or decreased excitability or conductivity. This phenomenon was discovered by Sechenov in 1862, which was very important because all reflex acts, without exception, always involve inhibition.

The inhibitory process always arises in connection with the excitatory process and is inseparable from the latter. This was the view of Pavlov and Wedensky. The most robust theory of inhibition is Wedensky's theory of *parabiosis,*[1] in which

[1] From the theory of parabiosis, the emergence of inhibition is interpreted as a result of a conflicting excitatory process: a first level of subthreshold stimulation produces local excitation; a higher level

inhibition is a modification of the excitatory process under which the latter becomes a stagnant and limited process. Pavlov described two types of inhibition: internal and external. The first is that which arises internally in the centers, such as the processes of dishabituation or reciprocal inhibition (when the act of swallowing inhibits inspiration), while external inhibition occurs at the first application of the stimulus [22, 23].

The Concept of Reflex In Latin, "reflexus"means that it goes back and forth. In physics, it could correspond to a ray of light that changes its direction by a reflecting surface. This term of reflex was first used by Descartes to describe the reactions of the organism to the stimulation of the sense organs in the treatise on the Passions of the Soul [24]. Before Pavlov, reflexes were considered only as reactions of the organism to the stimulation of receptors, which, in the first place, always originated equally in animals of defined species in response to the stimulation of a receptive field of a given reflex and, secondly, could be effected even in the absence of the upper parts of the CNS. Such reflexes were opposed to so-called "voluntary movements" that depended on the activity of the upper parts of the CNS [22]. For Pavlov, an organism can only survive as long as its activities are balanced by the excitations that come from the outside world. Reflexes are the elements of this adaptation or constant equilibrium [23].

Types of Reflexes According to Pavlov

In the first instance, reflexes can be classified as positive or negative, that is, excitatory or inhibitory; but they can also be external or internal depending on the origin of the stimulus. In a second instance, Pavlov developed an adittional classification of reflexes into innate or unconditioned and conditioned or acquired reflexes.

(a) Unconditioned reflexes *(UR)* can be carried out by the lower parts of the NS. As a rule, they lead to reactions that are similar in individuals of a given species: coughing, sexual reflexes, and defensiveness. And there is always a constant connection between the external agent and the organism's response. However, these reflexes are very few in number and are inadequate to ensure the survival of the organism, since, deprived of higher nervous activity, the animal can become an incapacitated who soon ceases to exist [1, 23]. In the act of feeding, an innate reflex is, for example, the secretion of saliva upon direct contact of food with the tongue´s receptors.
(b) Conditioned reflexes (CR) are temporary connections stablished through the signaling activity or function of the cerebral hemispheres, which arise when two cortical foci of excitation act successively (excitatory) or simultaneously

of stimulation causes the excitation to spread; but at a much higher level, the excitation stagnates and stops spreading. The ease with which this inhibition is generated depends on the lability of the center. The lower the lability, the easier it is for inhibition to develop. This phenomenon is not the same as fatigue, because while fatigue arrives a few seconds later, parabiosis develops in the course of prolonged activity. Fatigue is an absolutely normal condition, while parabiosis is a deviation from normal activity [22].

(inhibitory). They are acts formed during life that respond to a change in the external or internal environment. If the action of some neutral agent (which will be called a conditioned stimulus) coincides in time with the action of a stimulus (usually of greater intensity) that evokes an unconditioned reflex, then a conditioned reflex develops. For the creation of CR, the first condition is the repetition of this association (reinforcement). If this association is repeated, the neutral stimulus eventually becomes a signal stimulus. The second condition is that the indifferent or neutral stimulus must precede the action of the unconditioned stimulus by a few seconds (5–10 seconds). On the basis of each UR, countless CR can be formed, explaining organisms' ability to develop CRs for all physiological functions. This makes possible the almost infinite multiplication and extension of connections between the organism and its environment [1, 23]. In the act of feeding, an excitatory CR in a dog is, for example, the association of seeing the piece of meat (seconds beforehand) with the stimulus information from the direct contact of the food in the mouth (unconditioned stimulus). When this association is repeated several times, the presentation of the image of the piece of meat alone, even without direct contact of food in the mouth, later generates salivation (see Fig. 13.2).

(c) *Natural reflexes*: An example of this type is the salivatory CR, which associates visual stimuli (seeing the milk, seeing the piece of meat) or olfactory stimuli (the smell of the food) with the unconditioned stimulus -- direct contact of the food with the tongue´s receptors -- to produce salivation. After reinforcement/repetition, the conditioned stimulus alone (smell, image) will be able to trigger the salivation response.

(d) *Artificial reflexes*: These involve associating non-natural stimuli with the UR, such as pairing the sound of a bell or metronome with the unconditioned stimulus of a piece of meat placed directly in the animal's mouth to produce salivation.

(e) *Inhibitory reflexes*: While excitatory conditioned reflexes are those that trigger some action or response in the organism, inhibitory conditioned reflexes are those that can suspend or eliminate the response of a previously established reflex. An external stimulus can become inhibitory if it meets the following conditions: first, it must be neutral to the organism; second, it must be presented simultaneously with the conditioned stimulus; and third, it must occur in the absence of the unconditioned stimulus. For example, if one wishes to inhibit an artificial CR established between the sound of the metronome and the direct placement of the food in the mouth to elicit salivation, a neutral stimulus (such as gently touching the animal's skin) must be presented while the metronome is sounding, without the subsequent presentation of the food in the mouth (see Fig. 13.4).

Pavlov explored different types of inhibitory agents whose information can be channeled primarily through visual, olfactory, auditory, and tactile analyzers. When these inhibitory agents are applied systematically and repetitively, they can maintain their inhibitory power. This is called conditioned inhibition. These agents may end up exerting an inhibitory role on other conditioned reflexes [23].

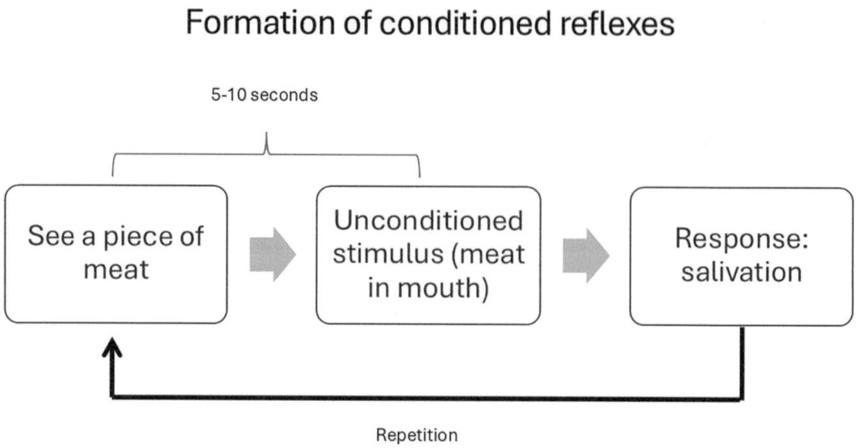

Fig. 13.2 Formation of an excitatory conditioned reflex through the "successive" presentation of stimuli. (Source: Own elaboration)

Another aspect to consider is that an inhibitory CR can also be subject to inhibition, leading to the reinstatement of the excitatory CR that it had previously suppressed.

(f) *Exteroceptive and interoceptive reflexes*: Exteroceptive reflexes correspond to stimuli from the external environment that trigger a response in the organism when paired with an UR or innate reflexes. These reflexes can be formed based on the stimulation of the different analyzers (visual, olfactory, tactile, auditory, taste and thermal). Interoceptive reflexes, on the other hand, can arise from the association of stimuli from interoceptors (muscular or visceral) with unconditioned stimuli to produce a specific response [22].

(g) *Second-and third-order reflexes*: Pavlov observed the occurrence of second- and third-order CRs in the study animals. For second-order conditioning to occur, the activity of the new neutral stimulus to be associated must have ceased at least 10 seconds before the onset of the conditioned stimulus. That is, if one wishes to associate the sound of a bell with the CR in Fig. 13.2, the bell must stop ringing at least 10 seconds before the piece of meat is presente to the dog's eyes. The same holds true for third-order reflexes [22, 23]. If the action of the neutral stimulus continues until the onset of the conditioned stimulus (previously formed), it will result in inhibition of the reflex.

The Generalization Process in the NS The generalization process consists of an irradiation of excitation in the NS that can be observed under the increase of stimulation of the receptors to a certain extent, since if stimulation is prolonged beyond certain thresholds, inhibition ensues. In the specific case of conditioned reflexes, when a conditioning is created for a certain agent, it happens that several similar agents can always evoke the same RC even if their action has not been reinforced by a US. According to Pavlov, generalization usually does not extend beyond the ana-

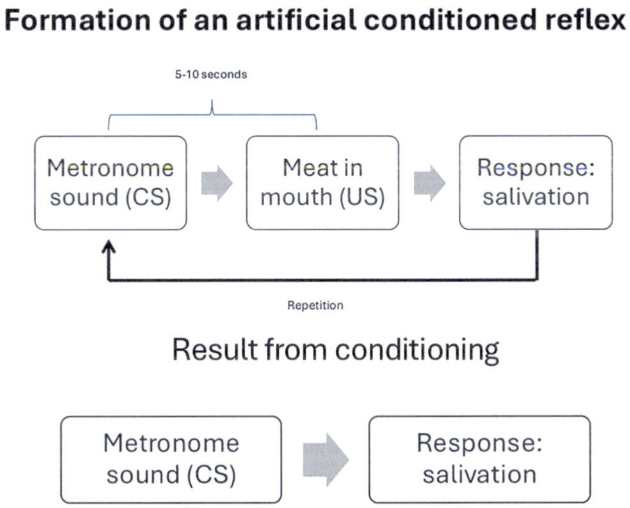

Fig. 13.3 Example of the formation of an artificial conditioned reflex with conditioned stimulus (CS) and unconditioned stimulus (US) until the result from conditioning. (Source: Own elaboration)

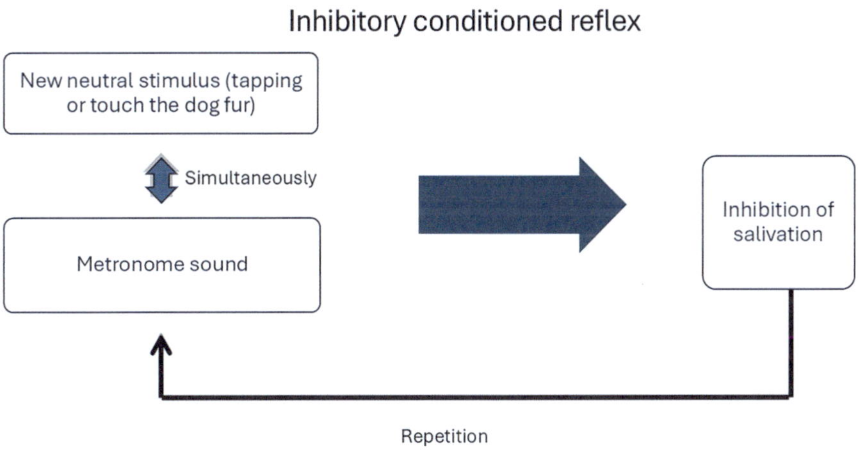

Fig. 13.4 An example of the formation of an inhibitory conditioned reflex. The new neutral stimulus is applied simultaneously to the metronome sound but without the presentation of US (according to Fig. 13.3). The final result is the inhibition of salivation. (Source: Own elaboration)

lyzer on which the stimulus was conditioned. Pavlov described it as follows: "If a special agent is connected with some physiological activity for the first time, the excitation produced by this agent radiates upon the given receptive center; therefore, it is not a point in the brain of the given analyzer, but the entire analyzer or some part of it" [22].

In the case of a pathological deviation, in which the reciprocal inhibition is altered, this can result in a greater generalization of reflexes, reducing effectiveness and altering other cortical functions [22].

The Process of Corticalization in the NS In the strictest sense, corticalization refers, in evolutionary physiology, to functions that were phylogenetically performed by lower portions of the NS but evolved to be carried out by the cerebral cortex [22]. However, in a broader sense, the concept of corticalization can also be employed to refer to how certain physiological or pathological functions and reflexes may initially be coordinated from lower portions of the NS, but at other times may undergo conditioning processes coordinated by the cortex. Bykov and Kurtsin [20] described several cases of corticalization of vegetative functions, in which reflexes that seemed so "autonomous" such as the secretion of digestive enzymes, could end up being conditioned to certain emotions, certain words, or concepts (see second system of signals). Another example of this can be the innate reflexes that take place within an embryological segment[2] (see Chap. 15), which can also be conditioned and coordinated from the cerebral cortex.

The First and Second Signal Systems Pavlov defined the first signal system as the one which enables the signaling of reality through stimuli from the receptors of the visual, auditory, tactile, olfactory, gustatory, and thermal analyzers. The information from these analyzers generates impressions in the cerebral hemispheres and notions of the natural world around us [22, 25].

The second system of signals is constituted by language, which is a signal of the first system. This system is an abstraction of reality and makes it possible to form generalizations [26]. This system establishes connections between objects or phenomena and the words by which they are designated, and the acts that derive as a consequence. Connections between verbal signals and real stimuli are formed according to the laws of elaboration of temporal connections. For example, when a child learns to pronounce the word "milk" (and almost simultaneously hears it), they associate it with the image of milk, its smell and its taste. Now, language not only allows to signal external stimulations, but also internal ones [22].

Language allows a person who had a traumatic experience with some object in reality to evoke the entire physiological response (for example, increased heart rate, sweating, etc.) just by reading, listening, or talking about that object. Another typical example is when a person is told to "imagine a few drops of lemon falling in their mouth," causing them to experience increased salivation without the actual presence of the lemon. Some words or expressions do not always trigger an action, but can generate a specific inhibition, such as when another person is told "watch out!," this could generate a temporary inhibition of movement.

[2] Such as the cutivisceral, visceromotor, or osteovisceral reflexes, which are rooted in embryology and originally constitute innate reflexes.

2.4 *The Dominant Center or Focus According to Ukhtomsky*

At the beginning of the twentieth century, the English physiologist Sherrington posed the question: given all the receptors, sensory pathways or centers active at a given time in the NS, how is it possible to explain that only a few take control? For example, in the case of movement, Sherrington believed that the simplest explanation was that the most excited center took the lead.

Ukhtomsky in 1904 began to study precisely in this direction, seeking to understand how a "dominant center"was formed, after the failure of an experiment in which the expected reaction (movement of a limb) never happened since the organism was prepared for another reflex activity (defecation). Any additional excitation that came in simply accelerated the vegetative process, whereas the motor reaction could only take place once the first process had ended.

Ukhtomsky understood that a dominant center is a focus of excitation in any division of the NS that modifies the activity of the nerve centers by attracting impulses toward itself that, in the absence of the dominant one, would elicit a different reflex. In other words, it is a constellation of centers with increased excitability at different levels of the brain, spinal cord, and autonomic nervous system that takes the lead to a large extent and predetermines the pattern of reactions currently occurring in the centers [22, 27].

These dominant foci align with Wedensky's theory of parabiosis, in the sense that they can manifest an excitatory or inhibitory state depending on the type of stimuli that reinforce them. If the stimuli are of mild to moderate intensity, they will induce excitation of the center, but if the excitation is very high, it ends in parabiotic inhibition. Likewise, these centers can inhibit other reflexes that are within the same pathway of action [22, 27].

There are four main characteristics that dominant centers exhibit [20]:

1. Increased excitability.
2. Excitation stability.
3. Sum of excitation.
4. Inertia.

With respect to the second characteristic, the tendency to stability of excitation is clear; however, a dominant focus can end its action when:

1. When the final result has been reached.
2. When another dominant focus has formed that is not compatible with the current one.
3. By direct inhibition from the CNS.

A dominant focus often leaves irreversible traces in the CNS that can be reactivated after its action has ended. It is as if a memory or traces of past actions are left behind. These memories cause the organism to respond to environmental stimuli according to the dominant ones that are most ready or prepared to take action [27].

Dominant foci are responsible for all perceptual, motor, behavioral, and emotional acts. It should be noted that emotions play a crucial role in living beings because they can elevate and reinforce excitement, which facilitates memory consolidation. An impression unrelated to any emotion is destined to be removed very quickly [27].

Likewise, dominant foci can also become pathological, influencing the functional dynamics of the other centers, extending the irritation to other related centers, or inhibiting the normal functioning of centers incompatible with their operation. These dynamics of the dominant foci often escape from a local domain to extend their influence even to sites anatomically distant from the initial dominant foci. For example, a pathological dominant focus originating in an anatomical segment affecting the viscera of the heart can, reflexively, extend its irritation to the viscera lung -- with which it shares an embryological origin -- but if the organism's history includes a site of less resistance due to prior trauma in the lower limbs, the irritation could radiate to that site, giving rise to pathological manifestations. Although the example mentioned so far covers only physical aspects (somatic and visceral), a pathological dominant can likewise be related to the emotional and mental sphere.

2.5 The Health-Disease Concept and the New Bases for a New Theory in Medicine According to Speransky

Alexei Speransky was born in 1888 in the city of Urzhum. He studied medicine at Kazan University, where he had as one of his professors the surgeon Alexander Vasilyevich Vishnevsky, and graduated with honors in 1911. By the beginning of World War I, Speransky began his military service, ending up as chief medical officer. After the demobilization, in 1918 he returned to the university, where he was elected as a prosector of the Department of Anatomy.

By 1920, he was elected professor and director of the Department of Surgery. However, around 1922, he entered into a crisis and conflict with the foundations of medicine, and decided to study physiology. That year he decided to go to Petrograd, to the Institute of Experimental Physiology, to study with Ivan Pavlov and soon became one of his most trusted collaborators, later participating in research with his mentor. One of Speransky's main interests was the study of neuroses, focusing on the study of pathology.

Speransky was a highly awarded scientist; in 1937 he received the Pavlov Prize by the USSR Academy of Sciences, and for the rest of his years he received the Stalin Prize and two orders of Lenin. During 1945, he headed the General Institute of Experimental Pathology of the Academy of Medical Sciences of the USSR [28].

Speransky became a visionary pathophysiologist who, thanks to his training with Pavlov and his personal journey as a researcher, proposed a "Copernican turn" in medicine's concept of the health-disease process [29]. By the time Speransky formulated his “Bases for a New Theory in Medicine” in 1936 [28], it is interesting to see how he conceptually anticipated proposals that today can only be clearly understood from the complexity sciences (from nonlinear dynamic systems and chaos theory applied to medicine) (see Chap. 7). His proposals, grounded in rigorous experimental bases from a logical and methodological point of view, invite nonlinear, irreversible, evolutionary, and integrative readings of physiological processes in medicine [30].

Speransky, like Pavlov, designed experiments very strictly so that an animal had to be healthy beforehand, with no history of trauma or prior irritation, in order to be subjected to an experiment. Animal observation was also carried out over an extended period (chronic experiments) that stretched far beyond the apparent recovery of the animal from an experimental injury. This allowed them to observe changes that did not happen immediately but took their time to manifest. For example, an experimental lesion could be induced in the sciatic nerve of the animal’s right hind limb, and over the course of days to weeks an ulcer would appear on the ipsilateral hind limb; however, a few weeks or months later, symmetrical ulcers might also develop on the contralateral limb. Likewise, pathological changes could be observed months later in the forelimbs, pelvic or abdominal organs, among others. All this was strictly recorded in the experimentation logs and analyzed at the time of concluding the experimental results. The experiments were also carried out on different animal species, replicated by other groups of fellow researchers, and many included both control groups and experimental groups.

The core conceptual elements of his proposal are the following [21]:

A. *On the role of the NS in pathology*: Unlike classical conceptions of disease pathogenesis, Speransky conceives the NS as a whole[3] that intervenes and organizes all the pathological processes of the organism without exception. Clinical manifestations arise from the expression of pathological reflexes organized by the NS.
B. *On the nature of irritation*: Irritation in the body is a process that has a reflex basis that is not restricted to a specific area of the body, since this reflex can extend to other nearby or distant areas depending on individual memories.
C. *About the irritant and irritation*: Irritants can be infectious, traumatic, toxic, physical, or chemical. The role of the irritation process in the body, in the vast majority of cases, is more important than the irritant itself. This irritation process depends on how the organism’s “terrain” is: it depends on its prior functional state or tone of the NS (excitatory, inhibitory), on its metabolic or physicochemical state, and on the organism’s previous memories. Speransky also demonstrated how, from any point int the organism, irritative information

[3] Speransky considers the NS as an indivisible unit. In his work, he expressed his disagreement with the division or classification that the analytic school imposed on the nervous system, dividing it into central, peripheral and autonomic NS [21]. This division is the result of an analytical rationality and methodology and does not mean that NS really operates in a divided way, nor that there are parts of it independent of each other or autonomous in reality.

can be generated and reflected to other parts of the same organism, regardless of the type of irritant and whether the information originates from a sensory, motor or autonomic branch.[4]

D. *Regarding the trophic function of the NS:* In the NS there is a trophic function[5] that is "ubiquitous" throughout the organism. This trophic function in the history of physiology, due to analytical methodologies, was attributed to the division of the autonomic or vegetative nervous system. However, many of Speransky's experiments demonstrate that it is easy to generate, from any point in the NS, the activity of mechanisms that generate physicochemical alterations in the periphery. The vegetative nervous system is merely a special case of those functional characteristics that are known as nervous trophism.

   If the nervous system satisfactorily provides trophism and, consequently, maintains the function of cells and tissues, then the body is in a state of health and high resistance to potentially pathogenic factors [28].

E. *Regarding dystrophies in the organism*: Within the framework of Speransky's theory, "dys-trophy" turns out to be the pathological alteration or deviation of this trophic function coordinated by the NS (neurodystrophy), thus affecting the tissues it innervates and giving rise to pathological reflexes and manifestations.

F. *On segmental extension and beyond the segment of neurodystrophies:* Speransky observed that neurodystrophies could exhibit several behaviors: they could be limited to a segmental sphere (encompassing other tissue and organic structures innervated by the same segmental nerve group—see Chap. 15) or they could follow a course that leads to the spread of neurodystrophy beyond the segment from which it began. It is important to mention that, within the framework of the segment, an irritation originating at one point of the segment will tend to become symmetrical, that is, to express itself in the contralateral tissues, in the case of paired structures. This was verified by Speransky and his collaborators through histological studies in which, after injury to some tissue or nerve of a specific segment, they observed morphological changes in the roots, ipsilateral and contralateral dorsal root ganglia 10–15 days later.

If the neurodystrophic process continues, or if further irritations are added to the pathological process, what will happen after observing ipsilateral and contralateral changes in the dorsal root ganglia and roots is that the inflammatory reaction will begin to spread in a non-uniform way throughout the spinal cord, reaching, in some cases, to the cerebral cortex[6] (disseminated encephalomyelitis). Speransky observed that it was very common that, if the pathological process had begun in the lumbosacral section (lower or hind limbs), the inflammatory

[4] Following Speransky's thinking, these classifications of nerves are also the result of an analytical process of thought, but they do not reflect reality. In academic practice, the object (the nervous system) is divided to facilitate its understanding, but this does not mean that in reality this object is divided.

[5] The word trophism comes from the Greek τροφή, which means "food". In medicine, it has been used to refer to the process and nutritional status of a tissue.

[6] Corresponding to a phase of corticalization or generalization of neurodystrophy.

process easily "jumped" to the cervicothoracic section (upper or front limbs). Otherwise, if the neurodystrophic process had begun in the cervicothoracic segment, its spread would eventually affecting the lumbosacral segment.

Other ways of extending irritation beyond the segment no longer depend on aspects that seem to have a biological or phylogenetic basis but depend on the system's history of irritations. That is, in a hypothetical case of an organism that has experienced an initial irritation in the lower limbs, but this inflammation has apparently subsided and disappeared, when an irritation occurs or a "second hit" occurs elsewhere -- for example, in the trigeminal region (an extraction or a root canal in humans) -- the process in the lower limbs can reactivate and continue its pathological course, generating an inflammatory joint process or chronic pain in that limb.[7]

G. *On the sum of irritations and second hit*: According to Speransky, and as previously mentioned, irritations tend to accumulate. However, this is an aspect that depends on the time factor. In other words, it depends on how much time has elapsed between one irritation and the next. If two irritations occur very close in time, the pathological reaction to the first irritation can inhibit the reaction to the second. But if the irritations are distanced from each other for a certain time, it may happen that, although the body's reaction to a first irritation has subsided, once a second irritation is added (regardless of the place where it occurs), it acts as a "second hit," giving the first irritation a kind of "force" that restarts the initial pathological process, facilitating its clinical manifestation.

On the other hand, Speransky repeatedly observed that in animals, surgical procedures intended to prevent a pathological process from spreading, what they really achieved was to increase and add to the pathological process. Thus, the surgical procedure, depending on when it occurs in the organism's history, can act as just another irritant, like any other trauma.

H. *Importance of irritations of the oral cavity in pathophysiological processes:* Speransky and collaborators demonstrated with several experiments how neurodystrophy could be generated from an irritation in the oral cavity of an animal, affecting other organs and structures of the organism. After performing an extraction of an animal's molar, leaving the alveolus exposed to irritating substances (chemical or infectious), he observed that, days to weeks later, the animal developed infections such as conjunctivitis, keratitis, otitis, sinusitis, caries of several teeth, and even pulpal necrosis. But he not only found segmental involvement in these experiments (within the trigeminal circuit), but also, in some cases, pneumonia or hemorrhages in the lung parenchyma and various gastrointestinal disturbances, including hemorrhagic ulcers.

I. *On the participation of NS in infectious processes*: Infectious diseases are also undergoing a reinterpretation in the light of Speransky's theory. Having experimented with a wide range of microorganisms and their derivatives (such as the

[7] These processes highlight the non-linearity of reactions or reflexes in the organism, as well as the total dependence of individual factors in the course of diseases.

rabies virus, diphtheria and tetanus toxin, streptococci, staphylococci, *Vibrio cholerae*, meningococcus, Koch's bacillus, *Treponema pallidum*, and *Salmonella typhi*), Speransky and his group of collaborators were able to conclude that, in a large proportion of cases, infectious disease was merely the "indicator" of an underlying neurodystrophic problem. In some cases, infections can also initiate the pathological process, but their role has been overestimated and isolated from the state of the nervous system. By affecting trophism, tissue nutrition is impaired and its physicochemical characteristics are altered, making the tissue a "culture agar" more or less suitable for the growth of microorganisms.

Although it is true that some infectious agents have some special tropism for certain organs or tissues, such as the lung tropism of the Kochs bacillus, Speransky demonstrated how this tropism could be modified by interventions in the NS that changed the dominant foci. For example, affecting the embryological segment related to the kidney (through the direct injection of the bacillus into the ovary or testicle) to first observe renal involvement in that body in 100% of cases before affecting the lung.

Another aspect observed by Speransky is that in infectious processes, even when the infectious agent has been completely eliminated or the toxin derived from an infectious agent has been completely neutralized by its antitoxin, the irritative and pathological process in the organism continues its course, unleashing qualitatively different clinical presentations depending on the infectious[8] agent. In this regard, Speransky recalled the teachings of Wedensky and Uktomsky, who stated that "the nerve is not an unusually labile apparatus, but rather one of variable lability, designed for the faithful reproduction of different forms of excitation rhythms" [21].

For this reason, Speransky insisted on the importance of focusing on the study of the irritation process, the pathological reflexes triggered by it, and its variables in the organism. Therefore, eliminating the infectious agent is no guarantee of destroying the pathological process, because it has ceased to be the direct cause of the disturbance that was triggered in the organism.

J. *Reinterpretation of the health-disease process*: By studying the irritative processes, the extent of irritation process in the organism, the sum of irritations, and the memories the organism retains of these irritations (which make it impossible to understand the dynamics of each organism without knowing its history), Speransky arrived at a new interpretation of the health-disease process (see Fig. 13.5) [21]:

> The very act of collision between the organism and the foreign agent escapes, in most cases, all observation and estimation, since these two quickly merge into one.

[8] As if some kind of information from the infectious agent had impregnated the NS, generating a change in its excitation rhythms.

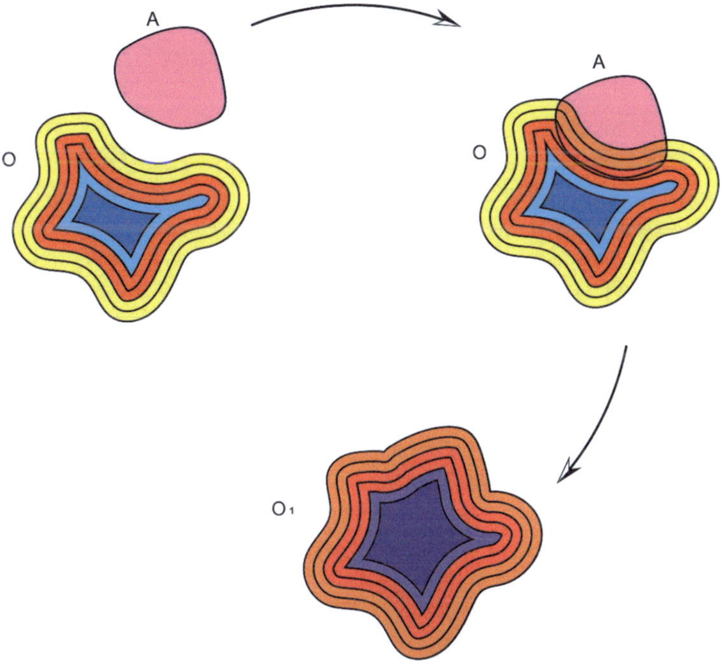

Fig. 13.5 Speransky's proposal on the process of agent-organism collision is shown in a graphic way. In the upper left image, the organism (O) and the agent (A) are shown in an initial stage; the upper right image illustrates the process of "collision" between O and A; in the image below, we can see an organism that differs from the previous one by several features in its pattern of organization, configuring, in agreement with Speransky, a new organism O1. (Source: Own elaboration)

> We are here not dealing here with a disease in the organism, but with a NEW organism[9] that is distinguished from the original by a number of constant or accidental features.
>
> Disease is not something foreign to the organism, but is part of it, combining with all the rest in a single whole.

In addition, Speransky demonstrated cases in which there was a natural resistance to infections, organisms that activated their natural mechanisms to avoid getting sick (also called the process of sanogenesis) [28]. However, when an alteration of this nervous system was generated through a non-specific irritative act, these natural mechanisms in that organism could be affected.

[9] Within the framework of the current chaos theory and nonlinear dynamic systems, Speransky would be referring to the occurrence of irreversible, dynamic, and evolutionary phenomena in the physiological and pathological processes of organisms.

2.6 On Therapeutic Interventions targeting the NS for the Treatment of Diseases in Organisms

Once the mechanisms of pathogenesis in the organism coordinated by the NS were revealed, Speransky also focused on discovering those mechanisms that could generate a change in this pathological dynamic. At the beginning of his research, he found that certain interventions in the organism could generate both delay or total arrest of the development of a pathological process after an irritation, as well as partial or complete recovery of a pathological process that had already been established.

Speransky found that interventions such as "pumping"[10] could change the pathological course of end-stage meningitis in children at Leningrad's Filatov Hospital, leading to a complete recovery in 71% of cases. In other cases, it prevented death and prevented the development of a pathological process after exposing rabbits to a high dose of diphtheria toxin. These results were reproduced with similar results with streptococci, staphylococci, cholera vibrio and salmonella typhi. Pumping was also able to modify the susceptibility of the organism to certain drugs, such as ether, preventing the induction of a narcotic state in animals exposed to this substance. In humans, other applications of pumping were used as a single or adjuvant treatment to treat Parkinson's disease, rheumatic diseases, exanthemic typhus, and quinine-resistant malaria, among others [21].

However, pumping was not the only therapeutic tool found by Speransky to change the course of pathological processes. Thanks to the research of his professor A. V. Vishnevsky, he learned about the therapeutic effects of local anesthesia. At that time, the anesthetic available was novocaine (better known today as procaine).

It was not the first time that the therapeutic effects of anesthesia on inflammatory processes had been explored; Spiess in 1906 had already found that both wounds and various types of inflammation recovered much faster with the use of local anesthesia. These facts were also verified by A. V. Vishnevsky at the same time [31]. Then, around 1923, there is a record of the creation of his method of anesthetic infiltration, which was later called "local anesthesia by creeping infiltratation"[11] [32]. This method began to be widely used in the treatment of inflammatory, infectious, and necrotic disorders, as well as in GI ulcers, intestinal obstruction, shock, and burns, among others [33].

Vishnevsky, along with his surgeon son Alexander Alexandrovich, began to observe complications secondary to intense irritation following surgical procedures, which resulted in poor wound healing, edema, and even necrosis of the tissues. Obviously, infection, sepsis, and shock were also observed. For this reason, they began to develop methods to reduce the irritations that were generated

[10] Pumping consisted of a procedure in which a lumbar puncture was performed, cerebrospinal fluid was extracted and then reintroduced, again and again, until the fluid obtained was bloody.

[11] This creeping method consisted of massive blockage of a large number of nerve elements and differed from truncal blocks.

intraoperatively. This led them to use local anesthetics in the postoperative phase under the name of "novocaine blocks," observing an improvement in phlebitis, acidosis, and pulmonary complications. Everything pointed to the valuable role of local anesthesia in a wide spectrum of inflammatory conditions. For many years, they used local anesthesia in acute and chronic inflammatory phenomena without any mention of complications. They also infiltrated the base of boils (the underlying tissue) to verify the decrease in inflammation and then used local anesthesia in acute and chronic osteomyelitis of the long bones by infiltrating the tissues [33].

Later, the Vishnevskys created the following kinds of blocking:

1. Novocaine blocks for the lumbar sympathetic chain, adrenal plexus, renal plexus, and neighboring sympathetic and cerebrospinal nerves.
2. Circular blocking of the limbs and blocking by planes.
3. Presacral, vagus-sympathetic block, and limited nerve block in situ.

After many years of carrying out these blockages, the Vishnevskys proposed an explanation of their mechanism of action in the organism, through the observation of their activity divided into two physiological moments [33]:

1. At first, exclusion or nerve block occurs, during which nerve impulses are interrupted.
2. In a second moment, nerve excitation occurs, during which trophic regulation of the NS takes place.

Soon, the Vishnevskys began to observe "remote" effects of novocaine blocks, prompting their colleagues Kirtzen and Zuberman at the Institute of Surgery to propose that novocaine exerts its action at a distance through the CNS, under conditions where humoral diffusion is not possible. According to the clinically evidenced experiences of the Vishnevskys and their collaborators, the regulatory function is not only manifested at the local level of the NS but at the general level. Here, by Ukhtomsky's law of dominance, the new irritation is captured primarily by the diseased or sensitized foci, both central and peripheral.

Speransky had the opportunity to use the knowledge of his colleagues and also used novocaine in experimental models in which he administered tetanus toxin to rabbits and dogs, finding that if he mixed the toxin with the anesthetic and injected it into the animal's subcutaneous tissue, the development of the disease was delayed or prevented in more than 50% of cases. Later, he adopted the scheme of novocaine blocks to achieve therapeutic effects in affections of the digestive organs, the organs of the face, and even in septic processes, as documented in the appendices of his main work [21].

Speransky argued that anesthesia, like pumping, could have a therapeutic effect by acting as a weak irritant. Weak irritants, according to the Vishnevskys, have the ability to improve tissue metabolism and increase their vital and defensive capacity by modulating the inflammatory process [33]. In other words, anesthesia can function as an agent that favors eutrophic mechanisms in the organism. Speransky thought that this weak irritant could also trigger a reorganization of the organism: Assuming that a part P is separated from the organism O, it will not result in an "O minus P" situation because the elements of O will have reorganized in a different

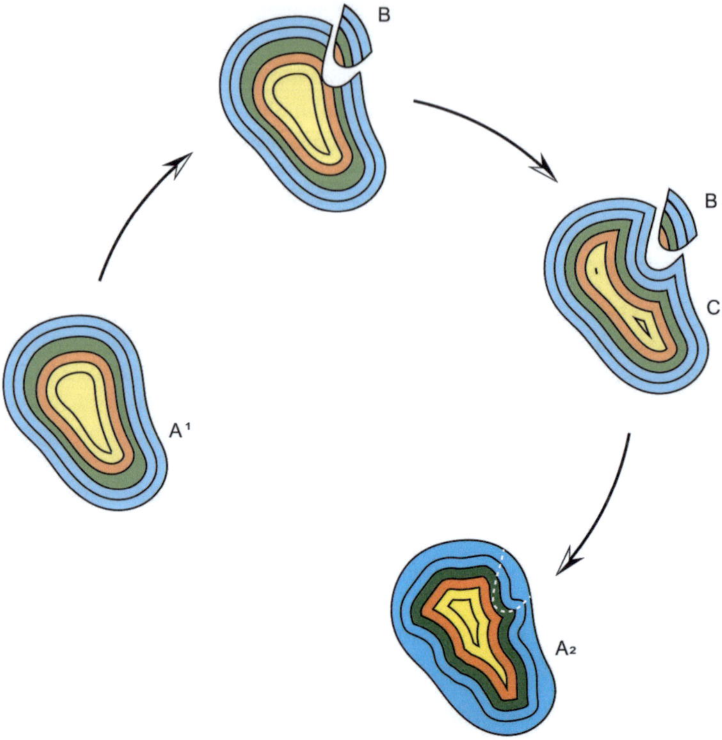

Fig. 13.6 Speransky's proposal on the reorganization of the organism as a complex system, subsequent to the anesthetic action, is illustrated. The organism is in a state A1, and part B is anesthetized. Next, the organism is reorganized without part B, constituting a new organism C. By the time the anesthetic effect is over, part B is integrated back into that organism, but in this process both the organism's interpretation of part B changes, as well as globally, thus constituting a new organism A2. (Source: Own elaboration)

way, until they form the structure O1. Once part P is reintegrated into the organism, the latter is reorganized again, forming the O_2 system (see Fig. 13.6).

2.7 *Corticovisceral Pathology*

The problem of the relationship between the cortex and organs was studied by the Pavlovian school for more than 30 years. Bykov generalized and systematized them in the work "The Cerebral Cortex and the Internal Organs." Corticovisceral pathology studies the disorder of the functional relationships between the cortex and the organs. Its foundation is the reflex theory of Sechenov, Wedensky, and Pavlov; its starting point is Pavlov's doctrine of "experimental neuroses" and it is inspired by Speransky's findings on considering the reflex mechanism in the genesis of pathologies.

One of the first experimental neuroses in animals to be induced and studied was in 1916 using a circle and an ellipse. The circle was part of a CR, and the ellipse was presented without reinforcement. But the researcher was changing the angulation of the ellipse so that it progressively resembled the circle, until at one point the dog could no longer differentiate between one and the other, and entered a state of generalized excitement. In Pavlov's laboratory, Petrova found that animals suffering from neuroses developed tachycardia, dyspnea, alopecia, trophic ulcers, and organ tumors, among other pathological conditions.

Anokhin states that the basis of neurosis is the conflict between two integral activities, between two systems of stimulation; it is the overtension due to two rival activities. The origin of these neuroses is based on signaling that comes first from the external environment and, secondly, from the internal environment of the organism. They also have a great influence when an external and interoceptive disturbance converge. Whereas when information comes solely from interoceptive signaling, it has a lower impact.

Ukhtomsky in this regard stated that:

> The cerebral cortex acts as a mediator between two isolated and independent data sets. Each one is regulated by its own laws in space and time. However, the life of an organism depends on how quickly one series adapts to another, according to the specific meaning of their encounter [20].

Pavlov considered that in human beings the analogue of experimental neuroses would be the adverse or traumatic conditions of human life (going through misfortunes, loss of loved ones, and suffering constant abuse, among others).

Organ disorders can arise as a result of a neurosis that generates a functional weakening of cortical cells and lability of nervous processes, especially internal inhibition. This leads to an alteration of cortico-subcortical relationships with consequences for the vegetative system and viscera. However, visceral diseases can also be generated by the CR route as a result of the formation of a temporary connection that can have both and general effects. First, the visceral disturbance is limited to a functional disorder. Then, depending on the degree of alteration and duration of the disorder, organic lesions are created. This alteration can persist in a vicious cycle, in which the cortex persistently transmits pathological signals to the viscera, until cortical activity returns to normal.

For example, Bykov and Kurtsin (1968) mention in their work that some researchers combined an acoustic stimulus with the injection of camphor, forming a CR with the acoustic sound. When the sound was heard again, epileptic contractions appeared in the animals, just as when camphor was injected. In another experiment, the researchers injected dysenteric toxin into dogs in a room. Kazantsev pointed out a single injection was sufficient for the animal to develop the entire symptomatic complex of the dysenteric process in the room where the injection had been administered. Via CR, it is possible to generate many morbid phenomena such as hypertension, cardiac dysfunction, a diabetic state, secretory and motor alterations of the digestive system, and different blood disorders.

However, not only can pathological phenomena be created through CR, but they can also be suppressed. There was a case of a patient with bronchial asthma that always occurred at the same time of night. At the indicated time, they instructed her to set an alarm clock. Then, asthma attack occurred every time the alarm sounded. Days later, she suspended the alarm and the asthma attack did not occur again.

In humans, through the second system of signals, multiple vegetative disturbances can be induced and positive influences can be exerted on existing ones. Experiments have been described in which various emotions or hypnotic states modify cardiovascular status and other visceral reflexes, such as nausea or increased digestive secretions. For example, the suggestion under hypnosis that three glasses of water are being ingested resulted in an increase in the elimination of up to 500 mL of urine during the first hour afterward [20].

2.8 Functional Systems According to Anokhin

Pavlov's theory of RCs leaves a gap in explaining why living organisms are concerned with creating corrections for their behavioral errors. That is, goal-directed behavioral acts do not end after the action, as the reflex theory indicates, but continue until they achieve that satisfy the dominant needs. In addition, the activity of organisms is sometimes not limited to the external stimuli, as there are also internal stimuli, genetics, individual experiences, etc.

Pyotr Anokhin's theory of functional systems (FS), although at the same time inspired by Pavlov's theory of CR, emerges as a proposal to overcome its limitations. The FS are units of the organism's integrative activity, comprising a complex of multiple systemic organizations connected by their dynamic relationships. They are "dynamic, self-organizing, self-regulating central/peripheral organizations." These systems interact and cooperate in achieving adaptive outcomes that are useful for the system and for the organism as a whole. Some control the internal environment; others control behavior and their interaction with the environment and their companions. Some FSs that control metabolism are genetically determined, while others arise during ontogeny according to the needs of the environment [34].

FS are also characterized by forming mechanisms that anticipate current events and correct the results:

> Any deviation from an important critical level of a physiologically important factor leads to an immediate mobilization of numerous apparatuses of the corresponding FS with the aim of restoring the adaptive outcome that is vitally essential [34].

They selectively involve various organs and tissues within their activity under a principle of cooperation, which means that no element is a passive part of the FS but actively interacts with other elements of the FS to facilitate the achievement of the adaptive result. In the light of this new conception, the organs would not have fixed functions but rather dynamic ones that vary according to the FS to which they belong.

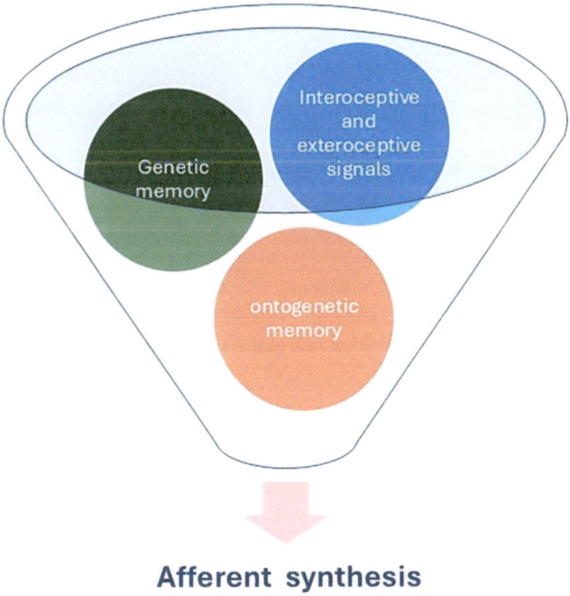

Fig. 13.7 Afferent synthesis. (Source: Own elaboration)

All FS, regardless of their complexity, have a basic architectural or functional structure that is composed of several stages [34]:

1. *Afferent synthesis*: At this stage, the CNS synthesizes excitations caused by internal needs, external stimuli, and other triggers, with the constant use of genetic and individually acquired memory (see Fig. 13.7).
2. *Decision-making*: This restricts the degrees of freedom of the FS's activity and selects only one line of action of the effector capable of satisfying the needs required by the organism.
3. *Acceptor of action results*: Efferent action formation is the stage of predicting (anticipating) the required outcome of the FS's activity. At this stage, the main parameters of the required result are programmed and a constant evaluation is maintained through feedback mechanisms.
4. *Efferent synthesis*: This is where an executive act is formed centrally and then executed by the peripheral effector elements recruited by the FS.
5. *Evaluation of the Result of Action*: It is permanent and is carried out through reverse afferentiation (feedback) generated by the appropriate receptors stimulated by external factors and through humoral signals received by the involved structures. In this process, reverse afferentiation with respect to outcome plays an evaluative role in the systemic self-organization of goal-directed behavior and acts as the first determinant of the self-regulation of all SFs (see Fig. 13.8).

Through the formulation of the notion of "reverse afferentiation," Anokhin established a recognized priority in the field of cybernetics in living systems. This reverse

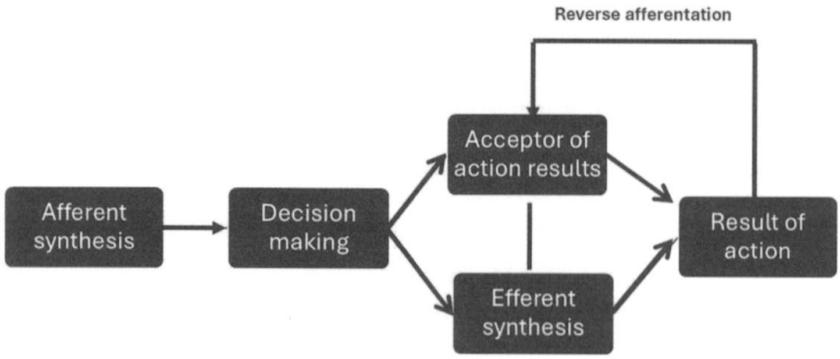

Fig. 13.8 Arquitectonic of functional systems. (Source: Own elaboration)

afferentiation had been introduced 12 years earlier than the concept of feedback by Norbert Wiener.

Another aspect to consider is that, at any given time, the activity of the organism is determined by a dominant FS in terms of its contribution to survival and adjustment to the environment. Likewise, after the satisfaction of a dominant need, the organism's activity focuses on another socially or biologically significant dominant need through the creation of a new FS. This process occurs all the time in organisms [34].

According to the theory of the FS, emotions have an essential biological value since they have the power to mobilize the intention and actions of the organism to satisfy emerging needs. Negative emotions usually induce the search for a support agent, whereas positive emotion accompanies the moment of achieving results and constitutes positive reinforcement. Positive emotions also have the characteristic of helping in memory retention, which includes the entire sequence of actions that made the goal be met [35].

Moreover, from this perspective, mental and emotional processes involve not only the brain but the entire organism, similar to the stance of "embodied cognition" aligned with Hegel's "neutral monism," which argues that the mental and physical levels are two aspects of a unified reality. In other words, the term "mental" characterizes the organization of activity not only in neurons but also in other anatomical structures of the organism [36].

2.9 *Application of the Concepts of Synthetic Physiology and Nervism to the Clinical Practice of Neuraltherapeutic Medicine*

2.9.1 In the Initial Assessment of a Patient

One of the first applications that arise from the concepts of synthetic physiology and Russian nervism to the practice of neuraltherapeutic medicine is that, when evaluating a patient in consultation, it is essential to bear in mind first and foremost that they are an indivisible being, with internal systems and elements that establish nonlinear and dynamic relationships and that they possess a history of events that have been stored as memories throughout the entire organism. These memories allow an individual to have a singular physiology (with unique CR and FS) and make their own life narrative the only reliable text to consult (see Chap. 20).

As will be seen in Chaps. 15 and 24, the analysis of a patient's life history, from the perspective of synthetic physiology, has two main axes:

1. Determine, in the context of URs that are based on embryological development, what is the level of reflex involvement of a given segment (whether trigeminal, cervical, dorsal, etc.). These reflexes tend to exhibit the least interindividual variability, indicating that the progression of an irritation within a segment could be more easily anticipated by understanding its embryological relationships (see Chap. 15).
2. Determine the temporal associations that originated in the history of an organism, including its body and psyche (through the second signal system and corticovisceral relationships). Clearly, those CRs formed from early childhood are of special interest, because they will set the pattern for the tendencies the organism will exhibit in adulthood, such as, respiratory or gastrointestinal processes in childhood. More easily, the oldest CRs are the ones that can become dominant foci. This does not exclude the possibility that more recent CRs may acquire such pathological dominance. Importantly, understanding such ancient reflexes could serve as a basis for identifying where post-trauma irritation is most likely to extend (beyond the segment) in adulthood (see Chap. 24).

2.9.2 In the Diagnostic Field

Precisely, due to the fact that RCs and FS are dynamic, changing during the life of the individual, this supports the position of neuraltherapeutic medicine in considering that lifelong diagnoses, such as hypertension, hypothyroidism, and diabetes, cannot be established. It can only be said that, for a certain time, an organism can have a certain number of pathological reflexes and a special pattern of organization, which can change partially or completely in the course of life, depending on how the system interacts with the new external information and its internal motivations and needs.

On the other hand, in the context of Speransky's theory, pathologies can have several stages of evolution: they may be at a segmental level, beyond the segment, or in a generalized process. It is important to remember that when considering the genesis and evolution of pathologies, the oral cavity should not be excluded, since many pathological foci or reflexes can originate as a result of infectious, traumatic, as well as chemical irritants (see Chap. 43) or electromagnetic irritants (see Chap. 17) generated by the presence of metallic materials within the oral cavity.

2.9.3 In the Therapeutic Field

Understanding that pathologies, in the light of Pavlov's theory of CR, are reflexes that were created at a given moment between UR and new stimuli that each organism integrated into its ontogenetic development, all physiological and pathological reflexes are potentially inhibitable, as Pavlov demonstrated. But this ability to inhibit a pathological reflex will vary according to the UR with which it was associated. For example, a CR associated with survival information may require many reinforcements to inhibit, whereas one associated with gastric secretion may be easily inhibited with just few repetitions.

Moving on to the action of procaine or local anesthesia, it could also be understood in the light of Pavlov's theory of CR with the following case: when a patient is experiencing pain, for example, in a limb, and at that very moment a weak stimulus is applied to the body, according to the Pavlovian rules of conditioned inhibition, this can lead to the inhibition of a previously established pathological reflex, as long as it is not reinforced by the UR (the cause that generated it). In the case of emotional trauma, evoking the exact memory that triggers the pathological reaction (panic, depression, anxiety, etc.) while applying a weak stimulus can also generate a conditioned inhibition (see Chap. 41).

Another important aspect in therapy that has a leading value is to be able to intervene in the identified pathological dominant foci, since, as a consequence of inhibiting a dominant center, other reflexes that are associated with it can be suppressed, facilitating the patient's recovery in a much shorter time (see Chap. 25).

In the case of acute or chronic infectious diseases, according to the findings of Vishnevsky and Speransky, neuraltherapeutic action can serve as an adjuvant to these processes. Subsequent studies in the literature have reported a broad-spectrum antimicrobial effect of procaine [37], which could support the therapeutic decision to administer it alone (in a few specific cases) or in combination with antibiotics. However, additional studies would be required to support these decisions in clinical practice.

2.9.4 Post-therapeutic Phase

Finally, in the post-therapeutic phase, due to the mechanisms of nervous inhibition and excitation, an organism may exhibit a transient increase in its excitatory process until a natural transmarginal inhibition is reached, rapidly or progressively suppressing the pathological symptoms. In other words, after an intervention with procaine, it is possible to observe a transient increase (in a matter of hours) of symptoms, which then subside over the following hours or days. The speed of these inhibitory changes will depend on several factors, such as the tone of the SN, the presence of other CR/FS that are active at the time of the intervention and the type of NS (which is determined both genetically and epigenetically), which can express different types of response to stimuli (rapid, slow, vigorous, or phlegmatic).

2.9.5 The "Interfering Field" in the Light of Synthetic Physiology

In the history of neural therapy in Germany (see Chap. 2), the occurrence of distant reactions from the site of initial application of procaine has been reported several times. It has also been mentioned that these changes can occur in a matter of seconds, for example, the immediate elimination of chronic pain with recovery of the functionality of a lower limb after the injection of procaine in an upper limb. This phenomenon was called at the time "phenomenon in seconds"and its occurrence was attributed to the existence (until then, hypothetical) of "interfering fields.".

It is interesting to see how synthetic physiology can provide, at this point, all the understanding and strenght of the experimental bases that underpinned the studies of Pavlov, Ukhtomsky and Speransky alike. In the first place, from the theory of CR, these "distant" associations are not the exception but the constant. The CNS has a permanent cortical coupling function that allows it to generate temporal associations that can relate, within the framework of individual histories, anatomical parts apparently distant from each other. If one of these cortical associations is therapeutically intervened upon, it is highly feasible that a change can occur within seconds despite the anatomical distance of the related elements. Since they are absolutely close when considering the representation of its elements in the cortex, the distance is only apparent. In this case, the factor that united them was a "synchronous discharge"in time, generating a non-local process.

For his part, Ukhtomsky offers a much clearer physiological scenario for the "interfering field," since his concept of dominant centers or foci provides a comprehensive and robust description of what is observed in clinical practice. There are traumas or irritating memories that at some point generate distant reactions that cannot be explained by analytical physiology. A dominant focus changes the functioning of other nerve centers, both favoring the "irritative excitation" of some and inhibiting others. For illustrative purposes, a patient, for example, after undergoing hernia surgery that included the placement of a foreign material in the abdomen (mesh), begins to manifest trigeminal neuralgia with no apparent cause. Obviously, within his life history, he had already had several lesions and irritations in the oral cavity and other branches of the trigeminal, but when the focus of dominance formed in the abdomen, it attracted to its "orbit" the focus of excitation of the trigeminal territory (which had remained subthreshold and was weaker than the abdominal). At the same time, it inhibit thyroid function, causing hypothyroidism in the patient that also began from abdominal surgery. Then, when procaine is injected in the abdomen, trigeminal neuralgia subsides, as well as a regulation of thyroid hormone secretion.

Speransky, in his research that began in 1923, also clearly identified the generation of processes at a distance from the site of initial irritation. As previously mentioned, this was supported by histological studies after the sacrifice of the animal. In fact, he called this type of phenomenon "extension of the dystrophic process beyond the segment."

Much remains to be explored and expanded, but synthetic physiology and Russian nervism undoubtedly paved the way for a greater understanding of the complexity inherent in health-disease processes.

Acknowledgements My sincere thanks to Jorge Kaczewer, coordinator and professor of the Higher University Course of Neuraltherapeutic Medicine and Neurofocal Dentistry, which is carried out together with the University of Rosario in Buenos Aires, Argentina. Jorge K. shared with me bibliographic material related to Russian Nervism, which facilitated the elaboration of this chapter.

I also express my gratitude to Jorge Iván Salazar Marín. Professor of the Neural Therapy area of the Master's Degree in Alternative Medicine, Faculty of Medicine, National University of Colombia, for his invaluable contributions during these years in the field of Russian Nervism that include both bibliographic materials and knowledge transfer.

In memory of Miguel Martínez, who was a professor and coordinator of the Master's program in Physiology at the Faculty of Medicine of the National University of Colombia. He was my guide and reading companion, instilling in me a motivation for critically examining the history of physiology and always reminding me of the importance of building bridges in knowledge.

References

1. Bykov K, Konradi G. Fundamental concepts of physiology. In: Bykov KM, editor. Text-book of physiology. Moscow: Foreign Languages Publishing House; 1960. p. 15–45.
2. Sarmiento LD. History of institutionalization of neural therapy in Colombia [master's thesis] [Bogotá]: Universidad Nacional de Colombia; 2014. 72 p. [Spanish] Available at: https://repositorio.unal.edu.co/handle/unal/49642.
3. Pinilla-Bonilla LB, Rodríguez DC, Villamil-Villar WA. British and Russian Nervism: a comparison between two trends in history focused on nervous system. Méd UIS. 2024;37(1):33–40. [Spanish]. Disponible en: https://revistas.uis.edu.co/index.php/revistamedicasuis/article/view/15186
4. Canguilhem G. Constitution of physiology as a science. Palau A, translator. In: Kayser C, editor. Physiologie. Volume I. Paris: Editions Medicales Flammarion; 1963.
5. Guerlac H. Chemistry as a branch of physics: Laplace's collaboration with Lavoisier. Hist Stud Phys Sci. 1976;7:193–276. https://doi.org/10.2307/27757357.
6. Leon A. Laplace-Lavoisier Collaboration. Gen Sci J 2022 May [Internet]: 1–21. Available at: https://www.gsjournal.net/Science-Journals/Research%20Papers/View/9236.
7. Canguilhem G. The normal and the pathologic. Buenos Aires: Siglo veintiuno Argentina; 1971. [Spanish]
8. Stahnisch FW. François Magendie (1783–1855). J Neurol. 2009;256(11):1950–2. https://doi.org/10.1007/s00415-009-5291-3.
9. Rothschuh KE. The physiology. In: Laín Entralgo P, editor. Universal history of medicine. Barcelona: Salvat Editors; 1974. p. 59–97. [Spanish].
10. Navarro K, Pinilla L. The contributions of Henry head to neuroanatomical and physiological bases of therapy segment. Méd UIS. 2013;26(2):33–44. [Spanish]. Available at: https://revistas.uis.edu.co/index.php/revistamedicasuis/article/view/3919
11. Swash M. Henry head and the development of clinical neuroscience. Brain. 2008;131(12):3453–6. https://doi.org/10.1093/brain/awn258.
12. Grashchenkov NI. Relationships between British and Russian medicine and neurology, and the role of the National Hospital, Queen Square, London, in the Development of Russian Neuropathology. J Neurol Neurosurg Psychiatry. 1960;23:185–90.

13. Mirsky MB. Establishing the Golitsyn hospital: the contribution of professor Efrem Osipovich Mukhin (1766-1850). J Med Biogr. 2010;18(3):127–32. https://doi.org/10.1258/jmb.2009.009094.
14. Nikolenko VN, Litvinenko LM, Nikityuk DB, Klochkova SV. E. O. Mukhin—the nugget of Russian land (to the 250th anniversary). J Anat Histopathol. 2016;5(3):95–7. [Russian]. https://doi.org/10.18499/2225-7357-2016-5-3-95-97.
15. Sorokina TS. Formation of scientific physiology in Russia (First Half of the XIX Century) problems of social hygiene, health care and history of medicine 2015; 23 (4): 52—57 [Russian]. Available at: http://elib.fesmu.ru/Article.aspx?id=323262
16. Lisitsyn Yu. Glevob Ivan Timofeevich. In: Petrovsky BV, editor. Great Medical Encyclopedia (BME), 3rd ed. [Internet] [cited 2024 Dec 10]. [Russian]. Available from: https://бмэ.орг/index.php/ГЛЕБОВ_Иван_Тимофеевич.
17. Kofler W. I.M. Sechenov (1829–1905) and the scientific self-understanding for medical sciences. J Hist Neurosci. 2007;16:30–41.
18. Babkin B. Ivan Petrovich Pavlov (1849–1936). Nature. 1949;164:510–1. https://doi.org/10.1038/164510a0.
19. The Nobel Prize. Ivan Pavlov: the Nobel Prize in physiology or medicine 1904. [Internet] [Tue. 3 Dec 2024.]. NobelPrize.org. Available from: https://www.nobelprize.org/prizes/medicine/1904/pavlov/facts/.
20. Bykov KM, Kurtsin IT. Cortico-visceral pathology. 2nd ed. Madrid: Editorial Atlante; 1968. 849 pp. [Spanish]
21. Speransky AD. A basis for the theory of medicine. New York: International Publishers; 1943.
22. Konradi G. Activity of the nervous system. In: Bykov KM, editor. Text-book of physiology. Moscow: Foreign Languages Publishing House; 1960. p. 516–670.
23. Pavlov IP. Conditioned reflexes: lessons on the function of great hemispheres. 3rd ed. Madrid: Ediciones Morata; 2021. 433 pp. [Spanish]
24. Descartes R. Passions of the soul. 1st ed. Madrid: Biblioteca Nueva; 2005. 192 pp. [Spanish]
25. Delov V. Voice and speech. In: Bykov KM, editor. Text-book of physiology. Moscow: Foreign Languages Publishing House; 1960. p. 740–7.
26. Windholz G. The second signal system as conceived by Pavlov and his disciples. Pavlov J Biol Sci. 1990;25(4):163–73. https://doi.org/10.1007/BF02900699.
27. Zueva EY, Zuev KB. The concept of dominance by A.A. Ukhtomsky and anticipation. In: Nadin M, editor. Anticipation: learning from the past. The Russian/Soviet contributions to the science of anticipation, Cognitive systems monographs, vol. 25. New York: Springer; 2015. p. 13–35. https://doi.org/10.1007/978-3-319-19446-2_2.
28. Delitsyna NS, Magaeva SV, Karganov MY. Academician Alexei Dimitrievich Speransky. Moscow: Research Institute of General Pathology and Pathophysiology Publisher; 2019. 113 pp. [Russian]
29. Pinilla-Bonilla LB. Application of the Peircean research method to the work of Speransky. In: Oostra A, Zalamea F, editors. Cuadernos de sistemática Peirceana. Bogotá: Editorial Nomos; 2012. p. 93–114. https://www.unav.es/gep/bibliopeirceana.html.
30. Pinilla-Bonilla LB. Critical analysis of the theoretical-methodological procedures in the researches of A. D. Speransky supporting neural therapy from Peircean logic [master's thesis] [Bogotá]: Universidad Nacional de Colombia; 2010. 119 p. Available at: https://repositorio.unal.edu.co/handle/unal/6873.
31. Dosch P, Dosch M. Chronological survey. In: Dosch P, Dosch M, editors. Manual of neural therapy according to Huneke. 2nd ed. Stuttgart: Georg Thieme Verlag; 2007. p. 4–8.
32. Lazareva EV, Luzhkov BN. Aleksandr Vasilievich Vishnevsky – soviet surgeon, academician of the USSR Academy of Medical Sciences. Youth Innov Bull. 2012;1(1):181–2. [Russian]. Available at: https://new.vestnik-surgery.com/index.php/2415-7805/article/view/1177
33. Vishnevsky A. The Novocain blockade and balsamic Oleophorous antiseptics as a pathogenic therapeutic form. Buenos Aires, Cartago. 1958.

34. Sudakov KV. Theory of functional systems: a keystone of integrative biology. In: Nadin M, editor. Anticipation: learning from the past, The Russian/Soviet contributions to the science of anticipation. cognitive systems monographs, vol. 25. New York: Springer; 2015. p. 153–73. https://doi.org/10.1007/978-3-319-19446-2_9.
35. Vityaev EE. Purposefulness as a principle of brain activity. In: Nadin M, editor. Anticipation: learning from the past, The Russian/Soviet contributions to the science of anticipation. Cognitive systems monographs, vol. 25. New York: Springer; 2015. p. 231–54. https://doi.org/10.1007/978-3-319-19446-2_13.
36. Alexandrov YI. Cognition as systemogenesis. In: Nadin M, editor. Anticipation: learning from the past. The Russian/Soviet contributions to the science of anticipation, Cognitive systems monographs, vol. 25. New York: Springer; 2015. p. 193–220. https://doi.org/10.1007/978-3-319-19446-2_11.
37. Schmidt RM, Rosenkranz HS. Antimicrobial activity of local anesthetics: lidocaine and procaine. J Infect Dis. 1970;121(6):597–607. https://doi.org/10.1093/infdis/121.6.597. PMID: 4393033

Chapter 14
British Nervism

Laura Bibiana Pinilla Bonilla

1 Introduction

Although the term "Nervism"was originally coined in Russia by the physiologist Ivan Pavlov to denote the predominant or central role that the nervous system has in the coordination of the physiological and pathological processes of organisms, the title of this chapter refers to a similar trend that was generated in Great Britain, led especially by two authors, Henry Head and James Mackenzie [1].

Although many other authors contributed to this vision in medicine in Great Britain, it is beyond the scope of this chapter to carry out an exhaustive review of each of these authors, so the review presented will be centered on the two main authors of this school of thought.

Tracing the antecedents in history since the sixteenth century, it has been documented that Russia and England had exchanges between doctors and professors that had a special influence on the school of neuropathology developed in Russia. This fact was facilitated at the time by Peter the Great in Russia, who introduced the European system of medical education for his country [2].

But this did not only end there, since, during the nineteenth century and the first half of the twentieth century, a large number of short and long visits by scientists and doctors between the two countries were generated to exchange knowledge and participate in scientific events. Physiology in general, as well as physiology focused on the nervous system, has been of particular interest. The friendly relationships between Sir Charles Sherrington and Nicolai Wedensky have been a great example

L. B. Pinilla Bonilla (✉)
Faculty of Medicine, Master in Alternative Medicine, Neural Therapy Area,
Universidad Nacional de Colombia, Bogotá, Colombia

Integrated Health Services Subnetwork of the South, Research and Innovation Center,
Bogotá, Colombia
e-mail: lbpnillab@unal.edu.co

L. B. Pinilla Bonilla et al. (eds.), *Neuraltherapeutic Medicine*,
https://doi.org/10.1007/978-3-032-03257-7_14

of these exchanges. These exchanges continued afterward between Sherrington and Pavlov. Later, one of Pavlov's students, Leon Orbeli, was under Langley's direction in the Cambridge physiology laboratory. Orbeli also had the support of the National Hospital in England and of Gordon Holmes, co-investigator with Henry Head on central sensory pathways [2].

As a result of these relationships and exchanges, a trend emerged in the area of medicine and physiology with two main characteristics: the first has to do with the application of concepts from Darwin's theory of evolution to physiology and biology, and the second is the recognition of the relevance of the nervous system in the physiological and pathological mechanisms of humans and animals [2, 3].

The central axis of this chapter focuses, then, on the life and work of Henry Head and James Mackenzie around their conception of the nervous system as the central axis of the physiological and pathological mechanisms of the organism.

2 Henry Head

Henry Head was born in London in 1862. From the age of 8, he wanted to become a doctor. He studied at Cambridge University, where he obtained a degree in natural sciences. In 1884, he decided to study with Ewald Hering in Prague [4] for 2 years on respiratory physiology and color vision. He returned to London in 1886 to complete his medical studies at University College Hospital in 1890. He was subsequently appointed to work at the National Hospital, in Queen Square; then at Victoria Park Hospital for thoracic diseases; and at Rainhill Asylum in Lancashire, where he had the opportunity to delve into mental pathologies [5, 6].

As discussed in detail in Chap. 15, Henry Head published in the Brain Journal one of his most important works for the field of neuraltherapeutic medicine, which is the basis of what is currently known as visceral dermatomes and Head's zones [7]. After this work, he published two more complementary manuscripts along the same line [8].

In 1899, he was accepted as a Fellow of the Royal Society (See Fig. 14.1), proposed by John Langley and John Hughlings Jackson, among others. In 1896 he was appointed as assistant physician at the London Hospital. In this hospital he took over the professorship taught by Hughlings Jackson, who retired in 1894. Jackson's influence was very important and can be seen in his monograph on aphasia and speech disorders [5].

Head was also always interested in patients' life experiences, stress, and mental changes. In 1901, in fact, he published a manuscript in which he describes the mental changes associated with visceral diseases [9]. Among the clinical cases he presented for the London Hospital, his presentations on contractures and spasms of mental origin are recognized [5, 10].

In 1903, Head dared to be the subject of an experiment, in collaboration with William Halse Rivers, in order to understand the complexities of the peripheral nervous system. The experiment involved cutting the peripheral branches of Henry Head's radial nerve and then suturing them again. Head documented for four

Fig. 14.1 Formal portrait of Sir Henry Head looking right. (Source: G. C. Beresford. Wellcome Collection)

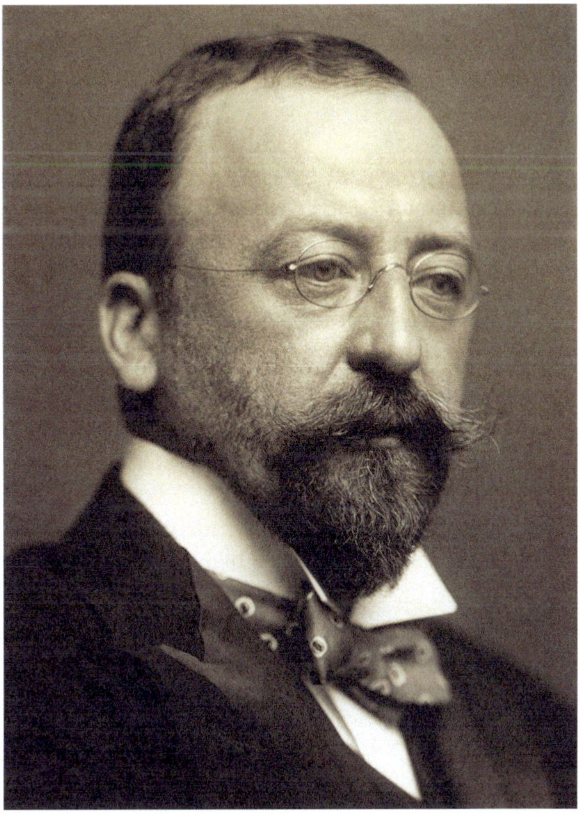

consecutive years the evolution and recovery of his sensitivity together with Rivers. From these experiments, he was able to discriminate between two types of sensitivity that he called protopathic and epicritic [6].

From 1908 to 1925, Henry Head was editor of Brain Journal. At the end of his years, he suffered from Parkinson's disease, although he remained mentally lucid until he died in 1940 [5] .

3 James Mackenzie

James Mackenzie was born in 1853 in Perthshire, Scotland. In 1874, at the age of 21, Mackenzie began studying medicine at Edinburgh University, obtaining his degree in 1878. In 1879, he was appointed as a physician at the Edinburgh Royal Infirmary Hospital. He later settled in the town of Burnley, in the northwest of England, where he remained until 1902. During those years, Mackenzie dedicated himself to studying the meaning of the signs and symptoms that patients suffered and, in addition, sought to understand the mechanism of these symptoms and their prognostic significance [11–13]. Driven by this interest, he began to delve into the changes in sensitivity that were expressed in visceral diseases [14] and, in 1906, he published a study on the participation of autonomic reflexes in the production of visceral pain [15].

When one of his young patients died in labor of heart failure, Mackenzie decided to investigate cardiac diseases with the help of a phlebograph or polygraph, a new instrument that had been developed at the time, with which he was able to study numerous traces from the pulse and relate them to the signs and symptoms of the patients. He even invented the term "extrasystole" and studied various types of arrhythmias, which contributed to the development of cardiology [12].

Mackenzie defended his ideas vigorously in London and became a well-respected professor and physician. In fact, he was elected a Fellow of the Royal College of Physicians, receiving the degree of knight (See Fig. 14.2) [12].

At the age of 65, in 1918, Mackenzie returned to practice medicine at St Andrews and became director of the St Andrews Clinical Institute. While he was director of this institute, he published one of his lesser-known works, in the British Medical Journal, in which he explained his theory on the altered reflexes of the nervous system, by which the symptoms of diseases were produced [16].

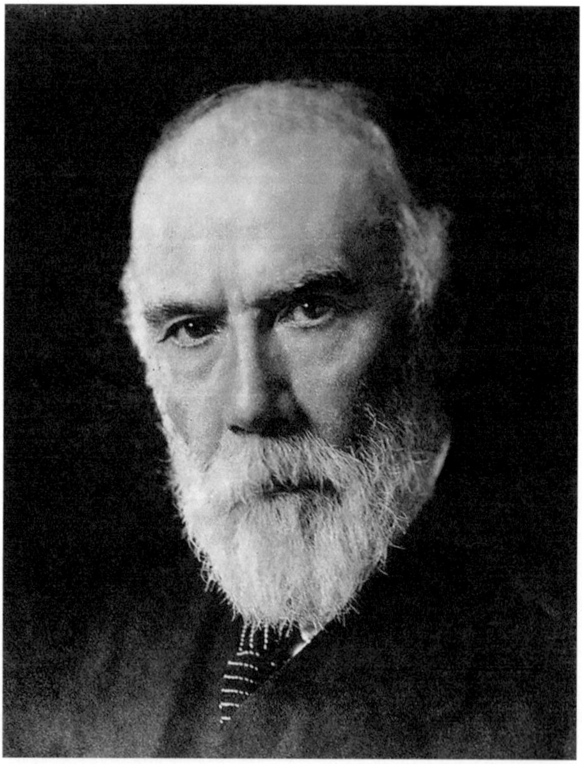

Fig. 14.2 Portrait of Sir James Mackenzie (1853–1925), cardiologist. Attribution 4.0 International (CC BY 4.0). (Source: Wellcome Collection. M0000151: https://wellcomecollection.org/works/dgrmwjg8)

Until the end of his years, Mackenzie criticized specialists who concentrated on diagnosing and treating only one organ while neglecting the entire body. He said that true medical science was to be based on the clinical observation of the whole human being, as he mentions in this passage:

> I fear the day may come when a heart specialist will no longer be a physician looking at the body as a whole, but one with more and more complicated instruments working in a narrow and restricted area of the body—that was never my idea [17].

4 Why Talk about British "Nervism"?

In a previous study conducted by Piñilla et al. [1], a comparative analysis of the Russian school of synthetic physiology or nervism, with the concepts developed by Henry Head and James Mackenzie was carried out, identifying seven areas of coincidence.

It is important to clarify that the proposals of British authors, which are focused on the nervous system and its role in the physiological and pathological processes of the organism, have been little known. Nonetheless, thanks to the characteristic approach of Neuraltherapeutic medicine, the recognition of the valuable proposals of these two authors in relation to the nervous system was facilitated from this area.

Next, an argument is made based on seven axes or conceptual categories [1] that allow us to understand the core of the thought of the British school of nervism.

4.1 The Reflex as the Basic Physiological Unit of the Organism

In his "Theory of disturbed reflexes in the production of symptoms of disease" [16], Mackenzie placed the reflex at the center of the pathophysiological mechanisms that generate a disease. The disease is then the expression of altered reflexes.

Articulated with his theory, there are visceromotor reflexes that generate symptoms in muscle tissues secondary to visceral alterations such as hyperalgesia or increased tone [13]. He also described that the alteration of these reflexes could manifest itself in the bone plane, generating sensitivity in ribs and vertebrae [14] (osteovisceral reflexes).

Meanwhile, Henry Head in his doctoral thesis "On disturbances of sensation with special reference to the pain of visceral disease" [7], describes how superficial reflexes are usually altered in cases of visceral disease, causing a stimulus on the skin, which under normal conditions should not generate any pain or discomfort, to be perceived as painful or as an exaggerated sensation to the touch perceived as tickling. Not only does it describe how cutivisceral reflexes are affected in the presence of disease, but it also describes other types of reflexes, such as the patellar reflex or other types of motor reflexes that are altered in the presence of visceral disease.

4.2 *The Role of the Nervous System as the Main Coordinator of the Body's Pathophysiology*

Mackenzie believes that the whole organism and the activities of the organs depend on reflexes that have their center in the nervous system. The harmonious interplay of these reflexes between the parts of this organism generates what is known as "health" [16].

Mackenzie defines mechanisms by which reflexes could be altered, including the action of the nature of the stimulus on the nervous system and internal aspects that modify the tone of the nervous system. In his own words:

> Symptoms, or, in other words, alterations in the reflex, may be referable to causes acting upon any part of the arc, but in practice they are found to be mainly, confined to alteration in A, the receptor; B, the nerve center or C, the effector [16].

For his part, Henry Head also identified the participation of the nervous system in the generation of the symptoms that were part of the diseases:

> For we must suppose that a sensory disturbance passes up the nerve fibres from the viscera to set up changes in the activity of that segment of the spinal cord in which they terminate; and that these disturbances of activity are referred to that portion of the skin which is supplied by the affected segment [7].

Likewise, it refers to the resistance of the nervous system as something decisive to define the progress of a disease .

4.3 *Physiological Continuity Between Viscera and Other Tissues of the Segment*

Between 1893 and 1896, Henry Head devoted himself to describing the pathophysiological continuity between viscera and skin. In the first manuscript, he showed the reflex changes in skin sensitivity presented by patients with visceral diseases below the clavicles [7]. In his next work, he presented alterations in skin sensitivity for the viscera above the clavicles, including the teeth,[1] and including the reflex sensitivity of the viscera from trunk to head [18]. In the third part of this work, he described, in more detailed semiologically terms, the pain of heart and lung disease [19].

For his part, Mackenzie describes in several sources the mechanism of visceral pain and explains the visceromotor reflex that occurs in the presence of visceral disease, generating muscle contractions that can be accompanied by hyperalgesia. He also described that in some cases of visceral disease, the vertebrae and ribs could be sensitive thanks to a reflex mechanism [13–16].

In Chap. 15, the integration of the contributions of these two authors to segmental physiology and semiology is proposed, based on the most recent knowledge of

[1] These were considered viscera as well, along with the group of the other viscera of the face.

embryology that provides all the support for the understanding of the segment with its cutivisceral, visceromotor and osteovisceral reflexes.

4.4 A Non-dualistic Stance on the Mind–Body Aspects

In 1901, Henry Head published a study in which he proposed a non-dualistic position with respect to the physical and mental clinical manifestations of individuals with visceral diseases. Head describes how subjects suffering from different acute or chronic visceral diseases can present mental changes such as depression, delusions of persecution, olfactory, auditory and visual hallucinations [9].

In the same way, James Mackenzie also described cases of visceral disease such as the "soldier's heart" which is characterized by dyspnea, fatigue, and palpitations produced by exertion and chest pain, along with an increase in heart rate. Because of this, Mackenzie said that neurosis is one of the main causes of this unhealthy process in the heart's viscera. He identified that these patients presented other mental changes such as apathy, irritability, memory loss, and generalized fatigue. And he also referred to mental changes associated with urinary and circulatory system conditions, among others [13] .

4.5 Forms of Extension and Generalization of Irritation of the Nervous System

In the section on generalization of general diseases that Henry Head described in his first manuscript [7], the ways in which an irritation or alteration in one organ or part of the body begins to spread to other parts of the organism. These are announced as rules and conditions for generalization. Summarizing what Henry Head has described; it can be concluded that the rules for generalization are as follows:

1. The irritation tends to become symmetrical, especially in organs that are bilateral.
2. When the disease remains untreated and there is decreased resistance to the nervous system, irritation can spread to contiguous areas of the same segment that were previously unaffected.
3. If the condition of vulnerability or diminished resistance remains, the irritation begins to spread beyond the segment, specifically to sites that, according to the individual's history, have been previously affected.
4. Finally, a stage may arrive that corresponds to generalized irritation.

Head also described some conditions that decrease the general resistance of the nervous system, such as :

1. Anemia.
2. Fever.

3. Menstruation.
4. Mental shock.

4.6 The Relevance of the Role of Teeth and the Oral Cavity on Systemic Health

Mackenzie devotes several sections of his manuscript on *Symptoms and Their Interpretation* [13] to describing odontalgia and the ways in which this condition can end up affecting other parts of the body via the nervous system. This includes the extension of the irritation to other contiguous parts of the initially affected site in the maxilla or jaw. Additionally, in his manuscript of the *British Medical Journal* [16], he described how a dental disease in a clinical case ended up affecting the development of a clinical manifestation secondary to angina pectoris.

Meanwhile, Henry Head, in the second manuscript published in 1894 [18], gave an exhaustive description of the clinical manifestation of dental disease, showing the areas of cutaneous hypersensitivity that are found in relation to each of the teeth. These areas of hypersensitivity project onto areas of the face and part of the head (see Chap. 15).

4.7 The Role of Personal History and the History of Irritations of the System

Henry Head described cases of specific resistance in which the individual history of each patient was decisive in defining the clinical manifestation. Citing the example of menstruation, Head explained that patients can present various clinical manifestations according to their history; that is, they may not only present skin hypersensitivity within the areas related to their segmental origin between T11 and L1, and between L5 and S3, but they may also present symptoms in other parts of the body. As examples, several cases of menstruating women are described, exhibiting supraorbital and forehead pain secondary to refractive error, pain in the upper thoracic area secondary to chronic lung disease, and pain in the solar plexus area secondary to gastric disease, among others [7].

Meanwhile, Mackenzie described several cases in which the individual's history makes a difference in the clinical manifestation and course of the disease. For the patient from the last section who had angina pectoris, the symptoms showed up not only in the heart area (in the thorax and ulnar aspect of the left arm) but also in the face because of dental disease. Another very illustrative case was about a woman with severe cardiac angina without any improvement with the established treatments. Mackenzie identified the pelvis as the source of her pathology. This condition was verified when, spontaneously, the patient had an abscess release in her pelvic area, generating immediate relief from angina with a favorable recovery [13].

5 Conclusions

By looking at the seven axes, or conceptual categories, suggested in this chapter, there are many reasons to believe that in Great Britain, a current grew that was a lot like Russian nervism, with the nervous system as the center of all pathophysiological processes.

The researches of the British Head and Mackenzie not only contribute to the clinical and semiological evaluation of patients, but also contribute to the understanding of the unity of the nervous system and the body–mind unity, reiterating the importance of life history and individualities.

References

1. Pinilla-Bonilla LB, Rodríguez DC, Villamil-Villar WA. British and Russian nervism: a comparison between two trends in the history of medicine focused on the nervous system. MED UIS. 2024;37(1):33–40. [Spanish]. https://doi.org/10.18273/revmed.v37n1-2024003.
2. Grashchenkov NI. Relationships between British and Russian medicine and neurology, and the role of the National Hospital, Queen Square, London, in the development of Russian neuropathology. J Neurol Neurosurg Psychiatry. 1960;23:185–90.
3. Bykov K, Konradi G. Fundamental concepts of physiology. In: Bykov KM, editor. Text-book of physiology. Moscow: Foreign Languages; 1960. p. 15–45.
4. Baumann C. Henry Head in Ewald Hering's laboratory in Prague 1884-1886: an early study on the nervous control of breathing. J Hist Neurosci. 2005;14(4):322–33.
5. Swash M. Henry Head and the development of clinical neuroscience. Brain. 2008;131(12):3453–6. https://doi.org/10.1093/brain/awn258.
6. Lenfest SM, Vaduva-Nemes A, Okun MS. Dr. Henry Head and lessons learned from his self-experiment on radial nerve transection. J Neurosurg. 2011;114(2):529–33. https://doi.org/10.3171/2010.8.JNS10400. Epub 2010 Oct 8. PMID: 20932092
7. Head H. On disturbance of sensation with especial reference to the pain of visceral disease. Brain. 1893;16(1–2):1–133.
8. Navarro K, Pinilla L. The contributions of Henry Head to neuroanatomical and physiological bases of therapy segment. Méd UIS. 2013;26(2):33–44. [Spanish]. https://revistas.uis.edu.co/index.php/revistamedicasuis/article/view/3919
9. Head H. Certain mental changes that accompany visceral disease: the Goulstonian lectures for 1901. Brain. 1901;4(3):345–429.
10. Brain R. Henry Head: the man and his ideas. Brain. 1961;84(4):561–6. https://doi.org/10.1093/brain/84.4.561.
11. Macnair WR. The beloved physician, Sir James Mackenzie: a biography. Arch Intern Med. 1928;41(6):924–5. https://doi.org/10.1001/archinte.1928.00130180157010.

12. Moorhead R. Sir James Mackenzie (1853-1925): views on general practice education and research. J R Soc Med. 1999;92(1):38–43. https://doi.org/10.1177/014107689909200115. PMID: 10319040; PMCID: PMC1297041
13. Mackenzie J. Symptoms and their interpretation, vol. 1. 4th ed. London: Shaw & Sons, Fetter Lane., 7 & 8; 1920.
14. Mackenzie J. Some points bearing on the association of sensory disorders and visceral disease. Brain. 1893;16(3):21–353.
15. Mackenzie J. The meaning and mechanism of visceral pain as shown by the study of visceral and other sympathetic (autonomic) reflexes. Br Med J. 1906;G30:1523–8.
16. Mackenzie J. The theory of disturbed reflexes in the production of symptoms of disease. Br Med J. 1921;1(3135):147–53. https://doi.org/10.1136/bmj.1.3135.147. PMID: 20770150; PMCID: PMC2414502
17. Mair A. Sir James Mackenzie MD 1853–1925. General Practitioner. London: Royal College of General Practice; 1986.
18. Head H. On disturbances of sensation with especial reference to the pain of visceral disease: part II. Head and neck. Brain. 1894;17(3):339–480.
19. Head H. On disturbances of sensation with especial reference to the pain of visceral disease: part III. Pain in diseases of the heart and lungs. Brain. 1896;19(2–3):153–276.

Chapter 15
Segmental Physiology

Jazmín Ariza-Tarazona and Laura Bibiana Pinilla Bonilla

1 Introduction

The understanding of segmental anatomy is based on the knowledge of metamerism, a term that refers to the segmentation, visible or not, that occurs from plants to vertebrates in their embryological formation (segmentation that begins from the third week of gestation in humans with the formation of somites) [1].

It is important to remember that during embryological development, some parts of a segment change position due to rotation and elongation, which can cause parts of it to be found with significant distances in some segments; as an example, the C8 segment has representation of the myotome in the ulnar area of the hand and also in the lumbar area [1].

In vertebrates, metamerism refers to a segment of the spinal cord and nerves associated with the extension of its branches (ventral, lateral, or dorsal). When spinal nerves innervate a segment of skin or subcutaneous cellular tissue, it is known as a dermatome; the muscle groups innervated by this spinal nerve are called myotome; the group of skeletal structures is called a sclerotome, and the viscera(s) innervated by this spinal nerve is called a viscerotoma or enterotome [1].

The importance of metamerism or segmentation lies in the fact that it is the explanation of the communication and interaction between the surface of the body

J. Ariza-Tarazona
Master in Alternative Medicine, Neural Therapy Area, Faculty of Medicine,
Universidad Nacional de Colombia, Bogotá, Colombia

L. B. Pinilla Bonilla (✉)
Faculty of Medicine, Master in Alternative Medicine, Neural Therapy Area,
Universidad Nacional de Colombia, Bogotá, Colombia

Integrated Health Services Subnetwork of the South, Research and Innovation Center,
Bogotá, Colombia
e-mail: lbpinillab@unal.edu.co

L. B. Pinilla Bonilla et al. (eds.), *Neuraltherapeutic Medicine*,
https://doi.org/10.1007/978-3-032-03257-7_15

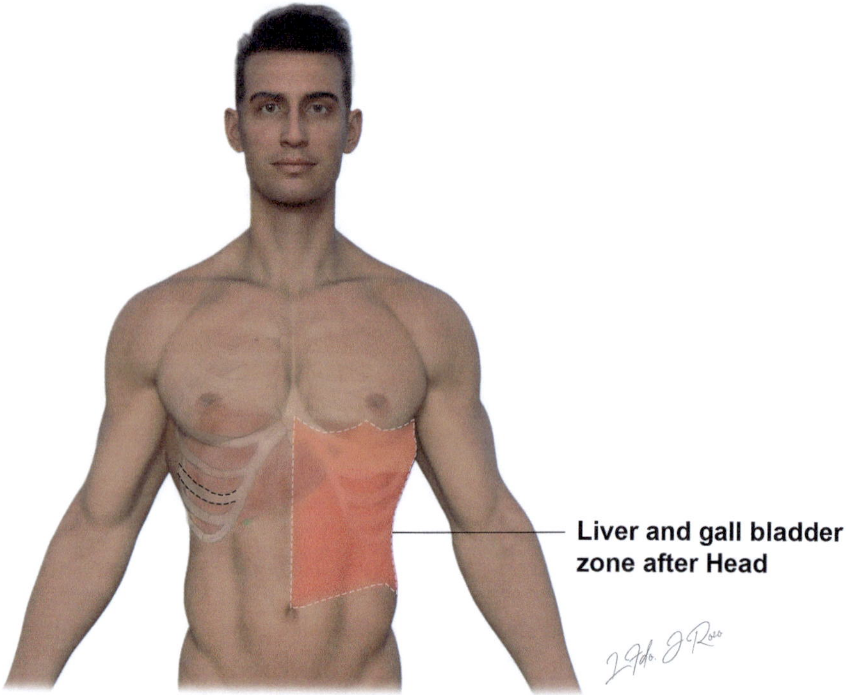

Fig. 15.1 Segmental relationships in the organism

and the internal environment [1] (see Fig. 15.1). This communication is bidirectional, in such a way that the stimulus or affectation in some part of the segment directs the information to the nerve center via afferent and creates a reflex as an efferent response, which can be proprioceptive or in the form of a multisynaptic reflex. This type of communication can be seen in the segmental reflexes within which are the cutaneous-visceral, osteo-visceral, viscero-visceral, and viscero-muscular (or viscero-motor) reflexes (see Fig. 15.2), which were described for the first time in history based on the research of Henry Head and James Mackenzie [2–4].

This chapter aims to provide from the brief biographies of those who were Henry Head and James Mackenzie, the explanation of the main parts of a segment (dermatome, myotome, and sclerotome), to the exposition of the segmental manifestations of each of the organs from the face to the pelvis.

1.1 Henry Head

Henry Head (1861–1940) was an English neurologist recognized for his studies on the Hering-Breuer reflex [5–7], aphasia [8, 9] and skin sensitivity related to visceral disorders [10–12], mainly. Specifically, the research on skin sensitivity published in the journal Brain in 1893 contributed to the recognition of his outstanding doctoral thesis within the framework of his studies in medicine [10].

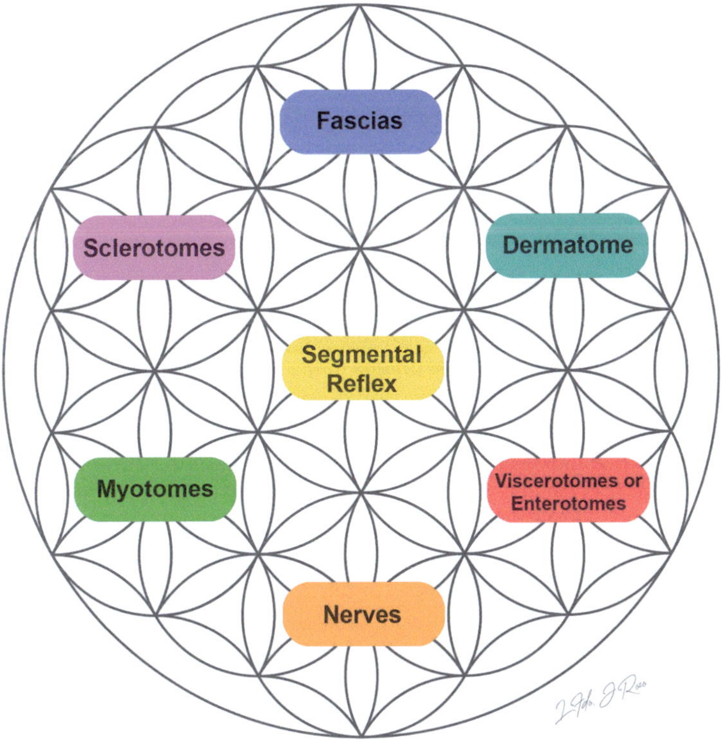

Fig. 15.2 Segmental relationships

Head identified that patients with visceral disorders such as gastric disorders generally had areas of skin hypersensitivity, with long paths and very well-defined borders that, later within his observations, he determined that they coincided exactly with the areas occupied by the skin outbreak of herpes zoster, which encouraged him to investigate at what level of the nervous system these areas belonged [10]. It is worth clarifying that, by this time, the concept of dermatome had not yet been postulated.[1]

Head was interested in determining the changes in sensitivity and temperature of certain areas of the skin that were associated with visceral diseases, a goal he achieved through the exploration of the skin with the blunt tip of a pin and with hot and cold sponges. In the areas of altered sensitivity, Head found well-defined edges that did not overlap, unlike Sherrington's findings that were based on posterior root injury, affecting the sensation of touch in the monkeys. Noting this difference in overlapping, Head postulated that these areas of the skin could be related to the distribution of spinal segments. In his first work, Head described 13 areas in total, from the infraclavicular area to the lower limbs that did not overlap and that

[1] The term is believed to have been first used by Otfrid Foerster in 1933 [13]

presented areas of maximum pain (peak). Although these 13 united areas covered a large area of the body surface, there was a zone of gap in the lower limbs that Head could not find by studying visceral diseases, so he proceeded to supplement it with cases of spinal injury reported by his colleagues Thorburn, Horsley, Oppenheim, Herter, and Star. In this way, he managed to complete the map from the clavicles to the feet, which was the basis for proposing a denomination of these areas in an anatomical and numbered way, such as "Dorsal 5," "Lumbar 1," "Sacral 2," and then move on to an abbreviated use of them, which for the example would be D5, L1, S2, respectively [10]. These areas would be recognized as dermatomes in later studies.

In a second part of his work, Henry Head described the areas of the skin that presented some type of alteration above the level of the clavicles. For this purpose, he used the study of diseases of the organs of the face and neck, including the teeth. These areas, unlike those of the first study, were mostly named according to their anatomical location instead of being numbered [11].

It is important to mention that Henry Head not only limited himself to describing the areas of the skin (which would later be recognized as dermatomes), but part of his study was dedicated to describing the set of areas of the skin altered by visceral diseases of each organ. As an example, he observed that when there was kidney disease, there were four sensitive areas of the skin that corresponded to levels from D10 to L1. Therefore, on the one hand, there are individual areas of skin (dermatomes), and on the other, there are zones that reveal sensitivity to a single organ and are related to a group of dermatomes (Head's Zones).

Although Head never explicitly spoke of "cutaneous-visceral" reflexes, when he explains why an area of the skin becomes sensitive in the presence of visceral disease, he describes that it is a "reflex" response whose base is the medullary segment [10]. That is why, subsequently, this use became widespread in some texts .

1.2 James Mackenzie

The renowned Scottish cardiologist James Mackenzie (1853–1925) had less recognition as a semiologist. Beyond the field of cardiology, Mackenzie problematized the classical conception of medicine, stating that the signs and symptoms that a doctor discovers in the semiological examination obey a reflex nature regulated by the nervous system, and considered that the key to a "new medicine" lies in this integrative axis based on the nervous system [3] (see Chap. 14).

Mackenzie fully agreed with Henry Head in observing the modification of the skin's sensory reflexes in the presence of visceral diseases (cutaneous-visceral reflexes). In addition to this, in his research he identified alterations in muscle sensitivity and tone (viscero-motor reflexes), as well as hypersensitivity in the joints and periosteum (osteo-visceral reflexes) as a reflex response to visceral disease [14, 15].

Mackenzie understood that when a morbid process in one viscera results in increased stimulation of the nerves passing from the viscera to the spinal cord, this increased stimulation affects neighboring centers located "within" the spinal cord, thereby affecting sensory, motor, and other nerves [15].

2 Dermatomes

A dermatome is understood to be the area of skin and subcutaneous cellular tissue innervated by a spinal nerve.

There are several maps of dermatomes described in history. It is considered that the first most complete map in humans described was that of Henry Head [13], although at the time, the word dermatome had not yet been considered. The diversity of the maps described is due to the fact that while the study was being conducted, the exploration was carried out with various methods, which generated marked differences, since some dermatomes were based on the exploration of touch such as Sherrington's (see Fig. 15.3), others reflected sensitivity, pain or autonomic responses.

Historically, it has been defined that a dermatome whose boundaries are anatomically established by dissection of the spinal nerve to the subcutaneous tissue is known as a subcutaneous dermatome, while a dermatome whose boundaries are based on clinical examination is known as an epidermal dermatome, the latter being those that provide information about the internal environment [1].

For practical purposes, the classification of dermatomes that will be adopted from now is inspired by the Austrian author Ingrid Wancura [1], which is based on segmental anatomy (Fig. 15.4):

The algetic dermatomes that were described by Henry Head (see Fig. 15.5) have important characteristics for Neuraltherapeutic medicine as follows:

- Provide information about interactions and the phenomenon of projection to the body surface.
- Hypersensitivity to clinical examination in visceral disease in most patients.
- It is based on the interaction of the spinal nervous system and the autonomic nervous system.

These characteristics provide information about visceral disease, which manifests itself as pain on the body surface, but also with other symptoms that are reflected as changes in temperature (coldness or increase in temperature) and in autonomic reflexes such as piloerection.

Each Head's zone could manifest hypersensitivity in points that Henry Head described as maximum points (MP) (see Fig. 15.5). These MPs are always the first ones appearing with a visceral disease and the last ones disappearing. These MPs could provide early information about visceral diseases, acting as prodromal signs and appearing even before any radiological or laboratory changes could be identified [1].

Dr. Henry Head carried out an exhaustive follow-up study in cases of herpes zoster (more than 300 patients), where he clinically followed each patient,

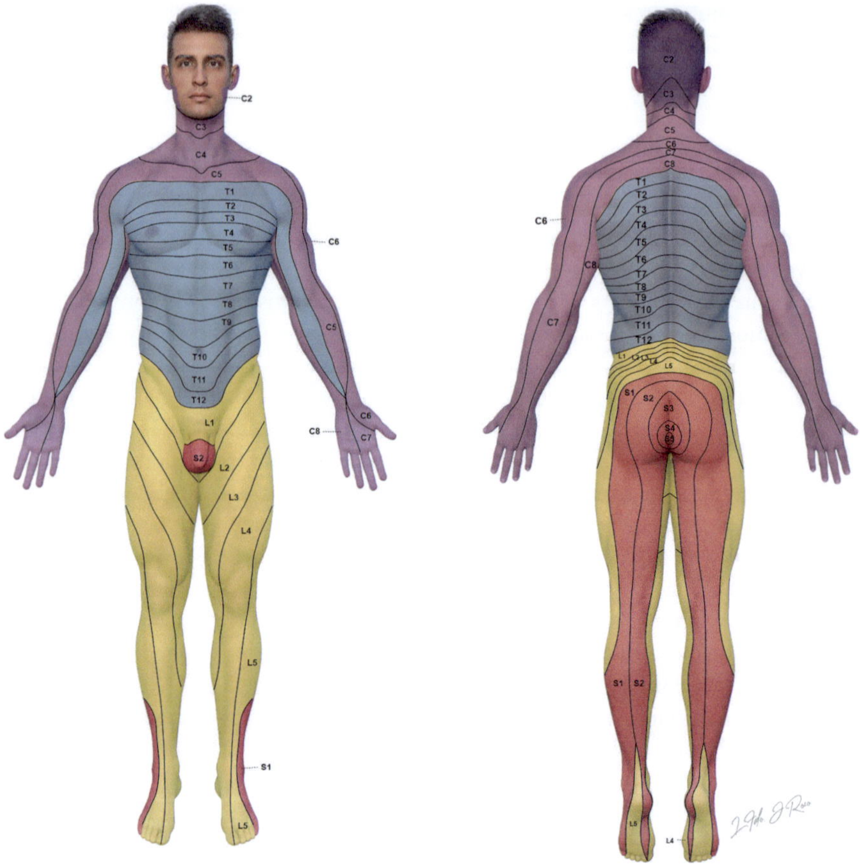

Fig. 15.3 Sherrington's dermatomes (adaptation)

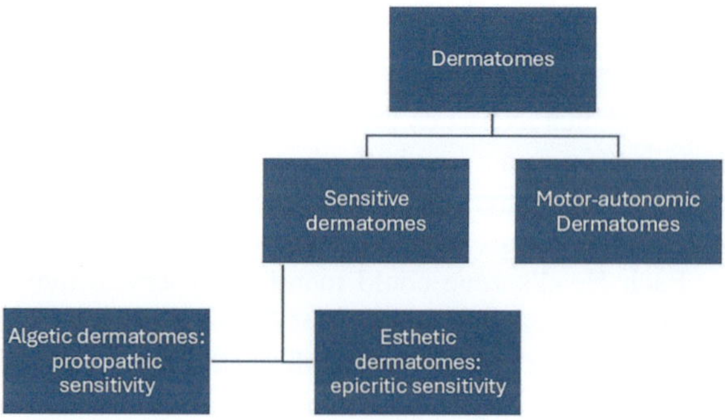

Fig. 15.4 Classification of dermatomes

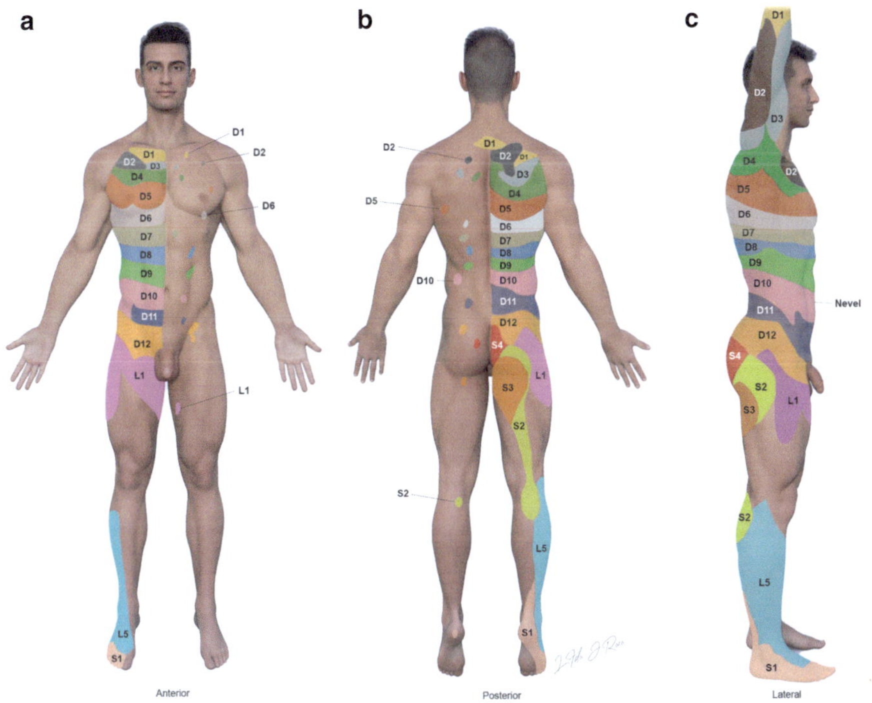

Fig. 15.5 Dermatomes (algetic) according to Head. Image **a**. Anterior view: on the right side dermatomes are shown; on the left side, maximum points after Head are depicted. Image **b**. Posterior View: on the right side, maximum points after Head are shown; on the left side, dermatomes are depicted. Image **c**. Lateral view, only dermatomes are shown

discovering that herpes zoster manifested itself in the dermatome that is related to a viscera [10], becoming an indicator of its pathology.

He then concluded that there are dermatomes that express visceral disease and are determined by examining the perception of pain (protopathic sensitivity), which have defined borders (and do not overlap like tactile dermatomes), making them suitable for determining the segmental boundaries in the skin in the case of visceral disease. In this way, it can be understood that the algetic dermatome and visceral organs share the same segmental spinal nerve [10]. Consequently, a visceral disease manifests itself in the algetic dermatome(s) as hyperalgesia in the so-called Head's areas.

3 Myotomes

James Mackenzie was one of the first authors to identify the reflex phenomenon which is the contraction of certain muscles as a result of information (pathological or irritative) from a viscera. On several occasions, Mackenzie cited how the muscles of the abdominal wall could be contracted as a result of gastritis, for example.

According to this author, in the presence of visceral disease, not only may the muscles be reflexively contracted, but they may also be hyperalgesic [16] or have a perception of decreased muscle strength [14]. From the semiological point of view, it is of enormous importance to know the segmental level of innervation of each muscle in order to understand its visceral correspondence.

Each spinal nerve influences a specific region of the striated muscles, which is called the myotome. Consequently, it is important to emphasize that myotome and muscle are not interchangeable concepts in this academic context [1].

Similar to the story of the discovery of dermatomes, in the case of myotomes, there are numerous discrepancies between the different maps described. These discrepancies are based on differences in exploration methods, which were mostly based on individual clinical experiences and, in a smaller percentage, were based on anatomical and electrophysiological examinations [17].

Some authors agree that the first explorations of dermatomes began with Herringham at the end of the nineteenth century [1, 17]. Herringham described the course of nerves in cadavers of fetuses, children and adults, identifying myotomes of the upper limb [18]. Although this method had many limitations, Herringham's work seems to have influenced the maps described later.

Some authors have also investigated myotomes by stimulating the roots during spinal surgery and, although it is a good method, it has the possibility that the electric current can travel to other roots. Other authors have investigated cases of single radiculopathy, presenting certain limitations, which have been tried to be overcome through MRI or surgery. In the case of manual muscle testing (MMT), there can also be confusion, since the movement of certain joints can be compound and require several muscles. Finally, electromyography (EMG) has also been tried, but the pain-related limitations of this approach are already known [17].

As a result of all these explorations, it has been found that almost all muscles are of plurisegmental origin, that is, they are innervated by several spinal nerves, such as the trapezius muscle, whose innervations come from three different levels of the cervical region (C2–C4) [1].

With regard to the determination of the segmental level, it is important to note that, when Herrigham performed the detailed dissections on the brachial plexus in 1886, he discovered some guiding rules about the innervation of the muscles, which are the following [18]:

1. "Of two muscles, or of two parts of a muscle, that which is nearer the head-end of the body tends to be supplied by the higher, that which is nearer the tail-end by the lower nerve."
2. "Of two muscles, that which is nearer the long axis of the body tends to be supplied by the higher, that which is nearer the periphery by the lower nerve."
3. "Of two muscles, that which is nearer the surface tends to be supplied by the higher, that which is further from it by the lower nerve."

Although these rules were described in the context of the study of the brachial plexus, their applicability to other segmental muscle levels has been verified [1].

3.1 Muscle Segments

In this section, the different groups of myotomes are shown organized by topographic area (head and neck, cervical, thoracic and lumbosacral segment). In the case of the head, although it is true that the embryological segmentation in this area is partly due to the formation of the rhombomeres [19] that give rise to the cranial nerves and are related to the formation of the pharyngeal arches (see Chap. 10), the information presented in this chapter will correspond to the classic numbering of the cranial nerves [20] (i.e., III–XII, and not R1–R8) (see Table 15.1).

It is important to mention that the segmental information that has had the highest degree of research and that is shown in Table 15.2, with clinically verified information, through EMG and Magnetic Resonance Imaging, has been that corresponding to the upper limb area (C5–T1) [17, 21–23]. The information related to the other segments such as the thoracic (Table 15.3) and lumbosacral (Table 15.4) segments has been constructed on the clinical experience of several authors [1, 17, 24, 25].

Note that the distribution of myotomes from the pelvis and the lower limb follows a very characteristic metameric sequence, as shown in Fig. 15.6, where the pelvic floor receives the most caudal segmental innervation in the human body.

Finally, it is important to note that although in the case of dermatomes according to Head there is a "gap zone" that for the upper segment is between C5 and C7 and for the lower segment is between L2 and L4, for the specific case of myotomes (and consequently, for sclerotomes), this gap is not evident given the wide distribution of muscle insertions.

Table 15.1 The myotomes of the head (cranial nerves) and neck (first 4 cervical segments) are shown, specifying the area of innervation and the action exerted by the segmental group

Myotomes of the head and neck part	III	IV	V	VI	VII	IX	X	XI	XII	C1	C2	C3	C4	Area	Action to assess
Extrinsic eye and sphincter of the iris	■													Eye	Hearing, eye movement, chewing, swallowing, and phonation
Superior oblique of eye		■												Eye	
Tensor tympani muscle			■											Ear	
Muscles of Mastication			■											Chewing	
Soft palate			■											Swallowing	
Mylohyoid			■											Swallowing	
Anterior belly digastric muscle			■											Swallowing	
Lateral rectus of the eye				■										Eye	
Muscles of facial expression					■									Face	
Stapedius muscle					■									Ear	
Stylopharyngeus muscle						■								Swallowing	
Cricothyroid and larynx							■							Phonation	
Palatoglossus/Palatopharyngeus							■							Swallowing	
Superior, middle and inferior Constrictor pharyngeal							■							Swallowing	
Trapezius								■						Neck	
Muscles of the tongue									■					Swallowing	
Back straight most of the head										■				Head	Circular movements of the head and neck
Straight back under the head										■					
Rectus capitis posterior major muscle										■	■				
Rectus capitis posterior minor muscle										■	■				
Sternohyoid										■	■	■	■	Hyoid and larynx	
Sternothyroid										■	■	■	■		
Sternocleidomastoid								■			■	■	■	Head	

Table 15.2 The cervical segment that is related to the muscles of the upper limb, specifying the area of innervation and the action exerted by the segmental group

Muscles of the cervical segment - upper limb	C2	C3	C4	C5	C6	C7	C8	T1	Area	Action to assess
Trapezoid	■	■	■						Shoulder	Inspire with the arm in abduction
Diaphragm		■	■	■					Diaphragm	
Elevator of the scapula		▒	■	■					Scapula	
Rhomboids			■	■					Scapula	
Deltoid			▒	■	▒				Shoulder	Raise your hand and request to speak
Supraspinatus			▒	■	▒				Shoulder	
Infraspinatus				■	▒				Shoulder	
Teres minor				■	■				Arm	
Biceps				■	▒				Elbow	Flexion of elbow
Brachioradial				■	▒				Elbow	
Extensor carpi radialis longus muscle				■	■				Wrist	Take the seat belt pilot and co-pilot in the car
Serratus anterior				■	■	■			Arm	
Subscapularis				▒	■	■	■		Arm	Fasten the seat belt of the pilot and co-pilot of a car
Extensor carpi radialis brevis muscle					■	▒			Hand/fingers	
Pronator teres					■	▒			Forearm	
Pectoralis Major					■	■	■	▒	Arm	
Pectoralis minor					■	■	■		Shoulder	
Teres major					■	■	■		Arm	
Flexor carpi radialis					▒	■			Wrist	
Triceps					▒	■	▒		Arm	Get ready to throw bowling ball, with the arm in extension
Latissimus Dorsi					▒	■	▒		Arm	
Extensor carpi ulnaris muscle						▒	■		Wrist	
Flexor carpi ulnaris muscle						▒	■		Wrist	Playing castanets, and moving the hands as in a Sevillana
Finger common Extensor						▒	■	▒	Hand/fingers	
Abductor pollicis longus						▒	■	▒	Hand/fingers	
Abductor pollicis brevis						▒	■	▒	Hand/fingers	
Extensor pollicis brevis						▒	■	▒	Hand/fingers	
Flexor digitorum profundus muscle (4)						▒	■	▒	Hand/fingers	
Extensor of the index							■	▒	Hand/fingers	
Abductor digiti minimi							■	▒	Hand/fingers	
interossei							■	■	Hand/fingers	
Flexor digitorum profundus muscle (1)							▒	■	Hand/fingers	
Flexor pollicis longus muscle							▒	■	Hand/fingers	
Pronator quadratus muscle							▒	■	Forearm	
Abductor pollicis brevis							▒	■	Hand/fingers	
Flexor digitorum superficialis								■	Hand/fingers	

Note: The black color represents a complete innervation of that segmental level, while the gray color corresponds to a partial innervation of that segmental level. In this table, the first thoracic segmental level was included to show the complete innervation of the upper limb

Table 15.3 The thoracic segment is shown specifying the area of innervation and the action exerted by the segmental group

Muscles of the segment thoracic	T2	T3	T4	T5	T6	T7	T8	T9	T10	T11	T12	Area	Action to assess
Transversus thoracis	■	■	■	■	■							Chest	Expiration
Rectus abdominis				■	■	■	■	▒	▒			Abdomen	Contraction
Abdominal external oblique					■	■	■					Abdomen	Rotates and flexes
Abdominal transverse						■	■	■	■	■	■	Abdomen	Contraction
Serratus posterior								■	■	■	■	Chest	Expiration

Note: Gray shows an area for which there is a discrepancy of concepts between different authors and/or that it is considered that the innervation could be partial

4 Sclerotomas

James Mackenzie, in one of his manuscripts published in the journal *Brain*, made one of the first references to the presence of osteoarticular sensitivity in the case of visceral diseases since 1893:

> Further, distinct tenderness may be found in pressure over certain vertebrae, and that when there is no increased sensitiveness of the tissues interposed between the vertebras and pressing thumb. These tender vertebras frequently afford very valuable evidence of the organ diseased [15].

In the same manuscript, published in 1893, Mackenzie mentions several clinical cases where he observes the correlations, for example, between vertebral sensitivity and heart disease, as well as identified the relationship between pain of the D6-D7 vertebrae and gastric disease. These two cases were verified post-mortem. This sign of vertebral sensitivity, in honor of the person who initially described it in the context of visceral disease, the authors of this chapter have proposed to call it "Mackenzie's sign."

Although these were very valid and novel observations, the path of research on the innervation of the musculoskeletal system has not become as developed [26] as evidenced in the history of dermatome and myotome research [27, 28].

Very similar to the history of dermatomes, which begins with the participation of an eminent neurologist, in the case of sclerotomes, the first most complete historical description of the association between the skeletal apparatus and segmental levels was made by the Swiss neurologist Joseph Jules Dejerine [29] in 1914. During his observations, Dejerine was able to first identify that superficial (cutaneous) sensitivity did not always correspond to deep (musculoskeletal) sensitivity. The second part of the work consisted of performing a detailed cadaveric dissection of the trajectory of each spinal nerve from its origin [26].

Table 15.4 The lumbosacral segment is shown specifying the area of innervation and the action exerted by the segmental group

Muscles of the segment lumbosacral	**T12**	**L1**	**L2**	**L3**	**L4**	**L5**	**S1**	**S2**	**S3**	**S4**	**Area**	**Action to assess**
Quadratus Lumborum	■	■	■								Lumbar	Lateral bending
Sartorius		▒	■	▒	▒						Hip/knee	Flexion, abduction, and adduction of the hip
Iliopsoas		▒	■	■	■						Hip	
Gracilis			▒	■	■						Hip	
Pectinuous			▒	■	■						Hip	
Adductor longus and brevis			▒	■	▒						Hip	
Quadriceps			▒	■	▒						Knee	Kick a soccer ball
Tensor fascia latae					▒	■					Hip	
Tibialis Anterior					▒	■	▒				Foot /Toes	
Gluteus medius					▒	■	▒				Hip	
Extensor digitorum longus						■	▒				Foot /Toes	Circular movements of the foot
Extensor hallucis longus						■	▒				Foot /Toes	
Extensor digitorum brevis						■	▒				Foot /Toes	
Gastrocnemius						▒	■				Knee/Foot	
Semitendinosus						▒	■	▒			Knee	
Semimembranosus						▒	■	▒			Knee	
Fibularis longus and brevis						▒	■	▒			Foot /Toes	
Posterior Tibial						▒	■	▒			Foot /Toes	
Flexor digitorum longus						▒	■	▒			Knee/Foot	
Flexor length of the hallux						▒	■	▒			Knee/Foot	
Gluteus maximus						▒	■	▒			Hip	Bring the foot towards the gluteus
Quadratus femoris						▒	■	▒			Hip	
Piriformis						▒	■	▒			Hip	
Biceps femoris long head						▒	■	▒			Knee	
Biceps femoris short head						▒	■	▒			Knee	
Soleus							■	▒			Foot /Toes	
Abductor hallucis							■	▒			Foot /Toes	
Quadratus plantae							■	▒			Foot /Toes	
Lumbricals							■	■	▒		Foot /Toes	Move fingers closer and further apart
interossei							■	■	▒		Foot /Toes	
Levator ani									■	■	Pelvic floor	Contraction of the perineum
Coccygeus									■	■	Pelvic floor	

Note: Gray shows an area for which there is a discrepancy of concepts between different authors and/or that it is considered that the innervation could be partial

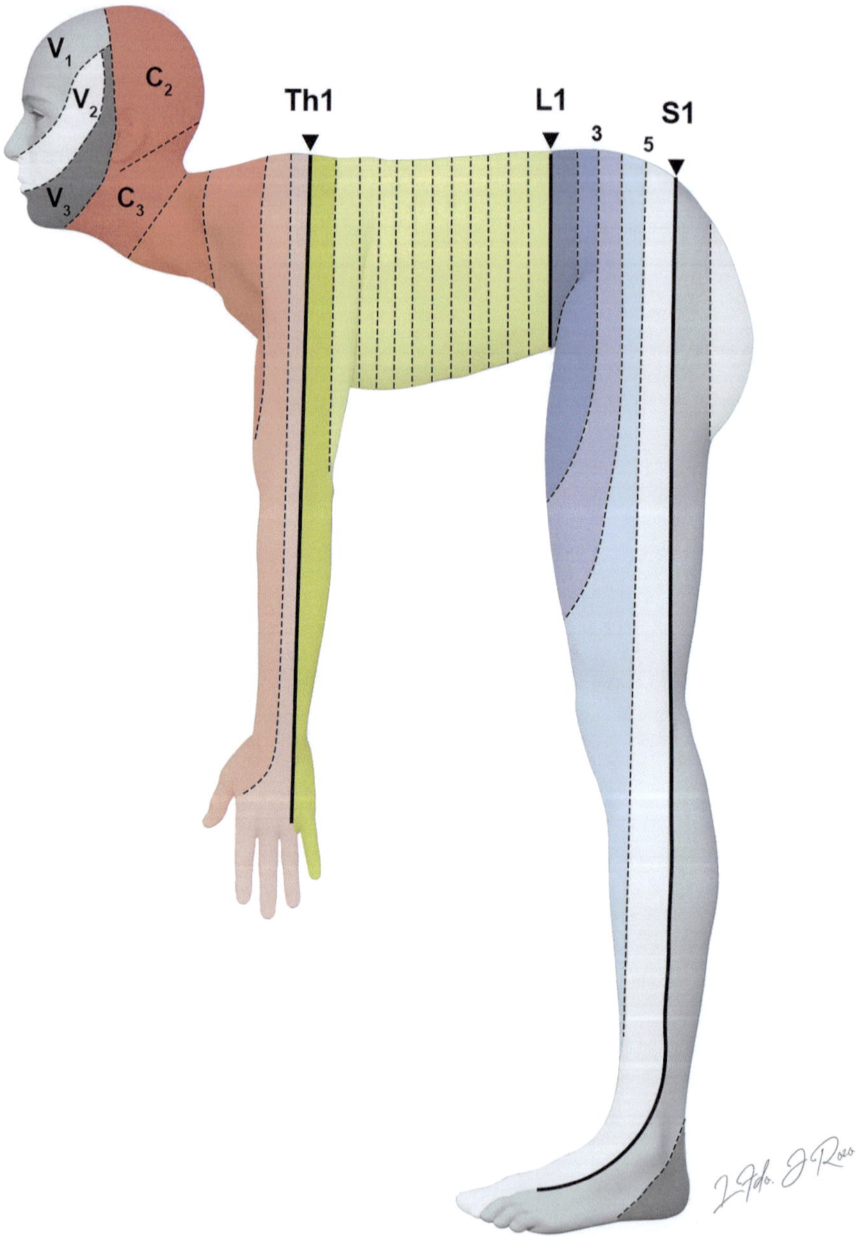

Fig. 15.6 From the pelvis to the caudal end, the distribution and metameric sequence is understood in the light of the position shown in the figure, where it can be seen that the anterior and medial aspect of the lower limb is innervated by upper lumbar levels. And in the case of the gluteal area and posterior aspect of the lower limb, it is innervated by the most caudal levels of the body

Later, Kellgren, in 1939 [30], found a similar map when examining the distribution of reported pain after injections with hypotonic saline solution in deep tissues such as ligaments, tendons, joint capsules, and muscles.[2] The term sclerotoma was not really defined until later, by Inman and Saunders in 1944 [31]. These authors analyzed the distribution of pain referred to non-bony tissues in patients with focal bone lesions and in a group of volunteers who underwent direct periosteal stimulation by scratching with a fine needle. They created a map of the segments of the spine that corresponded to the areas of referred pain for each stimulation point, similar to Kellgren's [26].

Subsequent research that included clinical studies to define areas of sclerotomes has questionable accuracy, and this led to its exclusion from the literature for many years. The only available animal study that has managed to verify the specific bone area innervated by a spinal nerve has been conducted by Gajda et al. in 2004 [32]. In this study, a retrograde tracer was placed under the periosteum of the rat's tibia and the neuronal bodies located in the dorsal root ganglia corresponding to the segmental levels L3 and L4 were marked [26].

New studies have been able to demonstrate, reliably, the sensory innervation of the spinal cord and the periosteum of long bones in murines [33], as well as the sympathetic innervation of the femur and mandible in mice [34].

4.1 Skeletal Segments

Figure 15.7 shows Dejerine's restored and modified map (where the peripheral nerve information was removed), showing the sclerotomic distributions of the head and neck area (Fig. 15.7a) innervated mainly by the trigeminal and cervical plexus branches.

Note that sclerotomes of the lower limb, in the specific case of the femur, do not follow a descending order. This is explained by the position and embryological sequence in which the metameres arose in the embryo (see Fig. 15.6).

4.2 Mackenzie's Sign

The evaluation of Mackenzie's sign is performed by applying firm pressure with the thumb on the spinous processes in a direction perpendicular to the plane of the table while the patient is in the prone position (see Fig. 15.8). This sign, as described by Mackenzie, can be an indicator of visceral disease. Likewise, during treatment with

[2] This highlights the idea that the use of the term "sclerotome" has acquired a certain ambiguity. On numerous occasions, it has been used to refer to the spinal segmental innervation of deep tissues, such as muscle, tendon, joint capsule, ligament, bone, and periosteum, however, this use of the term is inappropriate

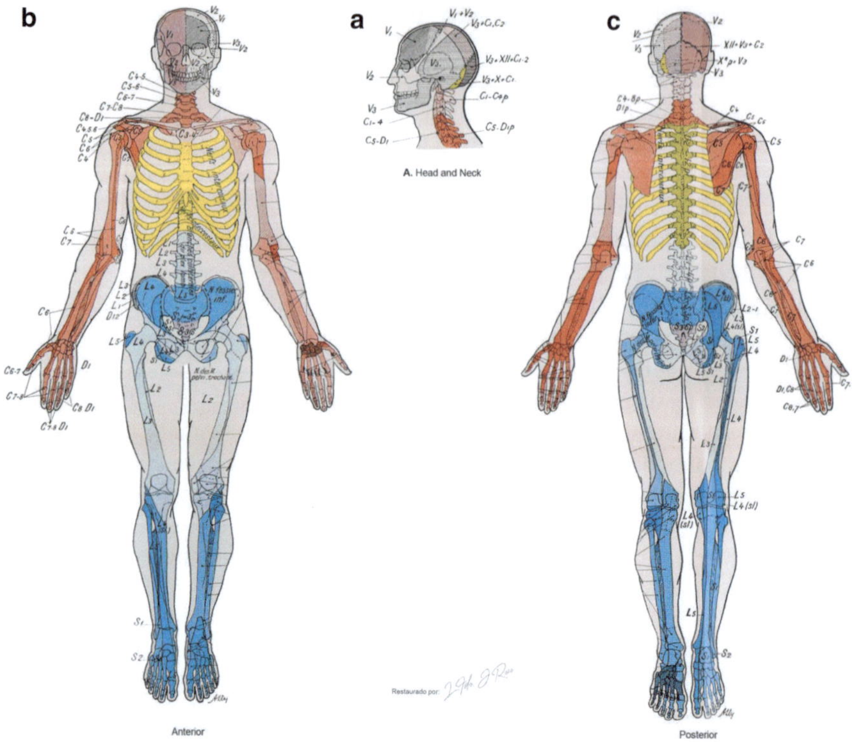

Fig. 15.7 The restored map of Dejerine's sclerotomes is shown. Figure (**a**) shows the head and neck area. In (**b**), the anterior view is observed, and in (**c**), the posterior view of the skeletal system is shown, showing the sclerotomes in relation to the upper limb (C4-D1), the pelvis (D12-S4), and the lower limbs (L2-S2) [28]

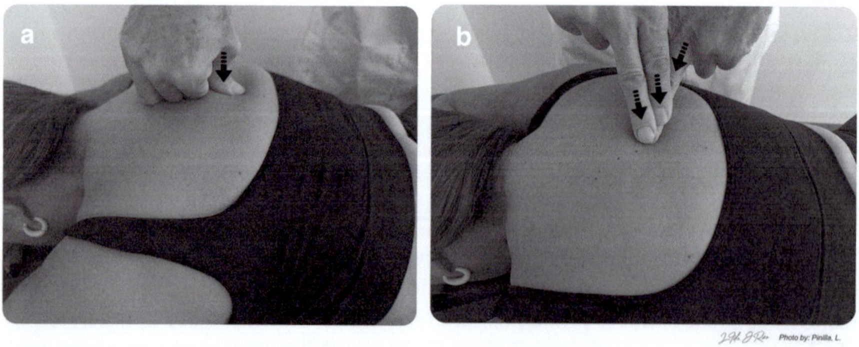

Fig. 15.8 Evaluation of Mackenzie's sign by exerting pressure with the thumb (**a**) and with the second and third fingers (**b**) (Photograph taken by: Samuel Bonilla)

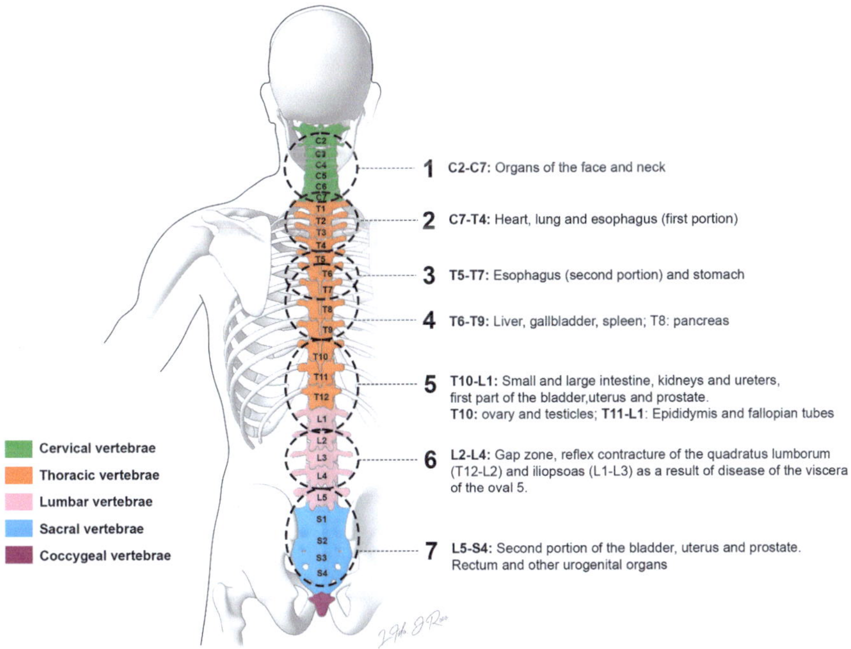

Fig. 15.9 The seven ovals representing the correspondence of the positive Mackenzie sign are shown. All ovals, except 6, show the segmental visceral correlation. In the case of oval 6, it correlates "indirectly" with the viscera of oval 5, given the insertions of the quadratus lumborum and iliopsoas muscles that present more cranial innervation, when they are in a state of contracture

Neuraltherapeutic medicine, it can be a diagnostic tool that allows evaluating the impact of a previous intervention, by verifying, for example, its subsequent disappearance when performing a therapeutic approach to the Head zone corresponding to the viscera of the same segmental level. Similarly, as will be seen in later chapters, sclerotomic levels can also be the object of direct intervention for therapeutic purposes.

Figure 15.9 shows the distribution of Mackenzie's sign based initially on Wancura's proposal [1] but modified by the authors of this chapter. This proposal is based on the observations made during 9 years of academic and clinical practice by professors Ariza and Pinilla.

5 Organs and Their Metameric Expression in Trunk and Limbs

Each organ, due to its embryological origin and metameric development, is related to an area of the skin, one or more muscle groups, skeletal structures, and can be related to other viscera with which it shares the same origin or segmental innervation. The evaluation of the skin component can be facilitated with the use of a blunt-tipped instrument, while the evaluation of deeper components is focused on palpation and the performance of certain clinical tests. In subsequent chapters, we will expand on the information about the physical examination and the diagnostic tools that can facilitate the evaluation of each of the components of a segmental level.

Next, the tissues and segmental relationships that each organ maintains through the nervous system will be specified, including Mackenzie's sign.

5.1 *Heart*

Viscera	Dermatome - Head's zone	Myotom	Sclerotome	Mackenzie	Viscero - Visceral
Heart (see Fig. 15.10)	Anterior: Covers segments from T1–T4. Posterior: From C7 to T7 (around the scapula). In the upper limb: Covers T1 and T2 levels. Cervical segments left predominance.	Rotator cuff, subscapularis, pectoralis major and minor, teres major, muscles of the upper limb and transverse thorax	Shoulder girdle, first 5 ribs, upper limb bones	Oval 2	Lung, Esophagus

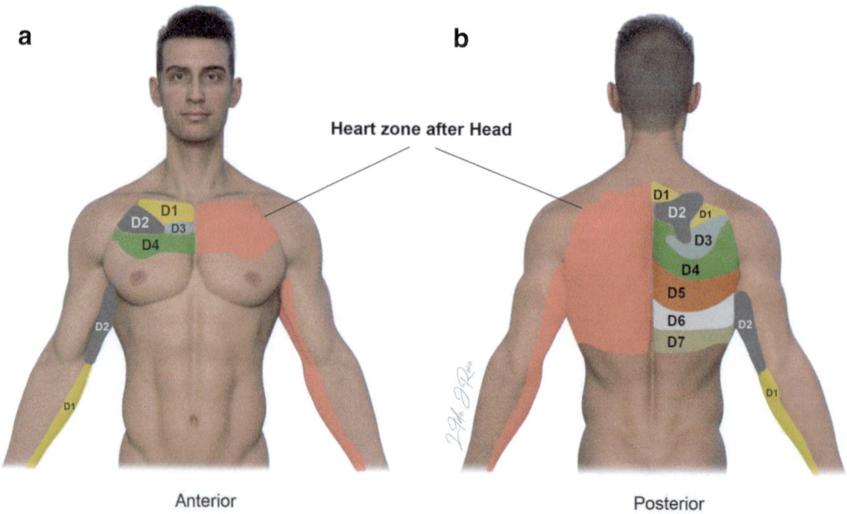

Fig. 15.10 Head's zone of heart. (**a**) Anterior view; (**b**) posterior view

5.2 Lung

Viscera	Dermatome - Head's zone	Myotom	Sclerotome	Mackenzie	Viscero-Visceral
Lung (see Fig. 15.11)	T1–T7 segments may have posterior sensitivity up to T8–T9 in case of pneumonia or tuberculosis. Cervical segments. Tenderness in the radial aspect may be found in the upper limb.	Rotator cuff, subscapularis, pectoralis major and minor, teres major, muscles of the upper and transverse limb of the thorax, rectus abdominis	Shoulder girdle, the first 7 ribs, upper limb bones	Oval 2	Heart, Esophagus

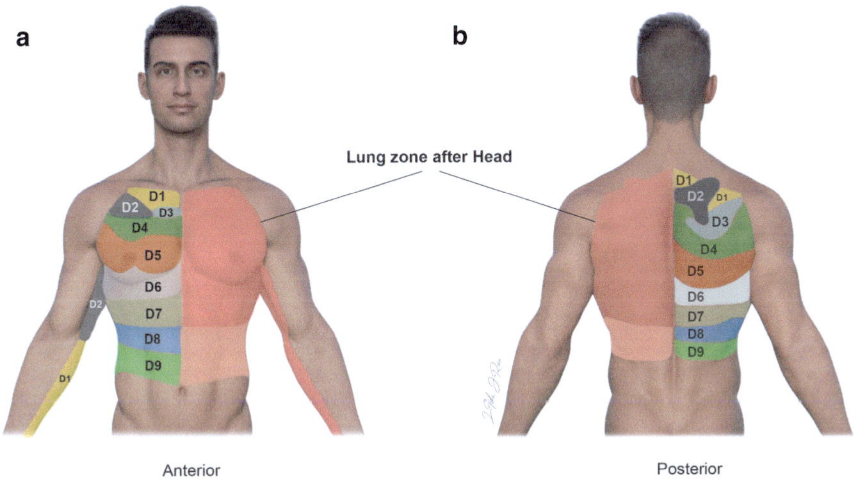

Fig. 15.11 Head's zone of lung. (a) Anterior view; (b) posterior view

5.3 Oesophagus

Viscera	Dermatome - Head's zone	Myotom	Sclerotome	Macken-zie	Viscero-Visceral R
Oesophagus (see Fig. 15.12)	Dermatomes Upper half T2–T5 Lower half: T6–T8 Peak: T5 with anterior axillary line	Transverse thorax Rectus abdominis T2–T8 Intercostals External oblique Transverse abdominis	Costal arches T2–T8 and their sternocostal joints	Oval 2 & 3	Lungs and heart

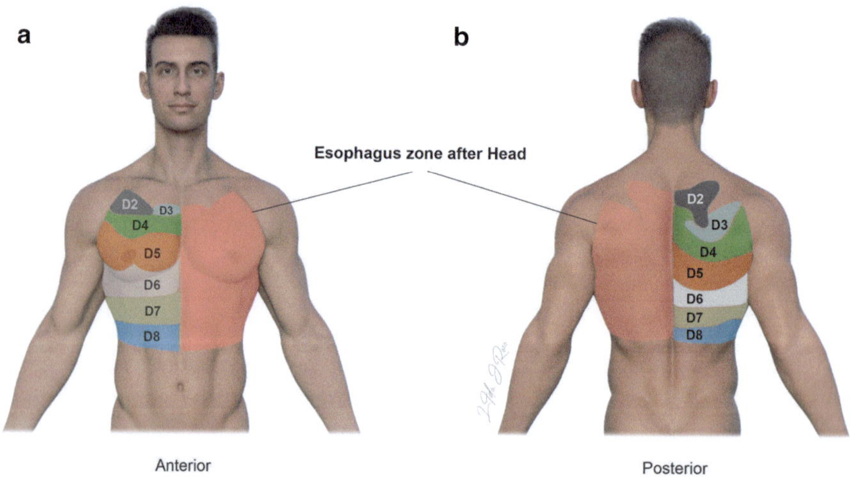

Fig. 15.12 Head's zone of the esophagus. (**a**) Anterior view; (**b**) posterior view

5.4 Stomach and Duodenum

Viscera	Dermatome - Head's zone	Myotom	Sclerotome	Mackenzie	Viscero-Visceral R
Stomach and duodenum (see Fig. 15.13)	Dermatomes S6–T9 (could T5) Scapulo-ensiform zone Bilateral trend Peak: T6–T8 ventral	External oblique M. Trapeze Paravertebral M. Rectus abdominis Transverse abdominis	Lower sternum Lower thoracic spine Right duodenal rib arches, left stomach and chondrosternal joint T7–T9	Oval 3	Duodenum, atria, and caudal esophagus

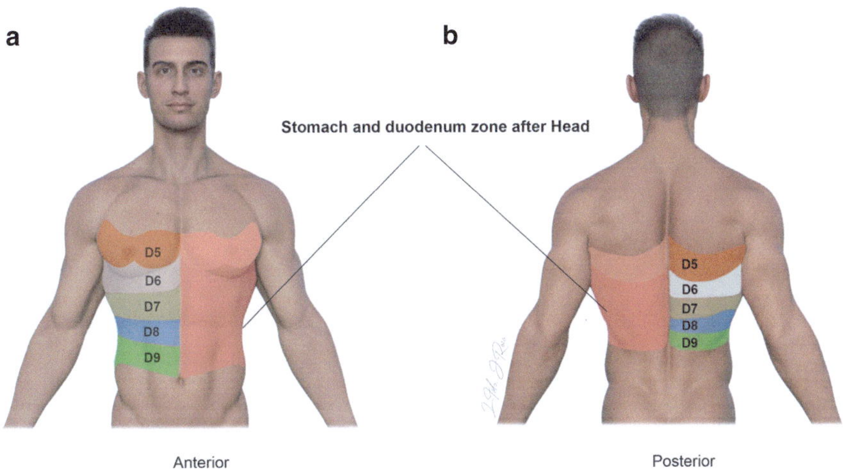

Fig. 15.13 Head's zone of the stomach and duodenum. (**a**) Anterior view; (**b**) posterior view

5.5 *Liver and Gallbladder*

Viscera	Dermatome - Head's zone	Myotom	Sclerotome	Mackenzie	Viscero-Visceral R
Liver and gallbladder (see Fig. 15.14)	Dermatomes Right T7–T9 liver Hepatomegaly T10 T7–T9 gallbladder (T6) Peak: S8	L4–L5 myotomes in Tibialis anterior and right peroneus Paravertebral Rectus abdominis External oblique. Transverse abdominis Intercostals T2–T8	T10–T12 and iliac crest Right rib arches T11–T12 Shoulder joint L4 medial malleolus and medial border of the foot. L5 lateral malleolus and 1 toe	Oval 4	Duodenum Pancreas Auricle

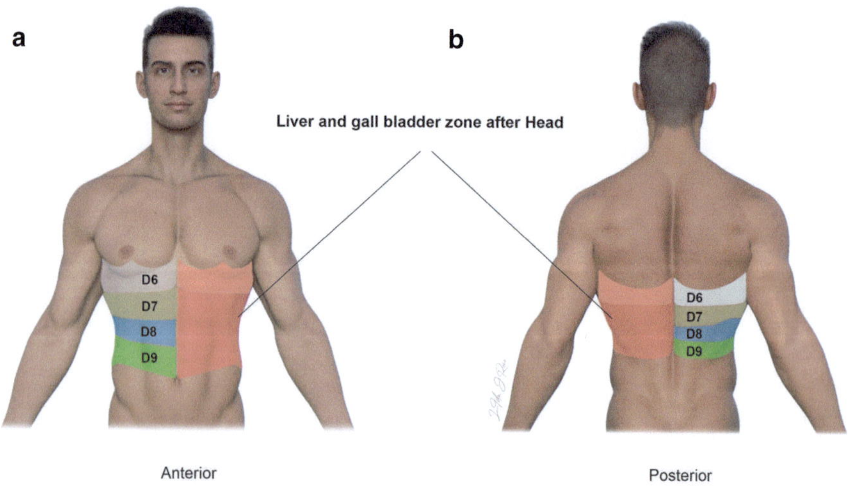

Fig. 15.14 Liver and gallbladder zone. (**a**) Anterior view; (**b**) posterior view

5.6 Pancreas

Viscera	Dermatome - Head's zone	Myotom	Sclerotome	Mackenzie	Viscero-Visceral R.
Pancreas (see Fig. 15.15)	Not described by Head, but related to the sympathetic innervation of T8 (possible T6 to T9). Maximum point T8 left	Rectus abdominis muscleExternal oblique Transverse abdominis Paravertebral muscle pain	Eighth left rib arch	Oval 4	Stomach Duodenum Liver

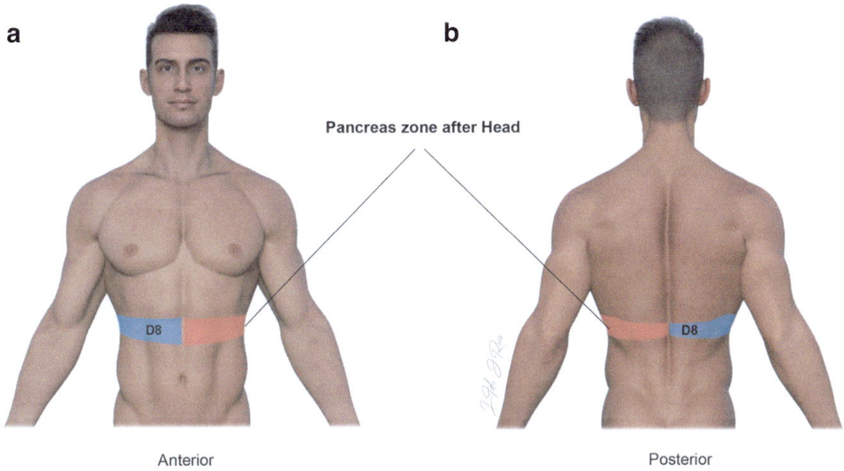

Fig. 15.15 Head's zone of the pancreas. (**a**) Anterior view; (**b**) posterior view

5.7 Spleen

Viscera	Dermatome - Head's zone	Myotom	Sclerotome	Macken-zie	Viscero-Visceral R.
Spleen (see Fig. 15.16)	T8, T9 left Possible (T6 to T11 in splenomegaly)	Rectus abdominis muscle External oblique Transverse abdominis Paravertebral muscle pain	Eighth left rib arch	Oval 4	Stomach Duodenum Liver

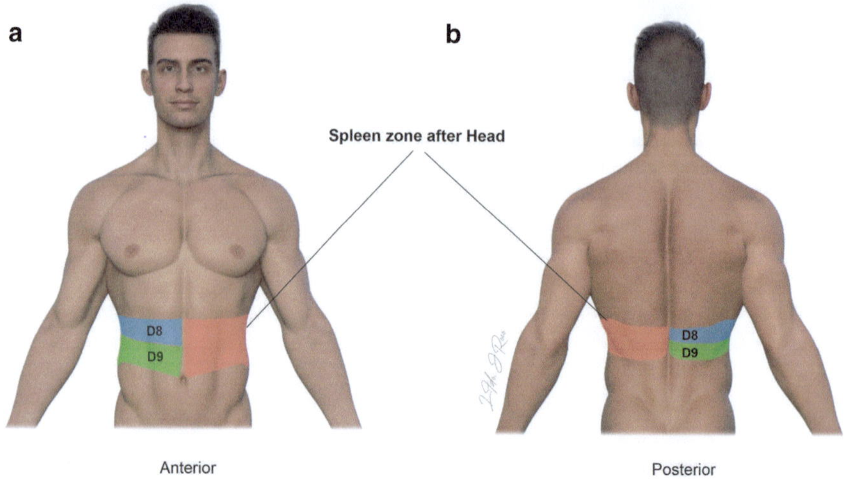

Fig. 15.16 Head's zone of the spleen. (**a**) Anterior view; (**b**) posterior view

5.8 *Jejunum and Ileum*

Viscera	Dermatome - Head's zone	Myotom	Sclerotome	Mackenzie	Viscero-Visceral R.
Jejunum, íleum (see Fig. 15.17)	Umbilical pain Possible(T9) T T10–T11–T12 Peak: T10 left jejunum T10 right ileum	Transverse abdominis Serratus anterior	Spinous processes of jejunum L1 Ileum L2 12 rib arch	Oval 5	Ovaries testicle kidney

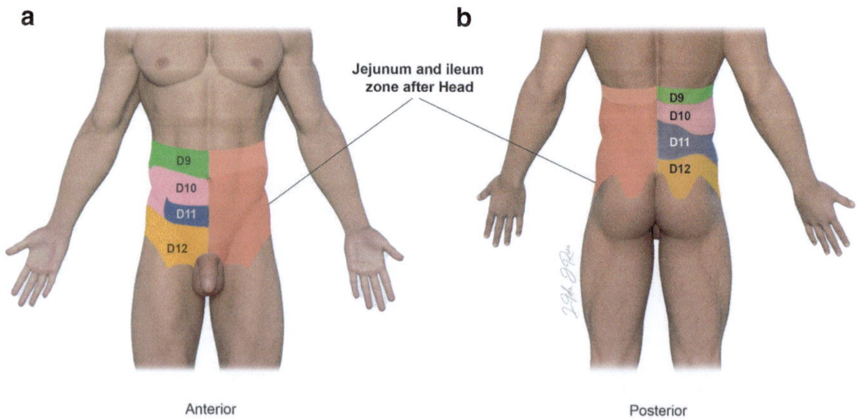

Fig. 15.17 Head's zone of jejunum and ileum. (**a**) Anterior view; (**b**) posterior view

5.9 Ascending, Transverse, Appendix, and Cecum Colon

Viscera	Dermatome - Head's zone	Myotom	Sclerotome	Mackenzie	Viscero-Visceral R.
Ascending, transverse, appendix, and cecum colon (see Fig. 15.18)	T11, T12, L1 Appendix: Ventral: T11 (Mc Burney point) Dorsal: to the right of the vertebral body of L2. Cecum, ascending colon and transverse: Ventral: T10 to L1 in a line between navel 6 and pubic symphysis Dorsal: To the right of the vertebral body L2	Transverse abdominis Serratus posterior Quadratus lumborum Sartorio Iliopsoas	Rib arch 12 L2 in the iliac crest or in the proximal third of the femur	Oval 5 and/or 6	Uterus, kidney, bladder, colon

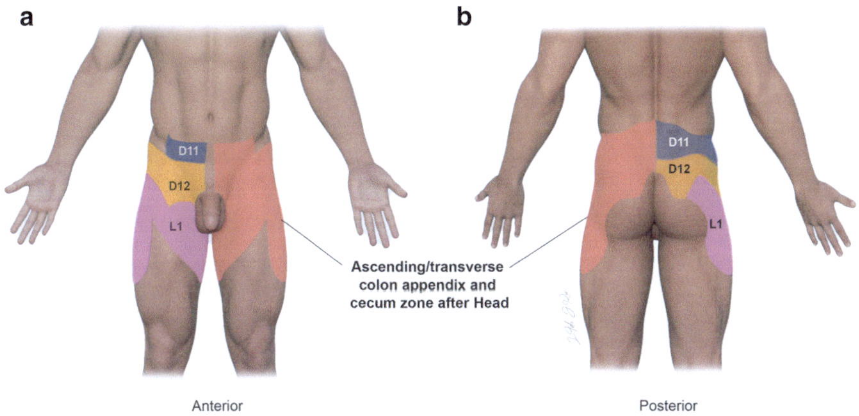

Fig. 15.18 Ascending colon, transverse, appendix and cecum area. (**a**) Anterior view; (**b**) posterior view

5.10 Descending Colon, Sigmoid and Rectum

Viscera	Dermatome - Head's zone	Myotom	Sclerotome	Mackenzie	Viscero-Visceral R.
Descending colon, sigmoid and rectum (see Fig. 15.19)	T11, T12, L1, L2 **Anterior**: Descending colon: Three fingers on pubic symphysis to the left side (T12) Sigmoid and rectus colon: to the left of the pubic symphysis (L2) **Back**: Descending colon: upper half of the sacrum, on the left side. Sigmoid and rectal colon: lower half of the sacrum on the left side and coccyx. Rectum: S2, S3, S4.	Transverse abdominis Serratus posterior Quadratus lumborum Sartorio Iliopsoas Gracilis Pectineus Long adductor Quadriceps	Rib arch 11 and 12 L2 in the iliac crest or in the proximal third of the femur	Oval 5 (6)	Uterus, kidney, bladder, colon

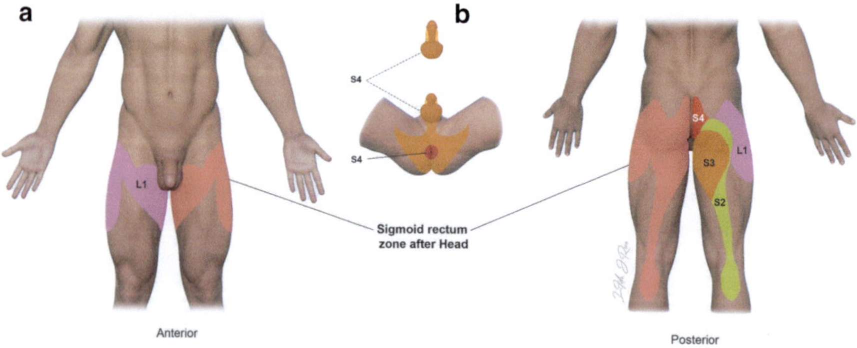

Fig. 15.19 Head's zone of the descending colon, sigmoid and rectum. (**a**) Anterior view; (**b**) posterior view

5.11 *Kidney and Ureter*

Viscera	Dermatome - Head's zone	Myotom	Sclerotome	Mackenzie	Viscero-Visceral R.
Kidney (see Fig. 15.20)	Kidney and ureters: T10–L1 Renal pelvis and ureter: T11, T12 and L1	Transverse abdominis Serratus posterior Quadratus lumborum Sartorio Iliopsoas Gracilis Pectineus Long adductor Quadriceps	Rib arch 10, 11 and 12 L2 in the iliac crest or in the proximal third of the femur	Oval 5	Uterus, bladder, colon, ovary, testicle

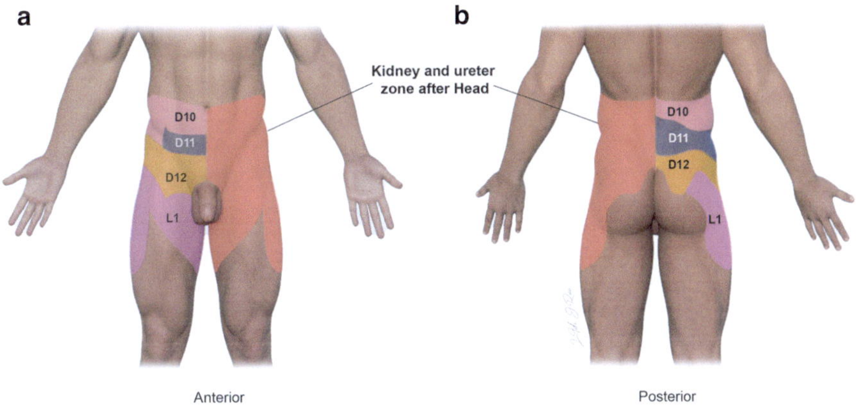

Fig. 15.20 Head's zone of the kidney and uréter. (**a**) Anterior view; (**b**) posterior view

5.12 Bladder

Viscera	Dermatome - Head's zone	Myotom	Sclerotome	Mackenzie	Viscero-Visceral R.
Bladder (see Fig. 15.21)	Double innervation: (T10) S11–L1 S1–S4	Rectus abdominis Muscular paravertebral Iliopsoas Lumbar Square Sartorius Posteroinferior serratus External, internal, and transverse abdominal oblique, Cremaster	Heel iliac ridges	Oval 5 and/or 7	Colon, kidney, appendix, ovary, uterus, rectum

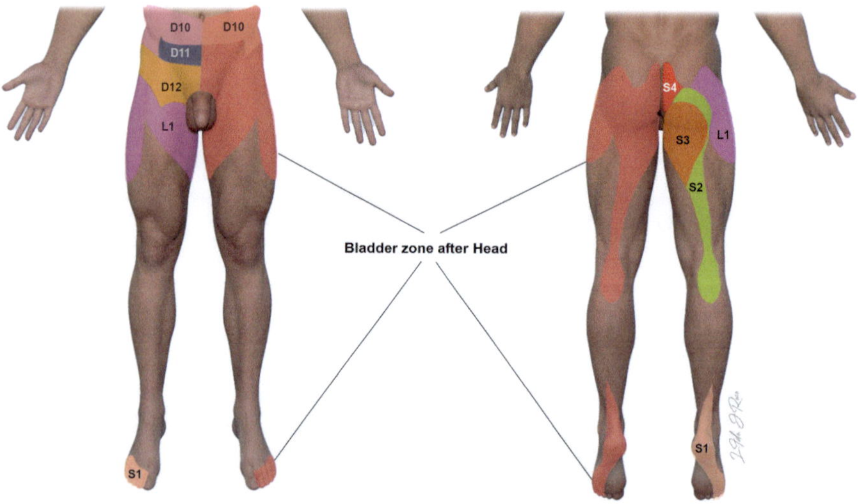

Fig. 15.21 Head's zone of the bladder. (**a**) Anterior view; (**b**) posterior view

5.13 Ovary, Testicles, Uterus, and Adnexa

Viscera	Dermatome - Head's zone	Myotom	Sclerotome	Mackenzie	Viscero-Visceral R.
Ovary, testicle, uterus, and adnexa (see Figs. 15.22 and 15.23)	Ovary and testicle: T10 Epididymis: T11–T12 (L1) Annexes T11-L1 Uterus: T10–L1 S2-S4 Cervix: Upper cervical canal: T11 and T12 Inferior: S3 and S4	Paravertebral, iliopsoas, Quadratus Lumborum, Serratus posteroinferior External oblique, internal and transverse abdominis Cremaster, rectus, transverse abdominal Gracilis, Sartorius **S1 and S2 myotomes:** Glutes and hamstrings include the gastrocnemius, soleus, and plantar muscles.	Pubic symphysis L2 vertebra L5-S1 iliac sacral points and greater trochanter. Anterior iliac crest and symphysis	Oval 5 and/or 7	Colon, kidney, appendix, ovary, uterus, rectum

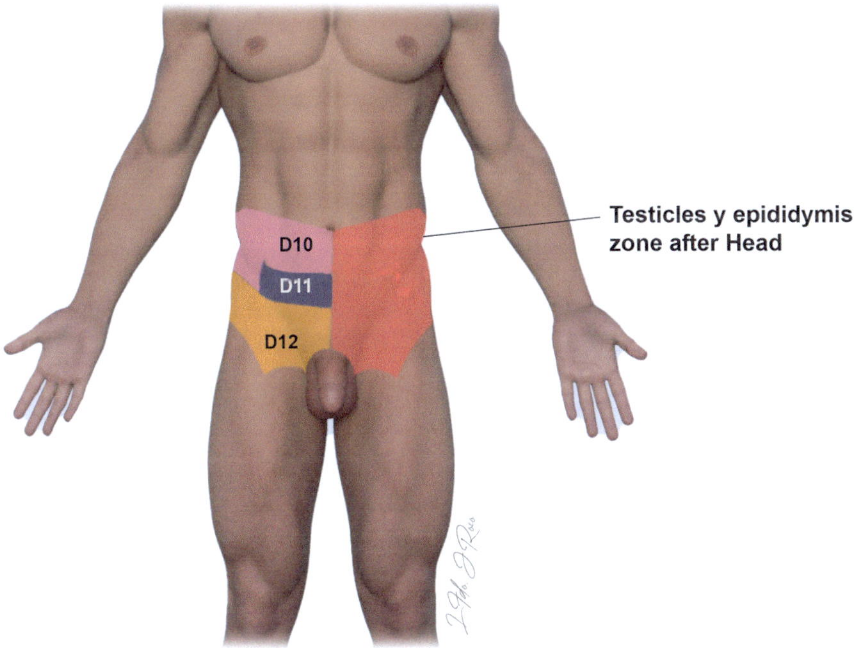

Fig. 15.22 Head's zone of the testicle

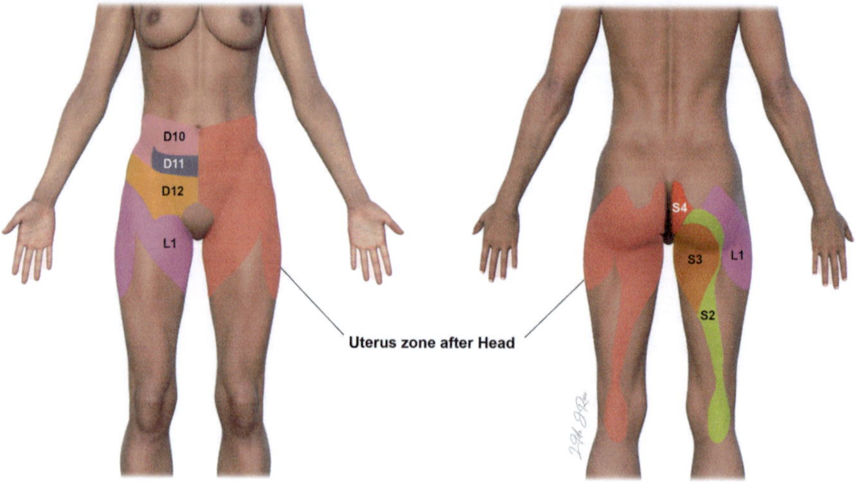

Fig. 15.23 Head's zone of uterus and ovaries

5.14 Prostate

Viscera	Dermatome - Head's zone	Myotom	Sclerotome	Mackenzie	Viscero-Visceral R.
Prostate (see Fig. 15.24)	T10–T12 (L5) S1-S3	Myotomes from L5 to S2 (piriformis, rotators, gluteus maximus)	T10–T12 rib arches in (free ends) Sclerotomes from L5 to S2 Iliac crest Vertebra T10, T11, L5, S1 to S3, Sacrum, ischial tuberosity, calves, soles, and hallux		

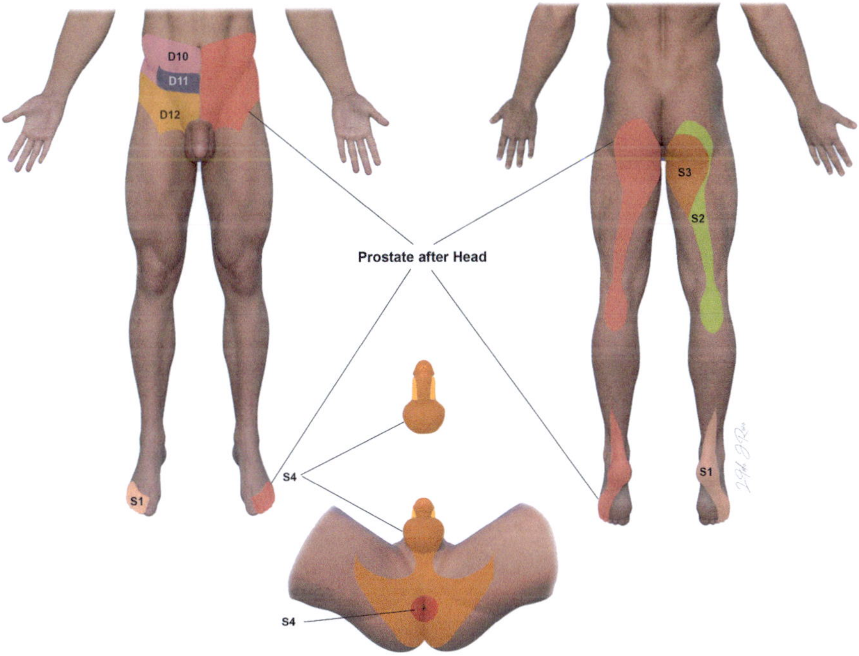

Fig. 15.24 Prostate Head's zone

5.15 Epididymis

Viscera	Dermatome - Head's zone	Myotom	Sclerotome	Mackenzie	Viscero-Visceral R.
Epididymis (see Fig. 15.25)	T11 & T12 inguinal ring skin Outer thigh Perineum	Scarpa-inner knee triangle	VertebraL5, S1 and S2		

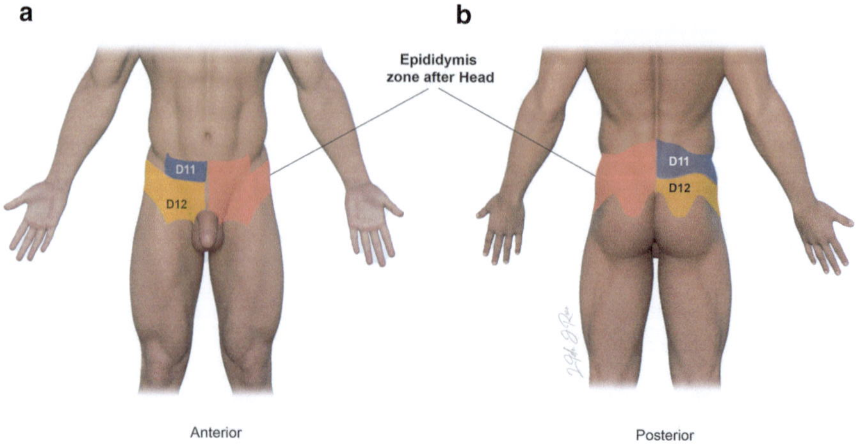

Fig. 15.25 Head's zone of epididymis. (**a**) Anterior view; (**b**) posterior view

6 Metameric Expression of the Organs of the Head and Neck (Including Teeth)

The information listed below shows graphically and tabulated the Head's zones of each of the organs, integrating the information with the associated myotomes, sclerotomes and possible segmental viscero-visceral reflexes. Myotomic and sclerotomic information regarding this group of organs is also based on knowledge of embryological development, from the formation of rhombomeres to those derived from pharyngeal arches [35–37].

6.1 Eye

Organ	Dermatome - Head's zone	Myotome	Sclerotome	Mackenzie	R. Viscero-Visceral
Eye (see Fig. 15.26)	Frontonasal, medioorbital, malar, frontotemporal, temporal, vertical	Tensor tympani muscle, muscles of mastication, soft palate, mylohyoid (trigeminal) Frontal, temporal, orbicular (facial)	Frontal, temporal, maxillary	C2–C3	Nose, teeth, ears, tonsils, sinuses, parotid

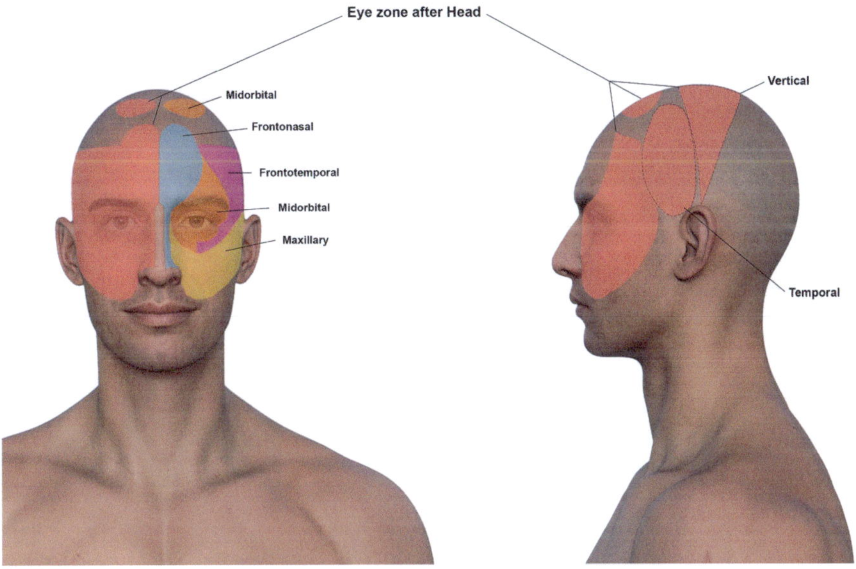

Fig. 15.26 Head's zone of the eye

6.2 Ear

Organ	Dermatome - Head's zone head	Myotome	Sclerotome	Mackenzie	R. Viscero-Visceral
Ear (see Fig. 15.27)	Vertical, parietal, hyoidea, mandibular,	Tensor tympani muscle, muscles of mastication, soft palate, mylohyoid (trigeminal)	Temporo-mandibular joint	C4–C5	Nose, teeth, eyes, tonsils, sinuses, parotid

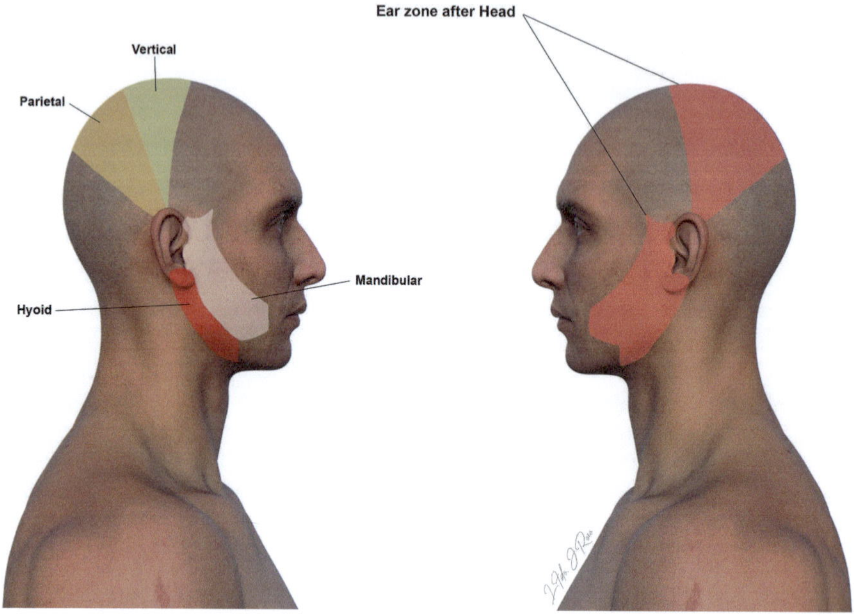

Fig. 15.27 Head's zone of the ear

6.3 Nose

Organ	Dermatome - Head's zone	Myotome	Sclerotome	Mackenzie	R. Viscero-Visceral
Nose (see Fig. 15.28)	Frontonasal, nasolabial, medioorbital	Tensor tympani muscle, muscles of mastication, soft palate, mylohyoid (trigeminal) Frontal, orbicular, procerus (facial)	The nasal bone, maxilla	C4–C5	Ears, teeth, eyes, tonsils, sinuses, parotid

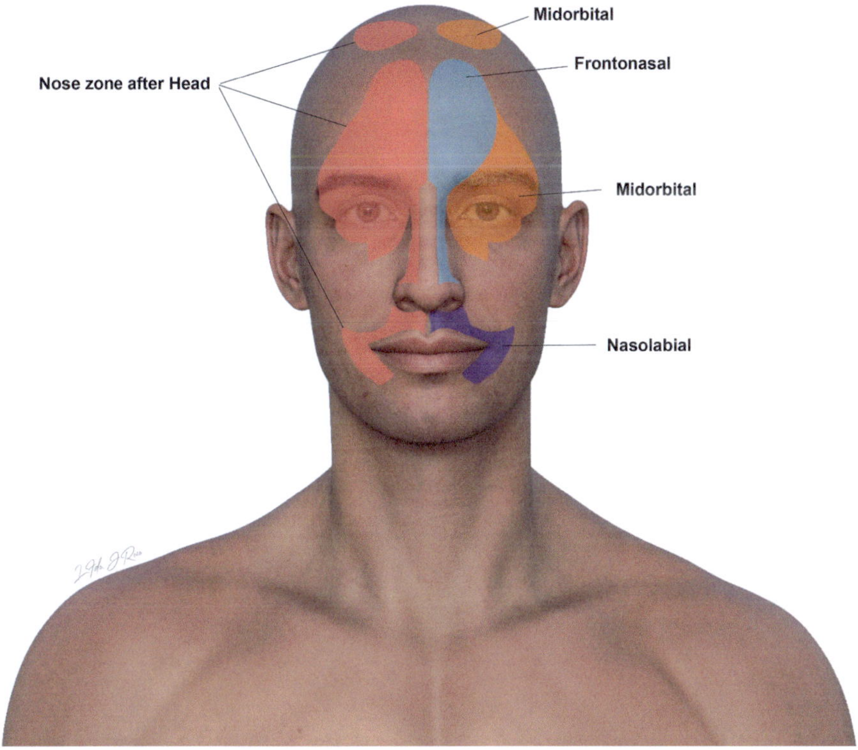

Fig. 15.28 Head's zone of the nose

6.4 Tonsils

Organ	Dermatome - Head's zone	Myotome	Sclerotome	Mackenzie	R. Viscero-Visceral
Tonsils (see Fig. 15.29)	Hyoidea	Stylopharyngeus (IX) muscles of mastication, tensor tympani muscle, soft palate, mylohyoid (V)	Hyoid bone, maxilla, temporomandibular joint	C4–C7	Tongue, ears, teeth, salivary gland, maxillary sinuses, nose, eyes

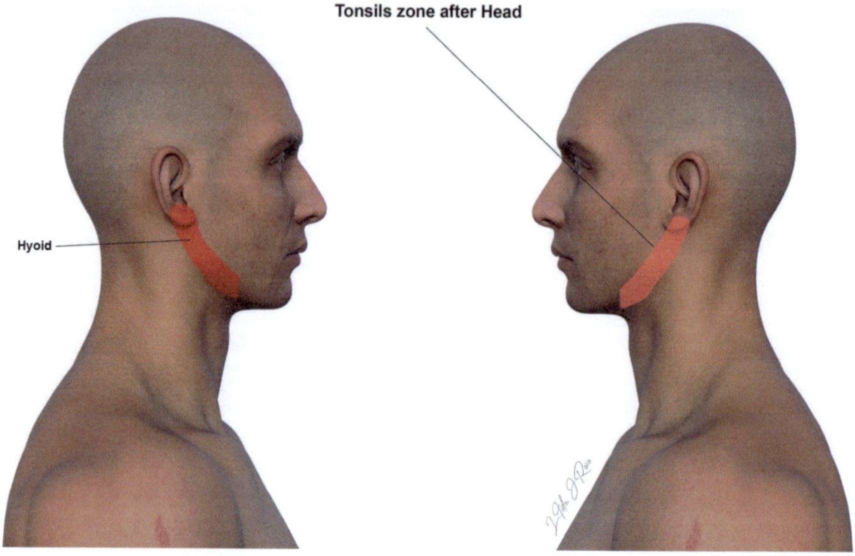

Fig. 15.29 Head's zone of tonsils

6.5 Tongue

Organ	Dermatome - Head's zone	Myotome	Sclerotome	Mackenzie	R. Viscero-Visceral
Tongue (see Fig. 15.30)	Hyoid, mental, laryngeal, superior, occipital	Tongue (XII)	Occipital bone	C2–C3	Teeth, tonsils, ears

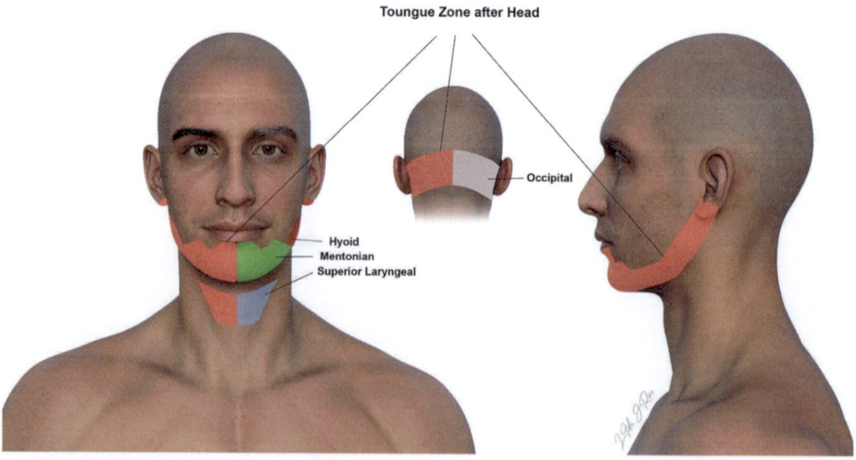

Fig. 15.30 Head's zone of the tongue

6.6 *Larynx*

Organ	Dermatome - Head's zone	Myotome	Sclerotome	Mackenzie	R. Viscero-Visceral
Larynx (see Fig. 15.31)	Laryngeal superior and inferior	Cricothyroid, palatoglossus and palatopharyngeus, constrictor of the pharynx	N/A	C2–C3	The right subclavian artery, thoracic aorta, left, parathyroid

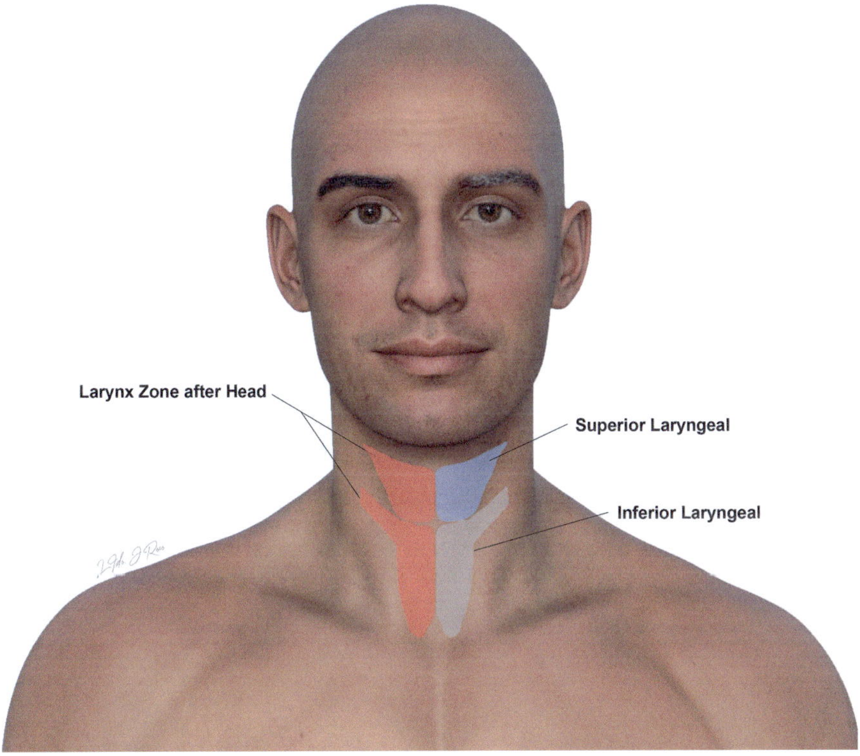

Fig. 15.31 Head's zone of the larynx

6.7 Upper Incisors

Teeth	Dermatome - Head's zone	Myotome	Sclerotome	Mackenzie	R. Viscero-Visceral
Upper incisors (see Fig. 15.32)	Frontonasal	Muscles of mastication, tensor tympani muscle, soft palate, mylohyoid (V)	Maxillary bone, temporomandibular joint	C4–C5	Nose, sinuses, ears, eyes, teeth

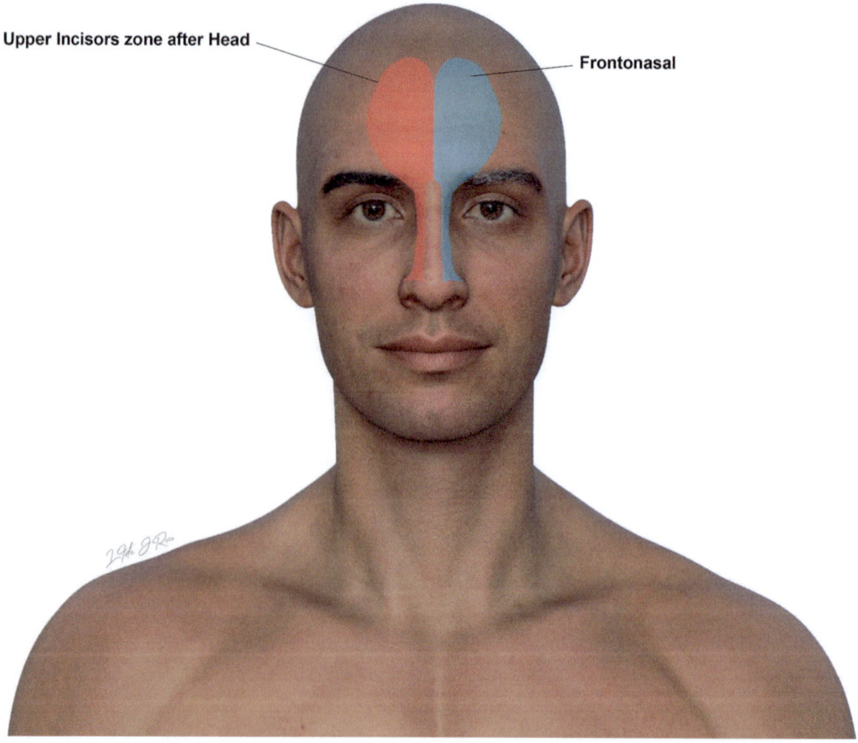

Fig. 15.32 Head's zone of upper incisors

6.8 *Canines and First Premolar*

Teeth	Dermatome - Head's zone	Myotome	Sclerotome	Mackenzie	R. Viscero-Visceral
Canine and first premolar (see Fig. 15.33)	Nasolabial	Muscles of mastication, tensor tympani muscle, soft palate, mylohyoid (V)	Maxillary bone, temporomandibular joint	C4–C5	Nose, sinuses, ears, eyes, teeth

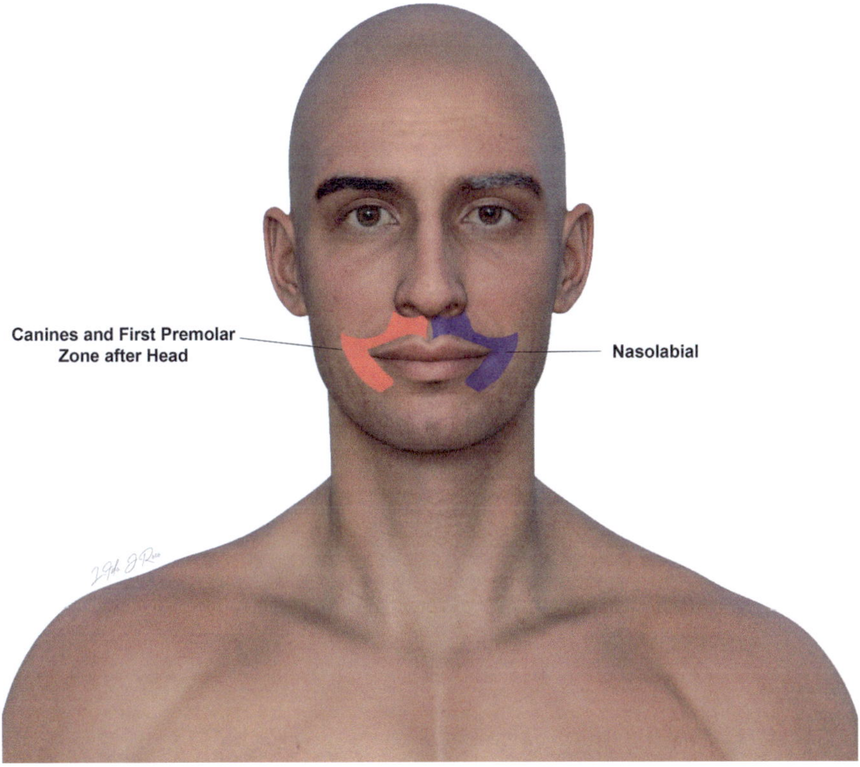

Fig. 15.33 Head's zone of canines and upper first premolar

6.9 Second Premolar and First Upper Molar

Teeth	Dermatome - Head's zone	Myotome	Sclerotome	Mackenzie	R. Viscero-Visceral
The second premolar and first molar upper (see Fig. 15.34)	Malar and temporal	Muscles of mastication, tensor tympani muscle, soft palate, mylohyoid (V)	Maxillary bone, temporomandibular joint	C4–C5	Nose, sinuses, ears, eyes, teeth

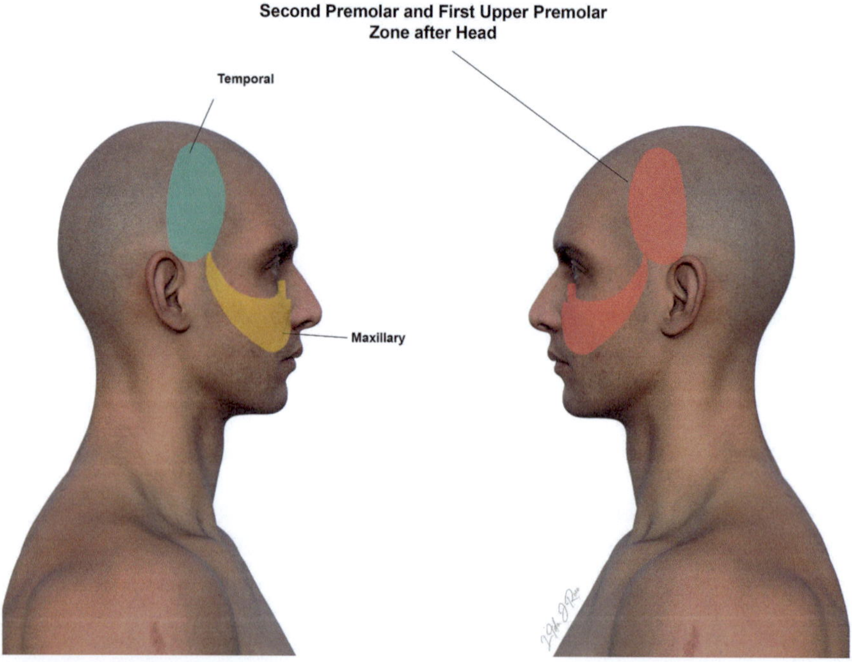

Fig. 15.34 Head's zone of the second premolar and upper first premolar

6.10 Second Molar and Upper Wisdom Tooth

Teeth	Dermatome - Head's zone	Myotome	Sclerotome	Mackenzie	R. Viscero-Visceral
Second molar and sup wisdom tooth (see Fig. 15.35)	Temporal mandibular joint (vertical)	Muscles of mastication, tensor tympani muscle, soft palate, mylohyoid (V)	Maxillary bone, temporomandibular joint	C4–C5	Nose, sinuses, ears, eyes, teeth

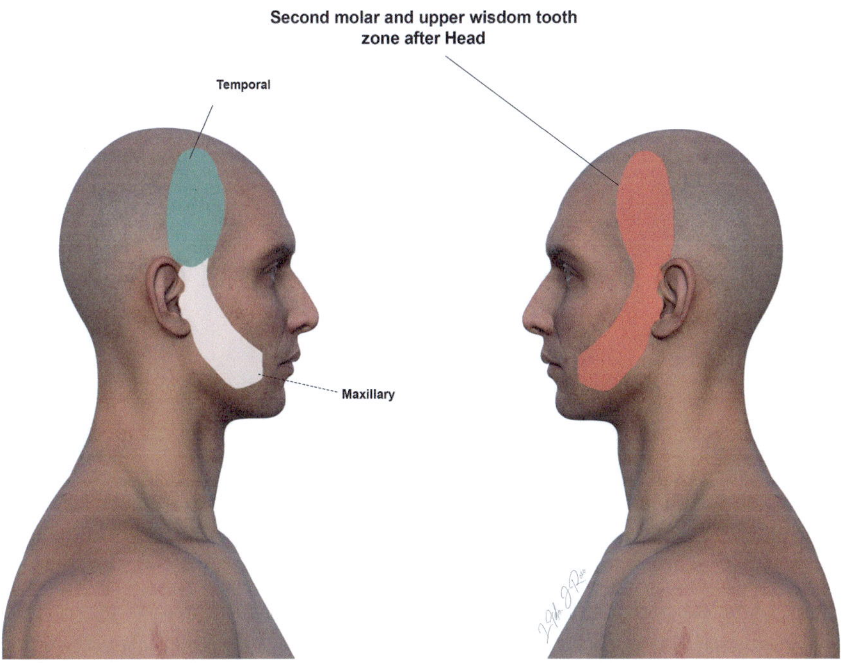

Fig. 15.35 Head's zone of the second molar and upper wisdom tooth

6.11 Incisor, Canine and Lower Premolars

Teeth	Dermatome - Head's zone	Myotome	Sclerotome	Mackenzie	R. Viscero-Visceral
Incisor, canine and premolars (see Fig. 15.36)	Mental (Hyoidea)	Muscles of mastication, tensor tympani muscle, soft palate, mylohyoid (V)	Bone of the jaw, temporomandibular joint	C6–C7	Tongue, ear, parotid gland, teeth

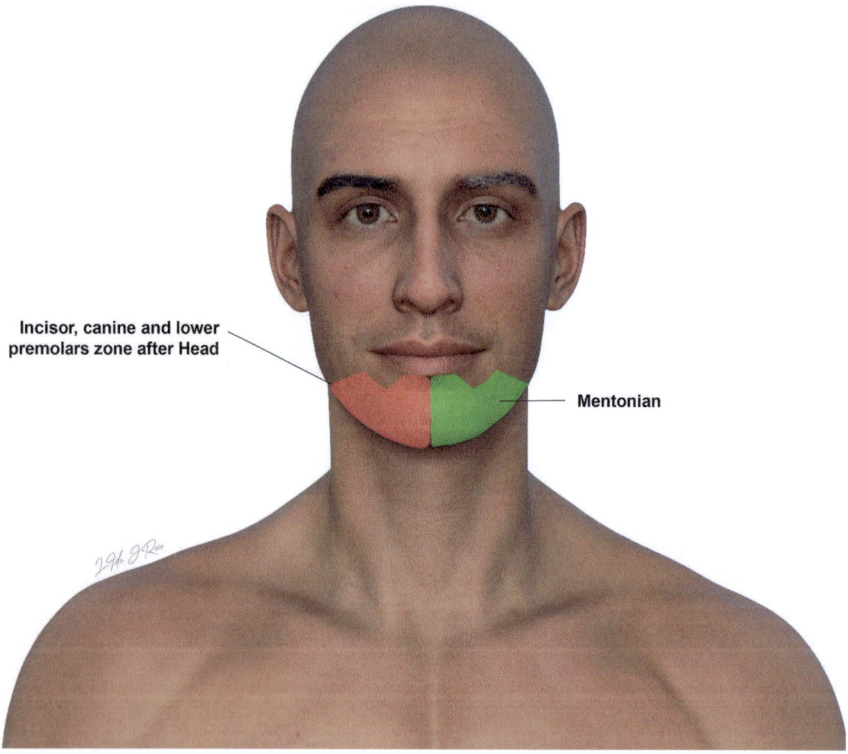

Fig. 15.36 Head's zone of incisors, canines and lower premolars

6.12 Lower Molars

Teeth	Dermatome - Head's zone	Myotome	Sclerotome	Mackenzie	R. Viscero-Visceral
Lower molars (see Fig. 15.37)	Hyoidea	Muscles of mastication, tensor tympani muscle, soft palate, mylohyoid (V)	Bone of the jaw, temporomandibular joint	C6–C7	Tonsils, tongue, ear, parotid gland, teeth

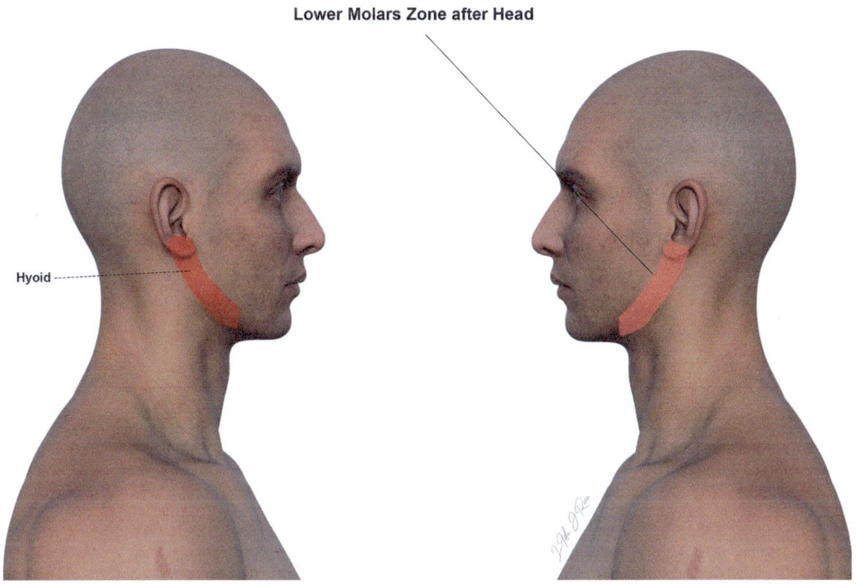

Fig. 15.37 Head's zone of lower molars

6.13 Lower Wisdom Teeth

Teeth	Dermatome - Head's zone	Myotome	Sclerotome	Mackenzie	R. Viscero-Visceral
Lower wisdom teeth (see Fig. 15.38)	Laryngeal superior	Muscles of mastication, tensor tympani muscle, soft palate, mylohyoid (V)	Bone of the jaw, temporomandibular joint	C6–C7	Tonsils, tongue, ear, parotid gland, teeth, larynx

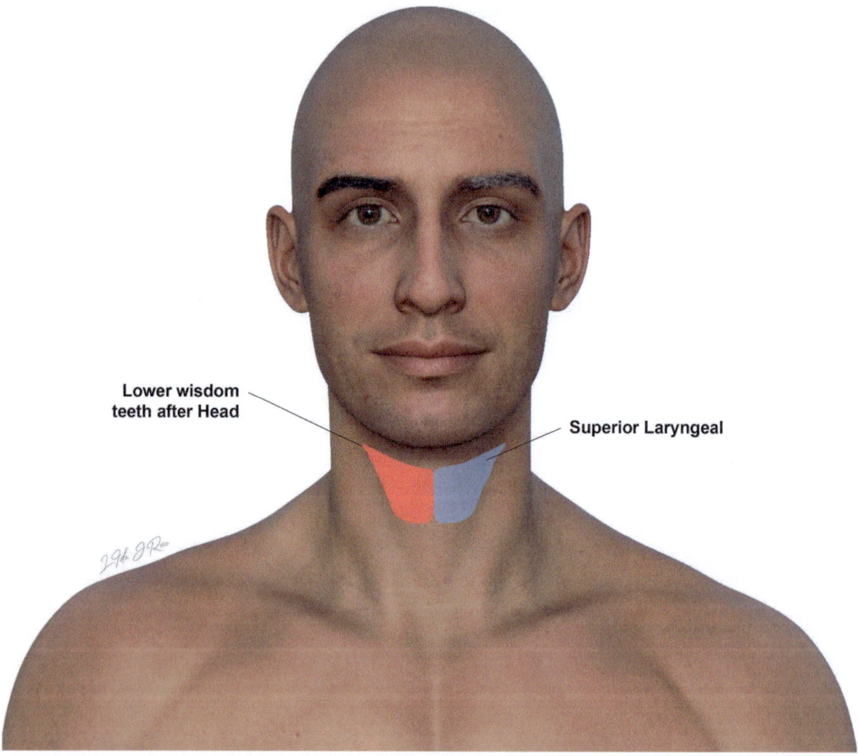

Fig. 15.38 Head's zone of lower wisdom teeth

7 Head Reflex Zones According to Henry Head

Head also described the existence of areas on the head, which manifested as pain and tenderness on the scalp or face and which also reflect visceral pathology, either local to the organs of the head, or in the organs of the thoracic, abdominal and pelvic cavities (Tables 15.5 and 15.6).

These zones have the following characteristics:

- Each organ of the head has one or more reflex zones.
- In herpes, it does not have the same corroborative value as in the trunk and abdomen.
- They do not overlap.
- The sensitive areas do not correspond to branches of nerve distribution but to areas that show evidence of visceral information that has been transmitted through the vagus nerve and its connections (see Chap. 31) or by transmission from visceral organs of the abdomen or thorax using pathways such as the phrenic nerve and cervical plexus.

Table 15.5 Head's zone on face and relationship with viscera of the head

Area	Pathologies
Frontonasal	Cornea, anterior chamber of the eye, top of the nose, upper incisors
Medioorbital	Hypermetropia
	Glaucoma
Fronto temporal	Thoracic viscera, iritis. In glaucoma associated with the temporal area. It is rarely found, only in diseases of the viscera of the head.
Temporary	Vitreous chamber (glaucoma), tooth decay, it is associated with the stomach.
Vertical	Eye
	Middle ear
	Disorders of the liver and gastric
Occipital	Abdomen, back of the tongue, pelvis
Maxilla	Sensitivity in iritis, increasing the tension of the anterior chamber vitreous, tooth decay of the upper jaw. The hard palate could be affected.
Mandibular	Last two molars
Hioidea	Ear, tonsils, lateral side of the tongue, teeth (lower molars)
Laryngeal superior	Lower molars and back of the dorsum of the tongue
Laryngeal inferior	Larynx especially vocal cords
Nasolabial	Lesions of the mucous membranes of the respiratory tract (frontonasal)
Mental	Odontomas
Esternomastoidea	Referred pain from viscera of the chest and abdominal
Esternonuchal	Only by visceral pathology of thorax and abdomen

Table 15.6 Head's zone on the face and relationship with thoracic and abdominal viscera

Reflexes on the head	Viscera
Frontonasal	Apices of the lungs, stomach, and liver
Medioorbital	Lung, heart (ventricles), arch and ascending aorta
Frontotemporal	Lungs (lower lobes) and heart (atria)
Temporary	The lung bases, and heart (atria) stomach (cardia)
Vertical	Stomach, liver, and first portion of small intestine
Parietal	Stomach, liver, and first portion of small intestine
Occipital	Liver, intestine, colon, ovary, testis, fallopian tubes, uterus, bladder (contraction)

References

1. Wancura-Kampik I. Segmental anatomy. 1st ed. Munich: Elsevier Urban & Fisher Verlag; 2009.
2. Navarro K, Pinilla L. The contributions of Henry Head to the neuroanatomical and physiological foundations of segment therapy. MÉD UIS. 2013;26(2):33–44.
3. Pinilla-Bonilla LB, Rodríguez DC, Villamil-Villar WA. British and Russian Nervism: a comparison between two trends in the history of medicine focused on the nervous system. MED UIS. 2024;37(1):33–40. https://doi.org/10.18273/revmed.v37n1-2024003.
4. Dosch P, Dosch M. Manual of neural therapy according to Huneke. 2nd ed. Stuttgart: Thieme; 2007.
5. Baumann C. Henry Head in Ewald Hering's laboratory in Prague 1884-1886: an early study on the nervous control of breathing. J Hist Neurosci. 2005;14(4):322–33.
6. Head H. On the regulation of respiration. Part I. Experimental. J Physiol. 1889;10:1–70.
7. Head H. On regulation of respiration. Part II. Theoretical. J Physiol. 1889;10(4):279–90.
8. Head H. Hughlings Jackson on aphasia and hindered affections of speech. Brain. 1915;38(1–2):1–27.
9. Head H. Aphasia and kindred disorders of speech. Brain. 1920;43(2):87–165.
10. Head H. On disturbances of sensation with especial reference to the pain of visceral disease. Brain. 1893;16(1–2):1–133.
11. Head H. On disturbances of sensation with especial reference to the pain of visceral disease: part II. Head and neck. Brain. 1894;17(3):339–480.
12. Head H. On disturbances of sensation with especial reference to the pain of visceral disease: part III. Pain in diseases of the heart and lungs. Brain. 1896;19(2–3):153–276.
13. Foerster O. The dermatomes in man. Brain. 1933;56(1):1–39. https://doi.org/10.1093/brain/56.1.1.
14. Mackenzie J. Some points bearing on the association of sensory disorders and visceral disease. Brain. 1983;16:321–53. https://doi.org/10.1093/brain/16.3.321.
15. Mackenzie J. The meaning and mechanism of visceral pain as shown by the study of visceral and other sympathetic (autonomic) reflexes. Br Med J. 1906;30:1523–8.
16. Mackenzie J. Symptoms and their interpretation, vol. 1. 4th ed. London: Shaw & Sons, Fetter Lane., 7 & 8; 1920.
17. Sonoo M. J Neurol Neurosurg Psychiatry. 2023;94:643–8.
18. Herringham WP. The minute anatomy of the brachial plexus. Proc R Soc Lond. 1887;41:423–41.
19. Namba K. Carotid-vertebrobasilar anastomoses with reference to their segmental property. Neurol Med Chir (Tokyo). 2017;57(6):267–77. https://doi.org/10.2176/nmc.ra.2017-0050. Epub 2017 May 1. PMID: 28458386; PMCID: PMC5495958

20. The University of British Columbia. UBC Neuroanatomy. Neuroanatomy.ca, The University of British Columbia. 2021. neuroanatomy.ca/. Accessed 21 Aug 2024.
21. Levin KH, Maggiano HJ, Wilbourn AJ. Cervical radiculopathies: comparison of surgical and EMG localization of single-root lesions. Neurology. 1996;46:1022–5.
22. Chiba T, Konoeda F, Higashihara M, et al. C8 and T1 innervation of forearm muscles. Clin Neurophysiol. 2015;126:837–42. S1388-2457(14) 00431-3
23. Furukawa Y, Miyaji Y, Kadoya A, et al. Determining C5, C6 and C7 myotomes through comparative analyses of clinical, MRI and EMG findings in cervical radiculopathy. Clin Neurophysiol Pract. 2021;6:88–92.
24. Higashihara M, Hatanaka Y, Ogawa G, et al. L3 and L4 innervation investigated from patients with single-root radiculopathy. Muscle Nerve. 2016;54:545.
25. Desai SS, Cohen-Levy WB. Anatomy, bony pelvis and lower limb: tibial nerve. [Updated 2023 Aug 14]. In: StatPearls [Internet]. Treasure Island: StatPearls; 2024. Available from: https://www.ncbi.nlm.nih.gov/books/NBK537028/
26. Ivanusic JJ. The evidence for the spinal segmental innervation of bone. Clin Anat. 2007;20(8):956–60. https://doi.org/10.1002/ca.20555.
27. Warwick R, Williams P, Dyson M, Bannister L, editors. Gray's anatomy. 37th ed. Edinburgh/New York: Churchill Livingston; 1989.
28. Greenberg SA. The history of dermatome mapping. Arch Neurol. 2003;60:126–31.
29. Dejerine J. Semiology of nervous system diseases. Paris: Masson. Reprinted in 1977 edition.
30. Kellgren JH. On the distribution of pain arising from deep somatic structures with charts of segmental pain areas. 1939. p. 35–46.
31. Inman VT, Saunders JB. Referred pain from skeletal structures. J Nerv Ment Dis. 1944;99:660–7.
32. Gajda M, Litwin JA, Adriaensen D, Timmermans JP, Cichocki T. Segmental distribution and morphometric features of primary sensory neurons projecting to the tibial periosteum in the rat. Folia Histochem Cytobiol. 2004;42:95–9.
33. Thai J, Kyloh M, Travis L, Spencer NJ, Ivanusic JJ. Identifying spinal afferent (sensory) nerve endings that innervate the marrow cavity and periosteum using anterograde tracing. J Comp Neurol. 2020;528(11):1903–16. https://doi.org/10.1002/cne.24862.
34. Thai J, Fuller-Jackson JP, Ivanusic JJ. Using tissue clearing and light sheet fluorescence microscopy for the three-dimensional analysis of sensory and sympathetic nerve endings that innervate bone and dental tissue of mice. J Comp Neurol. 2024;532(1):e25582. https://doi.org/10.1002/cne.25582.
35. O'Rahilly R, Müller F. The early development of the hypoglossal nerve and occipital Somites in staged human embryos. Am J Anat. 1984;169(3):237–57.
36. Toro-Tobon S, Manrique M, Paredes-Gutierrez J, Mantilla-Rivas E, Oh H, Ahmad L, Oh AK, Rogers GF. Pharyngeal arches, chapter 1: normal development and derivatives. J Craniofac Surg. 2023;34(7):2237–41. https://doi.org/10.1097/SCS.0000000000009374.
37. Meegalla N, Downs BW. Anatomy, head and neck, palatine tonsil (Faucial Tonsils). [Updated 2023 Jun 5]. In: StatPearls [Internet]. Treasure Island: StatPearls; 2024. Available from: https://www.ncbi.nlm.nih.gov/books/NBK538296/

Chapter 16
Communication in the Neuroimmune System

Lorenz Fischer

1 Introduction

Until a few years ago, the autonomic nervous system (ANS) and the immune system were considered to have separate functions. It has now become increasingly clear that the ANS and the immune system are inseparable and that immunological and inflammatory processes are controlled by the ANS [1–5]. There is even a bidirectional interaction ("cross-talk") between the ANS and the immune system, and that is why we use the term, "neuroimmune communication." The latter initially takes place rapidly and nonspecifically in the innate immune system and is important for maintaining homeostasis and economy in the organism, as well as for providing a protective response to injury or infection. Only later does the adaptive immune system "help" specifically, e.g., in the case of infections, with cell-mediated immunity (T lymphocytes) and humoral immunity (B lymphocytes, antibodies). Surprisingly, the nonspecific, "basal" processes in the neuroimmune system are the same for various causes such as mechanical trauma, infection, and psychological stress [5]. However, the neuroimmune system can also react excessively. This derailment often begins as an imbalance in the autonomic nervous system with sympathetic hyperactivity and turns into faulty neuroimmune communication. It is our opinion that it is the basis for numerous diseases [5], and that faulty communication occurs when the neuroimmune system is preloaded. If an event such as an infection or psychological or somatic trauma hits such a preloaded ANS, it can lead to a nonspecific overreaction with a "cytokine storm"and thus to excessive inflammation with tissue damage. The clinical picture—the disease—only appears at the end of this cascade and is

L. Fischer (✉)
Former Chair of Neural therapy (2002–2018), University of Bern, Bern, Switzerland
e-mail: fischer.lori@bluewin.ch

L. B. Pinilla Bonilla et al. (eds.), *Neuraltherapeutic Medicine*,
https://doi.org/10.1007/978-3-032-03257-7_16

dominated by the organ or organ system most severely affected. In the following, we would like to discuss the reasons for this overreaction.

Not all elements of neuroimmune communication are described in this short article. It only deals with important principles and serves as a basis for understanding the logical, nonspecific therapeutic interventions with local anesthetics (neural therapy).

2 The Integrative Function of the Autonomic Nervous System

Knowledge of the different levels of interaction in the ANS is important for understanding neuroimmune communication. The ANS consists of the sympathetic nervous system (SNS) and the parasympathetic nervous system (PNS) with the vagus as the main nerve. The ANS consists of a central (brain and spinal cord) and peripheral part. It coordinates organ functions with the help of the immune system, including inflammatory cascades and the endocrine and vascular systems. In doing so, the ANS tries to work according to the cybernetic principles of homeostasis and economy, depending on endogenous and exogenous factors. The ANS also plays a major role in controlling immune processes and the corresponding inflammatory cascades, as well as in regulating (micro)circulation and lymph flow (Fig. 16.1).

2.1 The Sympathetic Nervous System (SNS)

The SNS activates the body during stress. The SNS runs its efferents from the sympathetic centers in the brain, including the hypothalamus and rostral ventrolateral medulla (RVLM) [6, 7], via the nucleus intermediolaterales in the spinal cord, to the para- and prevertebral ganglia in the sympathetic trunk. From there, postganglionic fibers run into the interstitium ("basic system"), to the internal organs, and to the musculoskeletal system. Other vertical information pathways from the brain to the periphery are the hypothalamo-pituitary-adrenal axis (HPA), which influences the adrenal cortex, and the sympatho-adrenal (SA) system, which influences the adrenal medulla. Thus, we already see several "control elements" for the periphery, which in the interstitium includes immune cells as well as microcirculation. Sensory nerve fibers in the sympathetic trunk project from the periphery to the spinal cord and from there to the sympathetic centers (among others) in the brain, closing a reflex arc. A parallel path of the sympathetic nervous system running to the brain leads via cervical ganglia and perivascular plexuses.

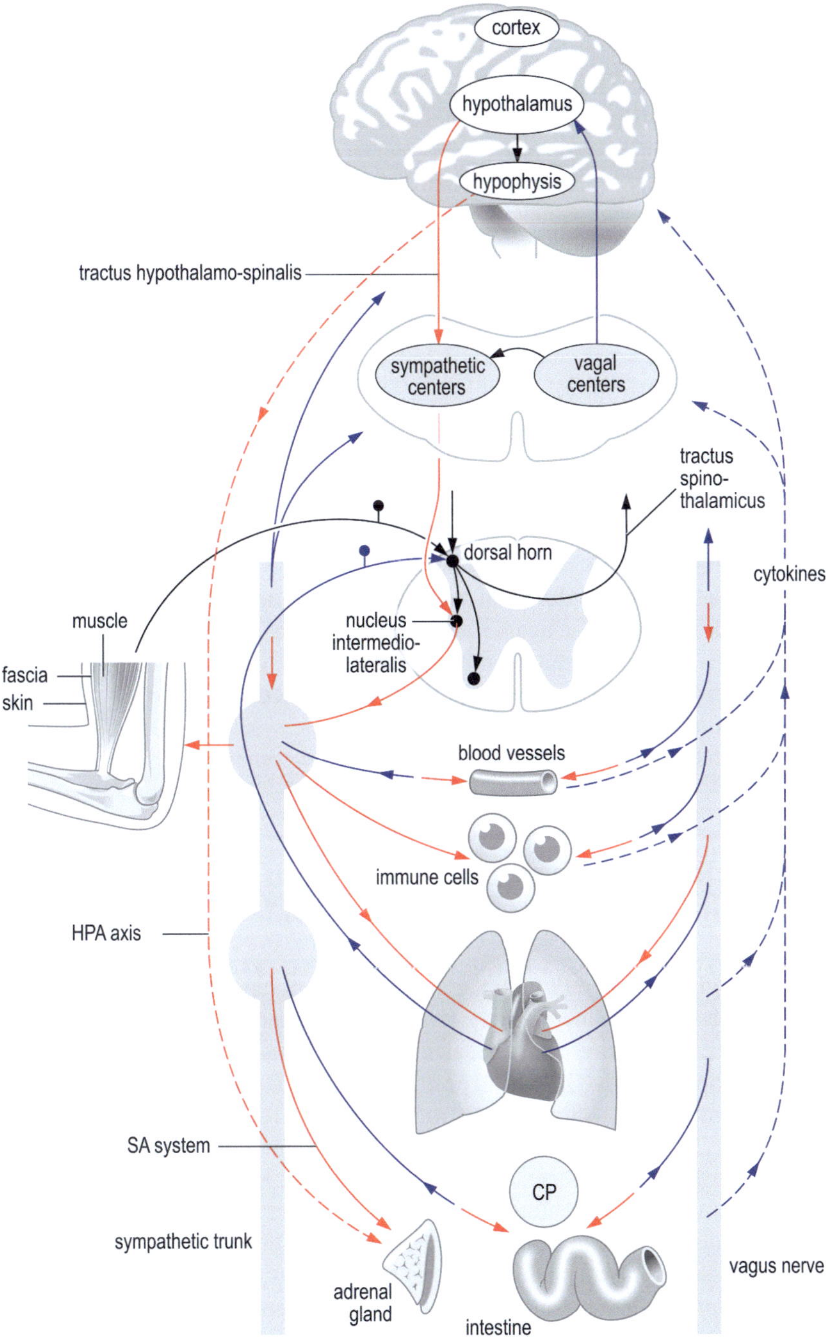

Fig. 16.1 Several negative and positive feedback loops form a complex system under the leadership of the ANS and give it a holistic character (for details, see text). Various efferent (red arrows) and afferent (blue arrows) "pathways" are shown in this figure. They are dependent on each other. For a better overview, the sympathetic and parasympathetic (vagal) systems were not drawn ipsilaterally. *CP* celiac plexus, *HPA* hypothalamic-pituitary-adrenal, *SA* sympatho-adrenal

2.2 *The Parasympathetic Nervous System (PNS)*

The PNS, particularly the vagus nerve, promotes relaxation and recovery. Efferent parasympathetic fibers of the vagus nerve originate in the brain from the nucleus ambiguus and nucleus dorsalis of the vagus nerve and form various plexuses together with the SNS (plexus pulmonalis, plexus cardiacus, plexus coeliacus, etc.). From there, the parasympathetic fibers continue into the periphery without switching and are only switched near the organs. The sensory nerve fibers in the vagus nerve take a "snapshot" of the state in the periphery and transmit this information to the brain stem, specifically, to the nucleus tractus solitarii (NTS).

2.3 *Interactions of Vagus and SNS in the Brain*

After receiving vagal action potentials, the NTS in turn establishes connections to the efferent vagal and sympathetic core areas mentioned in Sects. 2.1 and 2.2, as well as to integration centers such as the hypothalamus. The hypothalamus has connections to other areas of the brain such as the insula and the limbic system. After integrative processes, these again influence the hypothalamus and thus the sympathetic nervous system which transmits the information to the periphery. This means that stress and emotions, for example, also affect processes in the autonomic nervous system and therefore also in the neuroimmune system, so that the neuroimmune system can also be referred to as the "*psychoneuroimmune system.*".

3 How Do the Autonomic Nervous System and the Immune System Communicate with Each Other?

The interactions of the ANS with the immune system (and thus also inflammatory cascades) have become increasingly clear in recent years. Psyche, the somatic and the autonomic nervous system ANS, as well as the immune system, are inextricably linked in various negative [1–9] and positive [5] feedback loops. The ANS plays the main role in the coordination and control of immune processes (Fig. 16.1).

The central networks of the ANS are informed about peripheral inflammation and the state of the components of the immune system in the periphery via afferent nerve fibers (nociceptive neurons, as well as sensory nerve fibers in the sympathetic trunk and vagus nerve). In addition to this nervous information from the periphery to the brain, there is also a parallel humoral afferent information pathway. The information transmitters in this pathway are cytokines in particular. These are messenger substances that are produced by various cells such as immune cells or nerve fibers and promote the communication of immune cells with nerve cells in the regulation of inflammation. They originate from inflamed regions and from lymphoid organs.

This humoral and nervous afferent information brought from the periphery to the brain (after being processed in the brain stem and cortex, Sect. 2.3) has a significant influence on the strength of the efferent "response" that runs from the SNS, including the HPA axis, and from the vagus nerve back to the periphery. There, in turn, communication with the immune cells is "sought" [5–10].

With the help of sensory feedback processed in the brain, the ANS can not only control generalized inflammatory and immune responses via efferents, but also local inflammatory processes in the damaged tissue. The ANS can now have an activity-increasing or activity-reducing effect on the effector tissue. This simultaneously influences immune cells, inflammatory cascades, and microcirculation [5].

3.1 Bidirectional "Talk"

If the organism "demands" an immune response after a somatic or psychological trauma, an infection, etc., the nervous system and the immune system begin to "talk" to each other (Fig. 16.2). They inform each other via the aforementioned afferent and efferent pathways what "needs to be done at the moment" (e.g., more or less need for inflammatory substances in the periphery).

Efferent sympathetic nerve fibers influence mast cells, macrophages, fibrocytes, leucocytes, hematopoietic stem cells in the bone marrow, thymocytes, as well as lymphocytes in tonsils, bronchi, intestines, lymph nodes, and in the spleen [9]. Norepinephrine and other neurotransmitters of the SNS have an influence on immune cells, including T cells (cell-mediated immunity) and B cells (antibody production) [3]. Immune cells even express adrenoceptors for highly sophisticated communication [3]. Now, the SNS can very directly "command" the immune cells to produce more cytokines.

In contrast, fibers of the efferent vagus nerve inhibit the release of proinflammatory cytokines via acetylcholine receptors of the immune cells [11, 12].

This shows once again that the ANS, and thus the neuroimmune system, endeavors to keep the inflammatory response in physiological balance as far as possible with "accelerator and brake pedals."

The change in the concentration of immune and inflammatory mediators (cytokines, chemokines) is continuously registered by sensory neurons which transmit this information to the brain (Fig. 16.2). The centers of the ANS in the brain (Sects. 2.1 and 2.2) can now localize the inflammation or tissue damage in the periphery and reflexively initiate corresponding changes in the concentration of inflammatory mediators (efferents in Fig. 16.2). This precise localization would not be possible using the blood pathway alone. Inflammatory mediators such as cytokines and chemokines can therefore be described as neuromodulators [13, 14]. Interestingly, not only immune cells (macrophages, monocytes, lymphocytes, etc.) can produce cytokines, but also neurons of the central and peripheral nervous system, microglia, astrocytes, and vascular endothelial cells [15]. This opens up the possibility of integrating many systems that are positively coupled back to each other simultaneously

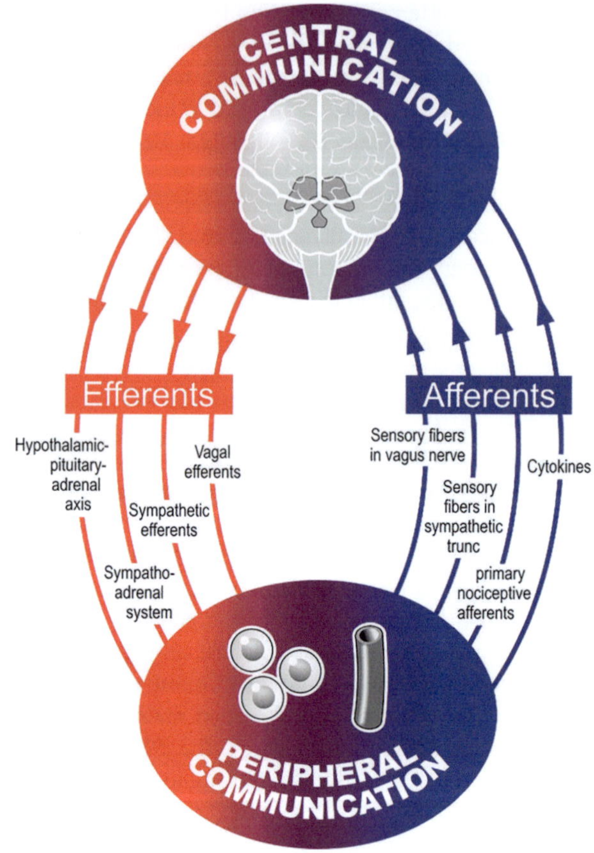

Fig. 16.2 In peripheral communication, nerve fibers, immune cells, blood vessels, and the endothelium a.o. are involved. They interact "bidirectionally" and "decide," for example, to produce a certain amount of cytokines or substance P. Their concentration is reported almost immediately via afferents to the brain, where vagal and sympathetic centers "talk" to each other and simultaneously interact with the limbic system, the hypothalamus, the pituitary gland, and the cortex. The result of this central communication is now communicated back to the periphery by means of the efferents shown (red). There, these "change requests" are fulfilled or adapted as required (peripheral communication) and immediately reported back to the brain (by means of the afferents shown in blue). Neuroimmune communication takes place both within the central nervous system and within the periphery, but also between the center and the periphery. (Modified from: Fischer L, Barop H, Ludin SM, Schaible HG: Regulation of acute reflectory hyperinflammation in viral and other diseases by means of stellate ganglion. A conceptual view with a focus on Covid-19. Autonomic Neuroscience: Basic and Clinical 237 (2022) 102903)

in the sense of an iteration [5] and can therefore communicate extremely quickly (which makes biological sense). The same applies to the fact that peripheral nerves (e.g., nociceptors) use in part the same mechanism for recognizing pathogenic molecular patterns (e.g., via toll-like receptors) as immune cells [14–16]. This also allows a very direct and immediate communication for the purpose of rapid provision of an immune response.

Many mechanisms run in parallel and simultaneously. Another example shows that during noxious stimulation (infection, trauma, toxin, etc.), nerve fibers themselves express proinflammatory neuropeptides, such as Substance P (SP) or Calcitonin Gene-Related Peptides (CGRP) [9]. However, these are also expressed by immune cells such as macrophages, lymphocytes, and mast cells [17]. This results in neurogenic inflammation with plasma extravasation and edema. Neuropeptides secreted by nerve fibers can in turn induce cytokine production in immune cells [18], thereby generating a further positive feedback loop [5].

The severity of an inflammatory disease is also closely related to the activity of sensory TRPV1-expressing neurons ("Transient Receptor Potential Channel," formerly also known as vanilloid receptor 1 or capsaicin receptor) in the sympathetic trunk and vagus nerve, as well as to the activity of sympathetic and vagal efferents in the lungs, which modulate inflammation and the immune system. All these neurons communicate with the immune system [19, 20], and when activated, they can release increased amounts of proinflammatory substances such as SP and cytokines. It is now apparent that this bidirectional communication allows the ANS and the immune system to become a functional unit.

4 Pathological Neuroimmune Communication

An adequate response of the neuroimmune system including "physiological" inflammation is protective. Interestingly, this response initially has the same nonspecific course, regardless of whether the trigger is a trauma, toxin, virus, bacterium or psychological stress, etc. [5]. In the following, we will discuss why a response of the neuroimmune system does not always involve a protective, physiological inflammation but can occur temporarily as hyperinflammation ("cytokine storm") with subsequent tissue damage. This acute form of pathological neuroimmune communication is clinically certainly most dramatic, which is why it has a special place in this contribution. The risk of acute "hyperinflammation" is increased in the case of chronic preloads (see Sect. 4.3) of the ANS which lead to an imbalance in the ANS.

Due to the chronic imbalance in the ANS and thus impaired neuroimmune communication, the immune system is weakened, which, in our opinion, also represents a risk factor for diseases such as cancer or autoimmune diseases, including neurodegenerative diseases (see Sect. 4.3).

4.1 *Imbalance in the Autonomic Nervous System (ANS) Can Lead to Acute and Chronic Inflammation*

In our opinion, a pre-existing imbalance in the ANS with dominance of the SNS plays the main role in a derailment. In general (with exceptions), a hyperactive SNS has a proinflammatory effect, while activated fibers in the vagus nerve have an anti-inflammatory effect [21]. In many acute diseases, tissue damage is caused not only by a specific agent, e.g., a virus, but also by an excessive immune response with consecutive excessive inflammation [5]. This is also referred to as *a "cytokine storm"* or *"hyperinflammation."* The much-cited "cytokine storm" is actually a consequence of a "sympathetic storm" (overview Sect. 5).

In addition to acute "hyperinflammation," the imbalance in the ANS can also lead to chronic inflammation and pain. We see this thesis confirmed by the results of our studies involving neural therapy, which in many cases works via a "reset" of the SNS [22–24].

4.2 *Clinical Consequences of Hyperinflammation*

Particularly in the early phase of hyperinflammation, life-threatening pathologies can be observed, such as *endothelial dysfunction, microcirculatory disorders,* and *coagulopathy*, which can lead to acute respiratory distress syndrome (ARDS), for example (Fig. 16.3). These pathologies are based on a pathologically increased activity of the SNS [25, 26].

We consider these consequences of hyperinflammation to be nonspecific, as they occur not only in severe courses of Covid-19, but also, for example, in influenza, severe craniocerebral trauma, autoimmune diseases in relapse, etc. [5]. The clinical and laboratory results of injections into the stellate ganglion using local anesthetics (neural therapy) are evidence of the leading role of the ANS, especially the SNS, in this hyperinflammation. This injection regulates neuroimmune communication in the brain and periphery [5], lowers proinflammatory cytokines, increases anti-inflammatory cytokines, and reduces pulmonary edema and endothelial dysfunction in general [26–31].

4.3 *Reasons for the Imbalance in the ANS as the Key to Causal Therapy*

Reasons for the imbalance in the ANS can be preloads such as psychological and emotional stress, obesity, untreated hypertension, so-called *"interference fields*"[32], *"first strike"*[33], *"shifted setpoint*"[34]. We refer to these preloads as *"neuromodulatory triggers*"[35]. The long-term therapeutic and prophylactic goal must

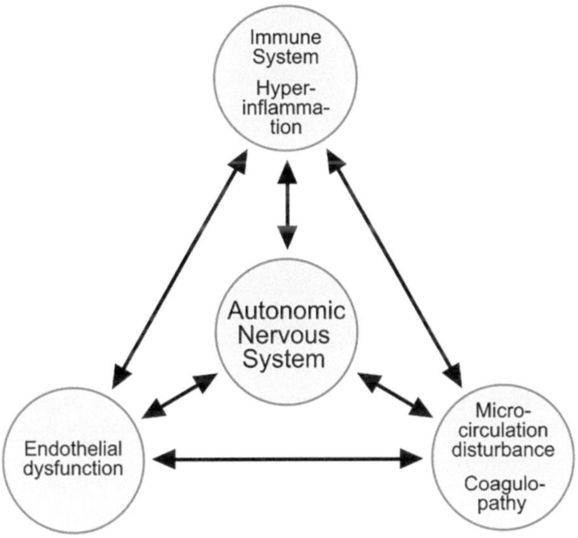

Fig. 16.3 Flow chart illustrating interactions between the hyperactive autonomic nervous system, the immune system with consecutive hyperinflammation endothelial dysfunction, and microcirculation disturbance, leading to coagulopathy. Arrows indicate the direction of influence between these components

therefore be to restore the balance between the hyperactive SNS and the vagus nerve [28]. In addition to compensatory measures that take into account the patient's life situation, this can be achieved by *injecting the stellate ganglion* with local anesthetics [5], by *stimulation of the vagus nerve* [34], or by treatment of "interference fields" (neuromodulatory triggers).

In the acute situation of "hyperinflammation" with "cytokine storm," neural therapy injections to the stellate ganglion with local anesthetics can be used, rapidly improving the inflammation and thus the clinical consequences of "hyperinflammation" [5] .

5 The Neuroimmune System: Chaotic and Holistic

5.1 *Chaotic System: Positive Feedback Loops*

In addition to the known negative feedback loops, we described several positive feedback loops that are interdependent in the neuroimmune system [5]. This makes the system holistic and highly complex. Each "part" is coupled back to the whole system [5]. The positive feedbacks (iterations) correspond in principle to *nonlinear mathematical chaos theory* described by Mandelbrot and Lorenz [36]. Such systems are very quickly adaptable. However, they are not stable and can, under certain circumstances, have a major impact even in response to minor pathological stimuli (e.g., in the neuroimmune system as a "cytokine storm"). This is particularly true if the SNS and thus the neuroimmune system is preloaded (also in line with chaos theory) [24].

5.2 Chaotic System: Self-Organization

Nonlinear (positive feedback) systems have the fundamental ability to *self-organize* in response to an internal or external stimulus. Self-organization is individual and unpredictable (indeterministic). The current state of the neuroimmune system has an influence on self-organization. In our opinion, (iterative) self-organization takes place as a constant physiological process in the neuroimmune system as a dynamic adaptation to external or internal influences. However, self-organization can also occur pathophysiologically, even as a hyperreaction (hyperinflammation) in the case of pre-existing preloads (see Sect. 4).

5.3 Chaotic System: Logical Therapeutic Implications

Thus, the analogous "ideal" therapeutic strategy in a hyperreactive, chaotic system appears to be to influence self-organization by means of preferably short-term impulses, so that it can approach a physiological balance again. This regulatory approach stands in contrast to long-term blocking in conventional medicine, which unfortunately also blocks physiological "parts" and is therefore associated with side effects. Of course, it is often not possible to do without it in practical medicine (individual consideration).

Nevertheless, neural therapy offers effective regulatory possibilities even in cases of hyperinflammation (see Sect. 4.3). After the "reset" by the local anesthetic, the neuroimmune system has the chance to reorganize itself [5]. We also see an explanation for the long-lasting effects of neural therapy in chronic inflammation or pain in this type of therapy that includes the reduction of pre-existing stresses (see Sect. 4.3) [22]. In the language of chaos theory, a better balance in the ANS creates the conditions for a better "initial state" of the neuroimmune system and leads to a more physiological self-organization. We were able to show [37] that a stellate injection not only influences the SNS, but also vagal fibers per diffusionem and via rami communicantes [37], as well as sympathetic and vagal centers in the brain. This improves the sympathetic-vagus balance, and the hyperactive immune system is measurably regulated [5]. The best possible physiological balance in a nonlinear (chaotic), holistic system is the best prerequisite for counteracting a hyperreactive derailment.

6 Conclusion

The new findings in neuroimmune communication are leading to a fundamentally new understanding of the pathophysiology of various diseases, particularly autoimmune diseases. The coordinating role of the autonomic nervous system (ANS), which is in close communication with the immune system and thus with the inflammatory cascades, is also becoming increasingly apparent. Therapy with local anesthetics (neural therapy) works to a large extent by influencing the ANS by means of "resets" which give the neuroimmune system the chance to reorganize. This is in line with a nonlinear, holistic view. The entire organism, including the psyche and emotions, is inextricably linked via the ubiquitous ANS and thus via the neuroimmune system.

References

1. Elenkov IJ, Wilder RL, Chrousos GP, Vizi ES. The sympathetic nerve—an integrative interface between two supersystems: the brain and the immune system. Pharmacol Rev. 2000;52(4):595–638.
2. Tracey KJ. The inflammatory reflex. Nature. 2002;420(6917):853–9.
3. Bellinger DL, Lorton D. Autonomic regulation of cellular immune function. Auton Neurosci. 2014;182:15–41.
4. Jänig W. Sympathetic nervous system and inflammation: a conceptual view. Auton Neurosci. 2014;182:4–14.
5. Fischer L, Barop H, Ludin SM, Schaible HG. Regulation of acute reflectory hyperinflammation in viral and other diseases by means of stellate ganglion block. A conceptual view with a focus on Covid-19. Auton Neurosci. 2022;237:102903.
6. Paton JFR, Spyer KM. Central nervous control of the cardiovascular system. In: Mathias CJ, Bannister R, editors. Autonomic failure: a textbook of clinical disorders of the autonomic nervous system. 5th ed. Oxford/New York: Oxford University Press; 2013. p. 35–51.
7. Ogundele OM, Lee CC, Francis J. Thalamic dopaminergic neurons project to the paraventricular nucleus-rostral ventrolateral medulla/C1 neural circuit. Anat Rec (Hoboken). 2017;300(7):1307–14.
8. Marvar PJ, Harrison DG. Inflammation, immunity and the autonomic nervous system. In: Robertson D, Biaggioni I, Burnstock G, Low PA, Paton JFR, editors. Primer on the autonomic nervous system. 3rd ed. London/Waltham/San Diego: Academic Press; 2012. p. 325–9.
9. Jänig W. The integrative action of the autonomic nervous system. 2nd ed. Cambridge: Cambridge University Press; 2022.
10. Kenney MJ, Ganta CK. Autonomic nervous system and immune system interactions. Compr Physiol. 2014;4(3):1177–200.
11. Ulloa L. The vagus nerve and the nicotinic anti-inflammatory pathway. Nat Rev Drug Discov. 2005;4(8):673–84.
12. Pavlov VA. Cholinergic modulation of inflammation. Int J Clin Exp Med. 2008;1(3):203–12.
13. Schaible HG. Nociceptive neurons detect cytokines in arthritis. Arthritis Res Ther. 2014;16(5):470.
14. Ji RR, Chamessian A, Zhang YQ. Pain regulation by non-neuronal cells and inflammation. Science. 2016;354(6312):572–7.
15. Galic MA, Riazi K, Pittman QJ. Cytokines and brain excitability. Front Neuroendocrinol. 2012;33(1):116–25.

16. Chiu IM, Heesters BA, Ghasemlou N, Von Hehn CA, Zhao F, Tran J, et al. Bacteria activate sensory neurons that modulate pain and inflammation. Nature. 2013;501(7465):52–7.
17. Stanisz AM. Neurogenic inflammation: role of substance P. In: Berczi I, Gorczynski RM, editors. NeuroImmune biology, Vol. 1: new foundation of biology. Amsterdam: Elsevier; 2001. p. 373–8.
18. Ansel JC, Brown JR, Payan DG, Brown MA. Substance P selectively activates TNF-alpha gene expression in murine mast cells. J Immunol. 1993;150(10):4478–85.
19. Chavan SS, Pavlov VA, Tracey KJ. Mechanisms and therapeutic relevance of neuro-immune communication. Immunity. 2017;46(6):927–42.
20. Nahama A, Ramachandran R, Cisternas AF, Ji H. The role of afferent pulmonary innervation in poor prognosis of acute respiratory distress syndrome in COVID-19 patients and proposed use of resiniferatoxin (RTX) to improve patient outcomes in advanced disease state: a review. Med Drug Discov. 2020;5:100033.
21. Schaible HG, Straub RH. Function of the sympathetic supply in acute and chronic experimental joint inflammation. Auton Neurosci. 2014;182:55–64.
22. Egli S, Pfister M, Ludin SM, Busato A, Fischer L. Long-term results of therapeutic local anesthesia (neural therapy) in 280 referred refractory chronic pain patients. BMC Complement Altern Med. 2015;15:200.
23. Fischer L. Antagonism and synergism in the autonomic nervous system—therapeutic usability. In: Thurneysen A, editor. Contrasts in medicine: the dialectics of health processes. Bern: Peter Lang; 2009.
24. Fischer L. Neural therapy. Neurophysiology, injection technique, implementation in practice. 1st ed. Stuttgart: Hippokrates; 1998. Fully revised 5th ed. Stuttgart: Thieme; 2019
25. Sheng Y, Zhu L. The crosstalk between autonomic nervous system and blood vessels. Int J Physiol Pathophysiol Pharmacol. 2018;10(1):17–28.
26. Chen YQ, Hu GX, Fu Q, Jin XJ. Effects of stellate ganglion block on blood pressure in spontaneously hypertensive rats. Zhejiang Da Xue Xue Bao Yi Xue Ban. 2012;41(1):65–8.
27. Liu MH, Tian J, Su YP, Wang T, Xiang Q, Wen L. Cervical sympathetic block regulates early systemic inflammatory response in severe trauma patients. Med Sci Monit. 2013;19:194–201.
28. Liu Y, Tao T, Li W, Bo Y. Regulating autonomic nervous system homeostasis improves pulmonary function in rabbits with acute lung injury. BMC Pulm Med. 2017;17(1):98.
29. Chen Y, Guo L, Lang H, Hu X, Jing S, Luo M, et al. Effect of a stellate ganglion block on acute lung injury in septic rats. Inflammation. 2018;41(5):1601–9.
30. Zhao HY, Yang GT, Sun NN, Kong Y, Liu YF. Efficacy and safety of stellate ganglion block in chronic ulcerative colitis. World J Gastroenterol. 2017;23(3):533–9.
31. Punj J. Multiple bilateral ultrasound-guided stellate ganglion blocks to treat acute vasculitis in a recently diagnosed patient of systemic lupus erythematosus. Indian J Anaesth. 2019;63(10):851–5.
32. Huneke F. The phenomenon in seconds according to huneke in neural therapy. Heidelberg: Haug; 1961.
33. Speranski AD. Basis for a new theory of medicine. Translated into German by Roques KR. Berlin: Sänger; 1950.
34. Tracey KJ. Reflex control of immunity. Nat Rev Immunol. 2009;9(6):418–28.
35. Engel R, Barop H, Giebel J, Ludin SM, Fischer L. The influence of modern neurophysiology on the previous definitions of "segment" and "interference field" in neural therapy. Complement Med Res. 2022;29:257–67.
36. Lorenz EN. Predictability: does the flap of a butterfly's wings in Brazil set off a tornado in Texas? American Association for the Advancement of Science 139th Meeting; 1972.
37. Puente de la Vega K, Gómez M, Roqueta C, Fischer L. Effects on hemodynamic variables and echocardiographic parameters after stellate ganglion block in 15 healthy volunteers. Auton Neurosci. 2016;197:46–55.

Chapter 17
Electromagnetism in Biological Structures: A Dimension to Take into Account in Medicine

Rodrigo Jaimes Abril

1 Electromagnetism and Biology

Bioelectric and biomagnetic phenomena are crucial to maintaining homeostasis in living organisms. For this reason, it is necessary and imperative to know, describe, quantify, and model these phenomena to establish adequate criteria for the diagnosis of the state of cells, tissues, organs, and organ systems and to propose alternative and relevant treatments to address the different pathologies that continuously occur in humans and animals.

Low-frequency (0–300 Hz) and high-frequency fields are generated in living organisms and are the basis of neuronal oscillations, circadian cycles and heart rhythms, cellular homeostasis, and the harmonious functioning of biological structures, such as in the brain and heart. Cooperative reactions of cell populations produce larger-scale fields than those generated by one or a few cells [1, 2].

Bioelectromagnetic fields (BEMF's) are produced at different scales (atomic, molecular, cellular, tissue, and organ) and are harmonized with the natural fields of the earth and the cosmos.

In general, in cells, molecules and macromolecules, tissues and organs, there is a heterogeneous distribution of electrical charges that creates Molecular Electrostatic Potentials (MEPs) and dynamic electric fields in space and time that interact in a complex way with each other and with external EMFs.

In structures such as ribonucleic acid (RNA) and deoxyribonucleic acid (DNA), MEPs can reach high values close to 1 V, which give rise to electric dipole moments that in turn generate intense electric fields around them, phenomena that make them more or less sensitive to external EMFs [1, 3].

R. Jaimes Abril (✉)
Master in Alternative Medicine, Neural Therapy Area. Faculty of Medicine, Universidad Nacional de Colombia, Bogotá, Colombia
e-mail: rjaimesa@unal.edu.co

L. B. Pinilla Bonilla et al. (eds.), *Neuraltherapeutic Medicine*,
https://doi.org/10.1007/978-3-032-03257-7_17

These may be additional reasons, to those of the spiral or coiled shape that DNA has, for which authors, such as Martin Blank, consider that DNA acts as a fractal antenna for electromagnetic fields (EMF) and radio frequency (RF) radiation, [4] Part VII.

Dielectric properties in living organisms are determined by the quantity, density, distribution, and transport of charges (positive and/or negative ions, electrons, and protons), by the electric potentials that create these charges, by the electric, magnetic, and electromagnetic fields and forces caused by the static, quasi-static, or moving position of these charges (electric current) with constant or variable speed. Likewise, the coupling of intra, extra, and intercellular signals, the transmission of electrical, chemical, and, in some cases, optical energy, which occurs constantly at the different levels of biological organization, as well as the amount of polar molecules (such as water, lipids, and tubulin) present in the different biological units or structures, are also important, among other factors [1, 3, 5].

These properties are expressed in cell membranes, organelles and cell nuclei, in the molecules and macromolecules that make up proteins, in the charge transport chains in the channels, in nucleic acids, in the cytoplasm, in the filaments and microtubules that make up the cytoskeleton, in the ion transporters and channels (from Ca^{+}, Cl^{-}, Na^{+}, K^{+}), in the pores and sodium (Na^{+}) and potassium (K^{+}) pumps found in the cell membranes of both excitable and non-excitable cells.

On a larger scale, properties are reflected, e.g., in electrical and chemical synapses, in the mechanisms of transduction and transmission of signals in the extracellular matrix or at the intracellular level, in piezoelectric effects in bones, in the movement of chromosomes during mitosis, and in the response mechanisms of cells and organisms to external stressors such as electromagnetic radiation (EMR), heat, pressure, and others.

The dielectric properties of the different functional units (membranes, proteins, organs, etc.) are described by relative permittivity ($\mathcal{E}$r) also called dielectric constant, by electrical conductivity (σ), by electrical capacity (C) also called capacitance, by magnetic permeability (μ), by membrane voltages and MEPs, by resistance (R) or impedance (Z), among other parameters. In the scientific literature on this subject, there is hardly any reference to inductance (L), a parameter that indicates the capacity to store energy in the form of a magnetic field, perhaps due to the difficulty of measuring it at molecular scales, but given the conformation of the DNA double helix and the α helices that form the polypeptides within the subunits of the proteins that cross the membrane in ion channels, it is to be expected that they have an important inductive behavior that would help to explain the response mechanisms of these structures to electrical stimuli that vary in frequency and intensity, such as EMFs.

Electric currents due to the movement of ions, electrons, and protons that originate in biological structures due to voltages and internal electric fields are another parameter to be take into account in the configuration of the electrical map of the organism or its parts. The quantum phenomenon of electron tunneling between biomolecules, synchronized with proton pumping, allows efficient transformations of energy into enzymes and other molecules [3]. Ohm's law for the electric field ($J = \sigma E$) can be applied to size them, and their direct or indirect measurement (e.g., in membrane ion channels or in the brain) accounts for their magnitudes which are usually in the range of micro, nano, or peak amperes.

Heterogeneity, related to the non-uniform distribution of electrical charges in molecules, cells and tissues, non-linearity related to the fact that the response to a stimulus is not always proportional to its intensity, and the anisotropy that has to do with the differentiated response of tissues with respect to the direction of the incident field, are common characteristics underlying these electrical and dielectric properties of tissues [6] and therefore, the classical equations governing EMF-biological matter interaction must be applied considering these properties for each biological entity.

To establish the dielectric properties of biological tissues and organs, they are considered as material with dielectric losses and magnetically transparent because the relative magnetic permeability (μ_r) is 1, i.e., it is assumed to be equal to that of vacuum [7, p. 503].

The dielectric properties of membranes as electrical capacitors are permittivity, capacity, conductivity, and capacitive reactance, all of which are described below.

In electricity, a device similar to a battery, which consists of two conductive plates between which there is a dielectric material (such as air or an insulating material or several combined) that when subjected to an electric potential difference, charges of different signs are deposited on either side, creating an electric field between the plates and storing energy in the form of electric field when they are charged, or returning that energy when discharged, it is called an electrical capacitor and its fundamental property is electrical capacity (also called capacitance).

There are parallel flat plate capacitors, cylindrical capacitors, and spherical capacitors. The earth and ionosphere make up a large spherical capacitor, and the membranes of the cells also behave as electrical capacitors with different characteristics depending on the type of cell. For example, axons, microtubules, and microfilaments can be modeled as cylindrical capacitors.

In the cell membrane, the charges are positive and negative ions of different elements, polar molecules or charged macromolecules that accumulate heterogeneously on either side of the membrane separated by the dielectric lipid bilayer creating a very intense electric field inside the membrane of the order of kV/m and even MV/m (10^7 V/m) [8] in a steady or resting state, magnitudes that are much higher than those recorded in urban environments or in the vicinity of lines, substations or high-voltage electrical machines. Membranes reach electrical potentials (or voltages) of the order of 100 mV [3, 9] on average and store energy in the form of an electric field that they give up, in part, when they are depolarized through ion channels, pores, or ion pumps.

Inside neurons, the density of magnetic field B caused by the currents of the action potentials is less than 10^{-8} T (0.01 μT) [8], which causes the earth's magnetic field, which is ≈50 μT [10], to dominate or suffocate it.

Whichever capacitor model is used to represent membranes, the capacity C depends on the geometry and is always directly proportional to the permittivity of its dielectric media (such as phospholipid layers in plasma, nucleus, mitochondria, cytosol, and microtubules.).

Table 17.1 shows membrane capacity and potential values for various classes of cells or tissues.

Permittivity indicates the polarization capacity of the polar molecules or the charged molecules that exist in the extracellular matrix, in the membranes and in the cytosol and, therefore, reflects the capacity of these structures to store energy in their electric dipoles that tend to orient themselves in the opposite direction to the incident EMF's, weakening their intensity in these structures and therefore, decreasing the electrical stress inside them. In other words, it is a measure of the bioelectrical response of tissues and organs given by the ability to provide opposition to the forces exerted by the applied external fields.

Dielectric permittivity ε_r and electrical conductivity σ in tissues and cells vary with the frequency of EMF's and with age [11]. Their variations can be observed in widely known works such as those of Gabriel [12] and Gabriel and Peyman [13], which are collected and processed in the IT'IS database [14]. In Matković's doctoral thesis [15] permittivity results are shown for brain tissues (white matter, gray matter, and cerebellum) of three species exposed to two types of commercial RF frequencies in the microwave range.

In all cases, as the frequency increases, the permittivity decreases. This means that an organ such as the brain, which has a relative permittivity of 9,190,000 at 60 Hz, 89.8 to 100 MHz and at 5 GHz has fallen to 41.1 (see the database of dielectric characteristics of the IT'IS foundation [14], at high frequencies the polarization capacity of your polar/charged molecules and cell membranes decreases when exposed to EMFs or external Electric Fields (EFs). Therefore, it stores less energy in its dipoles, making the internal electric field higher, thus allowing greater penetration of the incident electric field.

The above statement goes against what is maintained by some authors and organizations that issue non-ionizing radiation protection standards, who assign little

Table 17.1 Typical values of membrane potentials and capacitance for various cell classes

Cell or tissue class	Membrane potential [mV]	Capacity (C)
Non-proliferating cells[a]	$-50 < V < -100$	
Proliferating cells[b]	$-5 < V < -40$	
Adult stem cells	25	
Embryonic stem cells	−10	
Healthy lung, breast, and liver tumor cells		$0 < C < 140\ \mu F$[c] $20\ pF < C < 7\ nF$[d] $100\ pF < C < 7\ nF$[e]
Liver	$V < -40$	
Ribosomal outlet tunnel	$-8 < V < -22$	

Adapted from [3, 5]

[a]Of skeletal muscle, glia, neurons, fibroblasts, thyroids

[b]Thyroid and ovarian tumors

[c]Of normal and cancerous liver, lung, and breast cells in suspension

[d]Normal and cancerous liver, lung, and breast single cell

[e]Result of the interaction between both

penetration capacity into tissues at high frequencies, arguing that the energy at these high frequencies is absorbed mainly in the outer layers of the tissues. In addition, they indicate that, if it raises the temperature above the permitted levels, it would be more easily evacuated by radiation or convection mechanisms [7]. The induction of surface currents due to high-frequency EMFs is valid in materials that are good conductors of electricity, but as mentioned above, tissues are considered as dielectrics with losses and have a different behavior in the face of EMR.

On the other hand, the capacitive reactance X_c (which is the simile of the electrical resistance R of a conductive material, but in this case, represents the opposition of a capacitor to the passage of electric current), is a parameter that is also inversely proportional to frequency.[1] This variable has been little studied in biological structures and has even been very little taken into account to draw the electrical map of living organisms, especially humans. It is an indicator that justifies the increase of conductance and therefore of the current at high frequencies and the alteration of cellullar metabolism due to the entry or exit of ions to or from the cytosol in an abnormal way by the continuous or sporadic stress suffered by the cell due to exposure to artificial EMFs.

Similarly, it could be hypothesized about the inductive reactance X_L that the ion channels and pumps of the membrane may contain due to the spiral or α helix configuration that the polypeptides of the different protein subunits have when they cross it, in the DNA and in the microtubules and microfilaments that make up the cytoskeleton, among others (see configurations of these structures in [3, 16, 17]).

The X_L[2] has a behavior similar to that of the electrical resistance R of a conductive material, but this time it refers to the opposition to the current that would be presented by coiled structures such as those mentioned. As can be inferred from its equation, as the frequency increases, so does the X_L "Resistance,"which would imply that, exposed to high frequencies, ionic currents in the membrane channels or in microtubules and microfilaments would have more difficulty moving inside them. This would affect the conduction velocity of electrical signals, depending on whether this parameter takes precedence over the capacitive reactance, a little studied aspect, but it seems that the capacitive effect on membranes is stronger than the inductive one, at least at low frequencies.

Figure 17.1 shows characteristic values of some electrical parameters of the cells.

Considering capacitance C, capacitive reactance X_c, inductance L, and inductive reactance X_L to establish electrical models that explain the electromagnetic (EM) behavior of cells and tissues in the face of EMR is important and necessary to interpret the biological and health effects reported in the scientific literature and to apply

[1] For a parallel flat plate capacitor, $Xc = 1/2\ \pi f\ C$, where C is the capacitance and f the frequency, a ratio from which it can be inferred that it decreases with increasing frequency indicating that there will be greater conduction or displacement current through the ion channels or even through the lipid bilayer itself due to exposure to high frequencies rather than to low frequencies.

[2] For an electrical conductor (coiled) it is described by the equation $X_L = 2\ \pi f\ L$, where L is the inductance, which depends on its geometry and the magnetic permeability which is 1 in this case.

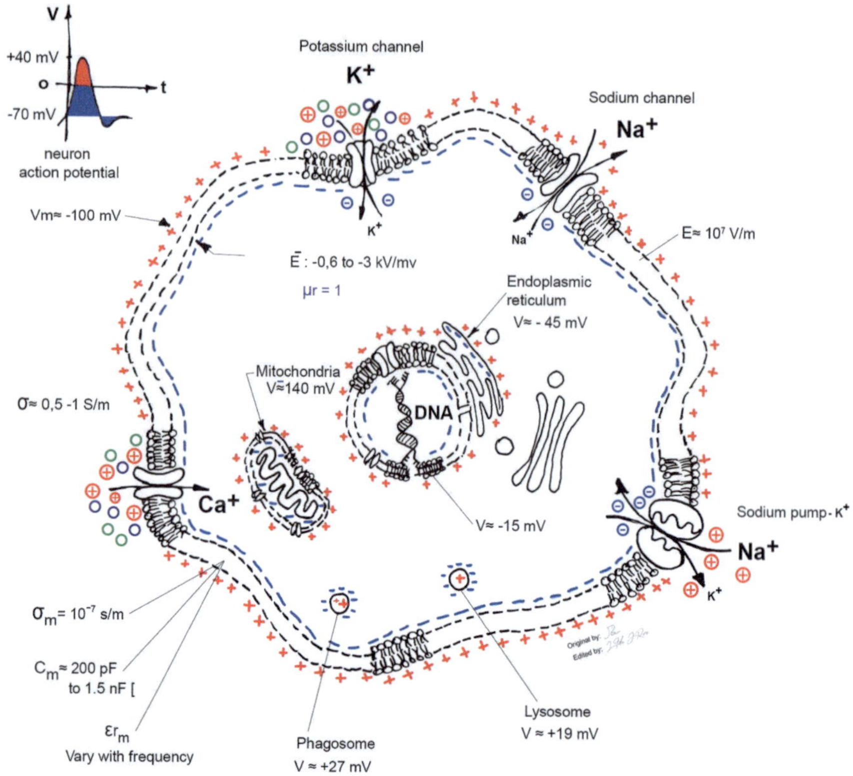

Fig. 17.1 Diagram of a cell membrane illustrating ion channels and organelles. Key features include potassium (K^+) and sodium (Na^+) channels, calcium (Ca^+) channel, and sodium pump. Organelles such as mitochondria, endoplasmic reticulum, and lysosome are labeled with their respective voltages. The diagram also shows neuron action potential with a graph indicating voltage changes over time. Various electrical properties and symbols are annotated, including electric field (E) in units of V/m ó kV/m, permeability (μr), and conductivity (σ) in units of S/m. The cell's DNA is centrally located. (Adapted from [3, 5, 18, 19])

this knowledge in the development of technologies for treatment, diagnosis, and prevention of diseases.

Some electrical models of the cell have been reported that combine capacities and inductances in parallel and resistors placed in series or in parallel with these elements [20–22]. These equivalent circuits are used to represent the electrical behavior of cells in a steady or rest state or in a transient state (response to some external stimulus), and must account for the phenomenon of resonance in them since they are electrical circuits very similar to those used to tune radio and TV frequencies in electronic equipment.

Thus, at certain frequencies the capacitive component may predominate and at others, the inductive component, and in the resonance condition, their reactances have equal weight. Memristors, which are newly discovered elements that must be taken into account in the circuits used to model biological units and which better explain their nonlinear behaviors in front of the EMRs, are mentioned later on. L and X_L parameters have not been taken into account in this study.

Al Ahmad et al., [5] found that healthy cells (lung, breast, and liver) in *in vitro* suspensions have higher permitivities and capacities than cancer cells of the same tissue type measured at frequencies between 0.1 and 10 kHz that are extremely low (ELF), indicating a greater capacity to store energy in the form of an electric field than their affected counterparts in that frequency range. Similar results were obtained for capacitances per cell measured at frequencies between 0.1 and 100 Hz. The interaction between both types of cells raised the C capacity of the set.

In contrast to the previous results, Hessinger et al., [23] analyzed several samples of liver cancerous tissue compared to healthy tissue exposed to point frequencies of 2.45 and 5.8 GHz and to a wide range of frequencies up to 26 GHz, reporting that the former have higher dielectric permittivity (real and complex) than healthy tissues in percentages ranging from approximately 20–60%. The explanation given for this parameter being higher in cancerous tissues than in healthy tissues is the higher sodium and water content of tumor cells and the dipole relaxation process that occurs at certain frequencies.

Electrical conductivity σ has a behavior contrary to permittivity in relation to frequency. As the frequency increases, the conductivity also increases indicating that there will be a greater movement of free charges such as ions (conduction current) and more rotation or vibration of the electric dipoles of polar molecules such as water or of charged macromolecules (displacement current) caused by the forces of the secondary electric field induced by the incident radiation. However, it is necessary to take into account the relaxation mechanisms that occur at certain frequencies that affect this parameter.

Thus, e.g., the conductivity of the brain goes from 0.1 S/m at 60 Hz to 4.19 S/m at 5 GHz (see the database of dielectric characteristics of the IT'IS foundation [14] indicating that there will be greater induced current and, therefore, a higher absorption of energy in the form of a magnetic field in this organ due to exposure to high frequencies.

Furthermore, analyzing the dielectric characteristics of drugs used in Neuraltherapeutic medicine and in other fields of medicine is relevant and necessary to evaluate their biocompatibility from the electromagnetic point of view (BEMC) and interpret their efficacy in treatments. This is the case of Procaine (also known as Novocaine) in percentages of 0.5% and 1% combined with Epinephrine, Bicarbonate, and Calcium, a compound with unique pharmacological effects proven by a rapid response from the body after its application.

Román, Jaimes and Osorio[3] studied the dielectric behavior of procaine in four different solutions based on the measurements of permittivity ($\mathcal{E}$r), capacity (C),

---

[3]Roman F, Jaimes R, Osorio Y. (2003). Acercamiento al comportamiento dieléctrico de la procaína y sus soluciones. Análisis de permitividad dieléctrica con la frecuencia. These results were never published but were presented at the 2003 World Meeting of Neural Therapy carried out in Bogotá, Colombia. See: https://www.terapianeural.com/congresos/46-congresos/109-colombia-2003-congreso-internacional-de-terapia-neural-resumenes

delta tangent (tg δ), quality factor (QF), and impedance (Z) and its variation with frequency under voltage and frequency conditions similar to those in the extracellular matrix. The results were surprising in terms of the high permittivity values found in all the solutions analyzed (between 4×10^6 and 12×10^6) and good quality factor, which characterizes them as excellent dielectric or insulating substances.

In this research, it was verified that all the parameters mentioned vary with frequency and with the voltage applied. Thus, εr, C, and Z decreased with increasing frequency, but at a voltage higher than 100 mV, the compounds lost their characteristics and became conductive, indicating a high susceptibility to electrical stress versus a good ability to store energy in their electric dipoles under normal physiological conditions. This gives rise to a deeper study of the electrical properties of drugs used in alternative medicine and conventional medicine and to hypothesize the mechanisms of action of procaine in the plasma membrane and at subcellular level.

Of particular interest from an electrical point of view are the microtubules (MTs) with their electrical potentials along them, their dynamics of electrical charge propagation in and out of the microtubule as ionic waves and with their electron hopping along tubulin monomers. These characteristics make them an electrical signal transport network between the cell membrane and the nucleus, enabling subcellular bioelectrical information processes typical of certain types of learning and memory, and they also play an important role in intercellular communication (e.g., in the brain) along with the actin filaments and microfilaments that make up the cytoskeleton [3, 24, 25].

Microtubules (MTs) are attributed key funtions in cell division and motility, intracellular transport and signals conduction in neurons, among others [24]. These authors propose, on a theoretical and experimental basis, that MTs behave like Memristors[4] which are one of the four fundamental elements of electrical circuits (the other 3 are resistors, capacitors, and inductances).

Perhaps because they are such recent elements and not fully developed, Memristors have not been taken into account in the analyses and models of electrical circuits used in engineering. At the biological level, these Memristors have been considered to explain and simulate several significant characteristics, given their ability to store a large volume of information and retain the memory of the history of the applied voltage and/or injected current, as well as the electric charge that has passed through it, related to the magnetic flux it creates.

In other words, memristors are non-volatile memory resistors and also exhibit capacitive and inductive properties that serve to hypothesize and investigate memory processes in cells, tissues, and organs such as the brain [24, 26]. An application of memristors to model the electrical properties of the skin was carried out by [27], in which it was demostrated that this element is able to simulate the observed

[4] Created in 1971 by Leon Chua, but its physical construction was only achieved until 2008 by Stanley Williams of Hewlett-Packard laboratories. [26]

nonlinearities and better describe the physics of skin capillaries, in a more precise way than if it had been done only with classical RLC circuits.

MTs have natural resonance at 8085 MHz [25], and experiments conducted by Bandyopadhyay (2010, 2011) mentioned in [25] show that there are resonances in conductivity in the 10 MHz range leading to electron transport in MTs using their quantum-mechanical properties. MTs have a high-frequency ε_r of 8.41 and a high-frequency polarizability of 2.1×10^{-33} C m^2/V (Mershin et al. 2006, mentioned in [25]) based on the crystal structure of tubulin.

The resonance between interacting biological macromolecules is crucial for their biological function, which is characterized by a specific frequency or wavelength for each function/interaction [17].

Figure 17.2 illustrates a proposed simplified view of the configuration of the electric field force lines distributed within an excitable eukaryotic cell in a resting

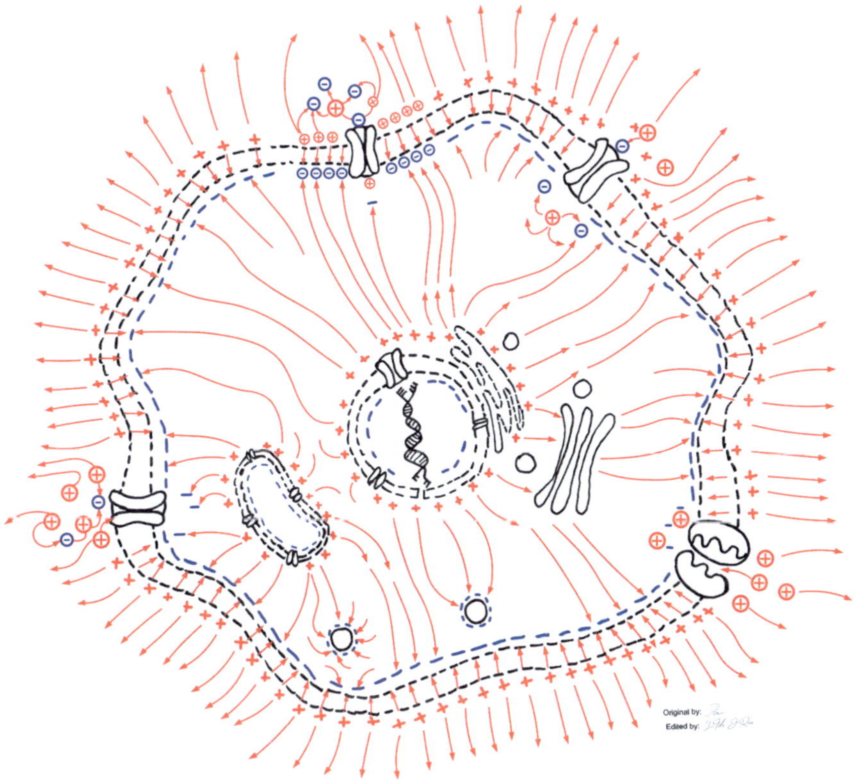

Fig. 17.2 Diagram of a eukaryotic cell showing various organelles and structures. The cell membrane is depicted with embedded proteins and ion channels. Red arrows indicate electric field lines of force acting on electrically charged particles, such as positive and negative ions, marked with red or blue circles and positive or negative signs, respectively. Key organelles like the nucleus, mitochondria, and endoplasmic reticulum are outlined. The nucleus contains a DNA helix. The diagram illustrates a simplified configuration of electric field distributed inside and outside an excitable eukaryotic cell in a resting state

state. These lines of force are directed from positive to negative charges, and any other charge (ions, electrons, or protons) is bound to be attracted or repelled by the electrostatic forces exerted in these force fields.

In general, the plasma membrane and the membranes of the organelles and the nucleus present high electric field strengths due to their thin thickness (on the order of 5–10 nm) and relatively high voltage (100 mV on average).

Currently, living beings are exposed daily, and usually simultaneously to different types of EMR, which, depending on their location with respect to the exposed subjects, constitute far-field exposures, as in the case of communications towers, radio and TV antennas, radars, transmission lines and distribution of electrical energy, etc. and near field, in cases of exposure to cell phones, modems, Bluetooth, and WiFi that are in close proximity to people.

Some sources emit transverse polarized plane waves characterized by the electric field E and the magnetic field B being uniform on flat surfaces, are in phase (i.e., reach their maximum and minimum points at the same time), are perpendicular to each other, and travel in a direction perpendicular to them. All types of low or high frequency EMFs carry energy through space and transfer all or part of it to subjects exposed to such fields by exerting radiation pressure on charged particles due to the momentum (the amount of motion) they carry [28]. The waves emitted by cell phone antennas and wireless mobile devices are more complex than uniform plane waves and are characterized below.

The set of diagrams in Fig. 17.3 shows the effects on the electric field configutation of the cells by far field and near field exposure to uniform plane waves.

EMFs exert forces on electrically charged particles that are in motion, which can be calculated with the Lorentz formula or also called the Lorentz Force. This equation states that the total force on the charged particle is the vector sum of the strength

Fig. 17.3 The image is a figure composed of three panels labeled a, b, and c. Panel a shows a graph with voltage (V) on the y-axis and time (t) on the x-axis, depicting two uniform plane wave waveforms labeled E (electric field) and B (magnetic field) emitted by an EMF source from ELF or RF radiation antennas. Depending on the intensity and frequency of these EMFs, the exposure of the cell to this type of EMF can induce forced oscillations in the ions and polar or electrically charged molecules near the ion channels or voltage-dependent channels, affecting their functioning, in addition to inducing voltages, currents, and electric fields in tissues and organisms as will be seen below. Panel b includes a graph with a negative waveform and an illustration of a cell with an electric field source labeled "Electric field source with negative electric charge." The effect of exposing a cell to the negative cycle of a wave that favors the process of hyperpolarization of the membranes due to the electrostatic forces that attract positive ions away from the membranes and repulsive forces on negative ions that push them away limiting the circulation of ions through ion channels. The cell components, such as the nucleus and mitochondria, are labeled, with red arrows indicating the direction of the electric field. Panel c features a similar cell illustration with a "Electric field source with positive electric charge,". The situation of exposing cell to the positive cycle of a uniform plane wave tends to depolarize the membrane due to the electrostatic forces that exert repulsion on the positive ions outside the membranes and the attractive forces of the negative ions making it easier for ions to flow through ion channels, which favors membrane depolarization of the electric field and the magnetic field ($F = q(v \, X \, B + E)$). In the case of ions and polar molecules or electrically charged molecules such as proteins in membranes, they not only respond to external electric and magnetic fields but also generate their own fields. In addition, they are also subject to nuclear forces and the force of gravity, which is why, to determine the integral, temporal, and spatial response, it is also necessary to consider Maxwell's equations, transport equations (such as Boltzmann's

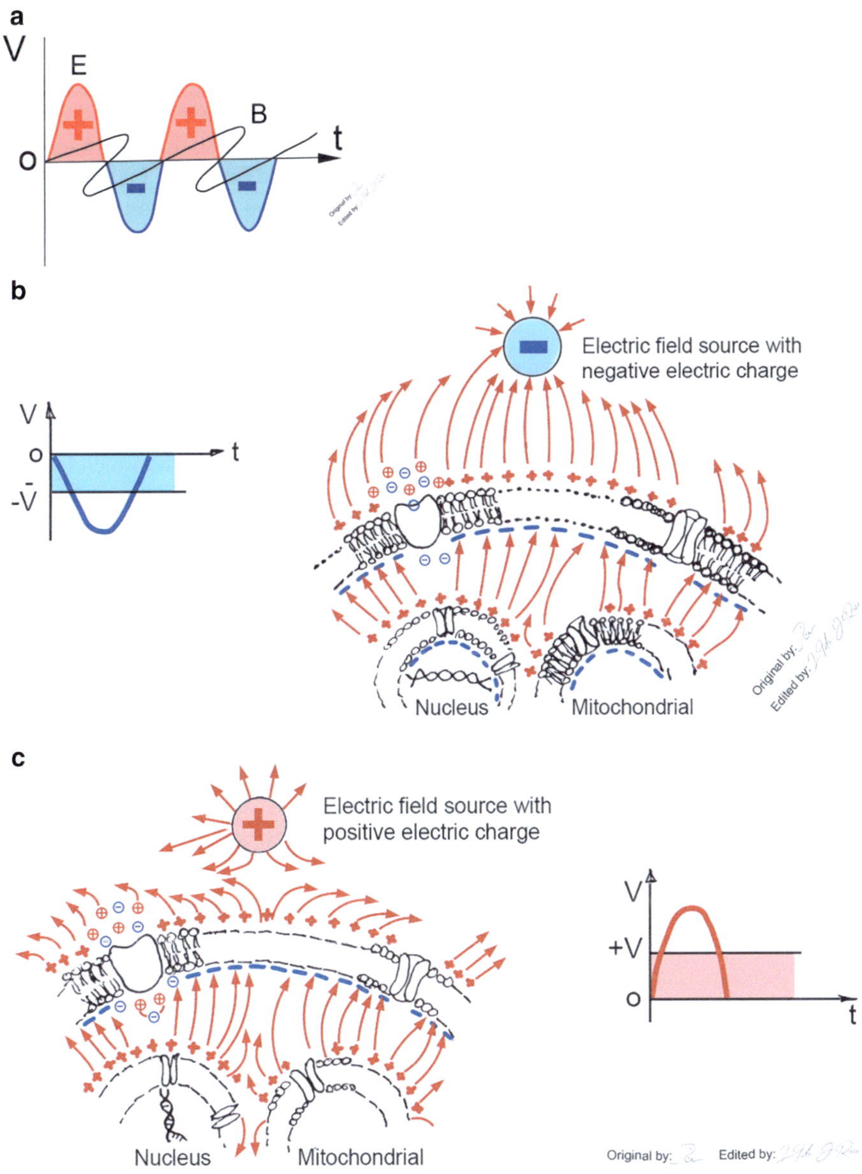

equation) and related equations in the areas of electrodynamics and magnetohydrodynamics, together with energy considerations, all of which is complex.

In Appendix, the equations for the calculation of the electrical, magnetic forces, and the electric and magnetic torques, and others related to the parameters discussed in this work, are given.

In this chapter, the question is raise as to why steady-state cells[5] potentials always tend to be negative, due to the higher concentrations of positive ions (mainly Na^+) on the outside of healthy cell membranes than on the inner side corresponding to the cytosol barrier? What main force drives ion conformations so that they always tend to create negative potentials in cell membranes and in the membranes of the organelles and the nucleus?

To answer this question, it is proposed that the natural electric field of the earth is the main cause of the resting potential of cells being negative, due to the mechanism of interfacial polarization or dipole polarization that occurs at these Extreme Low Frequencies (ELF from 0 to 300 Hz), an explanation that is complementary and coherent to that related to the mechanisms of ion diffusion, which prevails in the books and articles that deal with the subject as e.g., in 16.

Figure 17.4 illustrates a general configuration of the natural electric field (ionosphere-earth) and its EM action on the charges (ions) of the cell membrane that inducing the electrical membrane potential (voltage) o a cell.

When the intensity of the cloud-to-ground electric field reaches the values shown in the figure, the air does not resist this electric force and becomes conductive, generating atmospheric electrical discharges that carry high currents from the cloud to the earth or vice versa or between the clouds, causing high magnetic fields of a transient nature that are the cause of the so-called Schumann resonances. These resonances have an average frequency of 7.8 Hz [10] and have peaks in the frequencies of 8, 14, 21 Hz, etc. [30]. Important properties in the regulation of many biological functions and rhythms are attributed to these resonances.

The natural electric field, the natural magnetic field and the temperature caused by solar radiation, among other factors, cause ions pairs and ionic current densities to form in the atmosphere in the magnitudes indicated in Fig. 17.4 and permanent ionic currents and other charged particles that exist between the earth and the ionosphere which constitute the so-called global electrical circuit. [31]

It also alludes to the density of the earth's magnetic field, whose continuous lines of force go from the positive magnetic pole (which is located at the geographic south pole) to the negative pole (geographic north pole) and have values that vary geographically and daily depending on their interaction with the magnetic field of the sun and the radiations coming from it and from all parts of the universe. This magnetic field represents a protection for living beings since it traps most of the high-energy particles mentioned. In the tropics, the magnetic field density is on the

[5] When its dielectric properties do not vary over time. It corresponds to the resting potential in excitable cells (such as neurons) and the normal membrane potential in other cell types.

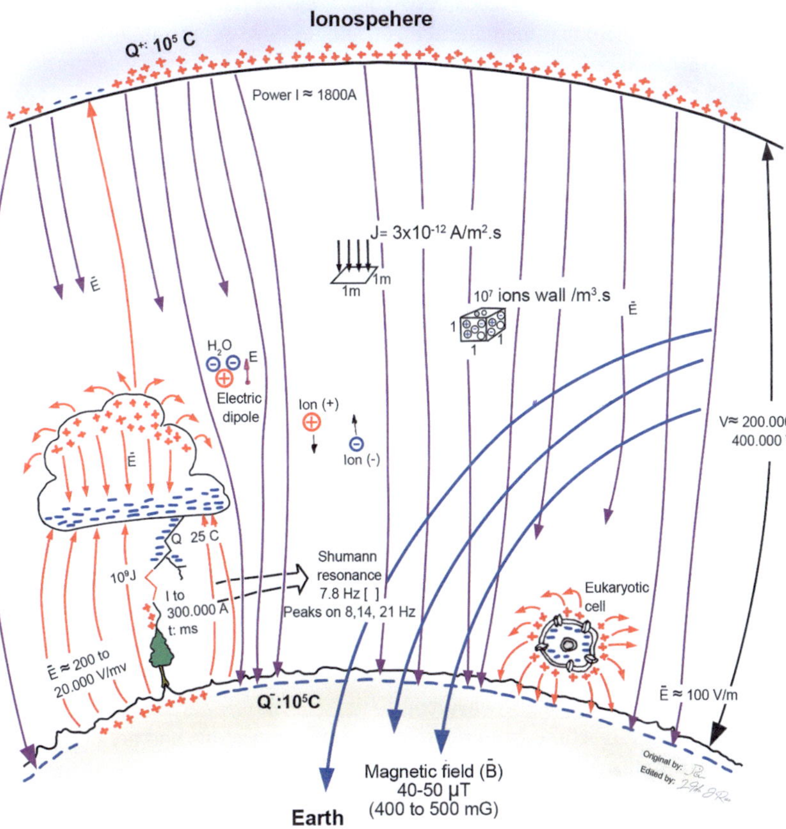

Fig. 17.4 Diagram illustrating the configuration of the earth's natural electric field directed from the ionosphere (positively charged) to the earth (negatively charged) and its action on electric charges, polar molecules and on the determination of membrane potentials of eukaryotic cells located near the Earth's surface. The electric field generated by storm clouds (such as cumulus-nimbus) that are negatively charged at the bottom and positively charged at the top is also shown generating a electric field of opposite polarity and more intense than that of the ionosphere-earth. A water molecule as an electric dipole, some positive and negative ions, and a eukaryotic cell are also shown with their respective electric fields aligned with the natural ionosphere-Earth electric field. The total electric current in amperes flowing from the ionosphere to the Earth, the surface current density per square meter per second (j), and the number of ion pairs per cubic meter per second that normally flow in the atmosphere are Also indicated. The lines with red or purple arrows indicate the lines of force of the electric field and the lines with blue arrows indicate the magnetic field density in μT in at Earth's surface. Schumann resonance frequencies are noted at 7.8 Hz with peaks at 8, 14, and 21 Hz. The units of the electric field E are given in V/m. (The values shown have been taken mainly from [29])

order of 50 μT (equivalent to 500 mG), but in general, the magnetic field density at the earth's surface can have values between 25 and 70 μT [10].

The magnetic field and the natural electric field have extremely low frequencies, and their variation between day and night is also low.

The electrical potential between the ionosphere and the earth varies between 200,000 V [10] and 400,000 V [29]. On a sunny day, the electric field near the earth's surface ranges between 100 and 500 V/m, but before a storm, it can reach values between 2000 and 20,000 V/m.

Other high-frequency radiations in the infrared spectrum, visible light, ultraviolet, γ, β rays, etc., are also part of the natural EM environment, but their characteristics are different from artificially created EM radiation by man and, therefore, their effects on biology and health are different.

Panagoupolos et al. [32, 33], establish the main differences between natural EMFs and man-made (artificial) non ionizing radiation NIR EMFs, which lie in the fact that the latter are polarized, pulsating and modulated, i.e., in addition to the high frequencies carrying information that are in the microwave range, there are ELF, ultra low frequency (ULF) and very low frequency (VLF) signals (between 0 and 30 kHz) that modulate their amplitude and contribute to establishing the so-called uplink and downlink links and have variability in time and frequency. This makes these radiations more bioactive than natural fields, although they do not induce significant heating in the tissues because they are low-intensity radiation.

The power radiated by broadcast (amplitude or frequency-modulated) and television transmitters is higher than that of cellular telephone base stations, but they use lower frequencies with longer wavelengths.

Natural radiations come from photon or atomic emissions and are not polarized, pulsating, or modulated, nor do they exhibit high variability like fields created by man-made circuits and antennas [32, 33].

A synthesis of the main features of the Earth's natural electromagnetic environment can be found in [10, 29, 30].

These natural electromagnetic conditions shaped and sustain life on the planet and affect the EM configuration of structures such as cells. In Fig. 17.4, the size of the cell has been exaggerated to see how the earth (which is negatively charged on its surface) attracks positive ions that are positioned outside the membrane and repels negative ions that are located inside the membrane, which induces the negative potentials that are always found in the membranes of all cells and the membranes of their organelles and the nucleus.

It is a cascade effect caused by the forces of the natural electric field which, because it is ELF and has relatively long periods (of the order of 100 ms), makes the ions have time to position and accumulate at the interfaces of the membranes and establish the aforementioned potentials, due to the mechanisms of interfacial and dipole polarization and the α and β relaxation zones that occur at low frequencies mainly. A detailed explanation of these polarization and relaxation mechanisms can be found in [9, 15].

2 Electromagnetism and Health

Living organisms have been born, grown, and evolved under the influence of natural forces incluiding the Earth's electric field which exists between the ionosphere and the Earth's surface and the Earth's magnetic field characterized by the Van Allen belts. Additionally, they are influenced by electromagnetic radiation (EMR) that comes from the sun and various parts of the universe.

However, since the discovery of electricity and with the evolution of electronics, communications, computing and information technology, large and small systems and devices for the generation, transmission, distribution and consumption of electrical energy have been designed, built and installed and wireless communication systems have been implemented using increasingly high frequencies and a diverse range of antennas and electronic equipment that generate and/or capture EMF's of which have strongly altered the natural electromagnetic environment.

In particular, since the last decade of the twentieth century, communication systems classified as CDMA, 1G, 2G, 3G (corresponding to the GSM system[6]), 4G (UMTS[7]), 5G, 6G, WiFi[8] and Bluetooth, Radars, low Earth orbit (LEO), geostationary orbit (GEO), and medium earth orbit (MEO) satellite technologies (network satellites that are used for communications and positioning at a global level) have been deployed exponentially, in all parts of the world. These communication systems are present in almost all rural and urban environments and form an increasingly dense network of artificial EMFs that are superimposed on natural fields.

On average, every 10 years there has been a change in wireless communication technologies in the world, a very short time to evaluate their impacts on biology and health, but in most countries, old and new systems and technologies coexist, intensifying electromagnetic pollution.

The Internet of Things (IoT) and artificial intelligence (AI) require these high-frequency communication systems (VHF, UHF, SHF, and EHF)[9] to increase the speed and amount of data transmitted, decrease latency times, and expand coverage. The trend is to raise the frequency significantly, reduce the radiation power of the modules (equipment and antennas) and increase their efficiency through technologies such as MIMO (Multiple Inputs, Multiple Outputs) antennas that do not irradiate the fields over wide areas, but focus the radiation beams or lobes to the sites where communication is established, concentrating power in those areas.

An emerging problem is that, in order to obtain the same or greater coverage of the service, it is necessary to considerably increase the number of base stations that will be closer to people, and, therefore, the energy demand will grow significantly

---

[6] Global System of Mobile Communication.

[7] Universal Mobile Telecommunication System.

[8] Wireless Fidelity.

[9] Very High Frequency, Ultra High Frequency, Super High Frequency and Extra High Frequency. See the electromagnetic spectrum.

in all parts of the world as well as the level of exposure of living beings to the fields produced by these devices and antennas.

However, the benefits widely recognized by society in general that these technical and technological developments have brought and that have allowed the innovation of sophisticated equipment, systems and apparatus for industry, commerce, transport, homes and in the medical field for the diagnosis and treatment of diseases, have also caused a very significant increase in potential risks for living beings in general and for health, in particular, caused by the exposure of people to the EMF's they generate.

The following are the most prominent biological and health effects reported in the scientific literature.

3 Biological and Health Effects of Extremely Low Frequency and Radio Frequency Electromagnetic Fields

Over the course of this century, extensive scientific knowledge has accumulated, indicating that there are fully identified and proven biological effects that occur at levels of exposure to EMFs and RF radiation (called low-intensity or non-thermal levels) well below the exposure limits established in the standards, some of which have health effects.

The following groups and projects publish the results of numerous studies on the effects of Non-Ionizing Radiation (RNI), most of which confirm a high effect/non-effect ratio:

- Bioiniciative [34].
- INTERPHONE [35].
- The World Health Organization's Electromagnetic Fields Project [36].
- La International Agency for Research on Cancer—IARC [37].
- La ICNIRP [38].
- The International Radiation Protection Association (IRPA)
- CERENAT.
- COSMOS study.
- La International School of Bioelectromagnetism "Alessandro Chiabrera".
- The group of scientists EMFscientist.org [39] calling for greater protection of the population from EMF exposure.
- The BioElectromagnetic Society BioEm [40] which merged the European Bioelectromagnetics Association (EBEA) and the American Bioelectromagnetic Society (BEMS) and has the official journal *Bioelectromagnetics*.
- The Inter-American Commission on Radiological Protection of Electromagnetic Fields CIPRACEM of Argentina and the SSM's Scientific Council on Electromagnetic Fields, advisory body of the Swedish Radiation Safety Authority [44, 45].

A broad and detailed list of the biological and health effects caused by exposure to man-made EMFs in the spectrum of Non-Ionizing Electromagnetic Radiation (NIR) including results of *in vivo* and *in vitro* experimental studies and epidemiological investigations have been reported [2, 4, 7, 33, 41, 43, 45, 46].

More recent reviews of the scientific literature on the biological and health effects of NIRs in humans, animals, and cells were conducted by [46, 47], who synthesized the results of several studies. The frequency ranges of the NIR analyzed were those of the sources commonly found in the environment, such as those of 50–60 Hz and the fields of wireless communication systems in the commercial bands of 3G and 4G, mainly.

Apollonio et al., [2] propose a multiscale methodology to model the interaction between exogenous EMFs and biological systems considering non-thermal mechanisms, starting at the atomic and molecular scale where EMFs can alter charge distributions, chemical states or energy levels and then, at subsequent scales, these changes can be detected and amplified to produce responses that could have consequences for the organism. This methodology, based on biophysics, complements the analyses of dosimetry-based models. This paper also makes a systematic review of several models proposed by other researchers.

Among the most outstanding short-, medium, and long-term effects contained in the aforementioned references are:

- Effects on gene and protein expression.
- Genotoxic effects. DNA alteration.
- Stress response of cells. Generation of heat shock proteins as a response mechanism. Oxidative stress through the action of free radicals.
- Effects on immune system function. Inflammatory and allergic reactions.
- Effects on neurology, behavior, memory, sleep, concentration, and learning. Headaches.
- Effects on the blood-brain barrier.
- Carcinogenic effects. Brain tumors, acoustic neuromas, glioma, meningioma, childhood leukemia, and breast cancer.
- Effects on melatonin production. Alzheimer's disease.
- Disruption in signal modulation at the cellular level.
- Effects on fertility and reproduction. Alteration of the quality and quantity of human sperm.
- Effects on fetuses and neonates.
- Effects on cell cycling, differentiation, proliferation, and apoptosis and on calcium metabolism.
- Effects on heart rhythm.
- Hypersensitivity to artificial EMFs.

It should be noted that, for some bodies in charge of establishing standards or guidelines for protection against exposure to NIR, such as ICNIRP, there are gaps in knowledge in areas such as the pain threshold and increases in body temperature and health effects from heating caused by RF EMFs, pain caused by contact currents, threshold of adverse effects due to thermal dosimetry on ocular structures and others. These should be investigated or deepened so that they are considered adequate evidence to establish thresholds for the appearance of health effects and establish appropriate exposure restrictions [48].

Furthermore, it is argued that the lack of clarity about the mechanisms of interaction Fields-Biological Structures that explain the reported effects, the insufficiency of evidence, the uncertainty in the dosimetry used, among other reasons, are arguments for not considering the results of many studies carried out and relevant in the development of the guidelines [48].

Among the immediate or very short-term effects produced by low-frequency or high-frequency EMFs are: the induction of voltages, fields, and electric currents of the same frequency as that of the incident field [6], interfacial, dipolar, atomic (also called ionic), or electronic electrical polarization phenomena may occur at the cellular level, molecular or atomic. Magnetic polarization phenomena and vibration or forced rotation of atoms and molecules can also occur, depending on the intensity and frequency of the applied fields and the conditions of the structural and functional units of the organism. A clear explanation of the mechanisms of polarization and relaxation processes ($\alpha, \beta, \delta, \gamma$) that occur in dielectric materials such as biological tissues, is found in the theses of Matković [15] and Sanchis [9].

Depending on the intensity of the above parameters and the exposure time, an increase in the absorption specific rate (SAR)[10,11] and temperature in tissues may occur when there is exposure to radiofrequency (RF) electromagnetic fields [49]. In fact, the two previous variables, together with the incident power density and the incident electric and magnetic field strengths, are the main variables taken into account by international organizations such as ICNIRP and IEEE to establish standards or guidelines that limit occupational or non-occupational exposure to artificial EMFs.

On the other hand, pulsed electromagnetic fields (PEMF) and/or amplitude or frequency modulated EMFs (such as those used in wireless communications) are known to be more bioactive than continuous or non-pulsed fields [50], hence they are widely studied to establish their negative effects on health or their therapeutic benefits at certain levels and frequencies.

It should be remembered that wireless communications systems such as 4G and 5G emit and receive signals (EMF) that not only correspond to the frequencies that carry the information such as microwaves but also involve low-frequency signals (modulators) that have a greater capacity to penetrate organisms [33]. Therefore, in the evaluation of the results of in vivo or in vitro experimental investigations that only take into account one type of frequency, the non-consideration of combined frequencies can lead to bias.

---

[10] Specific absorption rate (SAR)**:** Indicates the amount of energy absorbed in the unit of time per unit of mass. It is usually expressed in [W/kg] and is a fundamental dosimetric amount established in international guidelines and standards governing EMF exposure between 100 and 300 GHz.

[11] It is also defined as the amount of power absorbed from non-ionizing radiation (or amount of energy absorbed in the unit of time) per unit mass of a biological tissue and is evaluated on an average mass of 10 or 1 g. SAR is expressed in Watts per kilogram [W/kg]. [51–53, 66, p. 1222].

EMR fields impinging on biological structures can produce interference that amplifies or reduces their intensities at some points (called constructive or destructive interference) and induce parallel and coherent forced oscillations of polar molecules and charged molecules, especially mobile ions, in living cells and tissues, which can trigger biological effects [33].

The superposition of several EMFs that are linearly polarized and phase different (i.e., their maximum or minimum amplitudes do not coincide in time) can result in circularly or elliptically polarized EMFs, as is the case with the electric and magnetic fields of three-phase electric power transmission or distribution lines of 50 or 60 Hz.

The effects of interference and superposition of different fields with different frequencies and intensities occur in a combined exposure situation, which is the most common in all areas, causing their characteristics to change in time and space, creating transient peaks (hot spots) in the intensities of the EMFs that configure a complex and permanently dynamic exposure condition [32, 33].

The superposition can be of electric, magnetic, or EM field strengths or of wave intensities (i.e., powers, defined by the Poynting vector). In natural EMFs that come from different sources and are not polarized, the field strengths and strengths are added together and remain constant, but do not produce forced oscillations in critical biomolecules, although if the sources are many, the average field strength tends to be zero [32, 33].

Although natural EMFs typically have significantly higher intensities and energies of longer duration than non-ionizing artificial EMFs, the latter induce forced, coherent oscillations (motion in the same direction) in phase and in parallel planes with the polarized field applied in all charged polar molecules (such as water), and especially, in the free ions in and around all cells. These, in turn, exert higher resulting electrostatic forces on the sensors of the electrosensitive ion channels of the cell membrane than the mutual extinction forces on the same sensors due to their random thermal movements in all possible directions, activating them irregularly and thereby altering the electrochemical balance of the cell and generating biological effects [54].

It is these oscillations of the ions near the domains of the molecules that make up the electrosensitive ion channels of the membrane that cause them to open or close, altering the ionic configuration within the channel and not the incident electric field, since a very high field strength (in the order of 10^6 to 10^7 V/m, similar to that of the membrane electric field at rest) which is difficult to achieve under normal conditions of exposure to ELF and RF field strengths found in the environment [32, 55, 56].

At the molecular level, EMFs can produce conformational changes in proteins, leading to modulating biological processes [1]. Figure 17.5 shows a simplified scheme of near and far EMF waves radiated by a cell phone, by a base station and by a power line impacting a person.

At cellular level, EMFs are able to activate voltage-gated calcium channels, which open in response to changes in the electrical potential of the cell membrane, resulting in abnormal amounts of intracellular calcium ions [1, 57].

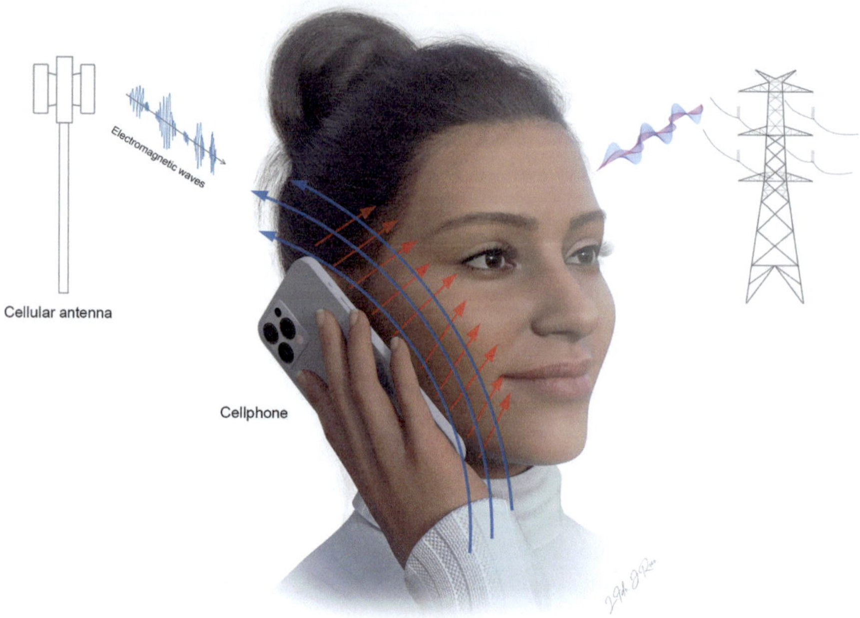

Fig. 17.5 Illustration of a person using a cellphone, with visual elements depicting electromagnetic waves. A cellular antenna is shown on the left, emitting waves labeled "Electromagnetic waves" towards the phone. Red and blue arrows illustrate the magnetic field and the electric field respectively emitted by the phone. On the right, a power line tower is depicted with wave patterns, indicating electromagnetic fields. The image highlights the daily exposure of a person to near-field and far-field radiation sources incident on a person's head and body, respectively

Exposure to specific EMR wavelengths in the visible and infrared spectrum can stimulate mitochondrial function and trigger protective cellular mechanisms, which is useful for developing therapeutic applications [58].

Several mechanisms of bioelectromagnetic signaling (generation, transmission, and transduction of signals) and cell-cell communication (CCC) that affect metabolism and energy transformation in cells and affect various types of pathologies are synthesized in [1, 59]. In conductive tissues, time-varying incident magnetic fields induce electric fields in them [1].

Zhen et al. [60] reviewed the existing literature related to the effects of magnetic (MF) and electromagnetic fields of different frequencies on iron metabolism in living organisms, finding that static magnetic fields, time-varying magnetic fields, pulsed electromagnetic fields (PEMFs), RF EMFs, and rotating polarized fields can increase, decrease or maintain the iron content in tissues and cells or alter its metabolism, depending on the frequency of the fields applied.

Cells activate heat shock genes and produce heat shock proteins very quickly and at a much higher rate than for heat itself, in response to electromagnetic stress, but these do not appear to have special genes that are activated to protect against electromagnetic stress, (Weisbrot et al. 2003) mentioned in [61] and repetitive stress leading to the continuous expression of heat shock genes can also result in the cancer induction (French et al. 2001) also mentioned by [61].

The World Health Organization (WHO) through the International Agency for Research on Cancer (IARC), has classified Extreme Low Frequency Magnetic Fields (ELF-MF) and RF fields as possibly carcinogenic to humans (Category 2B) based on the reported health effects of exposure to such fields [42] and the increased risk of gliomas, a type of brain cancer associated with the use of cordless phones [41, 62, 63, p. 151834].

One of the results that were taken into account for this classification were those reported by the INTERPHONE study [64] which showed considerable probability relationships (greater than 1.15) with a 95% confidence interval for glioma and meningioma in the tenth decile of the remembered cumulative call time, greater than 1640 h of cell phone use, being larger in the temporal lobe than in other lobes of the brain.

Other results considered were case–control studies conducted by the Hardell group in Sweden that reported a significantly increased risk of acoustic neuroma and malignant brain tumors even for exposures less than 5 years from the start of mobile phone use, and with fairly low levels of cumulative call time [7].

The SAR as one of the main dosimetric amounts established by ICNIRP and IEEE to establish guidelines or recommendations regarding human exposure to non-ionizing artificial EMFs, does not determine the biological effects caused by the EMR that caused it nor does it account for the characteristics of the incident fields and refers only to thermal effects, while the vast majority of the reported effects of environmental EMF's are not thermal in nature [50].

On the other hand, it is proposed to take into account more the parameters of EMFs such as frequencies (of carrier waves, modulation and pulses), the waveform, and the type of modulation, given the greater bioactivity of pulsed or amplitude-modulated fields than continuous or unmodulated fields of the same frequency and intensity.

The biological effects depend on the type of biomolecules that receive the radiation and the amount of energy they absorb over a certain period of time. For example, the damage is greater when energy is absorbed by nucleic acids (such as DNA) and enzymes than when radiation is absorbed by membrane lipids. However, it may happen that the effect on DNA is indirect, caused by the irregular release of free radicals into the cell due to conformational changes in membrane proteins that lead to an abnormal alteration of intracellular ionic concentrations, which triggers a cascade of intracellular events (including enzyme activity) that cause the abnormal release of these radicals [51].

The most recent protection guidance issued by ICNIRP [7] made some changes to the 1998 and 2010 standards to ensure that new technologies such as 5G cannot cause harm. However, a group of leading scientists committed to the study of the biological and health effects of non-ionizing EMFs consider that these standards do not adequately protect people or living beings since a considerable number of proven effects occur at values well below the limits established in them, which focus on thermal effects without giving relevance to the non-thermal. In addition, they call on the top leaders of the United Nations, the WHO, the United Nations Environment Programme (UNEP) and member countries to establish more protective guidelines and measures regarding the increasing and ubiquitous exposure of EMFs, promote precautionary measures and inform the general public of the health risks of such radiation [4, 39].

Several authors consider that there are "windows" of frequency or intensity where bioactivity reaches a maximum compared to the effects caused by lower or higher values of radiation parameters [6, 50, p. 6]: "The sensitivity of different biomolecules plays an important role in relation to the possibility of damage from a specific type of non-ionizing radiation, as well as a given SAR" [50].

4 Electromagnetism and Passive Metal Implants Used in Medicine

In recent years, the use of passive metal implants[12] (prostheses) in different parts of the body has increase to replace parts or support tissues fundamentally. At the same time, the general population has increased the use of devices such as cell phones, computers, modems, hearing aids, speakers, and baby monitors, which use Bluetooth or Wi-Fi technology to transmit data, voice, videos, and images through radio frequency links in the microwave range or in nearby bands. These devices emit high-frequency EMFs that represent near-field exposure (since they are used at distances of a few centimeters from the body) and therefore, the power received and induced can be greater than that transmitted by far-field sources such as communications base stations.

In orthopedic surgery, maxillofacial surgery, and neurosurgery, where passive implants are required, the characteristics of biological compatibility of the materials used (metals, ceramics, etc.) with the tissues or bones are usually taken into account. However, bioelectromagnetic compatibility (BEMC) analyses are generally not performed in the sense of considering that electrical currents, voltages, and fields induced by sources such as cell phones, are harmless to the functioning and homeostasis of the nervous, endocrine, and immune systems.

Frequency is a significant parameter because it influences the amount and density of power and energy absorbed by tissues. At wavelengths (λ) similar to the dimensions of the human body, organs and tissues, cells, individual molecules or conditioned metal implants, the resonance phenomenon occurs in which the greatest amount of absorbed energy or the Absorption Specific Rat (SAR) occurs [6, 7, p. 511, 11]. For molecular resonance phenomena, it is recommended to see the reference [17].

[12] They are those built of metallic or ceramic materials, which do not contain energy sources or electronic components that receive and/or emit signals that regulate biological functions as happens in active implants such as defibrillators, cardiac pacemakers, cochlear implants, etc.

Some reports, [11, 65, 66] focus on the effects of implants on tissue energy absorption by exposure to RF EMFs in the 900, 1800, and 2450 MHz frequency bands and with peak transmitted powers of up to 2 W, which are common to the powers transmitted by phones and WiFi devices, WiLAN, Bluetooth and laptops among others, but in general, the average transmitted powers are in the order of 100 mW or less for the latest generation phones.

The aforementioned studies report that linear metal implants can act as antennas that intensify the EMF near the implant and increase the absorbed energy (SAR) and temperature through the mechanism of redistribution of energy and heat in the tissues surrounding the implant, while circular implants act as magnetic induction loops. However, in the calculations and simulations carried out, the reference values established in the standards for these dosimetric parameters were not exceeded.

The induction of currents and voltages in passive metal implants and prostheses is produced by the capacitive and inductive couplings that are created between the sources of EM radiation that generate far- or near-field exposures (such as base stations, power lines, cell phones, modems, etc.) and the parts of the body exposed to these EMR sources [67].

If the capacitive coupling is strong, the voltages are higher and the energy is absorbed in the form of an electric field, but if the inductive coupling prevails because it occurs when the mutual inductance between the source and the implant is high, surface currents are induced in the implant or in the prosthesis which produce secondary EM fields (energy absorbed in the form of a magnetic field) that interact with the fields endogenous natural increased the energy absorbed [65]. When the source (e.g., a cell phone) is attached to the body, the capacitive coupling prevails, but if it is at a distance of millimeters, the inductive coupling prevails over the capacitive coupling [67].

For EM radiation fields where the electric field and the magnetic field oscillate synchronously, the two types of coupling mentioned occur with metal objects, but for ELF electric fields (such as those emitted by high voltage equipment, lines and appliances or some domestic or industrial equipment) the expected dominant coupling is the capacitive type, while for ELF magnetic fields (such as generators or electric motors) the resulting coupling will be inductive.

It is emphasized that the frequency and strength of incident fields, as well as the dielectric properties of tissues and cells, and the size, shape, and position of implants or prostheses with respect to the source and time of exposure, are determining parameters for assessing effects.

In oral restorative practices with implants or metal cores, bone-compatibility studies are usually carried out and dental and orthopedic procedures have been refined over time in the mechanical technique, but very little is considered bioelectromagnetic compatibility that considers the interaction or response of implants to sources of near-field EM radiation with resonant frequencies (such as those used in 3G communications systems, 4G, 5G, and 6G) for the dimensions of commonly used implants and prostheses. An electrical capacitive coupling model for dental implants was proposed by Osorio and Jaimes.[13]

International guidelines limiting occupational and non-occupational exposure to EMFs do not cover medical procedures using low- or high-frequency EMFs or the exposure of people who have metal implants that can alter or disrupt endogenous fields in the body with potential health consequences, because they are considered to be special situations of exposure where exposed personnel must be aware of the risks and take measures to mitigate them [7].

It should be noted that as the frequency of radiation increases, the current induced in metal implants becomes more concentrated on the outer surface. This is the so-called skin effect [68, p. 257].

Several studies related to the absorption of energy in the head due to exposure to radio frequency (RF) fields indicate that the specific absorption rate and current density are increased by the presence of metallic objects. This can produce short-term effects of a thermal or other nature, such as loss of balance, headaches, dizziness, high-frequency ringing (tinnitus), memory loss, involuntary movements, irregular heart rhythm, among others [69]. The measured or calculated SAR may exceed the limits established in the standards due to the presence of implants [66].

In particular, Safari and Abdolali, [69] found that the position of the implants in the mouth can raise the local SAR and the maximum SAR in the head and increase the current density in adjacent tissues due to the surface current induced in the implants by the RF fields emitted by cell phones at the 2G and 3G frequencies used in those simulations, which can affect the nervous system, causing loss of balance and dizziness. At the same time, these implants can affect the gain, dispersion, and resonance frequency of the telephone devices (i.e., the efficiency of the devices) due to reflection effects.

The shape of the implants plays an important role in the distribution of the SAR around them since the electrical flow (higher density of charges) is concentrated in the tips or thin edges, intensifying the local electric field, affecting the natural fields of the cells and tissue molecules around them and increasing the absorbed power.

The orientation of the implant with respect to the source of the external field is another factor to consider, since if it is parallel to the applied electric field vector (vertically polarized plane wave), there is greater induction.

When implants have nonlinear shapes, the mutual inductance depends on their geometric characteristics and their position with respect to the source. The greater the mutual inductance, the greater the interaction [70]. Larger implants or prostheses may disperse or reflect the incident field and cause a greater change in the distribution of the SAR.

Figure 17.6a,b illustrate the zones of electric field intensification induced in dental prostheses and implants exposed to radiofrequency EMFs.

[13] Osorio Díaz, Yosette and Jaimes Abril, Rodrigo. Implantes dentales desde la perspectiva de la inducción electromagnética. Paper presented at the II World Congress of Neural Therapy and Neurofocal Dentistry held in Bogotá, Colombia, in October 2016.

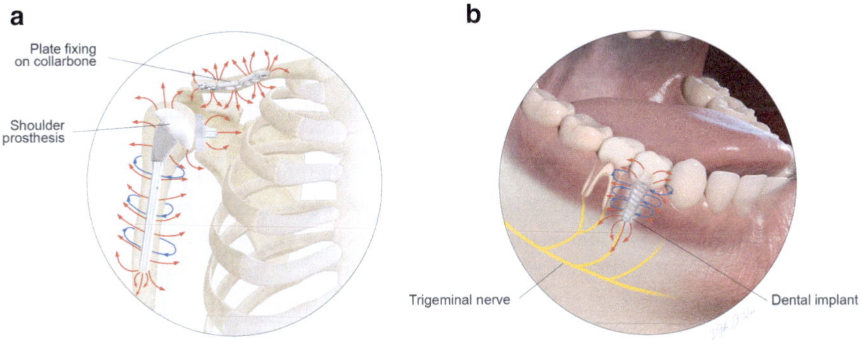

Fig. 17.6 Diagram showing two anatomical illustrations. Panel (**a**) depicts a shoulder with a prosthesis and a plate fixing on the collarbone, with red and blue arrows indicating the electric field and the magnetic field induced by exposure to external EMF sources. Panel (**b**) shows a dental implant in the mouth, highlighting the trigeminal nerve and the lines of force of the electric field (red) and magnetic field (blue) induced by exposure to an external EMF source such as a mobile device. Both panels focus on the intensification of the electric field induced in metallic prostheses and dental implants exposed to external radiofrequency EMFs, especially at the tips and edges

In general, the greater the relative difference between the dielectric properties, especially conductivity, of the two media, the greater the curvature of the electromagnetic field as it enters the medium with higher loss. Therefore, higher average SAR values can be expected in small volumes at the limit [70].

In the case of molecules, cells, tissues, organs, and the entire body, EM resonance occurs when there is a maximum transfer of energy from the source of EM fields with a frequency equal to or close to the natural frequency (or characteristic frequency) of biological structures, called the resonance frequency. This phenomenon manifests itself in an increase in the amplitude of the induced currents or voltages and in the powers absorbed by these structures.

When there is resonance, the responses in polarization, ionic currents, and absorbed energy are maximum, which can translate into heating or high SAR in some points near the metal parts or other side effects in tissues and cells, such as increased metabolism.

The resonance frequency (fr) of biological structures depends on the characteristic values of their capacitances (C), inductances (L), and electrical resistances.

For the exposure of biological structures to low-frequency magnetic fields, they are considered transparent and are therefore easily traversed by these fields. With regard to exposure to RF fields, it should be borne in mind that these can interact with hydrogen nuclei in the water present in the tissues, altering the alignment of their spins. This property is also used in nuclear magnetic resonance (NMR) diagnostic technology in which static or low-frequency but high-intensity magnetic fields are used to initially orient all the magnetic dipoles and then apply the resonant RF fields to the nuclei.

The materials used in orthopedics and dentistry for implants, stems, nails, screws, plates, rods, discs, wires, etc., are usually surgical stainless steel, titanium, titanium alloys, or Cr, Ni, Co, and Mo alloys. When an EM wave hits them (which are good electrical conductors) it causes the electrons on the surface to oscillate and produce a current of the same frequency as that of the incident wave, which, in turn, produces secondary EMFs acting, as well as antennas of weak radiation in the tissues [66, p. 1222, 70].

Whole-body resonance occurs when a person's height is similar to half the wavelength ($\lambda/2$) in free space, the person is standing and isolated from the ground, and the incident wave is flat and vertically polarized. This is a common exposure situation when radiation sources are far away from subjects, such as base stations (cell phone antennas, broadcast and TV antennas, and satellites), since most people wear insulating footwear. But if the person is in effective contact with the earth, the resonance occurs when the person's dimension is close to $\lambda/4$ and in this case, the SAR is greater [7, p. 511]. Above the full-body resonant frequency, SAR is not much different.

On the other hand, a resonant length observed for metallic objects such as implants with dimensions close to 0.42 λ (on average) and $\lambda/3$ at which the highest SAR is presented, have been reported by Matikka [11] and [65, 70] based on simulations or numerical studies carried out in several studies.

Table 17.2 shows the values of the frequencies at which EM resonance can occur in the whole body or in passive metal prostheses or implants and the corresponding resonant lengths.

Table 17.2 Whole-body or passive metal prostheses or implants EM resonance frequencies and corresponding resonant lengths

Frequency [MHz]	Wavelength λ of the incident field [cm]	Resonant length[a,b] $\lambda/2$ [cm]	Resonant length[c] $\lambda/3$ [cm]	Resonant length[a] $\lambda/4$ [cm]	Resonance in:
30	600	300	200	150	Whole body 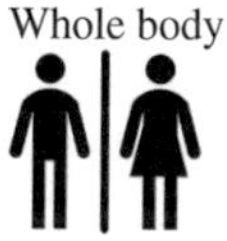
88	340	170	113	85	
100	300	150	100	75	
200	150	75	50	37.5	
800	37.5	18.8	12.5	9.4	Passive implants and/or metal prostheses
900	33.3	16.7	11	8.3	
1700	17.6	8.8	5.9	4.4	
1900	15.8	7.9	5.3	3.9	
2100	14.2	7.1	4.7	3.5	
2500	12	6	4	3	
2650	11.3	5.6	3.8	2.8	
3000	10	5	3.3	2.5	
3750	8	4	2.7	2	
5000	6	3	2	1.5	
6000	5	2.5	1.7	1.3	

Notes:
[a]Proposed resonant length in [7]
[b]Theoretical Resonant Length Proposed by [11]
[c]Observed resonant length reported by [11]

As shown in Table 17.2, frequencies between 30 and 200 MHz can produce whole-body resonance in people with heights between 200 cm (2 m) and 37.5 cm, respectively. The average resonant frequency is ≈104 MHz, which corresponds to waves emitted by FM radio antennas very commonly deployed in cities.

For frequencies between 800 and 6000 MHz, which correspond to the EMR spectrum emitted by cellular telephone devices and antennas (3G, 4G, 5G and 6G sub-Giga Hertz), cordless telephones, WiFi, WLAN, Bluetooth, MRI may occur in organs, implants and metal prostheses that have dimensions between 18.8 and 1.3 cm. Most dental implants and prostheses used in surgery and orthopedics are in this range of lengths.

Resonance in cells, organelles, microtubules, and molecules will occur at higher frequencies that have $\lambda/2$, $\lambda/3$, and $\lambda/4$ lengths similar to or equal to their dimensions.

For microtubules and molecules, and macromolecules, the work of Saha, Traddock and Tuszynski [25] and Cosic and Cosic [17] illustrates their resonant properties. Frequencies above 6 GHz using 5G and 6G wireless communications technologies are more likely to produce resonant effects on these biological structures and therefore more efficiently transfer energy from these radiations, with effects that have yet to be measured, evaluated or assessed.

5 Conclusions

In this work, the main electrical and dielectric properties of some functional biological units, such as cells and tissues, were analyzed. Its variation with frequency and its interaction with the Earth's natural fields and with artificial Electromagnetic Fields (EMFs) such as those generated by wireless communications systems and devices operating in different Radio Frequency bands were exposed. Similarly, its interaction with the extremely low frequency fields originated by electric power generation, transmission, and distribution lines, equipment, and appliances and devices used in the residential, commercial, medical, and industrial fields was also reviewed. This analysis must be taken into account by the medical community in the processes of diagnosis, treatment, and prevention of diseases and by the scientific and technological community for the design of systems and devices for medical use and medicines that are more compatible from the bioelectromagnetic point of view.

Several biological and health effects of non-ionizing electromagnetic radiation (NI EMR) reported in the scientific literature were discussed, some of which have been taken into account in establishing guidelines and recommendations on exposure for ELF and RF EMFs. The arguments of sectors of the scientific community that appeal for regulations to reduce the limits established, taking into account biology, in such a way that life and health are more protected, were presented. The thesis that EMFs are biologically active and can be harmful to health, depending on the frequency, intensity, time, distance, exposure situations, and conditions of the exposed subjects, among other factors, was corroborated.

The behavior of passive metal implants and metal prostheses as antennas that more efficiently capture Radiofrequency EMF was also analyzed, identifying the frequencies and lengths that can cause resonance and, therefore, induce great energy absorption in biological structures, altering the electromagnetic ecosystem of tissues and organs.

AI Use Statement No AI-assisted technologies have been used to write this chapter.

Funding No external funding has been available.

Conflict of Interest Statement The author declares that there is no conflict of interest.

Appendix: Related Equations

$$J = \sigma E\left[\mathrm{A/m^2}\right] \qquad \text{Ohm's Law for the Electric Field}$$

J: Current Density (A/m^2)
σ: Conductivity (S/m).

$$V = IR\left[\mathrm{V}\right] \qquad \text{Ohm's Law}$$

V: Electrical voltage or voltage (V).
I: Electric Current (A).
R: Resistance (Ω).

$$G = 1/R$$

G: Conductancia (S).

Electrical Polarization

$$D = \varepsilon E$$

E: Electric Field Strength (V/m).
D: Electric Flux Density (C/m^2).
ε: Permittivity (F/m).

$$\varepsilon = \varepsilon_0 \, \varepsilon_r$$

$\varepsilon_0 = 8.85 \times 10^{-12}$ Vacuum permittivity.
ε_r: Relative permittivity (dielectric constant).

$$\varepsilon_r = \varepsilon_{r'} - j\varepsilon_{r''}$$

$\varepsilon_{r'}$: It describes dielectric polarization, that is, the ability of a material to store energy in the form of an electric field in electric dipoles.
$\varepsilon_{r''}$: Describes losses in material exposed to EMF due to the conduction current of free ions or electrons, and to the displacement current due to the rotation or vibration of polar ions or molecules within the material.

$$P = \chi_e \varepsilon_0 E$$

P: Electrical Polarization.
χ_e: Electrical susceptibility

$$\lambda = c / f$$

λ: Wavelength [m].
c: Speed of light (≈300,000 km/s).
f Frequency (Hz).

$$\mathrm{B} = \mu \mathrm{H}$$

B: Magnetic flux density (T).
μ: Magnetic permeability.
H: Magnetic field strength (A/m).

$$\mu = \mu_0 \, \mu_r$$

μ_0: Vacuum permeability.
μ_r: Relative Permeability.

$$(F = q(v \, X \, B + E)$$

F: Lorentz forces. (for ion interactions).
v: Velocity of the charged particle.

$$T = m_e \times E$$

T: Electric torque (For interactions with dipoles).
m_e: Electric dipole moment.

$$T = m_m \times B$$

m_m: Magnetic Moment.

$$m_e = q \times d$$

q: Load quantity.
d: Distance separating the charges.

$$m_e = \alpha E$$

α: Electronic polarizability.

Resonant Lengths (for metal implants) in dielectric media:

$$l1 = \lambda / 3 = 0.33\lambda \qquad y \qquad l_{res} = c / \left(2\sqrt{\varepsilon r f}\right) \approx 0.42\lambda(\text{average})(11)$$

Note: The letters between ( ) indicate the units of those magnitudes.

References

1. Wang H, Zou W, Cao Y. Bioelectromagnetic fields as signaling currents of life. Radiat Med Prot 2024. Available from: https://doi.org/10.1016/j.radmp.2024.09.001.
2. Apollonio F, Liberti M, Paffi A, Merla C, Marracino P, Denzi A, Marino C, d'Inzeo G. Feasibility for microwaves energy to affect biological systems via nonthermal mechanisms: a systematic approach. IEEE Trans Microw Theory Tech. 2013;61(5):2031–45.
3. Funk RH, Scholkmann F. The significance of bioelectricity on all levels of organization of an organism. Part 1: from the subcellular level to cells. Prog Biophys Mol Biol. 2023;177:185–201.
4. BioInitiative Working Group. BioInitiative 2012. [Internet]. Available from: https://bioinitiative.org/
5. Al Ahmad M, Al Natour Z, Mustafa F, Rizvi T. Electrical characterization of normal and cancer cells. IEEE Access. 2018;6:25979–86.
6. Jaimes R, Nontoa C, Ortíz D. Efectos del Campo Eléctrico en los Seres Vivos [thesis]. Bogotá: Universidad Nacional de Colombia; Faculty of Engineering, Department of Electrical Engineering; 1987. p. 201.
7. International Commission on Non-Ionizing Radiation Protection (ICNIRP). Guidelines for limiting exposure to electromagnetic fields (100 kHz to 300 GHz). Health Phys. 2020;118(5):483–524.
8. Georgiev DD. Electric and magnetic fields inside neurons and their impact upon the cytoskeletal microtubules. In: Bandyopadhyay A, Ray K, editors. Rhythmic oscillations in proteins to human cognition. Springer; 2021. p. 51–102.
9. Sánchiz OA. Application of dielectrophoresis to the dielectric characterization of cells. Doctoral thesis. Madrid. 2008.
10. Cifra M, Apollonio F, Liberti M, García-Sánchez T, Mir L. Possible molecular and cellular mechanisms at the basis of atmospheric electromagnetic field bioeffects. Int J Biometeorol. 2021;65:59–67.

11. Matikka H. The effect of metal implants on the RF energy absorption and temperature changes in head tissues. Master's thesis. Kuopio: University of Eastern Finland; 2010. p. 105.
12. Gabriel C. Compilation of the dielectric properties of body tissues at RF and microwave frequencies [report]. London: Departamento de Física, King's College London; 1996. Report N° 19960322 04.
13. Gabriel C, Peyman A. Dielectric properties of tissues [report]. Mobile Telecommunications and Health Research Programme; 2005.
14. Baumgartner C, et al. IT'IS database for thermal and electromagnetic parameters of biological tissues [Internet]. 2024. [cited 2025 Jan] Available from: https://itis.swiss/virtual-population/tissue-properties/database/dielectric-properties
15. Matković A. Permittivity measurement of biological tissues and open-ended coaxial probe measurement method analysis. Doctoral thesis. Split: University of Split, Faculty of Electrical Engineering, Mechanical Engineering and Naval Architecture; 2024. p. 76.
16. Bear MF, Connors BW, Paradiso MA. Neuroscience: exploring the brain. Barcelona: Masson-Williams & Wilkins; 1998. p. 662.
17. Cosic I, Cosic D. Macromolecular resonances. In: Bandyopadhyay A, Ray K, editors. Rhythmic oscillations in proteins to human cognition. Singapore: Springer; 2021. p. 9–35.
18. Levin M, Stevenson CG. Regulation of cell behavior and tissue patterning by bioelectrical signals: challenges and opportunities for biomedical engineering. Annu Rev Biomed Eng. 2012;14:295–323.
19. Fennelly C, Soker S. Bioelectric properties of myogenic progenitor cells. Bioelectricity. 2019;18(1):35–45.
20. Elizondo Ángel E. Modelos eléctricos aproximados de tejido humano para análisis de respuesta ante influencia de ondas electromagnéticas a distintas frecuencias. Ciencia y Tecnología. 2014;14:49–62.
21. Scott AC. The electrophysics of a nerve fiber. J Biol Phys. 1976;4:166–91.
22. Park KS. Humans and electricity. Understanding body electricity and applications. Cham: Springer; 2023. p. 408.
23. Hessinger C, Reimman N, Hubner F, Schmidt S, Schuler M, Panahi B, Kaltenbach B, Polkowski C, Vogl TJ, Jakovy R. Dielectric contrast between normal and tumor ex-vivo human liver tissue. IEEE Access. 2019;7:164113–9.
24. Tuszynski JA, Douglas F, Freedman H, Sbitnev VI, Kim H, Santelices I, Kalra AP, Patel SD, Shankar K, Chua LO. Microtubules as sub-cellular memristors. Sci Rep. 2020;10:2108.
25. Saha A, Craddock TJ, Tuszynski JA. An investigation of the plausibility of stochastic resonance in tubulin dimers. Biosystems. 2012;107:81–7.
26. Nistala V, Sai M, Mathan N. Survey on performance of memristor. Int J Pharm Technol. 2016;8(3):16618–26.
27. Johnsen GK. Skin electrical properties and physical aspects of hydration of keratinized tissues. Doctoral thesis. Oslo: Faculty of Mathematics and Natural Sciences, University of Oslo; 2010. p. 48.
28. Tipler PA, Mosca G. Physics for scientists and engineers. 5th ed. New York: W.H. Freeman and Company; 2004. p. 1356.
29. Livanov D. The Earth's atmosphere. In: The physics of planet Earth and its natural wonders. Moscow: Springer; 2023. p. 123–57.
30. Hayakawa M, Hattori K, Ando Y. Electromagnetic phenomena and electromagnetic theory: a review. IEEJ Trans Fundam Mater. 2004;124(1):72–9.
31. Fernández Arroyabe PEA. Glossary on atmospheric electricity and its effects on biology. Int J Biometeorol. 2021;65:5–29.
32. Panagopoulos DJ, Johansson O, Carlo GL. Polarization: a key difference between man-made and natural electromagnetic fields in regard to biological activity. Sci Rep. 2015;5:14194.
33. Panagopoulos DJ, Karabarbounis A, Liolioulis C. Defining wireless communication (WC) electromagnetic fields (EMFs). In: Panagopoulos DJ, editor. Electromagnetic fields of wireless communications: biological and health effects. 1st ed. Boca Raton: CRC Press; 2023. p. 17–76.

34. Bioinitiative Working Group. Bioinitiative. 2006. [Cited 2024 Dec]. Available from: https://bioinitiative.org/. Accessed December 2024.
35. World Health Organization. The INTERPHONE study. 2011. [Cited 2025 Jan]. Available from: https://interphone.iarc.who.int/.
36. World Health Organization. The International EMF Project. 2005. [Cited 2025 Jan]. Available from: https://www.who.int/initiatives/the-international-emf-project.
37. World Health Organization. International Agency for Research on Cancer (IARC). [Cited 2025 Jan]. Available from: https://www.iarc.who.int/
38. International Commission on Non-Ionizing Radiation Protection. ICNIRP. [Cited 2025 Jan]. Available from: https://www.icnirp.org/
39. EMFscientist.org. EMF Scientist Appeal. 2015–2024. [Cited 2025 Jan]. Available from: https://emfscientist.org/index.php/emf-scientist-appeal
40. BioEM. BioEM. 2022. [Cited 2025 Jan]. Available from: https://bioem.org/
41. International Agency for Research on Cancer (IARC). Non-ionizing radiation, part II: radiofrequency electromagnetic fields, vol. 102. Lyon: IARC; 2013. p. 460.
42. International Agency for Research on Cancer (IARC). Non-ionizing radiation, part 1: static and extremely low-frequency (ELF) electric and magnetic fields, vol. 80. Lyon: IARC; 2002. p. 429.
43. Scientific Committee on Emerging and Newly Identified Health Risks (SCENIHR). Potential health effects of exposure to electromagnetic fields [report]. Luxembourg: European Commission; 2015. p. 288.
44. SSM's Scientific Council on Electromagnetic Fields. Recent research on EMF and health risk-Twelfth report from SSM's Scientific Council on Electromagnetic Fields, 2017. Report No.: 2018:09. p. 118. Available from: https://www.stralsakerhetsmyndigheten.se/en/publications
45. SSM's Scientific Council on Electromagnetic Fields. Recent research on EMF and health risk--Thirteenth report from SSM's Scientific Council on Electromagnetic Fields, 2018. Report No.: 2019:08. p. 95. Available from: https://www.stralsakerhetsmyndigheten.se/en/publications
46. Liu L, Huang B, Lu Y, Zhao Y, Tang X, Shi Y. Interactions between electromagnetic radiation and biological systems. iScience. 2024;27(109201):1–23.
47. Calvente I, Núñez MI. Is the sustainability of exposure to non-ionizing electromagnetic radiation possible? Med Clin. 2024;162:387–93.
48. International Commission on Non-Ionizing Radiation Protection (ICNIRP). ICNIRP. 2025 Jan. Available from: https://www.icnirp.org/en/publications/index.html
49. McIntosh RL, Anderson V, McKenzie RJ. A numerical evaluation of SAR distribution and temperature changes around a metallic plate in the head of a RF exposed worker. Bioelectromagnetics. 2005;26(5):377–88.
50. Panagopoulos DJ, Johansson O, Carlo GL. Evaluation of specific absorption rate as a dosimetric quantity for electromagnetic fields. PLoS One. 2013;8(6):1–9.
51. Panagopoulos DJO, Panagopoulos CG. Evaluation of specific absorption rate as a dosimetric quantity for electromagnetic fields bioeffects. PLoS One. 2013;8(6):1–9.
52. Institute of Electrical and Electronics Engineers (IEEE). Standard for safety levels with respect to human exposure to radiofrequency electromagnetic fields, 3 kHz to 300 GHz. New York: IEEE; 2006.
53. International Commission on Non-Ionizing Radiation Protection (ICNIRP). Guidelines for limiting exposure to time-varying electric, magnetic and electromagnetic fields (up to 300 GHz). Health Phys. 1998;74:494–522.
54. Panagopoulos DJ, Johansson O, Carlo GL. Evaluation of specific absorption rate as a dosimetric quantity for electromagnetic field bioeffects. PLoS One. 2013;8(6):1–9.
55. Panagopoulos DJ, Messini N, Karabarbounis A, Philippetis AL, Margariti L. A mechanism for action of oscillating electric fields on cells. Biochem Biophys Res Commun. 2000;272(3):634–40.
56. Panagopoulos DJ, Karabarbounis A, Margaritis LH. Mechanism for action of electromagnetic fields on cells. Biochem Biophys Res Commun. 2002;298:95–102.

57. Pall M. Electromagnetic fields act via activation of voltage-gated calcium channels to produce beneficial or adverse effects. J Cell Mol Med. 2013;17(8):958–65.
58. Hamblin MR. Shining light on the head: photobiomodulation for brain disorders. BBA Clin. 2016 Oct;1(6):113–24.
59. Su J, Song Y, Zhu Z, Huang X, Fan J, Qiao J, et al. Cell–cell communication: new insights and clinical implications. Signal Transduct Target Ther. 2024;9:196.
60. Zhen C, Zhang G, Wang S, Wang J, Fang Y, Shang P. Electromagnetic fields regulate iron metabolism in living organisms: a review of effects and mechanism. Prog Biophys Mol Biol. 2024;188:43–54.
61. Panagopoulos DJ. Gametogenesis, embryonic and post-embryonic development of drosophila. In: Spindler-Barth M, editor. Drosophila melanogaster: life cycle, genetics. New York: Nova Science Publishers, Inc.; 2012.
62. International Agency for Research on Cancer (IARC). Classifies radiofrequency electromagnetic fields as possibly carcinogenic to humans [Internet]. 31 May 2011. [Cited 2024 Oct]. Available from: http://www.iarc.fr/en/media-centre/pr/2011/pdfs/pr208_E.pdf
63. Moghnieh H, Rammal M, Barakeh R, Rachid E. Analysis of human head interaction in handset antennas using ground plane corrugation. IEEE Access. 2024;12:151834–45.
64. World Health Organization. The INTERPHONE study [Internet]. October 2011. [Cited 2025 Jan]. Available from: https://interphone.iarc.who.int/uicc-report-final-03102011.pdf
65. Virtanen H, Huttunen J, Toropainen A, Lappalainen R. Interaction of mobile phones with superficial passive metallic implants. Phys Med Biol. 2005;50:2689–700.
66. Virtanen H, Keshvari J, Lappalainen R. The effect of authentic metallic implants on the SAR distribution of the head exposed to 900, 1800 and 2450 MHz dipole near field. Phys Med Biol. 2007;52:1221–36.
67. Christ A, Fallahi A, Neufeld E, Balzano Q, Kuster N. Mechanism of capacitive coupling of proximal electromagnetic sources with biological bodies. Bioelectromagnetics. 2022;43:404–12.
68. Kraus JD. In: Elken AE, editor. Antennas. 2nd ed. Singapore: McGraw-Hill; 1988. p. 892.
69. Safari M, Abdolali A. Dental implants and mobile-phone use. IEEE Antennas Propag Mag. 2016. p. 2–10.
70. Virtanen H, Keshvari J, Lappalainen R. Interaction of radio frequency electromagnetic fields and passive metallic implants. Bioelectromagnetics. 2006;27:431–9.

Part V
Doctrine of Neuraltherapeutic Medicine

Chapter 18
Principles and Worldview of the Neuraltherapeutic Medicine

Edna Cecilia Garzón-Fuentes and Ivonne Astrid Díaz-Adarme

1 Introduction

As mentioned in Chap. 3, Neural Therapy in Colombia acquires a unique worldview, with its own doctrinal and philosophical body. This transformation allows it to consolidate itself as Neuraltherapeutic Medicine (NTM), a complex medical system, differentiated from other medical systems, including biomedicine [1–6].

To enunciate some principles of NTM, it is necessary to refer to its historical evolution (see Chaps. 1, 2, and 3). A series of significant events and experiences, framed in specific socio-historical contexts, allowed the consolidation of this novel body of knowledge and its recognition within the dimensions of a complex medical system (See Chap. 6) [2, 3, 5, 7, 8].

2 Epistemological Perspective

NTM marks ruptures with the ways of understanding and generating knowledge typical of hegemonic medicine, as well as with the way of understanding and interpreting life events [1, 2, 9–12]. These ruptures occur little by little through the different historical moments, gradually configuring their own epistemology.

Huneke Neural Therapy (TNH), which arrived in Colombia from Germany, already led to breaks and distances from the theories and concepts that framed medicine at the beginning of the twentieth century. Its astonishing clinical results do not find sufficient explanation from the conceptual frameworks of the time, leading to

E. C. Garzón-Fuentes (✉) · I. A. Díaz-Adarme
Master in Alternative Medicine, Neural Therapy Area, Faculty of Medicine,
Universidad Nacional de Colombia, Bogotá, Colombia
e-mail: ecgarzonf@unal.edu.co; iadiaza@unal.edu.co

L. B. Pinilla Bonilla et al. (eds.), *Neuraltherapeutic Medicine*,
https://doi.org/10.1007/978-3-032-03257-7_18

the exploration of other possibilities of interpretation of the facts. Initially, explanations were proposed based on the known segmental anatomical configuration of the nervous system, the electrical dependence of vital phenomena, and the totalizing integration provided by the vegetative nervous system [13–15]. These concepts were subsequently enriched by the contributions of the British physicians Henry Head and James Mackenzie, who identified neural reflex zones on the body's surface, in relation to the functioning of internal organs [14–26] (see Chap. 15). These explanations continue to be structured with the discovery and conceptualization of the "phenomenon in seconds" and the "interference field" (see Chap. 2), as well as with the incorporation of research derived from synthetic physiology or Russian nervism (see Chap. 13), and the research of Gustav Ricker [27] and Alfred Pischinger [28] (see Chap. 12). Also from the beginning, the proposals for the possible neural-therapeutic effects of procaine, beyond its anesthetic effects, were challenging [14, 15] as well as approaches to quantum physics, metaphysics and later to cybernetics [1, 13, 14, 29–34].

These findings and explanatory proposals necessarily led to the development of critical positions in the face of the analytical rationality of medicine, which segments the body into systems for its understanding and considers the separation between mind and body. There was also a critical stance against conventional diagnoses, considering that they did not contribute significantly to the understanding of the real processes observed in patients, nor to therapeutic decision-making [13]. This is how what the Huneke brothers called "a metamorphosis of thought" that configures "a neuraltherapeutic thought" takes place [13–15, 32].

"Neuraltherapeutic thinking" was enriched in Colombia, offering special contexts to Neural Therapy according to Huneke, initially from the effervescence of knowledge and practices that took place in the *Los Robles* school of thought with Dr. Germán Duque Mejía and later from the dialogue of knowledge that was developed around Dr. Julio César Payán, at the *Payanese* school of Neural Therapy (see Chap. 3).

In these spaces, at the same time as the previous conceptual frameworks of TNH were deepened, the perspective was expanded to include other areas of knowledge and practice that contribute to the comprehension of the daily changes and outcomes observed in patients. From the *Payanese* school, epistemological frameworks were extended and neuraltherapeutic thinking was projected toward broader social context, simultaneously demonstrating that alternative medicines represent distinct systems of thought and interpretations of reality, rather than merely differing tools from biomedical practices. In this way, an epistemological turn for Neural Therapy was consolidated in Colombia [2, 9, 35–39].

In the "new" epistemology that has been woven around neuraltherapeutic thinking, due to the evolution of the explanatory frameworks surronding Neural Therapy, some characteristic that are integrally related to each other can be identified :

- It is a dialogical, contextual, flexible and adaptive epistemology, which distances itself from the pretension of finding laws or unified knowledge applicable in a universal way, while avoiding extreme relativism or eclecticism [1, 2, 12, 40–43].

The preceding narrative illustrates the integration of novel explanatory frameworks and theories in the pursuit of theoretical approaches to comprehend the beneficial changes observed daily in patients following neural therapy, which surpass the explanatory capacity of conventional Western medicine. From the contributions of the *Payanese* school, the construction of an experiential, organic, dialogue, participatory, non-hegemonic, and non-deterministic knowledge was deepened, which recovers the space of the doctor's office as a space for daily research. In this way, a living school of maturation of thought was created, which moves in constant dialogue between the "inexplicable" improvements of the patients treated with the application of neural therapy, philosophical and academic reflection and what happens in the territory and in the community [1, 2, 9, 39] (see Chap. 3) .
- It has an integrative, synthetic, non-segmented viewpoint of the organism, which transcends the canonical analytical perspective of Western medicine. This new perspective reconciles the mind-body dichotomy and the division of the organism into systems, grounded in the understanding of the unifying function of the "vegetative" nervous system, which Ferdinand Huneke regarded as *"the link between matter and spirit"* [7]. The theories and experiments of Drs. Ricker and Pischinger are included as possible support [14, 15, 27, 28, 32, 44] along with theoretical postulates from biocybernetics and the theory of communication and information [29, 30, 45–47], theoretical biology [48–50] and electrical and quantum interpretations [51] including the approaches of Penrose and Hameroff regarding the existence of a quantum biological substrate of consciousness [52–55]. Some of these approaches from quantum physics, for some authors, are close to mysticism or offer interpretations that resemble the worldviews of native people who agree with the existence of an underlying reality more complex than the evident one [29–31, 46, 56–60] .

This unification is clearly seen in the contributions of Russian synthetic physiology, which describes an integrative and cohesive role of the nervous system, which makes the body's responses to any stimulus orchestrated from a whole and not by "parts"; implying that the classic divisions of the nervous system described are not operative in reality. From these concepts, it is understood that the nervous system acts in a network and has a modulatory and integrating role in the organism's information, in all adaptive processes, both pathological (inflammatory and infectious) and physiological, including mental and emotional processes [61–63] (see Chap. 13).

- From these approaches, the organism's ability to "become irritated" is recognized. It refers to the organism's capability to be upset and respond from its integrated totality to internal or external stimuli or "irritants," thereby modifying its physiological functions and the tone of the nervous system [61, 64]. The quotation marks are used because the word "irritant" or "irritation" is not taken in its usual sense of harmful or inflammatory stimulus but refers to information that the system incorporates dynamically and that has the capability to modify the organism [45, 61, 63, 65]. In this process, the phenomenon of "irritation" becomes relevant, that is, the processing of information in the form of a dialogue that occurs between the organism and the "irritant," beyond the specific characteristics of the latter .

- The understanding of the disease as a continuous, evolutionary, adaptive, and emergent process, which involves creativity and learning (see Chaps. 7 and 19). From this perspective, the view of health and disease as opposed and polar (static) states is overcome [1, 66, 67]. The so-called disease, in the words of Dr. Payán, *would be "the way in which an organism faces its conflicts at a given time"* [1].
- It is also characterized by the understanding of non-determinism in vital processes. It recognizes the presence of probability and irreversibility processes in the organism's responses [1, 41, 45, 48, 61], as well as the uncertainty and unpredictability of the quantum mechanical universe in complex adaptive systems [68] in which, in the words of Norbert Wiener, *"exact repetition is impossible"* [29]. From these contributions, the critical stance is accentuated in the face of the determining role of classical diagnosis in therapeutic decision-making in Western conventional medicine [10] (see Chap. 24) .
- Recognizes the inherent complexity of life processes in general and health/disease in particular. It incorporates components of the complexity paradigm, including complex thinking and the ability to relink concepts and knowledge that appear to be unrelated, opposed, or rejected [41, 69, 70]. Additionally, it incorporates approaches to the sciences of complexity (see Chap. 7) that, through a variety of perspectives, broadly speaking, strives to understand phenomena that transcend linearity and determinism [41, 68, 71–74]. The capability for self-organization in the biological, the relationships, links, and processes, as well as the properties that originate or evolve from these interrelationships, are the primary focus of their attention, rather than the "interacting elements" [49, 68, 75–80] .
- It is nourished by dialogic and participatory research methodologies. The new epistemology implies congruent research methods, where the hermeneutics of biographical accounts becomes relevant. In Neuraltherapeutic Medicine, the *dialogue of knowledge* and *Participatory Action Research (PAR)* have marked the path that has allowed the dialogic, participatory, non-hierarchical, and non-hegemonic construction of knowledge [38, 81–84] (see Chap. 46). These methodologies have left their mark on the linking of life history instead of the classic clinical history, as an epistemological tool and accompaniment in decision-making [2, 85, 86] (see Chap. 20).
- NTM involves the use and application of local anesthetics as neuraltherapeutic. That is, because of its properties different from anesthetic properties, including its ability to affect the tone of the nervous system and the trophism of tissues and therefore the course of pathological processes [13, 14, 53, 63, 87–89] (see Chap. 26).

- An ecological and biocentric dimension.[1] In Colombia, the integration approach is deepened, by involving the being more decisively with its environment, from a counter-stance against the separation of organism and environment, turning toward ecological, ecosystemic understandings of life and health [1, 2, 9, 37, 38, 59, 90, 91]. In the process, knowledge and wisdom of indigenous peoples are put into dialogue [1, 59, 87, 92] along with reflections and contributions from the thermodynamics of living beings or systems far from equilibrium [93, 94], chaos theory and the description of the behavior of nonlinear dynamical systems [3, 68, 78, 79], Ludwig Von Bertalanffy's systems theory [95], contributions from the self-eco-organization attributed to Edgar Morin [69, 96], and principles derived from quantum physics, among other areas [1, 2, 45, 48, 87].

3 Paradigmatic Perspective

From Thomas Kuhn's approaches, a paradigm refers to a specific perspective on reality, which would be supported by the network of concepts, beliefs, values, practices, explanatory models, and research methodologies that support this viewpoint [97–100].

From the epistemological point of view, it has been exposed in the previous section how the evolution of "*neuraltherapeutic thinking*" implies the inclusion of different frameworks of understanding that are linked in dialogue and tension with experience. These new insights, arising from both clinical experience with patients and the network of concepts and explanatory frameworks used to interpret them, progressively reshape the theoretical and practical assumptions that inform the formulation of research questions and the methodologies devised to address them. In this gradual evolution, Neuraltherapeutic Medicine underwent a paradigmatic shift, some of whose defining features can be outlined:

- It distances itself from the positivistic, deterministic, mechanistic paradigm of Western conventional medicine [1, 2, 12, 41, 56, 59, 92, 101], turning toward an ecological paradigm which provides a broad contextual, biocentric viewpoint and recognizes the complexity of vital events and living beings [1, 41, 56, 87]. Ferdinand Huneke, at the time, considered neural therapy as "*the polar complement so desperately needed by the inmense knowledge of our time, which is condemned to sterility until it can establish a connection with the living*" [56].
- It involves methods of knowing and understanding that are consistent with this new paradigmatic framework, which also entails a dialogic interaction between concepts and knowledge, and the singular contexts in which they are intended to be applied. It thus distances itself from conceptualizations with totalitarian,

[1] Biocentrism centers on respect for every living being and all forms of life. It implies an environmental and co-evolutionary ethics, distancing itself from anthropocentrism and theocentrism. It fosters cooperative and participatory relationships.

dogmatic, or universal pretensions in understanding vital processes, focusing instead on the processes and interrelations and on the subjects who embody and actively engage in these processes [2, 61, 87]. From this perspective, Dr. Payán proposes a reflective attitude when he uses the expressions *"sometimes"* and *"it depends*", combining them with various categorical statements. In this way, he invites us to understand the relative meaning within each specific context [1, 2, 87].

- Within this new paradigmatic perspective, with the overcoming of the dual or binary viewpoint between health and disease, there is the recognition of the vital processes of healing and disease, as interdependent adaptive processes, which imply flexibility, adaptability, creativity, and learning and that transcend any attempt at mechanical, causal, linear explanation [67, 102–104].
- The therapeutics is intented to stimulate the capacity and enhance the possibilities of self-regulation of the organism and not at standardized treatment according to certain diagnoses of disease [1, 2, 87] (see Chaps. 24 and 25).

4 Ethical-Ontological Perspective

The aforementioned epistemological and paradigmatic shifts entail changes in the dimensions, activities, and relationships of the being that embodies these processes:

- The perspective of individual health is transcended, actively linking community and ecological dimensions. By recognizing health/disease as a dynamic process, which is participatory, and contextual, community and collective dynamics of self-care and mutual care are promoted, as well as environmental and territorial health. Within these categories, all the constitutive relationships of the individual, cultural, family, socioeconomic, affective, access to food, etc., become relevant. These processes promote the reconnection of being with their environment in a broad sense, making them part and participatory [2].
- The dynamics and methodologies of dialogic and participatory action research allow different, solidary, non-hierarchical relationships to emerge between the human beings involved. This rethinking of the power roles inherent in relationships facilitates the emergence of a novel interpretation and significance in the roles of physicians and patients, as well as among the members of the communities concerned. The relationship is solidarized by promoting an active and participatory awareness of all actors [2] .
- The autonomy and action of the subjects in decisions about their health is promoted. From the critical recovery of history through the reconstruction of "Life History" as a guiding tool in therapeutic decision-making, the adaptive, learning and transformation capacity of reality in individuals and communities is recognized and promoted. These dynamics strengthen participatory awareness and capacity for action, consolidating autonomy, reducing dependence on external institutional or non-institutional powers [2] (see Chap. 20).

- The patient's voice is recovered. That is, the narrative of the subject in the role of patient is vindicated as relevant in the understanding of health/disease processes, their meanings and signifiers. As Santamaría describes it in Chap. 19, the biographical account is recognized as *"a comprehensive rather than an explanatory model of suffering"* [2] .
- It naturally leads to a rethinking of the meaning of "diseases" from this new conceptualizations o as an adaptive process. In this same perspective, the community experiences stemming from the earthquake (see Chaps. 3 and 46), promotes understanding crises as a learning opportunity [2, 90, 91] .
- Relationships and processes are invigorated within a constant invitation to foster dialogue as a pedagogical tool with great creative potential, even in scenarios of great disagreements and oppositions. Dialogue encompasses a wide spectrum beyond mere verbal exchange, including interactions among beings, groups, discourses, epistemological frameworks, various domains of knowledge, the organism in response to stimuli, and the relationship between reality and potential interpretations. This dialogue implies a worthy recognition of all agents, of all voices, without subordination. It does not imply that "anything goes" without any rigor. It implies that everything can be listened to and valued, trying to understand and respect its contexts and the logical frameworks from which it is sustained, even if they do not correspond to the dominant canonical logic [2, 39] .
- The *"Vital Disobedience,"* "Desobediencia Vital" is an expression proposed by Dr. Payán. Implies a critical, ethical, and political stance, and perhaps underpins the most profound transformation of the being on thepath of Neural Therapy[2] and perhaps underpins the most profound transformation of the being in the path of Neural Therapy. The synergy of these two simple words manages in a creative and poetic way (of *poiesis*[3]) to give a clear voice to and make it easy to remember the novelty and complexity of their approaches. This postulate suggests that life fundamentally embodies freedom, uncertainty, indeterminacy, creativity, learning, and evolution (in a non-deterministic creative context), as organisms continuously process diverse information (both endogenous and exogenous), thereby facilitating learning and adaptive mechanisms. Life then does not obey universal laws, predictions, determinisms, norms, or models of normality [1, 42, 92] .

In the account made in this chapter, an effort has been made to cover the most relevant characteristics in the historical evolution of "*neuraltherapeutic thinking*," from the Colombian perspective. Some features may be outside the description or may not appear to be explicitly included in the above. This is to be expected when it comes to philosophical reflection. The approaches described here seek to enhance the comprehension of the paradigmatic evolution of Neural Therapy in Colombia,

---

[2] The political refers to the quality that emerges in every human relationship, where it is necessary to dialogue about agreements and disagreements. It is essential to clarify that politics does not refer to sympathizing or not with parties or leaders of politics. https://revistas.unab.edu.co/index.php/reflexion/article/view/749/3950

[3] [106] https://ikusmira.org/p/poiesis-poyesis; [106]

recognizing its significant epistemological potential. The aim is to give, not a homogeneous and finished view, but a dynamic and evolutionary one of a process that is alive.

Finally, recalling the definition that Dr. Payán coined for Neural Therapy around the year 2000 and that was collectively ratified in the Declaration of Colombia of 2003, with the attendees of the World Meeting of Neural Therapy and Neurofocal Dentistry that year, could offer a compact view of what is narrated here.

Dr. Payán defines neural therapy as:

> A thought and practice of a medical, social, health type, rebellious and propositional at the same time, alternative and holistic in its conception, non-hegemonic, empirical and intuitive, dialectical, [dialogical], revolutionary, humanist, singular and unrepeatable in its practice; which restores to the living being its potentialities and capacities for healing and self-eco-organization, enabling in to relate harmoniously with itself, its social community and the universe. To achieve this, it delivers non-specific impulses to targeted areas of the patient's nervous system, according to their individual history" [1, 87, 105] .

References

1. Payán de la Roche JC. Vital disobedience, vol. 1. 3rd ed. Sabadell (Catalonia): Instituto de Terapia Neural; 2016. p. 1–200.
2. Garzón Fuentes EC. Neuraltherapeutic medicine in Colombia [Internet] [Master's thesis]. Bogotá: Universidad Nacional de Colombia; 2024. Available at: https://repositorio.unal.edu.co/handle/unal/87341
3. Beltrán EH, Vega JA. Neuraltherapeutic Medicine: an approach from complex medical systems. Universidad Nacional de Colombia. Editorial Universidad Nacional de Colombia; 2013. 1–159 p.
4. Salazar Marín JI. Neural therapy: from "orthodox" therapy to Neuraltherapeutic Medicine. In: Beltrán EH, Vega JA, editors. Neuraltherapeutic medicine: an approach from complex medical systems. 1st ed. Bogotá: Universidad Nacional de Colombia; 2013. p. 15–28.
5. Salazar Marín JI. Neural therapy: from "orthodox" therapy to a complex medical system [Master's thesis]. Bogotá: Universidad Nacional de Colombia; 2010.
6. Sarmiento LD. History and institutionalization of neural therapy in Colombia [Internet]. [Master's Thesis]. Bogotá. Universidad Nacional de Colombia; 2014. Available from: http://www.bdigital.unal.edu.co/43119/1/52145193.2014.pdf
7. Urrego Mendoza DZ, Martiletti A, Casas del Rio GH, Ruiz Díaz P, Vega Oviedo A. Alternative medicine: a vision from complex medical systems. 1st ed. Urrego Mendoza DZ, Vega Oviedo JA, editors. Bogotá: Universidad Nacional de Colombia, Faculty of Medicine. Medical Rationalities and Health Practices Research Group; 2011.
8. Urrego Mendoza DZ. Approach to alternative medicine as a complex medical system at the Universidad Nacional de Colombia. Revista de la Facultad de Medicina [Internet]. 2010 [cited 2022 Aug 31];58(2):155–6. Available at: http://www.scielo.org.co/scielo.php?script=sci_arttext&pid=S0120-00112010000200007&lng=en&nrm=iso&tlng=es
9. Cerón Villaquirán E. Neuraltherapeutic medicine, or the incessant metamorphosis of an incomplete school. Essay on the critical recovery of history and reflection on a corner of the Payan School of thought, origins of a new current [Internet]. Popayán; 2023 [cited 2025 Feb 6]. Available at: https://terapianeuralcolombia.com/images/articulos_ensayos/Medicina_Neuralterapeutica_HISTORIA.pdf

10. Payán de la Roche JC. Diagnosis, critiques, and possibilities [Internet]. [cited 2024 May 26]. Available at: https://terapianeural.com/articulos/14-del-concepto/41-el-diagnostico-criticas-y-posibilidades
11. Payán de la Roche JC. Biological medicine: a commitment to life. 1st ed. Buenos Aires: Salbe Ediciones; 2006. 1–2008 p.
12. Payán de la Roche JC. Neural therapy (TN): a paradigmatic proposal [Internet]. July 23, 2010. Available at: http://www.terapianeural.com/articulos/14-del-concepto/223-julio-c-payan-de-la-r
13. Huneke F. The phenomenon in seconds or the testament of a doctor. Translated by Dr. German Duque Mejía, editor. Vol. 1–3. Popayán: Editorial Los Robles; 1961.
14. Dosch Peter. Teaching book of neural therapy according to Huneke (procaine therapy). Volume 1 Theory and practice. Haug-Karl F. Haug, editor. Popayán: Los Robles; 1973.
15. Dosch P. Textbook of neural therapy according to Huneke (therapy with local anesthetics). 8th ed. Heidelberg: Haug Verlag; 1978.
16. Rodríguez Arias DC. British Nervism: comparative analysis of a trend in the history of medicine centered on the nervous system [Master's Thesis]. Bogotá: Universidad Nacional de Colombia; 2021.
17. Pinilla-Bonilla LB, Rodríguez DC, Villamil-Villar WA. British and Russian Nervism: a comparison between two trends in the history of medicine focused on the nervous system. MED UIS. 2024;37(1):33–40. https://doi.org/10.18273/revmed.v37n1-2024003.
18. Ariza Tarazona JS. Descriptive study of Henry Head's semiological contributions to neural therapeutic medicine: clinical cases. Monograph [Monograph presented as a partial requirement for the Master's degree in alternative medicine with emphasis on neural therapy]. Bogotá: Universidad Nacional de Colombia; 2017.
19. Navarro K, Pinilla L. The contributions of Henry Head to neuroanatomical and physiological bases of therapy segment. MÉD UIS. 2013;26(2):33–44. Available at: https://revistas.uis.edu.co/index.php/revistamedicasuis/article/view/3919
20. Mackenzie J. Symptoms and their interpretation. Vol 1. 4th ed. London: Shaw & Sons, 7 & 8, Fetter Lane; 1920.
21. Mackenzie J. Some points bearing on the association of sensory disorders and visceral disease. Brain [Internet]. 1893 [cited 2025 Feb 3];16(3):321–54. https://doi.org/10.1093/brain/16.3.321.
22. Wancura-Kampik I. Segmental anatomy. 1st ed. Munich: Elsevier Urban & Fisher Verlag; 2009.
23. Wancura-Kampik I. Segmentary anatomy – segmentary acupuncture. Revista Internacional de Acupuntura [Internet]. 2010 [cited 2025 Mar 3];70–4. Available at: https://www.elsevier.es/es-revista-revista-internacional-acupuntura-279-pdf-S1887836910700193
24. Mackenzie J. Remarks on the meaning and mechanism of visceral pain as shown by the study of visceral and other sympathetic (autonomic) reflexes. Br Med J [Internet]. 1906 [cited 2025 Mar 3];1(2374):1523. Available at: https://pmc.ncbi.nlm.nih.gov/articles/PMC2382104/
25. Head H. On disturbances of sensation with special reference to the pain of visceral disease. Brain [Internet]. 1893 [cited 2025 Mar 3];16(1–2):1–133. https://doi.org/10.1093/brain/16.1-2.1.
26. Head H. On disturbances of sensation with special reference to the pain of visceral disease: part II. Head and neck. Brain [Internet]. 1894 [cited 2025 Mar 3];17(3):339–480. https://doi.org/10.1093/brain/17.3.339.
27. Ricker G. Pathology as natural science – relational pathology. Berlin: Springer; 1924.
28. Pischinger A. The extracellular matrix and ground regulation: basis for a holistic biological medicine. North Atlantic Books; 2007.
29. Wiener N. Cybernetics and society. 3rd ed. Buenos Aires: Editorial Sudamericana; 1988. 181 p.
30. Von Foerster H. The seeds of cybernetics. Barcelona: Gedisa Editorial; 1991.

31. Payán de la Roche JC. General bases of biocybernetics applied to neural therapy [Internet]. [cited 2025 Feb 3]. Available at: https://www.terapianeural.com/publicaciones/16-articulos-y-publicaciones/de-las-teorias/125-bases-generales-de-la-biocibernetica-aplicadas-a-la-terapia-neural
32. Fisher L. Neural therapy according to Huneke; neurophysiology, therapeutic injection techniques. 3rd ed. Niño Ibarra MC, editor. Vol. 1. México; 2012. 1–261 p.
33. Rivera Rojas F. Medicine of Biocybernetic Regulations: Neuraltherapy. [Internet]. Asociacion Medicinas Complementarias; 1992 [cited 2025 Feb 3]. 1–170 p. Available at: https://www.iberlibro.com/9788488346018/Medicina-regulaciones-biociberneticas-neuralterapia-8488346018/plp
34. Payán de la Roche JC. 2nd Congress of neural therapy. In: Asociación de médicos y odontólogos de terapia biorregulativa AC. Popayán; 1994. p 1–55.
35. Fundación Para la Comunicación Popular FUNCOP, Centro de Información e Investigación sobre medicinas alternativas CIMA. Medicine, Ecology and Society: Critical Bases for Alternative Thinking. In: II National Colloquium on Alternative Medicines and Society 1990. Popayán: Ediciones FUNCOP; 1991.
36. Wilches Chaux G. (218) Health: an alternative vision (FUNCOP 1990) – YouTube [Internet]. 1990 [cited 2024 May 17]. Available at: https://www.youtube.com/watch?v=-pbjzaXZ6qU&ab_channel=GustavoWilches-Chaux
37. Wilches G. From the manual for a new user of planet earth. In: Medicine, ecology, and society critical bases for alternative thinking / II National Colloquium of Alternative Medicines and society 1990. Ediciones FUNCOP; 1991. p. 66–77.
38. Cerón Villaquirán E. Participatory action research and Neuraltherapeutic medicine [Internet]. 2023 [cited 2024 Jun 23]. Available at: https://www.terapianeuralcolombia.com/images/articulos_ensayos/investigacion-accion-participante-y-medicina-neuralterapeutica.pdf
39. Cerón Villaquirán E. From Dialogue of knowledge to dialogue of ignorances. Reflections to Politicize pedagogical action and Pedagogize political action* [Internet]. Bogotá; 2011 [cited 2024 May 18]. Available from: http://www.sustentabilidades.usach.cl/sites/sustentable/files/paginas/04-03.pdf
40. Andrade LE. Hegemonic Science and Epistemic Plurality. Revista Universidad Nacional de Colombia [Internet]. 2023 [cited 2025 Feb 27];2(5). Available at: https://revista.unal.edu.co/detalle/ciencia-hegemonica-y-pluralidad-epistemica
41. Schnitman DF. New paradigms, culture, and subjectivity [Internet]. Buenos Aires: Paidos; 1994 [cited 2024 Jul 23]. 5–463 p. Available at: https://www.academia.edu/54346557/Nuevos_paradigmas_cultura_y_subjetividad
42. Cerón Villaquirán E. From vital disobedience to epistemic disobedience – essay on theoretical biology and health. Popayán: Ediciones Popayán Positiva; 2018. 7–89 p.
43. Cerón Villaquirán E. Jump into the void, your wings will spread. Another epistemological view of health. In new epistemic approaches for research. Revista Red Pensar [Internet]. 2012 [cited 2025 Mar 3];1(2):43–55. Available at: https://editorialparmenia.com.mx/media/wysiwyg/pdf/REDpensar7.pdf
44. Barop H. Bases of neural therapy according to Huneke: Ricker's relational pathology. In: International meeting of neural therapy [Internet]; 2000. Available at: http://terapianeural.com/publicaciones/15-articulos-y-publicaciones/bases-clasicas/60-bases-de-la-terapia-neural-la-patologia-relacional-de-ricker
45. Andrade LE. In: Biologia D, editor. The demons of Darwin. Semiotics and thermodynamics of biological evolution. 2nd ed. Universidad Nacional de Colombia; 2003.
46. Lombardi O. Shannon's information: theoretical basis, conceptual articulations, and interpretations. 2020 [cited 2025 Feb 7]; Available at: http://www.apeironestudiosdefilosofia.com/
47. Shannon CE, Weaver W. The mathematical theory of communication [Internet]. The University of Illinois Press, Urbana; 1964 [cited 2025 Mar 3]. 1–125 p. Available at: https://monoskop.org/images/b/be/Shannon_Claude_E_Weaver_Warren_The_Mathematical_Theory_of_Communication_1963.pdf

48. Ramírez F, Balbín OA. Biologists Far from Equilibrium: New Evolutionary Metaphors of Theoretical Biology G, editor. Universidad Nacional de Colombia; 2004.
49. Goodwin B. The leopard spots: the evolution of complexity. Barcelona: Tusquets Editores S.A; 1998. p. 1–308.
50. Margulis L, Sagan D. Microcosmos. Four billion years of evolution from our microbial ancestors. [Internet]. 1st ed. Vol. 1. Barcelona: Tusquets Editores S.A.; 1995 [cited 2025 Mar 3]. 6–313 p. Available at: https://ia802803.us.archive.org/15/items/lynnmargulisdorionsaganmicrocosmosbiologyrepubblicanesimogeopoliticoteoriaendosi/Lynn%20Margulis%20Dorion%20Sagan%20Microcosmos%20Biology%20Repubblicanesimo%20Geopolitico%20Teoria%20endosimbiotica%20Massimo%20Morigi%20neomarxismo.pdf
51. Capra F. The Tao of Physics. 3rd ed. Málaga: Sirio; 2000. 480 p.
52. Hameroff S, Penrose R. Consciousness in the universe: a review of the "Orch OR" theory. Phys Life Rev. 2014;11(1):39–78. https://doi.org/10.1016/j.plrev.2013.08.002.
53. Cruz Y, Fayad R. Microtubules and neural therapy: proposal for a promising investigation. Rev Med. 2011;19(1):82–92. https://doi.org/10.18359/rmed.1228.
54. Hameroff S, Nip A, Porter M, Tuszynski J. Conduction pathways in microtubules, biological quantum computation, and consciousness. Biosystems. 2002;64(1–3):149–68. https://doi.org/10.1016/s0303-2647(01)00183-6.
55. Hameroff S, Penrose R. Orchestrated reduction of quantum coherence in brain microtubules: a model for consciousness. Math Comput Simul. 1996;40(3–4):453–80. https://doi.org/10.1016/0378-4754(96)80476-9.
56. Beltrán Dussán EH. Neuraltherapeutic medicine. Academic training based on competencies [Master's Thesis]. Bogotá: Universidad Nacional de Colombia; 2013 [cited 2025 Feb 17]. Available at: https://repositorio.unal.edu.co/handle/unal/21635
57. Payán de la Roche JC. Biological medicine: a non-compromised medicine. 1st ed. Bogotá: Ediciones AMO; 1986. 1–268 p.
58. Kineman JJ, Kumar KA. Primary natural relationship: Bateson, Rosen, and the Vedas. Kybernetes. 2007;36(7–8):1055–69. Available at: https://www.emerald.com/insight/content/doi/10.1108/03684920710777838/full/html
59. Garzón Fuentes EC. Neuraltherapeutic medicine. Contributions from alternative medicines in the perspective of decolonial knowledge. In: Pachamama, wisdom and territories: supporting the Pluriverse with the Llauto of our ancestors [Internet]. Cali; 2022 [cited 2024 Jun 19]. Available at: https://terapianeuralcolombia.com/publicaciones-articulos/articulos
60. Wilber K. Quantum issues. Mystical writings of the world's most famous physicists. duocédima. Wilber K, editor. Barcelona: Kairós; 2011. 1–317 p.
61. Toscano de La Torre F, Pinilla Bonilla LB. The principles of neural therapy from the foundations of nervousness to current neuroscience. Salud UIS J [Internet]. 2012;44(2):57–65. Available at: http://www.scielo.org.co/scielo.php?script=sci_arttext&pid=S0121-08072012000200008
62. Pinilla-Bonilla LB. Critical analysis of the theoretical-methodological procedures in the researches of A. D. Speransky supporting neural therapy from Peircean logic [Master's Thesis]. Bogotá: Universidad Nacional de Colombia; 2010. 119 p. Available at: https://repositorio.unal.edu.co/handle/unal/6873
63. Speransky AD. Foundations for a new theory of medicine. Vol. 1. Buenos Aires: Psique Editorial; 1954. 7–507 p.
64. Bykov K, Konradi G. Fundamental concepts of physiology. In: Bykov KM, editor. Text-book of physiology. Moscow: Foreign Languages Publishing House; 1960. p. 15–45.
65. Andrade Pérez LE. The informational perspective in the philosophy of nature. El Bosque University; National University of Colombia; 2022. 1–434 p.
66. Cardozo AM, Pinilla Bonilla LB, Andrade E. Rethinking the concept of illness from evolution and emergence. In: Beltrán Dussán EH, Vega Oviedo JA, editors. Neural herapeutic medicine: an approach from complex medical systems. Bogotá: Faculty of Medicine, National University of Colombia; 2013. p. 73–82.

67. Cardozo Pabón AM. Illness as an evolutionary and emergent process. [Internet] [Master's Thesis]. Bogotá: National University of Colombia; 2011 [cited 2024 Jul 25]. Available at: https://repositorio.unal.edu.co/handle/unal/20508
68. Gell-Mann M. The quark and the jaguar: adventures in the simple to complex. Barcelona: Tusquets Editors; 1994. p. 346.
69. Soberanes Arauz MA, Mo. Edgar Morin and complex thinking. In: XXVII Congress of the Latin American Sociological Association VIII sociology days of the University of Buenos Aires, Latin American Sociological Association, Buenos Aires [Internet]. Buenos Aires; 2009 [cited 2025 Feb 25]. p. 1–16. Available at: https://www.aacademica.org/000-062/1134
70. Morin E. Introduction to complex thinking. 1st ed. Vol. 1. Barcelona: Gedisa; 2011. 1–176 p.
71. Maldonado CE. Complexity as indeterminacy . Philosophy Journal of the University of Costa Rica [Internet]. 2024 [cited 2025 Feb 24];LXIII(167):19–1. Available at: https://revistas.ucr.ac.cr/index.php/filosofia/article/view/59257/62787
72. Maldonado CE, Gómez Cruz NA. The world of complexity sciences: a state of the art. Research document No. 76. Bogotá: Editorial Universidad del Rosario; 2010. 1–96 p.
73. Beltrán Bermúdez C. The world of complexity sciences. Innovar [Internet]. 2012 [cited 2025 Mar 3];22(45):157–9. Available at: http://www.scielo.org.co/scielo.php?script=sci_arttext&pid=S0121-50512012000300014&lng=en&nrm=iso&tlng=es
74. Maldonado CE. Information theory and complexity. The third scientific revolution. 1st ed. Gallego Cataño MA, editor. Vol. 4. Bogotá: Editorial Universidad del Bosque; 2020. 4–127 p.
75. Fischer L. Basis of neural therapy. Self-organization in biology [Internet]. [cited 2025 Mar 1]. Available at: https://www.terapianeural.com/articulos/16-de-las-teorias/74-bases-de-la-terapia-neural-autoorganizacion-en-la-biologia
76. Kauffman SA. Investigations: Complexity, self-organization, and new laws for a general biology [Internet]. Tusquets, editor. Tusquets Editores; 2003.
77. Kauffman SA. The origins of order: self-organization and selection in evolution [Internet]. New York: Oxford University Press; 1993. Available at: https://books.google.com.co/books?id=j7mq5QNszLwC
78. Prigogine I. The end of certainties. 5th ed. Santiago de Chile: Editorial Andrés Bello; 1997. 227 p.
79. Prigogine I. Just an illusion? Barcelona: Tusquets Editores; 1972.
80. Torres JLM. Currents of complexity: convergences and divergences. Eidos. 2020;32:359–85.
81. Cendales L, Mejía MR, Muñoz J. Pedagogies and methodologies of popular education "The road is made by walking." Vol. 1. Bogotá: Ediciones desde abajo; 2016. 1–250 p.
82. Figueiredo G d O. Participatory action research: an alternative for social epistemology in Latin America. Res J 86. 2015;39:1–20.
83. Ortiz M, Borjas B. Participatory action research: Fals Borda's contribution to popular education. Espacio abierto Venezuelan Sociol J [Internet]. 2008 [cited 2024 May 23];17(4):615–27. Available at: https://www.redalyc.org/pdf/122/12217404.pdf
84. Eljach M, Corredor CE, Jaramillo Salgado D, Rosero Morales JR. Fals Borda and the persistence of utopias. Popayán: Editorial Universidad del Cauca; 2009. 9–141 p.
85. Chárriez Cordero M. Life stories: a qualitative research methodology. Griot J Univ Puerto Rico. 2012;5(I):50–67.
86. Cotán Fernández A. Research-participation and life stories, the same path. In: III Conference on Life Stories in Education. University of Seville; 2012.
87. ACOLTEN/MNT, CONETSO JCP. Neural Therapy/Neural Therapeutic Medicine (MNT) in the context of the pandemic [Internet]. 2020. 84 p. Available at: https://acolten.com.co/wp-content/uploads/2020/07/LA-TERAPIA-NEURAL-MEDICINA-NEURALTERAPEUTICA-MNT-EN-CONTEXTO-DE-PANDEMIA_compressed.pdf
88. Gallego Jiménez JA. Possible effect of procaine as a neuraltherapeutic in the human erythrocyte membrane in vitro. [Internet]. [Master's Thesis]. Bogotá: National University of Colombia, Faculty of Medicine; 2010. https://repositorio.unal.edu.co/handle/unal/6838

89. Vischñevsky AV, Vischñevsky AD. Novocain blockade and oleo-balsamic antiseptics as a form of pathogenic therapeutics. Buenos Aires: Cartago; 1958.
90. Wilches-Chaux G. Tools for the crisis: disasters, environmentalism, and professional training. SENA. National Learning Service. Popayán: National Learning Service. SENA; 1989.
91. Wilches-Chaux G. At the edge of chaos [Internet]. Pensar, Institute of Social and Cultural Studies; 2000. 136 p. Available at: https://books.google.com.pe/books?id=SXu6AAAAIAAJ
92. Garzón Fuentes EC. Tribute to Dr. Julio César Payán De la Roche [Internet]. Terapianeural.com; 2017. Available at: http://www.terapianeural.com/articulos/20-y-mas/383-homenaje-al-dr-julio-cesar-payan-de-la-roche
93. EL PAIS. Ilya Prigogine, Nobel prize in chemistry and father of the "Theory of Chaos." EL PAIS Necrological Agenda [Internet]. 2003 [cited 2024 Jul 23]; Available at: https://elpais.com/diario/2003/05/29/agenda/1054159209_850215.html?event=go&event_log=go&prod=REGCRARTGENTE&o=cerrgente
94. Prigogine I, Stengers I. The new alliance. Metamorphosis of science [Internet]. 2nd ed. Madrid: Alianza Casa Editorial; 2004 [cited 2025 Mar 2]. 1–360 p. Available at: https://archive.org/details/prigogine-stengers.-la-nueva-alianza.-metamorfosis-de-la-ciencia-2004
95. Von Bertalanffy L. General systems theory. Fundamentals, development, and applications [Internet]. 7th ed. Mexico: Fondo de Cultura Económico; 1989. Available at: https://cienciasyparadigmas.files.wordpress.com/2012/06/teoria-general-de-los-sistemas-_-fundamentos-desarrollo-aplicacionesludwig-von-bertalanffy.pdf
96. Barberousse P. Theoretical foundations of Edgar Morin's complex thinking. Educare Electron J. 2008;12(2):95–113.
97. Kühn TS. The structure of scientific revolutions. 1st ed. Mexico City: Fondo de Cultura Económico; 1996.
98. Espinoza Verdejo Alex. The philosophical turn in Thomas Kuhn's thought on the incommensurability of scientific theories. Interciencia [Internet]. 2019 [cited 2024 Feb 23];44(11):653–9. Available at: https://www.redalyc.org/articulo.oa?id=33962174008
99. Bird A. The philosophy of the history of science of Thomas Kuhn. Discusiones Filosóficas. 2012;13(21):167–85.
100. Kuhn TS. The structure of scientific revolutions. 2nd ed. Mexico City: Fondo de Cultura Económico; 2004.
101. Aguilar MT. Descartes and the machine body. Pensamiento [Internet]. 2010 [cited 2025 Feb 26];66(249):755–70. Available at: https://revistas.comillas.edu/index.php/pensamiento/article/view/2491/2192
102. Varela F, Maturana H, Uribe R. Autopoiesis: the organization of living systems, its characterization and a model, Biosystems, vol. 5; 1974. p. 187–96.
103. Maturana H, Varela F. Of machines and living beings: Autopoiesis, the organization of the living. 5th ed. Chile:Editorial Universitaria; 1994. 71 p.
104. Herrero Uribe L. From mechanism to complexity in biology. Rev Biol Trop [Internet]. 2008 [cited 2025 Feb 7];56(1):399–407. Available at: http://www.scielo.sa.cr/scielo.php?script=sci_arttext&pid=S0034-77442008000100030&lng=en&nrm=iso&tlng=es
105. Declaration Colombia. In: World meeting of neural therapy and neurofocal dentistry [Internet]. 2003 [cited 2024 May 21]. Available at: https://acolten.com.co/publicaciones/https://terapianeuralcolombia.com/publicaciones-articulos/articulos
106. Zambrano Unda HM. The notions of Poiesis, praxis, and techné in artistic production. 2019 [cited 2025 Mar 4];7:40–6. https://doi.org/10.26807/cav.v0i07.221

Chapter 19
Disease as a Vital Process

Margarita Santamaría

1 Introduction

Michael Faraday (1791–1867), an English scientist, was 48 years old when a health event forced him to take a break from his career begun at a young age [1]. According to the notes of his doctor, Peter Mere Latham (1780–1875) had symptoms that consisted of headache, memory loss, and vertigo; in the physical examination, the doctor only documented a slight strabismus in the right eye. Being a character of profound importance in the development of different scientific disciplines, the ailments manifested by Faraday sparked interest from doctors and biographers in the rise of positivist medicine, as they attempted to provide a causal explanation for the suffering of this English scientist.

Alfred Stock (1876–1946), a German chemist, attributed the symptoms presented by Michael Faraday to mercury poisoning in 1925 [2]; previously, in 1915, other investigators suggested that the symptoms were secondary to cerebral atherosclerosis. This argument was based on the observations made by the neurologist Henry Bence Jones on transient ischemic attacks in the territory of the vertebrobasilar artery [2]. In 1973 [3], psychiatrist Edward Hare proposed amnesic syndrome as an explanation for memory complaints by reviewing letters sent by Faraday. Oppenheim [4] in 1991 attributed his afflictions to a possible depressive condition, and Larner [1] in 2021 proposed a Functional Cognitive Disorder (FCD) as an explanation for the clinical picture (FCD-).

Historical and medical debates on the clinical picture of the English scientist allow us to establish how the concepts of disease are mobile and dependent on the historical, economic, and cultural context in which they develop. The concept of disease obeys the purposes proposed to the therapeutic act; that is, if the concept of

M. Santamaría (✉)
Faculty of Medicine, Universidad Nacional de Colombia, Bogotá, Colombia
e-mail: sesantam@unal.edu.co

L. B. Pinilla Bonilla et al. (eds.), *Neuraltherapeutic Medicine*,
https://doi.org/10.1007/978-3-032-03257-7_19

disease consists of the alteration of a physiological (or pathological) variable, then the treatment will focus on fixing this particular variable. Conversely, if the perception of a disease aligns with the understanding of the individual undergoing treatment, it cannot align with the normalization of a specific variable but rather with the complexity of the individual seeking assistance.

Placing a goal on the medical act can change the notion of transforming the patient into the sum of their organs and functions, placing their biographical process at the center, and acting accordingly. "We need a concept of disease in order to decide who is entitled to treatment and to economic rights, who is to be exempted from social duties and who is morally accountable, and to decide what is the subject matter of medical science. Furthermore, a strictly, consistently, and coherently defined concept of disease could help the health care system face its basic economic, social, epistemological and ethical challenges, and could clarify the goal and limit of medicine" [5].

Neuraltherapeutic medicine places the suffering person at the center of its theoretical and practical reflections; its concept of disease incorporates a vital, complex, dynamic, and emergent approach to suffering. In this sense, the biographical account narrates the process of becoming ill and comes to life as a comprehensive rather than an explanatory model of the pathology.

2 Visions of the Concept of Disease

Different conceptions of disease have influenced the treatment decisions for human suffering or pain throughout the history of medicine. The concept of disease seems too obvious since it is easy to differentiate a sick person from a healthy one at first glance; however, the definition of disease turns out to be more complicated and debatable. For example, is it valid to say that a person who has a gene associated with Alzheimer's disease is sick? Should someone with a cholesterol of 250 mg/ml be considered sicker than someone with a cholesterol of 199 mg/ml, solely based on the definition of dyslipidemia? When efforts and resources are based on individual and collective health, the vicissitudes of medical knowledge do not prove to be futile. Focusing on variables in the therapeutic effort can lead to the disaggregation of a patient into systems and organs with multiple pathologies, depending on the thoroughness of their examination. This can result in the patient leaving the consultation with a list of multiple medications, some of which have contradictory therapeutic or adverse effects. From this perspective, clinical judgment focuses on accurately labeling the disease and, as Foucault suggests, places the patient in parentheses [6] .

Two general visions of disease can be defined throughout history; on the one hand, disease is conceived as an external entity that lands on people, causing havoc, and therefore, as an enemy, it must be attacked by all means. On the other hand, the second view proposes to observe the disease as a process of the interaction of the organism with the internal and external environment; it is not passive in the face of the information it receives but is an agent in constant relationship with itself, other people, and what surrounds it. At present, the first vision of the disease is led by the biomedical model; the second vision is under construction and is proposed from neuraltherapeutic medicine.

The biomedical model posits a comprehensive understanding of the world through reductionism, drawing inspiration from classical physics. As the first characteristic of the biomedical model, reductionism proposes the analysis of the whole from the sum of its parts, thereby composing the upper levels in the hierarchy from the sum of the lower ones. Thus, societies comprise minds and bodies, which in turn comprise systems, organs, tissues, cells, and genes. Disease is then understood as the compound of abnormal functions at the microscopic and molecular level, which can be treated through pharmacological interventions.

This vision, guided by an analytical epistemology, has carried out a microscopic analysis that has made the human genome known in detail, unraveling molecular mechanisms of multiple pathologies. The paradox is that despite the enormous techno-scientific advance in medicine, humanity is facing a pandemic of chronic conditions (obesity, diabetes mellitus, hypertension, etc.) [7]. The belief that the whole is the sum of its parts has resulted in the nebulous and routinely invisible interrelationships at both the microscopic and macroscopic levels. Biomedicine has made progress in reducing mortality; this is an undeniable fact; however, it generates doubts about the quality of life of patients whose existence is medically prolonged.

Recognized in the United Kingdom, oncologist D.W. Smithers exposes the flaws in the definitions of cancer as a cellular disease. Using an organicist and systemic approach, he illustrates the risks associated with reductionism in cancer research and medical practice through an analogy: "A lifetime of study of the internal-combustion engine would not help anyone to understand our traffic problems. The causes of congestion can be many. A traffic jam is due to a failure of the normal relationship between driven cars and their environment and can occur whether they themselves are running normally or not" [8] .

The second characteristic of the biomedical model is the medicalization of society, which corresponds to the treatment of existential and vital events as medical issues. Initially, a sanitary halo surrounded birth, disregarding the advancements in maternal mortality, appropriating ancestral and natural female labor, and placing it under the control of male doctors. The recognition of the practice of reifying birth has led in recent decades to promoting humanized childbirth as a strategy to place pregnant people at the center of the vital process of birth [9]. Death, the ultimate event of all living beings, has also migrated to hospital institutions; the farewells generated by rites of passage and the acceptance of human finitude have become cloistered in clinics, and even more isolated in Intensive Care Units. Of course, deaths can be avoided, and the hospital institutions since the seventeenth century ceased to be the place where one did not come out alive—hospices—to become centers of "cure of diseases" from which, sometimes, you can walk out [6–10].

The third characteristic of the biomedical model's conception of disease is dualism, which refers to the separation of mind and body. The foundation of dualistic thinking in medical science was provided by the French philosopher Rene Descartes (1595–1650), who, by identifying the human body as a knowable object, extracts it from the power of the medieval church. This view points to the materiality of the body along with the possibility of studying it as an object, while the mind is composed of the thinking substance—the soul. For Descartes, the body has an extensive substance; it is in a place in space and does not require that there be thinking beings around it. Conversely, the mind requires thought to exist, making it intangible, ethereal, and lacking a fixed location in space [11]. Nonetheless, the progenitor of dualism possessed a considerably more intricate perspective compared to his adherents from nearly four centuries after his birth. His correspondence with Princess Elizabeth of Bohemia reveals her inquiry into the process by which the soul interfaces with the body, enabling the activation of its constituent elements. Descartes' unpersuasive elucidation drew a comparison between the intangibility of gravity and its ability to move objects [12].

The Cartesian approaches granted knowledge of the body to men outside of religious mandates, but they also initiated the dissociation between mental and physical illnesses prevalent until then in conventional medicine. This vision generates a schism between the diseases of the body and indifference to the experience of suffering, as well as the impact of illness on the social and cultural life of individuals. In another sense, it disdains interventions that do not pass through the physical body and that can be effective in alleviating suffering [13].

The epistemological model of biomedicine separates the body from the mind, assigns the mind to psychologists, and treats the body, or soma, as the object of medicine. This dualistic vision is one of the fundamental characteristics of the biomedical model that forms a schism with the vision of mind–body unity of other non-hegemonic medical models [14].

The separation of subject and object, the fourth characteristic of the biomedical model, positions the sick person as a passive recipient of the interventions performed on his or her body; the disease becomes the object of medicine and the exclusive task of medical technology, while the person suffering becomes the recipient of the treatments. The health professional exercises authority in the doctor–patient relationship, which is vertical. This relationship synthesizes the other characteristics of biomedicine in its therapeutic potential; diluting the patient into isolated organs fragments their biography, eliminates their potential as an agent or interlocutor, and reveals only a set of organs that respond positively to statistical normality [15].

Francis Peabody's classic 1927 article [16] highlights society's urgent call to humanize medicine, emphasizing the need to care for sick people rather than diseases. This fragmentation of care has led medicine to have a technocratic vision of the organs isolated from the life experience of those who suffer and to prioritize compliance with protocols and guidelines over the singular care of individuals, families, and communities .

The fifth characteristic of the biomedical model is its observation of the environment as a risk factor for disease, drawing a distinction between environmental care and human health care. Capitalism views the environment as an input for industry, serving as a supplier of raw materials for human use, with the only constraint being the availability of its resources. In biomedicine, nature assumes a dominant role, with viruses, bacteria, fungi, or animals posing a threat to human health. The focus is on the environment's detrimental impact on human survival, associating human-produced pollution with vector-borne diseases. Clinical trials uncover therapeutic technologies in pharmaceutical laboratories; modern scientific discourse discards nature, labeling those who utilize it as at best pre-modern. This vision has placed the possibility of healing people solely in the hands of the big pharmaceutical industries, and from there it has promoted its paradigm of normal science, as Kuhn has said [17] .

3 Disease as a Vital Process

Engel [18] proposed a new biopsychosocial model in 1977, which aims to contextualize the patient's suffering beyond the altered organic conditions. In his classic article, Engel states: "The existing biomedical model does not suffice. To provide a basis for understanding the determinants of disease and arriving at rational treatments and patterns of health care, a medical model must also take into account the patient, the social context in which he [sic] lives, and the complementary system devised by society to deal with the disruptive effects of illness, that is, the physician role and the health care system. This requires a biopsychosocial model" [18, p.132].

Critics have questioned the implementation of this model. One criticism stems from the fact that the body–mind dualism persists as distinct entities, with various disciplines intervening in it. This approach maintains a biomedical perspective in medicine, which other disciplines like social work or psychology complement [19]. Furthermore, despite attempts to rectify this with multidisciplinary teams, the care of the individual patient remains fragmented, with the clinical-doctor–patient encounter still rooted in a vision that maintains the division into organs and parts, body and mind. Biographical and emotional data continue to be secondary adjuncts in people's experience of getting sick [19].

As previously discussed, biomedicine considers disease as an external entity that settles upon the helpless individual and wreaks havoc upon them. Neurotherapeutic medicine departs from this conception of disease, emphasizing the person who suffers as the protagonist of a process they have constructed from their life experience. This conceptual construction emphasizes the importance of the suffering subject, their narrative within the experience of illness, and the possibility of change. For neuraltherapeutics medicine, it is not possible to place a label as an unchangeable diagnosis since the process of falling ill is dynamic, indeterminate, and above all, unique to each person seeking help. Julio César Payán (see Chap. 3) [20] summarizes the vision of neuraltherapeutics medicine as follows: Disease, then, is not the opposite of health, but the vital process through which that being, composed of mind and body as a whole, seeks and maintains its own harmony with itself and with its environment [9, p. 17].

The discursive theme of the war against diseases changes, as it is not a fight against the external enemy; on the contrary, the proposal is to reflect on the process that has generated the symptoms and discomfort in the individual. A specific disease diagnosis does not define the person suffering; their identity process undergoes modification, and the disease serves as a reminder of the fragility of organisms [21]. According to Payán: "The disease is then interpreted as a vital event, as an individual adaptive process, and not as something external to the organism itself." It could be argued that the process of falling ill represents the way an organism resolves its conflicts at a specific moment. Logically, the role of the doctor and the patient is to seek the causes of the conflict, and they cannot be satisfied with merely silencing the way the being is expressing it. Thus, infections, bacteria, and viruses reflect that conflict, not cause it [9, p. 17]. Speransky, a Russian physiologist and disciple of Pavlov, demonstrated how the prior state of the organism (its nervous system) determined infection by various microorganisms, proposing that, contrary to the traditionally accepted view, microorganisms mostly could act as indicators of an underlying process and are not always the initiators of a pathological process [22].

The construction of knowledge about the human being in the process of becoming ill is nourished by the approach of complex systems, taking into account the concepts of nonlinear dynamics, evolution, and emergence; different from the biomedical paradigm for which the disease is determined, analyzed, and treated from a cause–effect relationship. Cardozo's research [23] illustrates, using the Peircean logic methodology, the concepts of evolution and emergence in neuraltherapeutic medicine. It emphasizes that a disease is a process that encompasses both 'functional novelty, irreducibility, and the organism as a whole', as well as structural novelty, irreversibility, and the ability to acquire habits' [23]. The interrelations and experiences (i.e., information) that organisms possess during illness produce multiple options, positioning them in a nonlinear dynamic [24]. Linear dynamics proposes predictable trajectories, with a cause–effect relationship and proportionality between the input and output magnitude in a given phenomenon. In the biomedical paradigm, a linear relationship is evident, which follows the sequence: etiological agent/risk factor – diagnosis – medication – cure. On the contrary, nonlinear dynamics shows us that in complex systems, small changes produce unexpected, unpredictable, and large effects [24, 25]. Biomedicine has recognized these processes of nonlinear dynamics in neural networks [26, 27], cardiovascular systems [28], and respiratory systems [29, 30].

Systems with linear dynamics have fixed, well-defined boundaries; for example, it's not a problem to know what is and isn't part of a car. Complex systems often have blurred boundaries. An item's membership in a given system is subject to change, and an agent can be a member of multiple systems at the same time. This can complicate problem-solving and lead to unexpected actions in response to change [25]. In conventional medicine, this complexity has been observed in the treatment of chronic diseases, which cannot be reduced to pharmacological interventions given the multiplicity of elements that come together in their treatment [31]; other examples can be found in the recent medical literature on cancer or sepsis [32–35].

By synthesizing classical mechanics and linear dynamics, we can compare the human body to a clockwork mechanism, where each part is clearly defined and distinguishable from the others. On the other hand, biological systems exhibit nonlinear dynamics, possess diffuse boundaries, and allow an element to be part of multiple systems simultaneously, such as connective tissue. Consequently, even minor changes in the initial conditions of an organism can lead to unpredictable and significant consequences.

Individual elements, free to act in unpredictable ways, form complex adaptive systems; their interconnected actions can alter the context for other elements [36]. The human body is made up of a network of elements in constant exchange of information; an example can be observed when the nervous system receives information about the amount of food and responds with the feeling of satiety, emitting neurotransmitters interacting with the endocrine system (e.g., leptin) and, through feedback loops, also shaping eating behaviors.

4 Experience of the Process of Getting Sick

Faraday's history reveals that his ailments did not fully align with the hypotheses proposed for his illness; there was no certainty of his exposure to toxic levels of mercury, nor did he meet all the parameters of mercury poisoning. The progressive deterioration of cerebrovascular disease did not support the hypothesis, as Faraday continued to be productive in the field of electromagnetism many years later. These challenges in medicine illustrate how disease processes behave as complex adaptive systems, with interconnected elements that have the freedom to act in different ways, leading to unpredictable outcomes.

Concepts about the disease or its process are valuable when they contribute to the treatment of individuals. This understanding has as its starting point the identification that those who experience the disease cannot be equated to defective cars that go to the mechanic for repairs. Because humans are more than organs, medicine cannot be reduced to biological vision alone [37, 38]. When a living being falls ill, it impacts and influences them on various levels that extend beyond their physical form, including families, communities, societies, cultures, the environment, and the cosmos.

Observing only the quantitative dimensions of a human being can lead to mechanistic reductionism. To understand (more than explain) human illness and suffering, the qualitative dimension must be incorporated. Edmund Pellegrino, an American philosopher, highlights this point: "Medicine is the most humane science, the most empirical of arts, and the most scientific humanities" [39]. Understanding the suffering of a disease in order to treat it is, above all, a profound philosophical reflection that pertains to the practice of medicine.

Neuraltherapeutic medicine explores phenomenology as a way of understanding the process of becoming ill. Anatomical and physiological knowledge, as well as the biographical process and people's lives, nourish it. This perspective alters the perception of disease as a dysfunction, situating it within the historical, social, political, and cultural framework. For neuraltherapeutic medicine, the process of getting sick offers the possibility of observing life differently and acting in different ways with oneself and others [21].

Illness is not opposed to health but constitutes a *continuum* of the passage of life in all spheres of the individual. For instance, persistent knee pain extends beyond issues with ligaments, muscles, or bones; it results in the inability to move, reliance on assistance for mobility, anxiety about falling, and constraints on daily activities.

This contextual view of the process of getting sick does not intend to relativize or minimize the suffering it generates in people. The therapeutic process consists of accompanying the process of getting sick, relieving suffering, and carrying out the joint search with the patient for their self-eco-organization; the collective search for good living is used. This is the main epistemic, ethical, and practical reason for neuraltherapeutic medicine.

5 Conclusions

Neuraltherapeutic medicine seeks to rescue the singularity of the human being, understanding this as the infinite contained in a finite space. Despite its foundation and nourishment in Western medicine, neuraltherapeutic medicine finds its potential in the divisions the biomedical model has created in the treatment of individuals with pathological conditions.

Neuraltherapeutic medicine, in its construction of the concept of disease, has managed to understand that the processes of disease are complex, indeterminate, and respond to nonlinear dynamics in which small interventions can cause great transformations or disturbances. Similarly, observing the diverse interrelationships that human beings surround themselves with restores medicine's humility toward the body in front of us, a body that feels, suffers, elaborates thoughts, and immerses itself in a network of family, community, political, social, cultural, and cosmic relationships. This chapter invites us to continue elaborating on the knowledge of pathological processes from diverse perspectives. These perspectives provide greater theoretical strength to accompany people's suffering, which ultimately becomes a global interrelation in the healing process of humanity.

Acknowledgment for the contributions to the conceptual and formal review to Vladimir Camilo Carrillo Guerrero, District Secretary of Education, Bogotá D.C.

References

1. Larner AJ. Michael Faraday's "loss of memory" revisited. J Hist Neurosci [Internet]. 2021 [cited 2024 Jun 7];30(2):155–62. https://doi.org/10.1080/0964704X.2020.1814978.
2. O'Biren J. Faraday's health problems. Bull Hist Chem. 1991;11:47–50.

3. Hare E. Illnesses of the past. Proc R Soc Med. 1974;67:617–8.
4. Oppenheim J. "Shattered nerves": doctors, patients, and depression in Victorian England. New York: Oxford University Press; 1991. 127 p.
5. Hoffman B. Complexity of the concept of disease as shown through rival theoretical frameworks. Theor Med Bioeth. 2001;22:211–36.
6. Foucault M. The birth of the clinic: an archaeology of medical Gaze. Buenos Aires: Siglo XXI; 1981. 304 p.
7. Vos T, Lim SS, Abbafati C, Abbas KM, Abbasi M, Abbasifard M, et al. Global burden of 369 diseases and injuries in 204 countries and territories, 1990–2019: a systematic analysis for the Global Burden of Disease Study 2019. The Lancet [Internet]. 2020;396(10258):1204–22. https://doi.org/10.1016/S0140-6736(20)30925-9
8. Smithers DW. Cancer: an attack on cytologism. The Lancet [Internet]. 1962 [cited 2024 Sep 21];279(7228):493–9. Available from: http://www.thelancet.com/article/S0140673662914757/fulltext
9. Rodríguez-Almagro J, Hernández-Martínez A, Rodríguez-Almagro D, Quirós-García JM, Martínez-Galiano JM, Gómez-Salgado J. Women's perceptions of living a traumatic childbirth experience and factors related to a birth experience. Int J Environ Res Public Health [Internet]. 2019 [cited 2024 Sep 21];16(9). Available from: /pmc/articles/PMC6539242/.
10. Flores-Pons G, Íñiguez-Rueda L. The biomedicalization of death: a review. Anales de Psicología [Internet]. 2012 [cited 2024 Sep 21];28(3):929–38. Available from: https://doi.org/10.6018/analesps.28.3.156171
11. Skirry J. Descartes, René: mind-body distinction. In: Internet encyclopedia of philosophy [Internet]. [cited 2024 Sep 20]. Available from: https://iep.utm.edu/descartes-mind-body-distinction-dualism/
12. Correll J. Descartes' dualism and its influence on [Internet]. SUURJ Seattle Univ Undergraduate Res J. 2022 [cited 2024 Sep 20];6:11. Available from: https://scholarworks.seattleu.edu/suurj
13. Duncan G. Mind-body dualism and the biopsychosocial model of pain: what did Descartes really say? J Med Philos [Internet]. 2000 [cited 2024 Sep 20];25(4):485–513. Available from: https://pubmed.ncbi.nlm.nih.gov/10916180/
14. Anjum RL, Copeland S, Rocca E. Rethinking causality, complexity and evidence for the unique patient a causehealth resource for healthcare professionals and the clinical encounter. Cham: Springer; 2020. 241 pp.
15. Canguilhem G. The normal and the pathological. Mexico: Siglo XXI; 1982. 242 p.
16. Peabody FW. The care of patient. J Am Med Assoc [Internet]. 1927;88(12):877–82. Available from: https://jamanetwork.com/journals/jama/fullarticle/245777
17. Kuhn T. The structure of scientific revolutions. Mexico: Fondo de Cultura Económica; 1971. 314 p.
18. Engel GL. The need for a new medical model: a challenge for biomedicine. Science [Internet]. 1977 [cited 2024 Aug 6];196(4286):129–36. Available from: https://pubmed.ncbi.nlm.nih.gov/847460/
19. Farre A, Rapley T. The new old (and old new) medical model: four decades navigating the biomedical and psychosocial understandings of health and illness. Healthcare (Switzerland). 2017;5(4)
20. Payan JC. Vital disobedience [Internet]. 1st ed. 2005 [cited 2024 Jul 13]. Available from: https://www.terapianeural.com/
21. Carel H. Phenomenology of illness. New York: Oxford; 2016. 248 p.
22. Speransky AD. A basis for the theory of medicine. New York: International Publishers; 1943.
23. Cardozo Pabón AM. Illness as an emergent evolutionary process [Internet] [Master's Thesis]. Bogotá: National University of Colombia; 2011 [cited 2024 Jul 25]. Available at: https://repositorio.unal.edu.co/handle/unal/20508
24. Goldberger AL. Nonlinear dynamics for clinicians: chaos theory, fractals, and complexity at the bedside. Lancet. 1996;347(9011):1312–4.

25. Plsek PE, Greenhalgh T. Complexity science: the challenge of complexity in health care. BMJ. 2001;323(7313):625. Available from: https://www.ncbi.nlm.nih.gov/pmc/articles/PMC1121189/
26. Ashwin P, Fadera M, Postlethwaite C. Network attractors and nonlinear dynamics of neural computation. Curr Opin Neurobiol. 2024;84:102818. Available from: https://www.sciencedirect.com/science/article/pii/S0959438823001435
27. Kołodziej M, Waliszewski P. Neuronal fractal dynamics. In: Di Ieva A, editor. The fractal geometry of the brain [Internet]. Cham: Springer; 2024. p. 191–201. https://doi.org/10.1007/978-3-031-47606-8_9.
28. Trzebski A, Śmietanowski M. Nonlinear dynamics of cardiovascular system in humans exposed to repetitive apneas modeling obstructive sleep apnea: aggregated time series data analysis. Auton Neurosci [Internet]. 2001;90(1–2):106–15. Available from: https://pubmed.ncbi.nlm.nih.gov/11485276/
29. Alassafi MO, Khan IR, AlGhamdi R, Aziz W, Alshdadi AA, Dessouky MM, et al. Studying dynamical characteristics of oxygen saturation variability signals using Haar Wavelet. Healthcare (Basel) [Internet]. 2023;11(16). [cited 2024 Aug 31]. Available from: https://pubmed.ncbi.nlm.nih.gov/37628478/
30. Gheorghita M, Wikner M, Cawthorn A, Oyelade T, Nemeth K, Rockenschaub P, et al. Reduced oxygen saturation entropy is associated with poor prognosis in critically ill patients with sepsis. Physiol Rep [Internet]. 2022 [cited 2024 Aug 31];10(24). Available from: https://pubmed.ncbi.nlm.nih.gov/36541282/
31. Wang Y, Xue H, Esposito L, Joyner MJ, Bar-Yam Y, Huang TTK. Applications of complex systems science in obesity and noncommunicable chronic disease research. Adv Nutr. 2014;5(5):574–7.
32. Uthamacumaran AA. A review of complex systems approaches to cancer networks. Complex Syst [Internet]. 2020 [cited 2024 Oct 10];29(4):779–835. Available from: https://arxiv.org/abs/2009.12693v4
33. Swanton C, Bernard E, Abbosh C, André F, Auwerx J, Balmain A, et al. Embracing cancer complexity: hallmarks of systemic disease. Cell [Internet]. 2024 [cited 2024 Oct 10];187(7):1589–616. Available from: http://www.cell.com/article/S0092867424001752/fulltext
34. Sloot PMA, Kampis G, Gulyás L. Advances in dynamic temporal networks: understanding the temporal dynamics of complex adaptive networks. Eur Phys J Spec Top. 2013;222(6):1287–93.
35. Schuurman AR, Sloot PMA, Wiersinga WJ, van der Poll T. Embracing complexity in sepsis. Crit Care [Internet]. 2023 [cited 2024 Oct 10];27(1):1–8. Available from: https://ccforum.biomedcentral.com/articles/10.1186/s13054-023-04374-0
36. Sturmberg JP. Health and disease are dynamic complex-adaptive states: implications for practice and research. Front Psychiatry [Internet]. 2021 29 [cited 2024 Dec 22];12. Available from: https://pubmed.ncbi.nlm.nih.gov/33854446/
37. Sturmberg JP. Evidence-based medicine – not a panacea for the problems of a complex adaptive world. J Eval Clin Pract [Internet]. 2019 [cited 2024 Dec 22];25(5):706–16. Available from: https://wiley.unalproxy.elogim.com/doi/full/10.1111/jep.13122
38. Choi W. Is it useful to understand disease through Husserl's transcendental phenomenology? Hum Soc Sci Commun [Internet]. 2024 [cited 2024 Oct 10];11(1):1–10. Available from: https://www.nature.com/articles/s41599-024-02756-5
39. Pellegrino E. Humanism and the physician. Knoxville: University of Tennessee Press; 1979. p. 248.

Part VI
Diagnostic System in Neuraltherapeutic Medicine

Chapter 20
From Medical History to Life History

Ivonne Astrid Díaz-Adarme

1 Why Life Story?

As narrated in Chap. 18, during the transformative axes of neural therapy toward neuraltherapeutic medicine (NTM), the theoretical incorporation of some disciplines caused clinical encounters with patients to undergo gradual transformations. This undoubtedly contributed to a shift in the way of approaching the patient's anamnesis and his or her medical history, the order of the same, and the inclusion of other topics necessary to understand the life of the patient, his or her environment, his or her identity, and contexts. These scenarios favored the understanding and incorporation of phenomenology [1] in the patient's narrative and, therefore, affect the clinical conceptions of the neuraltherapist for therapeutic decision-making.

As evidenced in Chap. 3, Payán de la Roche [2], almost 30 years before the concept of narrative medicine was documented [3], expresses the need to understand the nosological explanations that patients make for their diseases, framed within their socio-historical worldviews, as well as the factors that relativize the experience of their disease(s) and the tools they have used to face them. This self-reflexivity also determines a therapeutic field in itself [4].

On the other hand, neuraltherapeutic medicine, by not focusing merely on the body as a biological system and having a monistic approach [5], that is, that all physical change is related to a mental change in a synchronous way [6], requires a broad clinical analysis. This takes into account perspectives of corporeality beyond biomedical terms, where cultural inscriptions can be "mapped" [7] to highlight the clinical significance of a gender perspective [8], the different ways of inhabiting the body [9], and how these determine the social identity that generates diverse cultural forms of well-being, health, and disease.

I. A. Díaz-Adarme (✉)
Faculty of Medicine, Universidad Nacional de Colombia, Bogotá, Colombia
e-mail: iadiaza@unal.edu.co

L. B. Pinilla Bonilla et al. (eds.), *Neuraltherapeutic Medicine*,
https://doi.org/10.1007/978-3-032-03257-7_20

2 What Does the Life Story Contain?

Although one of the characteristics of the neuraltherapeutic medicine approach is its heterogeneity [10], and there are several possible clinical approaches, some characteristics are listed that allow us to speak of life history (LH), which complement the classic clinical history usually used in conventional medical training.

LH includes the usual sections of a medical history, such as personal history, family history, review by systems, pharmacological aspects, habits, etc., which also constitutes a regulatory requirement, but additionally:

- The use of fluent and simple language without technicalities is encouraged, where neuraltherapist, although specifically questioning, respects the direction of the patient's narrative, emphasizing events relevant to their life experience, such as recurrent illnesses, surgeries, emotional changes, job losses, or events that the patient considers to be determinants of their health [11].
- In this narrative, the doctor delves into their social environment, social groups of belonging, family composition, beliefs, and others that allow them to characterize their socio-historical environment and the relationship with it.
- As for the documentation, there are some suggestions for carrying out the life history [12]; however, another characteristic of the NTM is the freedom that the physician has to give his/her own body to his/her files, as long as they are adjusted to have enough elements to correctly address the neural theraphy and that allows him/her to make a comparison of the patient between controls. This includes all aspects of a patient's life, such as changes in physical and mental symptoms, changes in habits, and changes in the way of relating with others, that is, the integral evolution of the patient.
- Life history takes into account the chronology in the appearance of symptoms in order to weave their possible embryological counterpart (innate or unconditioned reflexes) and memory networks that have developed throughout life, where semiology is decentered and de-hierarchized in order to perceive other possible relationships and conditioned reflexes acquired throughout its ontogeny (see Chap. 13).
- For NTM, the life history always includes the history of the oral cavity, that is, dental pathologies, dental processes, implants, surgeries, type of bite, etc., since it is considered that the vast majority of dystrophies that generate pathologies are in the mouth [13, 14].
- It is vital to interpret nonverbal language and forms of corporeality that, as already mentioned, evidence cultural inscriptions and nonbiomedical nosological causes, difficult to address from mere clinical or quantitative data [4].
- The understanding of the patient and their family about their individualization is encouraged, since each life story is unique and incomparable with other people even if they share demographic spaces or age groups.
- The NTM, without having conceptualized it at that moment, through dialogue, it favours "rhizomatic thinking" as referred to by Deleuze and Guattari. A rhizome does not follow linearities; it is heterogeneous and allows any point to be con-

nected with another, since it has no center or root. This allows us to think from multiplicity and complexity, favoring the unraveling of the network of dynamics, and it generates a horizontal doctor–patient relationship since it does not favor authoritarian or vertical models because it is anti-hierarchical [15].

- LH includes questions related to determining cognitive, values, and praxis aspects of the patient with respect to their health-disease status. It also looks at how the patient has adopted the diagnoses from biomedicine and whether these have affected their identity, expectations, and treatment goals.
- In the LH of NTM, the approach from the gender perspective is transcendental, since different bodies are inhabited according to sex, gender, and age. Therefore, the historical conceptualization of the female body or diverse bodies affects the experience of health and disease [16, 17]. Likewise, there is sufficient epistemological evidence regarding the production of knowledge from a patriarchal approach [18], aspects that are not touched on in medical training (at least until a few years ago); therefore, it is important for the neuraltherapist to observe these differences [19].
- Developing the life history requires time; linking life data in a medical consultation of less than 45 min would be difficult, as it does not allow for the generation of trust, dialogue, or comprehensive approaches, especially if it is a first meeting [10].
- It has already been mentioned, in view of the monistic nature of NTM, and in conceiving the disease as an emergent process [20] (Chap. 19) for the life history, mental symptoms, causal relationships, as well as scenic or anecdotal descriptions of the patient, have as much relevance as clinical scales and criteria. The emergence of the human relationship arises from the dialogue of knowledge and "ignorance" between the neuraltherapist, patient, and family, avoiding classifying or prioritizing the symptoms described [21].
- Therefore, delving into detailed accounts of the patient's vital moments can create *"a therapeutic action map"* [4], not only to make sense of the disease or symptom, but also so that the NT drives the patient toward his or her own order, even if this does not necessarily coincide with the physician's intentions [22].
- It is important that therapeutic decisions are noted, as well as the relationships that the neuraltherapist makes of them for guidance in subsequent controls.
- The way to develop the anamnesis of the life history is dialogical and friendly, that is, the doctor "translates" the patient's communicative skills and directs the dialogue in such a way that they understand the intention of knowing their contexts. This would help connect moments or events related to their health-disease that can hardly be deduced with the classic data of a medical history. This conversation also recognizes their experiential wisdom and respects their otherness [23].
- In the construction of the life history during the NTM meetings, it is evident that the therapeutic decisions are joint, that is, they respond to a neuraltherapeutic logic, but they occur from the patient's freedom to access and accept it [24].
- In HL, while international classification manuals and guidelines are used for medical diagnoses, the focus is mainly on the total number of symptoms,

dystrophies, and observations that the patient reports. In the words of Payán de la Roche: "What is treated is not the disease, but the patient." Therefore, the objective is to document vital processes without labeling them because they disobey schemes or protocols [14, 22].

3 The Role of the Neuraltherapist Physician in Life History

Regarding the "doctor–patient solidarity relationship" [10], which is discussed in NTM, in a research work developed at the National University of Colombia, it was evident that the aspects that were enunciated constitute a starting point to achieve less imposing and, therefore, less hierarchical medical relationships. This is the main focus on which the neuraltherapist reintegrates the patient as an *active* subject of their therapeutic process and, therefore, allows them to reconstruct their subjectivities, delimit their therapeutic objectives, and identify the topics that they consider to affect their morbid processes. This goes beyond the clinical interpretation of the treating physician. This is, undoubtedly, a guiding factor in the type of neural therapy that the patient requires in each session.

Although in the first NTM consultation it is about reconstructing the patient's life history, due to time and the construction of the doctor–patient relationship, it would be impossible for it to be complete. Therefore, in each new consultation, it is about nourishing this life history with data that emerges and that the patient considers relevant or that the therapist gradually discovers. Every intervention includes NT nonlinearity and evolutionary irreversibility, as well as other concepts from NTM (see Chaps. 13 and 18). This makes it understandable that the body system changes from one experience to the next.

Likewise, it is important to emphasize that the life history is not only obtained during the anamnesis, but also at the end of the consultation, with a family member and very often in the middle of the physical examination, as explained in Chap. 21 in the examination of the patient the following are identified: scars, mouth with metals, implants, temperature changes, etc., which allow us to address and expand the life history, locating these findings where the neuraltherapist considers pertinent.

For the neuraltherapist, getting a comprehensive approach to the world that surrounds the patient is a challenge since they must have explored their own scholastic and metaphysical imprint [14], understand their social origin in order to transcend their prejudices and beliefs, which may be imposed in the attitudes and practices of their professional practice [22–25]. Additionally, as mentioned in Chap. 3, during the training, they recognize other epistemological supports, which are not opposed to their medical training; on the contrary, it resignifies [24].

The professional in NTM, in the exercise of interpreting the patient's life history, has recognized other rationalities that, from the social sciences, have contributed to the worldview of neuraltherapeutic medicine.

- It leaves human relationships outside the obsolete term of "being objective," because it considers the *interbeing*[1] [26] as a relational bridge with their patients, families, and other colleagues, two-way dynamics, where the therapist also undergoes a transformation with each patient and, therefore, changes their relationship with the world.
- The neuraltherapist understands that relativization is the rule. What Payan disseminated as "it depends and sometimes" is a call not to dogmatize NTM and that the professional allows himself the possibility of amazement at life and the emergent phenomena that occur in the practice of NTM inside and outside the office [27].
- It takes into account in the process of constructing knowledge and in its therapeutic relationships the concept of "senti-pensar"[2] to which Fals Borda referred, which, with regard to NTM, would be exposed as a non-dual exercise to find coherence between the use of medical rationality (technological advances) and inferential processes from perception or "the heart." This is linked to his vision of "participatory action research" [28], since for NTM, the medical act constitutes in itself an exercise of this participatory research, whose main researcher is the patient.
- One of the objectives of making the history of a patient's life is to have enough elements to understand the sociocultural fabric in which the patient's socio-historical environment develops: their social production of the body and therefore their cultural affiliation, beliefs, and the relationships they make with the nosology of disease beyond biomedical causes and, therefore, the development of the social contingencies that mitigate them [25].
- The neuraltherapist recognizes the complexity of the human being and, therefore, will avoid being categorical or imposing in their postures, understands their role as a companion, and is not afraid of the unknown or of amazement. They also allow themself the rights to tenderness, laughter, and so many others described by Payán de la Roche during his life [29].

[1] Interbeing: a term taken up by the author Maureen Murdock in her book The *Wise Woman: The Heroine's Journey,* which refers to the fact that "we are all one and coexist in a continuum of life". This is what Sandra Payán, Neuraltherapist, takes up in the community health gazette, where she resignifies and integrates this concept as part of the terms to make a call towards the biocentric paradigm, and therefore, it is pertinent in NTM and its epistemological conception.

[2] "Senti-pensar" is a term popularly used by the riverside inhabitants of the Colombian coasts (and some Colombian ancestral settlers), for whom, within their worldview, they are interconnected in the use of their thoughts (reason) and feelings (heart) in a synchronous way. Therefore, they do not leave aside their intuition or emotionality, nor their intellectual capacity. This allows them to live better with the rhythm of the nature they inhabit, far from the Western duality. It ended up being taken up again by Fals Borda in his academic production and later by Eduardo Galeano. Although there is no literal translation of the term due to its cultural connotation, the approximate translation "feel-think" or "feeling-thinking" will be used for the rest of the book.

4 Conclusions

- The use of life history in neuraltherapeutic medicine constitutes a particular form of approach from solidarity and empathy, generating valuable personal data that go beyond the collection of clinical events and that weave a complex and unique narrative from which the neuraltherapist chronologically links the events related to the health and disease of each patient.
- Through their life history, patients who consult NTM understand the importance of their body mapping, their individuality and the paths that have determined their individual, environmental, and collective health, regaining their autonomy in their process.
- The life story advocates for a doctor–patient relationship based on solidarity, mutual respect, gratitude, and acceptance of life's uncertainty.
- Neuraltherapeutic medicine develops in medical practice a research process where we *interbeing* with the patient and their family, and amazement is allowed at life through encounters called Life Stories.
- Finally, life history is a call to prioritize singularity over protocols or management guides, which, although they have some use, cannot replace human relationships, individual relativity, and the search for particular orders.

References

1. Charon R. Narrative medicine: honoring the stories of illness. New York: Oxford University Press; 2006.
2. Payán de la Roche JC. Biological medicine: a commitment to life. Buenos Aires: FisicalBook; 2006.
3. Charon R. Narrative medicine: a model for empathy, reflection, profession, and trust. JAMA. 2001;286(15):1897–902.
4. Díaz IA. Contributions of urban folk healing in Bogotá, towards a neural therapist and towards neural therapy (TN). Case study. Master's thesis. Bogotá: Universidad Nacional de Colombia; 2014.
5. Toscano De La Torre F, Pinilla Bonilla LB. The principles of neural therapy from the foundations of nervism to current neuroscience. Salud UIS. 2012;44(2):57–65. Available at: https://revistas.uis.edu.co/index.php/revistasaluduis/article/view/2591
6. Bykov K, Konradi G. Text-book of physiology. Moscow: Foreign Languages Publishing House; 1960.
7. Deleuze G, Guattari F. A thousand plateaus. Madrid: Editorial Pre-textos; 1996.
8. Lugones M. Gender in dispute. Feminism and critical theory: essays by women in Latin American thought. Buenos Aires: Editorial Tinta Limón; 2002. p. 143–59.
9. Grosz E. Volver al cuerpo: philosophy, body, and gender. Madrid: Ediciones Cátedra; 2001.
10. García Montealegre F. Approaches for a proposal of integrated health care from neural therapeutic medicine. Master's thesis. Bogotá: Universidad Nacional de Colombia; 2022. Available at: https://repositorio.unal.edu.co/handle/unal/81944
11. Towards a philosophy of medical practice. Dordrecht: Kluwer Academic Publishers; 2001.
12. Segura Chaves P. Design of a clinical history model for neural therapy in accordance with current regulations in Colombia. Master's thesis. Bogotá: Universidad Nacional de Colombia; 2010. Available at: https://repositorio.unal.edu.co/handle/unal/70491

13. Adaros J. Physical examination for the interfering field (based on the book "a physical examination for neural therapy? From Godoy to linearity"). Neural Ther. 2018; Available at: https://www.terapianeural.com/images/stories/teoric/JULIO_ADAROS_-_UN_EXAMEN_FISICO_PARA_EL_CAMPO_INTERFERENTE.pdf
14. Payán de la Roche JC. Vital disobedience, vol. Vol. 1. 3rd ed. Sabadell: Instituto de Terapia Neural; 2016. p. 1–200.
15. Deleuze G, Guattari F. A thousand plateaus: capitalism and schizophrenia. Valencia: Pre-Textos; 1980.
16. Grosz E. Volatile bodies: toward a corporeal feminism. Bloomington: Indiana University Press; 1994.
17. Fausto-Sterling A. Sexing the body: gender politics and the construction of sexuality. New York: Basic Books; 2000.
18. Harding S. The science question in feminism. Ithaca (NY): Cornell University Press; 1986.
19. Orduz Quintero C. Gender perspective of neural therapeutic medicine: practices, perceptions, and attitudes of neural therapists in Colombia in the last two decades (2002–2022). Neuraltherapeutics. Master's thesis. Bogotá: Universidad Nacional de Colombia; 2023. Available at: https://repositorio.unal.edu.co/handle/unal/85724
20. Cardozo Pabón A. Illness as an evolutionary and emergent process. Master's thesis. Bogotá: Universidad Nacional de Colombia; 2011. Available at: https://repositorio.unal.edu.co/handle/unal/20508
21. Payán de la Roche JC. Jump into the void. Your wings will spread. Bogotá: McGraw-Hill; 2001.
22. Payán JC. The medical act in the face of the holistic. Terapianeural.com. 2006 July 10 [cited Jan 2025]. Available at: https://www.terapianeural.com/articulos/14-del-concepto/120-el-acto-medico-ante-lo-holistico
23. Echandia Bocanegra F. Analysis of the articulation of neural therapeutic medicine with primary health care in the alternative health center La Nueva Esperanza in Popayán, Cauca from 1987 to 2005. Case study. Master's thesis. Bogotá: Universidad Nacional de Colombia; 2024. Available at: https://repositorio.unal.edu.co/handle/unal/85949
24. Payán de la Roche JC. What is neural therapy? Colomb Sci Technol. 1995;13(1):20–4.
25. Fries C. Bourdieu's reflexive sociology as a theoretical basis for mixed methods research, an application to complementary and alternative medicine. J Mixed Methods Res. 2009;3(4):326–48.
26. Murdock M. The wise woman: the heroine's journey. Madrid: GAIA Ediciones; 1991.
27. Payán JC. The new paradigms of alternative medicine. In: International meeting of neural therapy; 1998; Barcelona, Spain. Available at: https://www.terapianeural.com/articulos/22-memorias-de-los-encuentros/98-los-nuevos-paradigmas-de-la-medicina-alternativa.
28. Fals Borda O. Double history of the coast. Volume II: president Nieto. 2nd ed. Bogotá: Universidad Nacional de Colombia; 2002.
29. Garzón Fuentes EC. Neural therapeutic medicine in Colombia. Master's thesis in alternative medicine [Internet]. Bogotá: Universidad Nacional de Colombia; 2024 [cited 2025 Feb 6]. Available from: https://repositorio.unal.edu.co/handle/unal/87341

Chapter 21
Physical Examination in the Practice of Neuraltherapeutic Medicine

Jazmín Ariza-Tarazona and Laura Bibiana Pinilla Bonilla

1 Introduction

The science that studies signs, better known as semiotics, was originally founded by the mathematical logician Charles Peirce [1]. Thanks to Peirce, currently, in the medical context, medical semiology is known as a discipline that focuses on the study of the signs and symptoms presented by patients, on clinical observation and intentional inquiry, establishing an interpretation and a meaning that leads to a practical determination in the medical act for diagnostic and therapeutic purposes [2].

For years, medical semiology has been considered the fundamental axis of medical practice, but it has been displaced and overshadowed by technological advances, especially in the biomedical context. Without wanting to affirm that these advances in medical science are not useful, the clinical semiological exercise cannot be replaced by them. Even though technology advances considerably and artificial intelligence could establish diagnoses and propose a specific therapy, there are non-algorithmic inferential processes that are based on clinical experience and that are closer to a perceptual judgment. Charles Peirce called this logical perceptual process "abduction" [3]. These abductive processes occur during the observation and perception of the patient, which is properly achieved by using the physician's senses: palpating, sniffing, observing, and listening.

J. Ariza-Tarazona
Master in Alternative Medicine, Neural Therapy Area, Faculty of Medicine, Universidad Nacional de Colombia, Bogotá, Colombia

L. B. Pinilla Bonilla (✉)
Faculty of Medicine, Master in Alternative Medicine, Neural Therapy Area, Universidad Nacional de Colombia, Bogotá, Colombia

Integrated Health Services Subnetwork of the South, Research and Innovation Center, Bogotá, Colombia
e-mail: lbpinillab@unal.edu.co

L. B. Pinilla Bonilla et al. (eds.), *Neuraltherapeutic Medicine*,
https://doi.org/10.1007/978-3-032-03257-7_21

In other contexts, as mentioned in Chaps. 20 and 46 on life history and on social and community contributions, these processes that include perceptual processes may be closer to feeling-thinking, a term coined by Fals Borda and inspired by the fishermen of the Colombian coast [4].

In Neuraltherapeutic medicine, these processes where abduction or feeling-thinking arises are of immense richness for the doctor's work. Much of this exercise is based on performing an excellent physical exam.

2 General Considerations

The physical examination occupies, within the consultation of neuraltherapeutic medicine, an important space, because the individual's body expresses what has often not been presented as symptoms.

The physical exam begins from the moment the patient enters the office. There one can perceive the posture, the way of ambulation, limitations, attitudes, and facial expressions that will provide information enrichment. The emotional aspects of patients, which are usually part of the semiological exercise of observing and listening during consultation, will be discussed extensively in Chap. 22.

The physical exam also includes the evaluation of vital signs such as heart rate, respiratory rate, blood pressure, temperature, and oxygen saturation.

In accordance with what was discussed in Chaps. 10, 14, and 15, and inspired by the evaluation carried out by the neurologist Henry Head [5] to determine the areas of the skin that presented increased sensitivity secondary to visceral diseases (called algetic dermatomes) [6], the authors of this chapter suggest the use of the mechanical algesimeter or algometer. Particularly when assessing a dermatomic level, this is a useful tool for the evaluation of superficial sensitivity. On the other hand, if deeper levels are to be evaluated, such as spinous processes [7] or other musculoskeletal tissues, the physical examination should preferably be performed through the hands of the therapist, in direct contact with the patient's tissues (Fig. 21.1).

The mechanical algesimeter, also known as an algometer, is a device that generates a pressure of 4 kg/cm^2, or the pressure to whiten the nail bed of the thumb. The standardized procedure for examining tender points by this method has been described in several pathologies involving pain [8, 9].

The approach presented in this chapter will be done topographically from head to toe, for greater ease, emphasizing the importance of a complete approach, but its organization and approach are left to the discretion of the physician.

3 Head and Face Exam

Regarding the head, it begins by assessing the scalp and skull through palpation, looking for lesions, areas of pain, and scars. Subsequently, the algometer will evaluate the areas of hypersensitivity in the scalp that provide information on the viscera

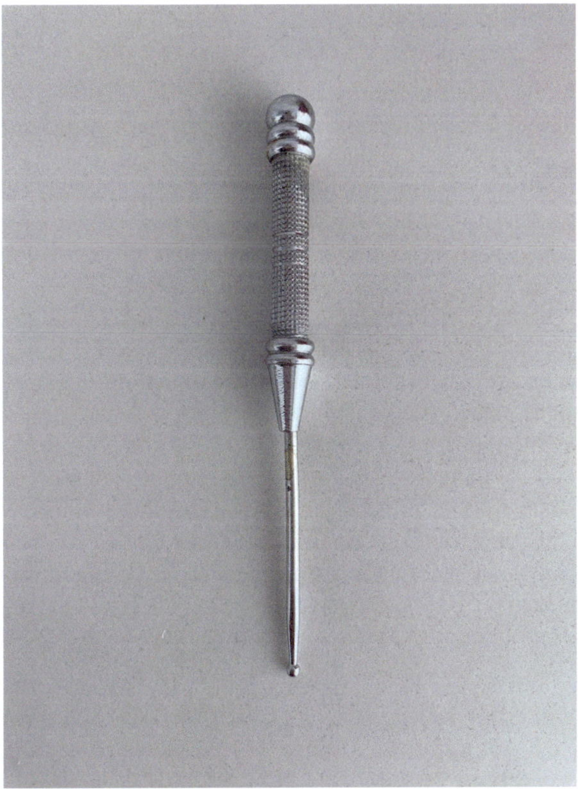

Fig. 21.1 Mechanical algemeter or algometer

reflex in the head, according to Henry Head [10] (see Chap. 15). It is also important to search for local injuries resulting from trauma, for example, or examination of the nerve roots distributed in the scalp, namely V1, C2, and C3.

On the face, check the supraorbital, infraorbital, nasociliary, auriculotemporal, mental, mastoid, maxillary nerve, lower dentary, and other main branches of the trigeminal nerve for tenderness or pain when touched. Also, check the neck for Adler's sign [11] and Mackenzie's sign (oval 1) reflexes (Chap. 15).

The examination of the mouth must be exhaustive due to the information derived from it. It is examined with inspection and palpation of the mucous membranes and gums in search of lesions, pain in the dental apexes, or sensitivity in extraction scars. Horizontal percussion (evaluation of periodontal tissues) and vertical percussion (evaluation of the dental apex), which is performed with the tongue depressor on each tooth. Gingival recession is evaluated, teeth are counted, the presence of mercury amalgam is identified, the presence of dental prostheses and the type (fixed or removable) is noted, the revision of the tongue is done, and the sensitivity of the tongue is assessed. For more information on the examination of the oral cavity, see Chap. 43.

4 Neck Exam

In the neck and the rest of the body, it is suggested to start with inspection, where the presence of lesions, telangiectasias, varicose veins, and changes in skin coloration, as signs of trophism, will be determined.

Deep palpation follows superficial palpation to avoid altering the examination's response or hiding signs. It begins with the assessment of autonomic reflexes (changes in temperature, in piloerection, or in sweating as a search for autonomic reflexes in visceral diseases) (see Chap. 14). This test can be done with the palm of your hand. In addition to the superficial sensitivity test, the mechanical skin algesimeter test is used to find out how sensitive the Head's zones are as a sign of visceral disease. From the neck to the extremities, this information is very important, since many visceral pathologies begin with the expression of changes in the autonomic reflexes in the area of the dermatome related to a viscera or in the Head's zone. Within the exam, an examination of their viscera, such as the thyroid, lymph nodes, and the presence of masses, should be performed.

During a neck exam, it is important to look for the Adler-Langer sign, which is pain when pressure is put on the area of the lateral processes of the cervical vertebrae. This can be a sign of the following problems: C1 is related to the maxillary sinus and nose, C2 is related to maxillary teeth, C3 is related to mandibular teeth, C4 and C7 are related to tonsils/ear [11].

5 Chest Exam

Inspection of the chest includes examination of symmetry, position with respect to the axis of the body, and superficial examination, as explained above. The thorax will first be checked for fasciae. This evaluation is done with the rolled clamp or Kibler test [12], which involves lifting the skin with the index finger and thumb and moving it cranially to seek any retraction or gelosa in the tissue. Subsequently, the examination is continued with the mechanical algometer, looking for sensitivity in areas of skin, which may or may not correspond to the Head's zones. Deep structures such as muscle and osteoarticular structures should also be examined in order to determine possible correlation with myotomes, sclerotomes, and bone areas with pain due to fracture scars, osteosynthesis, trauma, sprains, dislocations, etc. In the evaluation of Mackenzie's sign, correlation is found with the viscera of the thorax at the level of ovals 2 and 3 (see Chap. 15).

6 Abdomen Exam

In order to check the abdomen, the same steps are taken again and again: superficial palpation, superficial sensitivity testing with the mechanical algesimeter, rolled clamping, and deep palpation in the abdomen (to find megalys, pain, or areas of deep tension). Sclerotomas related to the abdominal area correspond to the costal arches and vertebral area related to ovals 4 and 5 of Mackenzie's sign (see Chap. 15).

The abdominal area is a place that has a great semiological richness since it is easier to access the planes of the fascia and perceive discrete contractures, tensions, and gels that are especially important for both the diagnostic and therapeutic fields.

7 Pelvic and Sacroiliac Examination

In this area, the assessment by planes (from dermatomes to sclerotomas) is continued as previously mentioned in the other areas. On the bone plane, for example, it is important to search for painful points in the pelvic girdle: iliac bones, pubic symphysis, hip joint, sacroiliac joint, sacral foramina, joints of the spine. These structures are frequently altered as the expression of pelvic visceral pathology, Mackenzie's sign, ovals 5 and 6 (Chap. 15).

8 Examination of the Spine and Back of the Body

The examination of the posterior region (dorsum) follows the same scheme as described above: inspection, superficial palpation, examination of deep sensitivity with a mechanical algesimeter, deep palpation, and examination of the spine in search of Mackenzie's signs. Supplementary information on this anatomical area can be found in Chaps. 34, 36, and 37.

9 Extremities

In both the upper and lower limbs, the evaluation is done in planes from dermatomes to sclerotomas. It is important to pay attention to the classical semiological examination, where the findings of the extremities are frequently interpreted as somatic information. From an approach that applies embryology and integrates the research of Henry Head and James Mackenzie, the examination of the extremities, on the contrary, provides, for the most part, visceral information (see Chap. 15).

10 Evaluation of the Effect of Neuraltherapeutic Intervention Through the Head's Zones and Mackenzie's Sign

The evaluation of superficial or dermatomic sensitivity with the mechanical algesimeter, after the superficial or deep neuraltherapeutic intervention, is a great ally to evaluate whether the therapeutic approach carried out has managed to manage the irritative foci in this organism. Likewise, Mackenzie's sign is also an ally for the evaluation of the post-intervention effect. This sign's negativization may lead the therapist to the conclusion that his intervention has been sufficiently targeted at the necessary foci.

For instance, if a patient has a problem with the trigeminal, a therapist may decide, after looking at the patient's medical history and physical exam, to infiltrate some odontons and branches of the trigeminal. Prior to the intervention, the physical examination of this patient showed increased skin sensitivity in the Head's zone of the eye (frontonasal area, medioorbital, frontotemporal), as well as sensitivity in the area of the temporal and vertical head due to inflammation of the temporomandibular joint. Evaluation of the neck showed a positive Mackenzie's sign, especially in the C2–C3 vertebrae. After these infiltrations (of some odontons and branches V1 and V2), the evaluation of the Head's zone of the eye, temporal and vertical, as well as Mackenzie's sign, becomes negative, representing a good indicator of management.

References

1. Oehler K. An outline of Peirce's semiotics. In: Krampen M, Oehler K, Posner R, Sebeok TA, von Uexküll T, editors. Classics of semiotics. Topics in contemporary semiotics. Boston: Springer; 1987. p. 1–21. Available from: https://doi.org/10.1007/978-1-4757-9700-8_1
2. Goic A. On the origin and development of the book Medical Semiology. Rev Med Chil. 2018; 146(3):387–90. Available from: https://doi.org/10.4067/s0034-98872018000300387
3. Sebeok TA. Sherlock Holmes and Charles Peirce: the method of research. Barcelona: Editorial Paidós; 1994. 100p.
4. Fals Borda O. Double history of the coast. Volume II: president nieto. 2nd ed. Bogotá: Universidad Nacional de Colombia; 2002.
5. Head H. On disturbances of sensation with special reference to the pain of visceral disease. Brain. 1893;16(1–2):1–133.
6. Wancura-Kampik I. Segmental anatomy. 1st ed. Munich: Elsevier Urban & Fischer Verlag; 2009. Chapter 1, p. 1.
7. MacKenzie J. Some points bearing on the association of sensory disorders and visceral disease. Brain. 1893; 16(3):321–53. Available from: https://doi.org/10.1093/brain/16.3.321
8. Okifuji A, Turk DC, Sinclair JD, et al. A standardized manual tender point survey: I. Development and determination of a threshold point for the identification of positive tender points in fibromyalgia syndrome. J Rheumatol. 1997;24(2):377–83.
9. Sinclair JD, Starz TW, Turk DC. The manual tender point survey [booklet and DVD/CD]. Salem: National Fibromyalgia Research Association; 2003.

10. Head H. On disturbances of sensation with special reference to the pain of visceral disease: Part II. Head and neck. Brain. 1894;17(3):339–480.
11. Fisher L. Neural therapy: neurophysiology, therapeutic injection techniques. 5th edition. Stuttgart: Georg Thieme Verlag; 2019. p. 208.
12. Dosch P, Dosch M. Manual of neural therapy according to Huneke. 2nd ed. Stuttgart: Thieme; 2007.

Chapter 22
Diagnostic Approach of Mental and Emotional Aspects

Leonardo Morales-Hernández and Laura Bibiana Pinilla Bonilla

1 Introduction

The approach and treatment of emotional and mental aspects in medicine in general represents a challenge for the practice of medicine itself. In the World Health Organization (WHO) and Pan American Health Organization (PAHO) World Report on Mental Health published in 2022, it was found that nearly one billion people were living with a mental disorder in 2019; 1 in 100 deaths were by suicide, 58% of them committed by people under 50 years of age. Likewise, 31% of these people have been diagnosed with anxiety disorders and 28.9% with depressive disorders. By 2020, during the pandemic, these percentages of anxiety and depression increased by close to 25% [1].

The biomedical approach, although it has prevented many deaths from mental health disorders, has focused mainly on care based on the biochemical suppression of symptoms. Approaches with exclusively empirical analytical methodology, which only consider materialistic and mechanistic elements, when they are oriented toward a profound transformation of the root cause of mental health problems, are clearly insufficient in Western medicine [2].

L. Morales-Hernández (✉)
Universidad Nacional de Colombia, Faculty of Medicine. Master in Alternative Medicine, Neural Therapy Area, Bogotá, Colombia

Santa Clara Hospital, Psychiatry Department, Bogotá, Colombia

L. B. Pinilla Bonilla
Faculty of Medicine, Master in Alternative Medicine, Neural Therapy Area, Universidad Nacional de Colombia, Bogotá, Colombia

Integrated Health Services Subnetwork of the South, Research and Innovation Center, Bogotá, Colombia
e-mail: lbpnillab@unal.edu.co

L. B. Pinilla Bonilla et al. (eds.), *Neuraltherapeutic Medicine*,
https://doi.org/10.1007/978-3-032-03257-7_22

When we talk about the root cause, we are not referring here only to alterations in brain neurotransmitters, since this is the consequence of a process of having a cause in that individual. Individual understandings and experiences, in the best scenario, can be stored and integrated in adaptive ways. However, not all individuals interpret the world and what happens to them in adaptive ways. There are experiences that can be configured as traumatic or in a state of conflict in the psyche of human beings.

Paraphrasing Baita, trauma refers to the consequence of exposure to situations of certain characteristics that:

> Exceed our ability to cope, or situations for which our possibility of completing the action of surviving, although successful, at first glance if we go walking, does not fail to remind us of its effects… it leaves us in a kind of "evil spell"… It is possible that we do not even remember that danger of the past, and even so, we continue to suffer – without understanding why – incomprehensible discomforts: nightmares, irrational fears, impossibility of doing certain things, aversion to certain places, or people, or tastes, or smells…. [3]

Although there is a wide range of mental disorders related to traumatic experiences, such as acute stress disorder, post-traumatic stress disorder, complex post-traumatic stress disorder, borderline personality disorder, dissociative symptoms, psychotic disorders, and somatoform disorders, there are many other relationships of traumatic events with different mental health disorders with which they overlap [4].

This chapter will develop around the FADEt technique, developed by the authors in 2015, whose acronym stands for *Fast Desensitization of Emotional Trauma.* This new technique is a synthetic scheme of diagnostic and therapeutic approach, which integrates conceptual elements of complexity, synthetic physiology and Russian nervism; neural therapy (neuraltherapeutic medicine), classical psychotherapy and new proposals in the area of psychology.

The present technique is part of an "incidental, unexpected" finding, while a patient was approached by means of a psychotherapeutic technique inspired by neuro-linguistic programming (NLP), hypnosis and eye movement desensitization and reprocessing. It was a patient suffering from depression and anxiety for more than 25 years, with a history of benzodiazepine abuse. More than five sessions were carried out where the techniques described were applied; however, although only the same memory network was being worked, a change in the perception of it had not yet been achieved, that is, a therapeutic result had not been obtained. In one of the sessions, since the patient reported having a lot of chest pain when she recalled the traumatic event of youth, it was decided to apply a few papules with procaine under a neuraltherapeutic scheme for pain management. Suddenly, not only did the patient show immediate relief from the symptoms, but additionally a change was observed in her facial expression, in her affective tone (the crying suddenly stopped), and the patient indicated feeling much better. In the following follow-up after this session, the patient had manifested global changes in her self-perception, had experienced the emergence of a new life purpose, had felt the sensation of no longer needing benzodiazepines, and began an assisted process of voluntary discontinuation of antidepressants.

Faced with the possibility that this case had been due to mere individual idiosyncrasy or that it had been a random event, the authors of this chapter began to test this technique in different types of patients and in the author's themselves in their personal therapy, finding similar results. Currently, some cases, collected over more than 10 years, are in and will be published in Chap. 41.

The first part of this chapter will deal with the epistemological bases of this proposal, based mainly on the approaches of Gregory Bateson. The second part aims to articulate the elements of some theories from the Nervism school, as well as to introduce the reader to classic and new psychotherapeutic tools such as hypnosis, systemic therapy, brief strategic therapy (BST), eye movement desensitization and reprocessing and NLP, which provide important elements for the understanding of this proposal.

The fourth part will briefly expose systemic conceptualization by levels. The fifth part refers to the interview scheme proposed by Morales to make an adequate approach to the case. The last part of this chapter concludes with a reflection on what is worthy of cure in each patient.

2 Epistemological Framework

In order to understand a new way of addressing the same problems that have arisen many times in humanity, such as mental illnesses and emotional disorders, it is important to broaden epistemology, that is, the conceptual or epistemological framework of how we understand the world. It is a matter of dimensioning in a different way the conditions presented by the people who attend in search of clinical help.

A century-old phrase by Freud that goes like this:

> Of the many teachings that Master Charcot lavished on me in his time at the Salpêtrière, there were two teachings that left a deep mark on me. The first, that we should never tire of looking at the same phenomenon many times (or feeling its effects); the second, that we should not worry about the contradiction of both parties when one has worked sincerely. [5]

This phrase summarizes to a large extent the way to investigate and expand epistemology and in the same way to expand the logical frameworks of understanding. To this end, this paper will use a leading author in epistemology who had a deep imprint on what can be called *complex thinking and systemic thinking*, that is *Gregory Bateson*. In his book, Spirit and Nature, many important elements are raised to understand this form of epistemology.

For Bateson, the universe is living and in it prevails "general" situations and what he, at that time, called "spiritual," which means that something is orienting the systems and their function; while the human race uses a thinking form based on "singular and materialistic." Bateson proposes an important key that is "*the pattern that connects*," [6] that is, to find some principles in nature that are placed there and that characterize it, for example, in anatomy, as an aesthetics of nature; this could also be called "meaning" which corresponds to the relations between the parties.

Briefly, it can be said that a system is made up of parts that interact mutually and that acquire rules in their process of functioning. The parts have a way of functioning in the way they connect with each other as elements of a system, and this allows patterns to be found. An example of a pattern is found in nature, already described by Hippocrates, such as the *vis medicatrix naturae,*[1] that is, this tendency that living systems have for their self-correction and healing, which integrate the parts and allow a change to be made, can be called a "meta-pattern," where the interacting parts are relating to each other. And it is important to understand that this is a process related to certain memory when the processes of healing or healing occur.

Humans analyze the phenomena through the language, reducing the phenomenon to signs, making it quantifiable or nominable. This mechanism is an artifice used by human brains or human cultures to understand what happens in nature.

> Language[2] goes far beyond the attribution of signs to different concepts, as it involves the use of syntax to logically relate words and express feelings… it makes it possible for us to go beyond thinking exclusively about the things in sight in our immediate present… to think about our thinking, to evaluate the future and to meditate on the past, words are abstractions of reality.[3] [7]

But the phenomenon that is happening there happens in reality, in those living systems. It could be said that the system, including its parts—the nervous system, the body, the psychological part, to name a few components that interact as a whole—has a history. A story, a memory, and the symptom are presented as a narrative, that is, as a form of communication.

The body and the symptom tell a story that in a given context acquires meaning. And this allows, if one understands history or narrative memory, to make changes in this organism. Hence the importance of being able to break or have different epistemological schemes to understand this mind, spirit, intention, energy, or pattern that connects. For example, it can be understood from different approaches as the scheme of neurology, psychoneuroimmunology or some other comprehensive approach.

In this sense, all communication requires a context and "without context there is no meaning." All phenomena have a form of communication and language is a form of it. It could be said that there are situations in which that communication was lost. We can take as an example the phenomenon of cancer, in which that intracellular or intercellular communication of some cells in general with the system is lost and the functioning loses the physiological form that corresponds to it. In other words, "growth and differentiation must be controlled by communication." That is to say,

[1] Vis medicatrix naturae, is a phrase attributed to Hippocrates that can be translated as "nature is the physician of diseases". Although it is not written directly in his texts, it is a fundamental principle of his entire theoretical and practical approach.

[2] Although language is not an exclusively human quality and has similar characteristics in bonobos and other higher primates, there is a great difference with other species.

[3] In the words of Jorge Luis Borges, "language is an effective ordering of that enigmatic abundance of the world."

the structure has a way in which it works and communicates and, from there, there is a guideline of how it should work.

In anatomy and in physiology there is something that Bateson called a *transforma* [6], a message that has a grammatical contextual configuration that allows us to make sense of a "supreme dignity" that the system has at that moment. The symptom is a message, a communication of a dialogue of meanings with a memory and history that has a sense in its attempt to solve it, even if it achieves exactly the opposite.

Continuing in the sense of epistemological principles, it can be said that in complex thinking and in the model as Bateson expounded, there are presuppositions or principles, as well as found in science in general and in religion, in the different ways of understanding, which propose this way of understanding the universe, life and in this case people and their ailments or diseases.

In general, science tries to take old principles, revises them and sometimes creates new ones, and in that process it does not necessarily arrive at something final, but is constantly being reevaluated. A phenomenon that frequently occurs in science is that many times those who practice it (the scientists themselves) are not aware of the very principles or assumptions that guide them.

Bateson exposes them as follows: the first principle is that "science never proves anything, that is, the fact that it is tautologically valid does not mean that it is true" [6]. There will always be a limitation in the levels of perception and the liminal, that is, sensory levels of the observer, which makes the person come to conclude certain principles in the hope that he/she will find the simplicity to understand them (in the manner of Occam), although it is not always achieved. In the same way, predictions are sought, which is not necessarily achieved in many fields. Science seeks to make sense of its presuppositions, science investigates, not proves.

The second principle used by Bateson is based on Alfred Korzivsky's phrase that states "*the map is not the territory, the name is not the thing named.*" It can be said that models or maps are changing in time and in history, and the symbolic status that these maps or those models of understanding or paradigms reach allows them to transform, understand, and explain reality but only in circumscribed moments. As an example, a presupposition of a culture or historical period may be influenced by imperialist or colonialist interests, whether religious or economic, that are imposed on others, which does not guarantee its validity, regardless of its hegemonic acceptance [2].

In line with the above, reality or phenomena happen, and what is built to understand them is a *paradigm, map, or model of understanding* that can say that the world is in a certain way, but there may be other different views of expressing it or different ways of describing its functioning.

The third precept that Bateson speaks of is *that there is no objective experience* [6], that is, that all experience is subjective, since humans make a map that is based on the sensory organs, on the functioning of the brain,[4] with the limitations and the good things it has, and finally from that background are located the perceptions and interpretations. As Maturana says, "objectivity must be considered in parentheses," in the book objectivity an argument that obliges [8]. The West or the civilization of the West has deep roots in the illusion of objectivity [6], but in reality, we have many limitations according to both our brain conditions and our conditions of perception and maps.

Another precept that the author uses is "*the processes of image formation are unconscious*," what does he mean by this?

That what we can verify is the behavior of people and not the processes that happen within their mind or brain, since the information we have about these processes is insufficient despite the extensive research that is done in the field. That is, *a narrative is constructed from a perceptual map* and from this the information is organized with these foundations.

At this point, reference can be made to Jacques Lacan, who speaks of the real, the symbolic, and the imaginary [9]. The real is that part of nature that may never be fully understood. That symbolism is mediated by the illusion of the construction of a map (or what he calls an otherness) and that is culturally imposed and shared by many, which does not mean that it becomes real. Their model of understanding is shared and depends on historical eras and hegemonic conditions. And the imaginary is already the construction that each of these observant subjects personally makes.

What relationship can this have in the way in which different people are treated therapeutically?

According to the map that is built, people perceive the world and the information is observed from there. It can be said that the process of therapeutic intervention consists largely of the intertwining (transitional space[5]) of these models between this treating person and the people or communities to be treated.

When the narrative of the querent can be aligned with that of the observers, it becomes feasible to enhance and transform the situation based on the information available. This involves many factors such as metanarratives, the ways in which I explain it, neurological phenomena, previous meanings, map transposition and connections that are being made. People's narrative is the explicitness of their perceptual map—in the words of Giorgio Nardone the reactive perceptual system— [10] and the contextual information that the observer has.

Continuing in the same direction, the narrative represents the explanation of the perceptual map, and the information that the observer can extract from said narrative and share with him will be the condition that will allow him to understand and possibly transform the situation of the individual or consultant.

[4]Although the concept I am going to issue may seem reductionist, we are actually communities of primates trying to understand the universe in all its infinite complexity. Our tools may be quite small for the size of the task. How would other species or communities of species interpret us?

[5]Although Winnicott spoke of transitional space in more emotional terms, space has many other cognitive, behavioral, and communicational elements, among others.

At this point, it is worth making a parenthesis to quote what Aristotle called causes (material, efficient, formal, and final), trying to explain the nature of objects. Aristotle's formal cause "updated" would correspond to *information* [11]. Sufficient information,[6] together with its inherent significance, is conveyed through a narrative expressed both verbally and non-verbally, which the therapist interprets throughout the session within the context of a common map.

In the same way that Eugenio Andrade explains [11], science in the West was based mainly on the first two Aristotelian causes, that is, on the material and the mechanical (efficient), attending only to these quantifiable elements; but there are many other elements such as the information that shapes matter (meaning) and meaning that correspond to the last two Aristotelian causes. In this way, in the nature of living beings there is a vital, organicist principle that allows them to self-organize. That is, a syntax with information that gives order to matter and a semantics that gives it meaning and significance, which although it has material bases, corresponds to the formal and final Aristotelian causes [2].

It is what Bateson could say as the "eye of the spirit or of the mind that is seeing," it is to have a model that allows us to understand and enter into transformation [6]. The ability to transform does not consist in being a map but in being (one could say) a *non-map* (like a Joker) that can be coupled to various situations. In this case, the challenge would be to be able to move between the different maps or narrative forms presented by patients or communities in order to carry out the transformations there, that is, there would not be a single, final and valid map, but it is the interfaces between them that allow effective communication and approach to transformations through the information that is delivered to people.

In fact, in the therapeutic act what is "delivered to people"—or to their system—either with phrases (as is done in psychotherapy), with homeopathic substances (as is done in homeopathy), with needles in specific points (as in acupuncture) or with procaine in neural therapy according to medical rationality, it is information that allows the transformation to be carried out according to the map that the person has. This map is not only a mental construction, but also a bodily, neurological and integral map that each of them has written in their memories.

What these therapeutic practices seek is to achieve comprehensive health care [12] that responds to the needs of users according to their own system and according to a care system with an integral conceptualization.

The fifth precept used by Bateson, which may be useful in this introduction, is that "the division of the perceived universe into parts and wholes is convenient and may be necessary, but no necessity determines how it should be practiced" [6]. What the author is trying to say here is that in the end these divisions are artificial, they are in the mind of the observer and there are levels to understand it, but it does not mean that reality is necessarily like this.

Another principle is also very useful [6]: "nothing can come from nothing," that is to say that it is impossible not to communicate, everything is information, the one

[6] It could be understood as the information that shapes.

who creates the context is the receiver of the message, in this case the user, the patient who receives the message (whether it is an intervention with Neuraltherapeutic medicine or a few sentences or a certain stimulation and it is he who gives the context). When he is saying that nothing can be generated out of nothing, it means that there has to be prior information so that the system is being organized in the way it is being presented. It is important to remember that in living beings there are negative entropic processes [13], which allow systems to increase their internal organization. This process occurs through stochastic learning, according to Bateson, which allows the system to change its memory banks.

Memory processes (which in some simplistic way can be called memory neuronetworks) are the ones that are transformed when people are treated. This memory, which does not refer only to a conceptual-cerebral memory, is also a neurological memory, an immunological memory, even a genetic memory, that is to say that what is worked on are chains of meaning.

These processes of memory associations will produce effects on matter, on people's health according to the complexity of the association of the information that has been recorded and the way it is manifested. What is sought with the FADEt intervention strategy, as with any comprehensive intervention, is to be able to provide the system with transformative information, a therapy that changes the system of meanings in an integral way.

In order to understand this way of intervening, another relevant aspect is to take into account that linear logic is a deficient model of cause and effect [6] and that the words of stability and change actually describe a part of our perceptions; in reality, the phenomena follow a logic of much greater complexity (See Chap. 7).

3 Fundamental Concepts

3.1 Synthetic Physiology and Functional Systems

As mentioned in Chap. 13, a current called synthetic physiology arises in the East that has its bases in Russian Nervism. Unlike the analytic school of physiology, which is better known in the West, the synthetic physiology school emphasizes the coordinating and integrating role of the nervous system in all physiological and pathological aspects of an organism [14]. This school maintains a monist position,[7] that is, it considers that the mind and the body are aspects of the same reality, which is the human being, without divisions [15]. In a first stage of development, this school bases physiological processes mainly on the theory of conditioned reflexes proposed by Pavlov [16], understanding the concept of reflex as a dynamic,

[7] Toscano and Pinilla (2012) define monism as follows: "Every change at the physical level correlates with a change at the mental level. It is not a deterministic causal relationship, since it is a synchronous phenomenon."

non-linear, and associative response that involves the organism as a whole. In a second stage of development, the theory of conditioned reflexes evolves into the theory of functional systems proposed by Anokhin, which involves important elements such as the self-correction of physiological functions facilitated by reverse afferentation (better known today as *feedback*[8]) and anticipation. Functional systems originate, from this perspective, not only as a response to environmental challenges but also to the individual's motivations and internal needs [17].

In this school, a reinterpretation (Copernican turn) of the health-disease process as a complex, dynamic, self-organizing, and evolutionary process also emerges [18, 19]. This approach is close to the most recent conceptions proposed by the sciences of complexity.

Within the framework of this school, the concept of neurosis takes on special relevance as a foundation for understanding the origin of pathologies of both the body and the psyche. According to Anokhin, when two conflicting pieces of information are presented in an individual's life, a neurosis is constituted. Conflicting information can come from both external and internal signals. Pavlov mentioned that these conflict situations, which generate neuroses, came in human beings from adverse life situations that were interpreted as traumatic. In the cerebral cortex, when presented with this conflicting information, processes arise that seek to regulate and adapt to the situation. Ukhtomsky argues that the interpretation that the organism gives to this conflict situation is decisive in the life of an organism [20].

The process through which the organism gives meaning or purpose to its existence or to the events that happen externally can be based on the theory of functional systems. Within the framework of this theory, a functional system is created with the purpose of fulfilling a physiological function (such as respiration, digestion, among others), as well as it can arise as a compensatory mechanism for information from the external environment that is a challenge for the body. Each functional system operates by recruiting all the necessary elements from the periphery to obtain an adaptive result. Likewise, it is permanently evaluating the results which generate positive and negative emotions that support the body's decision-making, through a feedback process, which also allows the functional system to be restructured and reorganized in the event that the anticipated result has not yet been obtained [21].

Anokhin argued that, in the specific case of a collision between two systems of stimulation with two contradictory information, this can lead to the "emotional" escape of one toward one of the predominant vegetative pathways in human being thanks to the particularities of their constitution and their biography. The nature of the emotion itself influences, generating a diversity of manifestations, where the escape of emotional stimuli can affect the vascular system, the heart, or the gastrointestinal tract, for example [20].

The predominant pathophysiological expression in each organism may also depend on its personal history. If prior to the emotional collapse, a person has had a

---

[8] As mentioned in Chap. 13, the theory of functional systems and their process of reverse afferentation are 12 years ahead of the conception of feedback proposed by Norbert Wiener, creator of cybernetics.

lot of irritations in the stomach due to bad eating habits and irritating foods, it is possible that this place becomes a site of less resistance that will cause them to be affected in the first place after an emotional event. Another illustrative case may be that of a woman who was forced to abruptly terminate her pregnancy feeling symptoms in the chest that she called "broken heart." Years later, when the same woman becomes pregnant again, throughout the gestation process she very frequently experiences cardiac arrhythmias such as ventricular extrasystoles. Finally, in the postpartum period, a situation of a breakup with the father of her child generates depression, appearing a process of atrial fibrillation that affects her quality of life more markedly. This is what is configured as a dominant functional system, inspired by the concept of focus or dominant center proposed by the physiologist Ukhtomsky (See Chap. 13).

3.2 Therapeutic Interventions Based on Pavlov's Theory of Conditioning

As discussed in Chap. 13, Pavlov discovers the mechanism by which a temporal association or learning (conditioned reflexes) is generated in the organism supported by the cerebral cortex that can have an excitatory or inhibitory nature. Pavlov's theory of conditioned reflexes not only allows us to understand how pathological reflexes can be created in the body but also exposes the basis for inhibiting the expression of previously established pathological reflexes. Many variables can be decisive in achieving this inhibition, such as the type of nervous system, the number of reinforcements or repetitions of this inhibitory process, the biological significance associated with the pathological reflex, the previously acquired conditioned reflexes, and the basis of innate reflexes that each organism has inherited genetically.

Despite all these variables, Pavlov described a simple and basic mechanism to understand how a process of conditioned inhibition was generated. This conditioned inhibition can be created by the presentation of weak, neutral stimuli that come from the visual, auditory, tactile, olfactory, or taste channels. When a pathological reflex is evoked and one of these stimuli is simultaneously presented, reflexes can be partially or completely inhibited after several periods of repetition [16]. In psychology, there are some approaches that have integrated the application of stimuli through one of the channels described for therapeutic purposes, such as neurolinguistic programming [22] or eye movement desensitization and reprocessing [23], among others. In the field of Neuraltherapeutic medicine, the application of stimuli to the skin or subcutaneous tissues is carried out, and this occurs simultaneously when a pathological reflex is active. This varied range of stimuli has allowed these different approaches to generate a modulation and reorganization of the dynamics of organisms, facilitating therapeutic processes. In the case of neuraltherapeutic medicine, the application of procaine has an additional effect to the stimulus generated from the point injection.

Some studies have shown, through electroencephalographic recordings and analysis of cerebral blood flow, that procaine increases cerebral flow globally and, to a greater extent, to the limbic system in a dose-related manner. Procaine was shown to have a double action on hippocampal excitability, since in addition to reducing recurrent inhibition, procaine reduced the response to excitatory input [24–27], while in an experimental model in rats, procaine was found to have the ability to inhibit conditioned fear. Based on these studies, it can be inferred that the action of the intervention with neuraltherapeutic medicine would have a dual action given by the application of the stimulus in the tissues while the pathological reflex is active and the pharmacological action of procaine with a regulatory effect on the limbic system.

For these reasons, the FADEt technique developed by the authors of this chapter integrates not only the application of weak stimuli by the visual, tactile, and auditory pathways as agents of conditioned inhibition, but also resorts to the dual action of neuraltherapeutic intervention.

3.3 Process of Restructuring Networks of Meaning: An Explanatory Model of the FADEt Technique

The notion of ontogenesis, understood as the transformations that take place in living organisms from fertilization to the moment of death, involves two important variables, which are genetic memories with their innate reflexes and epigenetic factors that include extrinsic and intrinsic variables (See Fig. 22.1). Epigenetics, since its conception by Conrad Waddington, corresponds to the study of hereditary changes in the function of genes that cannot be explained by the DNA sequence [28, 29].

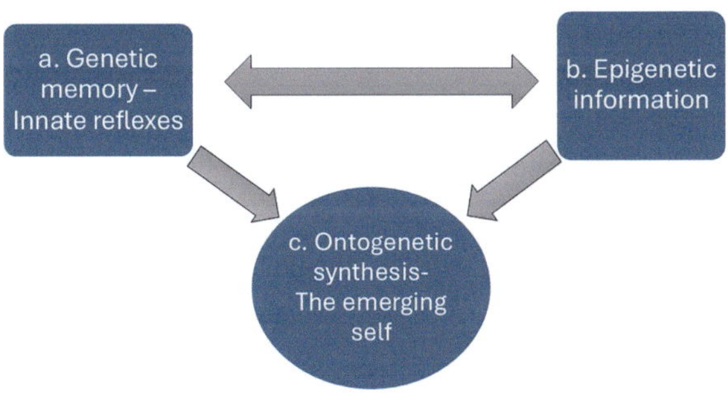

Fig. 22.1 The figure illustrates how ontogeny is a process of synthesis from which "being" constantly emerges, and which is determined by both genetic/innate reflexes and by epigenetic factors involving extrinsic and intrinsic variables. Genetic and epigenetic factors can influence each other during this ontogeny. (*Source*: Own elaboration)

More recently, it has been understood that epigenetic phenomena are mediated by DNA methylation and chromatin modifications. Among the extrinsic factors that generate epigenetic changes are environmental toxins, dietary components, and temperature alterations, among others. It has also been identified that some social factors such as maternal prenatal psychological stress, poverty, migration, urban housing, alcohol, and substance abuse could generate epigenetic changes [30].

On the other hand, there are also intrinsic factors that introduce a factor of chance, creating changes during ontogeny [29]. Part of these intrinsic factors may be determined by the memories or reflexes conditioned or acquired individually by organisms during their development. Individuals permanently establish interpretations about their own experiences and about the world around them. Anokhin, within the framework of the theory of functional systems, has generated a proposal for the conception of meaning for organisms:

> The conception of 'meaning' (…) in the perception of the external world, for example, it is obviously a variant of coincidence between the stored conditioned excitation and the return afferents, which are 'significant' in relation to this stored excitation. [31]

On the other hand, in Anokhin's view, it is the "purpose" or "anticipated end result" that acts as a guiding focus for both individual functions and global functional processes necessary for adaptation and conservation in the organism [21].

In coherence with the theory of functional systems, both the notion of meaning and that of purpose correspond to absolutely individual emergences, which depend on the synthesis that is generated from the exteroceptive, interoceptive, genetic information, and the memories acquired during the history of each individual (see Chap. 13).

Inspired by the theory of functional systems, the following is an explanatory theoretical model based on the experience of the two authors on the process of transformation of networks of meaning that occur during the therapeutic process of patients through the FADEt technique.

It is based on the fact that the conception of "being" or "self" is constructed from the interpretative synthesis of the experiences lived by each individual in his or her history (See Fig. 22.2). Experiences that the organism interprets as similar are stored in a common memory network. The element of similarity can usually be given by similar emotions or cognitions. For example, experiences that happened at different stages of the life of the same individual but that have in common the emotion of sadness under an interpretation of being abandoned can be stored in the same memory network.

In this way, memory networks can be configured in an individual's psyche that turn around different experiences, both positive and negative, with their respective meanings, such as, for example, the memory network of abandonment, the memory network of self-improvement, the memory network of unworthiness, the memory network of self-confidence, among others.

The therapeutic approach in this case focuses on the intervention of the individual's traumatic memories that, being under a conflict situation, are generating symptoms or pathological reflexes in the patient. As will be seen in Chap. 41, the approach

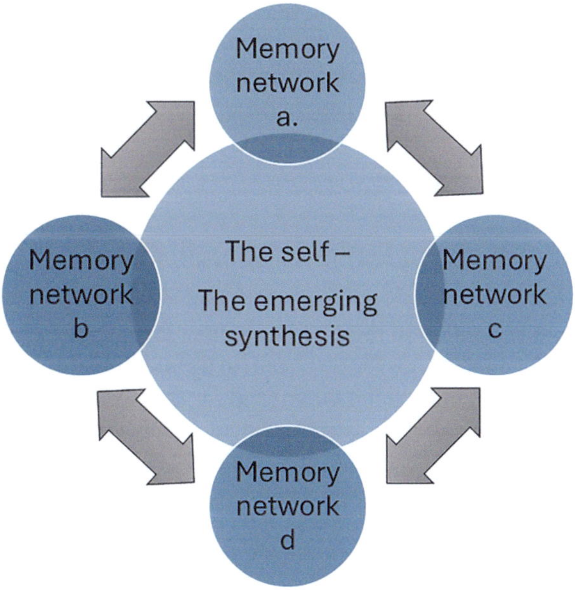

Fig. 22.2 The peripheral circles represent the memory networks that store interpretations of lived experiences with their corresponding meaning. These memory networks relate to each other and influence each other. The central circle represents the interpretative synthesis from which the global conception of "being" emerges. (*Source*: Own elaboration)

can be carried out in both acute and chronic situations. When the acute situation is addressed under this technique, it could generate temporary or permanent relief of the patient's symptoms, depending on whether the memory network that was intervened was a dominant focus or a secondary focus. If it is a primary or dominant focus, a relief of pathological reflexes (mental or physical) will be observed as a consequence.

In the case of a secondary focus, the root memory network or the dominant focus is searched. As a metaphor, the focus should not only be on the branches of the tree but also on the root. Generally, as emphasized in Chap. 13, these primary networks are anchored to traumatic memories of childhood or at some previous time in the patient's history. In addition, not only a single memory network that exhibits an adaptative disorder must be treated, but ideally all those that are necessary to generate a global transformation of the individual's psyche.

Once all the memory networks "worthy of being cured" are addressed (as will be seen later in this chapter), patients can not only observe more adaptive and spontaneous behavioral changes that manifest themselves in their daily lives, but also a change in their self-perception, that is, a change in the notion of "who they are" and their "purpose." Free from the negative conditioning generated by non-adaptive memory networks, free from the negative symptoms and pathological reflexes that these networks generated, within the framework of a global transformation of the networks of meaning that generate a new interpretative synthesis, the subject is free to define who he wants to be and, in many cases, even, to define a new life purpose.

These therapeutic processes, although are relatively quick compared to the classic approaches of psychotherapy, obviously take time. In the case of an individual memory network that is intervened, the authors' empirical experience has shown that it is possible to achieve complete desensitization in one or two sessions. It is difficult to specify how long it will take to observe global changes with a sense of restructuring of the being, since these are very individual aspects; however, it is possible to affirm that it could take a period of 2–6 months with a weekly or biweekly frequency of sessions.

4 Psychological Conceptualization

The evaluation of the patient requires that they be considered at different levels of understanding, on the one hand, in the individual psychology with all its history and meanings and, on the other hand, in the psychological interrelation that they have with themself, with their immediate family environment, with their community and with the social, cultural, and economic context in which they live.

From this way of understanding it, it is necessary to have multiple tools or models to be able to understand the complexity of the person and the phenomena that they present within their health.

4.1 Brief Presentation of Some of the Psychotherapeutic Elements That Make Up the FADEt Proposal

The following exposition seeks to briefly present for the reader an overview of the psychotherapeutic elements that the authors consider necessary to understand the context of the intervention. The content is not exhaustive; the reader is expected to delve into other sources what he or she deems relevant.

4.2 Constructivist Systemic Approach and Family Therapy

The decision to observe "reality as a system" is the principle that underpins the way of understanding nature and human interactions from this approach. From this perspective, a context is defined in which there is an interrelation of elements or interacting parts with a series of conditions such as circular causality, communication, hierarchy, limits, rules and norms characteristic particularly of that system, with the clarity that considering a single isolated element does not allow us to understand the complexity of the whole.

Systemic family therapy, which was born in the clinical field with constructivist foundations, considers the symptom as a "message that communicates in an ambiguous way the discomfort of a system" (such as the family or the individual in its context). It seeks the definition of problems from the patient's or family's own perspective,[9] giving great importance to the *"narratives and meanings"* that a family has particularly constructed [33] focusing a large part of its therapeutic strategy on communication and language analysis [34].

An important complement to this approach was developed by Bronfenbrenner that consists of conceptualizing a system as constituted by levels in which it can be observed. In the same way, a problem can be approached from this perspective by levels. In this definition, dynamics are considered to have social levels in reciprocal relationships [35]. In this way, it allows the concepts of social systems to be defined at different levels (nimo, micro, meso, macro, exo, and chrono) (See Fig. 22.3), in what could be called a systemic model of health and mental health. This includes multiple elements at each level and the possibility of influencing each other [34]. In this scheme, the nimosystem is the individual; the microsystem, the family; the mesosystem, the community; and the macrosystem, society.[10]

The systemic approach works especially on the therapist-patient relationship, understanding that the contents and narratives *emerge in second-order cybernetics.*[11] In its strategies, it seeks contextual, ecological, and sustainable solutions, emanating from the patient and his family. These fundamentals are compatible with

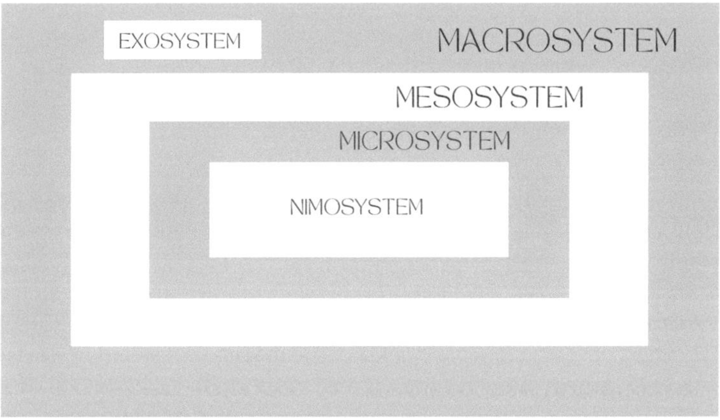

Fig. 22.3 Levels to understand the ecology of human development according to Bronfenbrenner. (*Source*: Own elaboration)

[9] The family is not the only thing that can be looked at as a system, in fact the original definition of systems is made by the biologist von Bertalanfy and can be applied at different levels such as the individual, the family, the community or society, depending on the type of problem or situation that is intended to be addressed [32].

[10] The exosystem refers to a subsystem that is located in the area of the macrosystem and that can have an influence on the area of the mesosystem. Similarly, chronus refers to time. They were not included in the present text for the sake of brevity and clarity.

[11] Second-order cybernetics refers to the observer being part of the phenomenon or in a simple way "what Peter says about John says more about Peter than about John". Applying this to the level of physics, it could be said that the way in which phenomena are observed also determines the way in which they behave, just as it happens with light with its qualities of particle and wave.

complex thinking and are used in the practice of interviewing and communication techniques with patients and families.

In the way in which the problem of the patients is addressed, a framework of understanding or joint narrative is constructed that allows different realities to be built with the patients, as evidenced in the following sentence: "psychotherapy becomes the art of replacing a construction of reality, which no longer fits, with another that in fact does fit correctly" [36], in other words, to move from an enslaving narrative[12] to a liberating narrative.

This type of approach, particularly in its narrative application, works especially with the meaning that people give to what "happens to them in life" or in their symptoms and situations, seeking that people come to "elaborate new categories of meaning, and to transform their own premises about the nature of meaning" [37].

Like the following two schemes, its foundations were largely developed at the MRI (Mental Research Institute) in Palo Alto and many principles shared with hypnosis and neuro-linguistic programming can be appreciated.

4.3 Hypnosis

For some authors, hypnosis was the fundamental basis for the development of many of the forms of psychotherapy that originated later [38]. Certainly, many of the authors who developed several forms of psychotherapy lived in part with these foundations.

Hypnosis can be understood as a special state of attention in which the person is absorbed in certain stimuli that allows the subject's potentialities to be developed to the fullest.

It can be said that when a person is highly concentrated on certain stimuli, they are in a trance condition that allows them to build their reality in a different way. The same can be observed in the elements of the medical consultation when there is a good therapist-patient relationship; it is also observed in social events when there is a shared feeling, or individually when the person learns to connect with oneself.

The professional who applies hypnosis techniques is called a hypnotherapist and, like any other therapeutic approach, has methods, objectives, techniques, and ethical elements.

In general, it can be said that it has three stages, which are absorption, ratification, and elicitation.

Some of the premises that are important from hypnotherapy are the following: "Where the problem arises, the solution is also found," "All hypnosis is self-hypnosis," "individuals function from their internal maps and not from their sensory

[12] The narrative corresponds to the explicitness of the perceptual map or the contextual information of the observer. It is a construction of meaning associated between the model of the observer and their reality. It is what Giorgio Nardone calls the reactive perceptual system.

experience," "the patient's resources lie in their personal history," " the person cannot give a non-answer" [39], among others.

4.4 Neuro-linguistic Programming (NLP)

Neuro-linguistic programming (NLP) is a derivative of the previous two. It was developed in the United States since the 1980s (Palo Alto, California), and its emphasis is on internal and external communication. It has practical applications that are easy to incorporate into the strategy of clinical interviews and therapeutic prescriptions [34].

It could be called "an advanced communication technology or techniques." Its foundations were basically developed from the observation of the authors Grinder and Bandler of the communicative strategies of three different great independent therapists: Virginia Satir, Milton Erickson, and Fritz Perls.

Among its main tools are anchors (positive or negative physiological perceptual associations that are presented to a stimulus and that are recorded in the unconscious), representation channels (people perceive the world differently visually, auditory or kinesthetically and their perceptual maps are different), eye movements are associated with the content of the mental process (known as ocular access keys),[13] communication is 95% analog and 5% digital and considers that language structures the neurology[14] of consciousness and allows rapport to be established between people [40].

The induction of *rapport*[15] *or empathy* is one of the key elements, implemented by the authors of this chapter, in the case-taking sessions and therapeutic work. This consists of communicating with the querent at the same level of verbal and nonverbal language. To do this, a permanent body check of the patient's forms of communication is used, such as their verbal content, their prosody, the movements of their face, arms, trunk, legs, their visual expressions and especially, their breathing. Thus, in a respectful way, the therapist responds with similar movements together, which allows a greater degree of communication and effectiveness in the process. It is a fluid dialogue with the whole body and in other words "the language that the therapist must speak is the language of the other" [34].

Neuro-linguistic programming allows a semiological reading of communication that is useful for the doctor or therapist and facilitates the deepening of the

[13] It refers to the fact that eye movements usually indicate how the person is connecting, whether it is more with their emotions, thoughts, memories or images at the time they are in contact with the therapist.

[14] That is why it owes its name "neurolinguistics".

[15] Rapport is a word that comes from the French language (rapporter: to carry something in return), In other words, what one person sends is returned by the other; in this context, it refers to synchronization or tuning.

information presented by the patient, especially that of an unconscious order, as well as the evaluation of its coherence.

4.5 Eye Movement Desensitization and Reprocessing

Desensitization and reprocessing through eye movements is a therapy developed since 1987 by Francine Shapiro (American psychologist). She performed a synclectic integration[16] of the best elements of multiple approaches previously developed. This technique manages to position itself in the therapeutic field of clinical psychology and psychiatry with 24 controlled clinical trials that demonstrate its effectiveness. This technique is recommended by the WHO, by the American psychiatric and psychological associations as an indication in post-traumatic stress disorder and anxiety disorders [23].

This technique has 8 phases [41], of which the following will be briefly presented:

1. Patient history and treatment planning, it is about making a very complete medical history, emphasizing possible situations that have produced trauma, or a memory associated with memory neuronetworks in a[17] non-adaptive way.
2. Prepare the person to be able to move on to the next stages with the strategies of physical position and breathing, the construction of the safe place, the selection of appropriate movements, and the use of specific metaphors.
3. Evaluation: The selection of the complaint or possible starting point (manifest target) is made to arrive through the "affective bridge" technique to the old traumatic contents (nodes or more unconscious). Selection of the work node in its components: perceptual income, negative belief, positive belief, and affective support of these beliefs.
4. Desensitization: A sentence is proposed that integrates the elements of step 3, and according to the indications, the stimulation and reprocessing movements are applied. This corresponds to bilateral brain stimulation movements according to the basic training manual and the author's original book [23].
5. Installation: A positive belief emanating from the user is selected.
6. Body examination: A body evaluation of the general condition is made.
7. Closing the session with emotional security for the patient.
8. Re-evaluation in the next session.

---

[16] By synclectic she refers to the systematic integration of different foundations, with diverse origins in a theoretical body that gives them coherence, different from eclectic, in which they do not have it.

[17] A memory neuronetwork is understood as the fundamental neural structures in learning that adaptively integrate the areas of the diencephalon and telencephalon in a broad way. In the pathological state, the circuits of the limbic system, especially the cerebral amygdala, become hyperactivated in non-adaptive ways.

Regarding the fundamentals described, it is proposed from the neurological point of view that anxiety and fear (one of the main factors of disturbance and disorder) have the nucleus ceruleus and the limbic system as brain anatomical referents, with a special relationship with the *cerebral amygdala*. The latter are hyperfunctional in people with severe disorders, especially those who have traumatic experiences (e.g., people with post-traumatic stress disorder), and thus establish a permanent autonomic connection with the sympathetic nervous system in relation to the hormone ACTH and the activation of the adrenal medulla with adrenaline [34].

This technique allows this hyperfunctional neuronetwork to be connected with other teleencephalic areas such as the anterior frontal cortex and other areas of language and thought, which allow information to be reprocessed, and thus changing the negative and limiting narrative or thought for an adaptive or liberating one.

Good framing, node detection, and bilateral brain stimulation movements can achieve this change for the subject's adaptation with desensitization and reprocessing of information in most cases.

4.6 The Games in Which We Participate

This is the title of the book that Eric Berne published in 1966, in which he develops the concept, applications, and therapeutic strategies of transactional analysis, which is fundamentally about human relationships and the different interactions with conscious and unconscious elements. However, the usefulness for the present work is the *reading of pathological dynamics* as a "game" [42] in which the actors repeat their actions recurrently with mutual discomfort that ends up generating suffering and symptoms.

The therapeutic strategy consists of recognizing this series of communications that are reiterated in the game and breaking them to change their pathological dynamics [43]; that is, to stop "playing" and live fuller relationships.

5 The Interview

The therapeutic interview is perhaps the main tool in which communication processes between the patient and the therapist take place. It is, therefore, a fundamental element for communication, interaction, and the dimensioning of the problem to be treated in each patient.

In a previous study carried out by Morales, a therapeutic interview model was developed [34] with which the patient was approached in a holistic way.[18]

[18] The term "Holistic" refers in this context to the intention of recomposing the whole by considering the 4 Aristotelian causes, understanding that any model of understanding is epistemologically limited.

It is important to bear in mind that each communication expressed by the user has a semiotics that is articulated in sound, visual, gestural, or other signals. As Cyrulnik says "speech modifies the biology of the human being… and confers on the sensory space a semantic value, a semantic territory." So, to speak, it is full of signifiers: each sign, communication, and even each molecule is a carrier of meaning [44].

The interview or the medical act in general, like almost all human patterns that have an importance in the field of human interaction and communication, have three stages: (1) a first stage that is the approach social stage or warm-up (social part), (2) a second stage in which the referring issue is worked on in depth (definition of the problem and its specific intervention) and (3) a third stage of closure in which it is expected to have responded to the expectations prior to that session and that the patient can continue his or her current life.

5.1 First Case Session, First Stage of the Interview

The aim is to make an empathetic connection with the patient, for which the presentation is made in a simple way, and in the same way, it is sought that he or she makes it. The goal at this stage is to learn about their life and life story. It is important to use a neutral topic that facilitates communication without alerting the person's defenses.

It could be very strategic to start life history with special emphasis on the genogram or Familiogram, which allows us to know the family relationships and the bonds that the person has established. To the extent that the person's relationships are known, the entry or exit of people from their circle can be established, some deaths or births of others. The connections (observation of non-verbal language) that they have in the face of these events, with themselves and with others could be compared.

Some questions are very practical for this:

What do you feel while you tell me that? Where do you feel it?
Put your hand where you feel it.

If possible, the subjective information is expanded with the following questions:

What is that body sensation like?
(using the visual analog scale)
On a scale of 0 to 10, where 0 is no disturbance or annoyance and 10 is the maximum disturbance, how annoying or disturbing is that feeling?

It is also possible that they describe the sensation through metaphors "heat, burn, compression, emptiness" or other metaphorical descriptions that in themselves are offering important information about the networks of meaning involved.

At this stage, each of the topics is not yet delved into, only a general map of the connections that the person has with others and with themself is being made. This prepares the ground to be able to enter the next stage where the problem will be defined more thoroughly.

> The response is permanently checked to define what was achieved and what failed as an effect of the interviewer-consultant interactions. To this end, the coherence between the levels of verbal and non-verbal language, the expression of symptoms, and the levels of disturbance are reviewed. [34]

The permanent establishment of rapport or empathy is sought.

> It is a dance of movements such as assent, laughter/smile, dialogue, assent and careful use of words on my part, thoroughly reviewing the type of words, tone and communicative style of the consultant. [34]

The tone of voice, the movements of the hands and trunk and the facial expression are moderated. Communications are directed especially toward the right side of the person, feedback and paraphrasing of the content is made, clarifications are requested, it is nodded or denied bodily, the hands accompany the dialogue, the person's breathing is reviewed and emulated. This attitude is maintained throughout the interview [34].

This first stage is a *staging* of the verbal and non-verbal communication tools that the interviewer has in interaction with the person. On this depends the achievement of trust or empathy to give continuity to the process.

5.2 Second Stage of the Interview

In this stage, we delve directly into what brings the patient into the therapeutic space. Many times, the reason for consultation does not really correspond to what the patient identifies as a problem after delving into this stage with strategic questions, and it is very important to define it because this will guide the intervention route.

In medical training, it is taught that the reason for consultation is definitely the first thing that is inquired about the patient and the objective of the medical act. However, without establishing a previous empathy, the reason for consultation and the expression of the problem could be left with many blind spots. The person is hardly going to reveal their intimacy and to present the interior of their real fears, problems, or difficulties with someone to whom they have not established trust.

Although there are different ways to get to know the background of the patient's situation, this structure of practical questioning allows it to be done in an organized way, specifying the reason for consultation with a scheme that directly or indirectly contains the following questions:

"1. What is the problem? 2. How is this a problem? 3. What has been done to solve it?"

Each of these questions allows the therapist to explore the narrative contained in the person's reference map or belief system. In the first question, it is clearly specified what he/she identifies as a problem. In the second, it asks what is really the context or the way in which the person understands it from their perceptual framework in an integral way, in which we are including the different physical, emotional, and behavioral symptoms, among others. This question can obviously be accompanied by many others that allow us to unveil the internal narrative of the person, with its accompanying fantasies and metaphors.

The questions accompanying this second question are fundamentally: what?, how?, when?, where does it happen?, according to whom is it like that? How did they know?, since when does they learn that?, what improves the symptoms?, what makes them worse?, and what would happen if this were resolved?, among others.[19] That is to say, they are woven together until the problem is clearly established.

When the problem has been clearly established in the person's own terms, feedback is given and the person will say "yes or no," depending on how the problem has been understood. It is convenient to issue this feedback within a scheme such as the following: "correct me if I am wrong, the problem is the following…".

The third question refers to what has been done to solve what they understood as a problem. It is common to observe that what patients do to solve this problem can become a new problem. In other words, they create attempted solutions that not really solve the initial problem.[20]

The conversation should include information about past treatments, the narrative (positive or negative) he or she has about those treatments, what has worked, and what expectations he or she has regarding "our therapeutic space and what we can commit to" [34].

This type of exploration is part of the strategic systemic approach and allows establishing a whole plan for evaluation and definition of goals within the process.

This construction can be better understood in Chap. 20, where it is referred to as the "life history" in Neuraltherapeutic Medicine. This term refers to establishing the occurrence of a person's symptoms or illnesses in relation to the events that took place in their biography.

In this second stage, psychotherapeutic or therapeutic interventions are implemented directly, if at all possible, in accordance with the understanding of the problem. It is possible that the formulation of the questions allows us to enter the intervention phase, or it is also possible that an important association has been found between an event experienced as traumatic and the cognitive, emotional, and somatic symptoms that the person presents, so it would be necessary to carry out the intervention in a comprehensive way at that time (See Chap. 41).

---

[19] The question "Why?" does not appear within the interrogation scheme. The reason for this is that usually the answer would arise from a pre-established framework that triggers the person's defenses, while the other questions allow us to get to the heart of the problem in a more ecological and comfortable way for the person.

[20] A good example of attempted solutions that end up complicating situations further is the use of substances or addictions to solve a problem of anxiety, insecurity or difficulties in relationships, where they do not solve the initial problem and become a new problem to be solved.

5.3 *Third Stage of the Interview*

As will be discussed in detail in Chap. 41, once the intervention stage is over, where the different therapeutic elements have been moved, a closure is carried out that allows consolidating learning elements, not only cognitive but also physical, in a comprehensive way so that the person can continue their life and their usual activity.

The process of mutual feedback is carried out with the consultant presenting the way in which it was approached and how a continuity of the intervention process will be maintained. The formulation of medications is made in case it makes sense within the process. Finally, strengthening the therapeutic alliance with the consultant and defining a consensual treatment plan [34].

5.4 *Next Sessions*

A similar scheme is followed to that carried out in the first session where the first part is about strengthening the therapeutic alliance, inducing rapport with different elements in a shorter way, and reviewing the changes achieved so far.

The second stage also delves into the problem with the question of: *What else needs to be healed now?*. According to what has been investigated, more specific interventions can be carried out by reviewing the emotional, cognitive, behavioral, or narrative contents, always comparing the relationship and coherence between verbal and non-verbal language. Always, it is important to strengthen the bond, promote self-observation, and awareness of the contents [34].

The therapeutic process is reviewed in accordance with the goals established for the third stage; the session, whether full or not, is concluded with the individual's emotional safety and psychoeducation of work-at-home instructions.

6 What Is Worth Healing

Psychiatry, current or hegemonic focused on drugs, generally underestimates the symptoms and only seeks to silence them. This criticism was declared by Sigmund Freud and Hahnemann[21] regarding the medicine of their time.

The meaning of symptoms is what Freud deepens in psychoanalysis [45] and what, in some way, many other authors have also sought. What is worthy of a cure

[21] Hahnemann criticized Hippocratic medicine focused on the humors and how it tried to silence the symptoms that people presented, without finding a real solution for them. Hahnemann, on the other hand, always sought to find a meaning in the symptom, looking for the substance (vegetable, animal or mineral) that induced something similar to the symptom (a kind of metaphor) and, on this, he bases his therapeutic scheme.

can be unraveled when the meaning of the symptoms is understood, both in their content and in the way in which they are produced. To do this, it is necessary to distinguish between the digital and the analog [36], as well as the interrelation between these two parts. In the same way, it is important to understand that the symptom itself is acting as a defense, presenting attempted solutions that are articulated to find a solution without actually succeeding in doing so.

Defenses are persistent attempted solutions in a reentrant circuit, where the neurological and the significant participate, converted into a habit that makes sense within the system of representations of each person or their culture.

The meaning of the symptom is just that: an attempted solution [10]; it is like deciphering any myth—the hero, Oedipus, or any other significant cultural reference—that is personal or can be culturally represented, taking its metaphors full of meaning and managing to make a transformation on them.

In the unconscious system of each person (or the reactive perceptual system narrated by Nardone), the codes are structured in metaphors or language games not only verbally but also in images, thoughts, emotions, and bodily sensations (to give some items of orientation). Language becomes a route to address these codes and thus creates a joint understanding map or navigation routes between the patient (consulting system) and the doctor or therapist (system with a supposed knowledge), whether institutional or circumstantial. To do this, it is essential to create a transitional space in which the patient's system of perceptions and the therapist's system of perceptions intersect.

To expand on the above, what has been called in medicine obsessive neurosis, obsessive-compulsive disorder, or obsessive-compulsive traits will be used below as an example, regardless of the classification system used (there are different examples of this in literature, in people's everyday lives, and in some popular television comedies).[22]

In the acts that a person with these characteristics presents (obsessive-compulsive), words have power and language becomes a trap in which significant fields and habits are repeated over and over again—what was called the omnipotence of words. Rites are constituted as a defense against the anguish that is generated, in a repetitive way, without review of the results produced. In other words, these rites unsuccessfully seek to manage, with repetitive acts, the anguish that paradoxically is increasing.

What is worthy of healing consists of finding in the memory networks of the patient's system the problems that appear to be central and then unraveling their meanings.

The approach is a metaphor in itself because it confronts the symptoms with their meanings. It uses the language of that system or context and introduces itself—in the manner of a fabric—into the patient's meanings and what they interpret as a

[22] The example can be seen in series such as Adrian Munk or Sheldon (Big Bang Theory) in television programs.

problem (the symptom and the problem contain in themselves the counter-logic of their healing).[23]

The approach through this strategy locates a different "codon of meaning".[24] This is information that *transforms the pattern that connects* with sustained defense (reentrant). Also, this allows the reorganization of the system[25] with the different significant roots that organize it in the subject's memories, whether these are emotional, cognitive, neurological, or immunological, among others.

As Freud explained at the time, in behaviors and rituals all the content of the meanings is placed in the patient's memory and the important thing is to decipher and use them.

The meaning of the symptoms and, therefore, what is worthy of healing has to do with the patient's intimate life, with their body, with their life history, with the previous dispositions and the significant learning that were fixed in that memory, including the epigenetic. This fixation refers to an interpretive system of memory fixed in time that is apparently isolated from the other conscious meanings of the system and that, when it finds new connections, it transforms and manages to change its processing (reactive perceptual system). The patient must come to self-transform their "whole memory," where the integral therapist is only a helper in the process, a well-informed advisor.

References

1. World Health Organization. World mental health report: transforming mental health for all [Internet]. World Health Organization; 2022. Available from: https://www.who.int/publications/i/item/9789240049338
2. Morales L. The reconstruction of the integral concept of health and community music therapy. Investigaciones en Seguridad Social y Salud. 2018;20(1):27–40.
3. Baita S. Puzzle: an introductory guide to trauma and dissociation in childhood. Buenos Aires: The Author; 2015.
4. Van der Hart O, Nijenhuis E, Steele K. The tormented self: structural dissociation and the treatment of chronic traumatization. Bilbao: Desclée; 2008.
5. Freud S. Letter to the journal "Le disque vert.". In: Freud S. Complete works. Buenos Aires: Amorrortu editors; 1976.
6. Bateson G. Mind and nature. Buenos Aires: Amorrortu; 2011.
7. Quian Quiroga R. Things you would never believe: from science fiction to neuroscience. Barcelona: Debate; 2024.
8. Maturana H. Objectivity: an argument to oblige. Santiago de Chile: Dolmen; 1997.

[23] There is a clear allusion to Milton Ericsson when he states that the symptoms carry the solution within themselves.

[24] This is a metaphor of "codon of meaning" in which viruses or genetic engineering through introducing a change in the genetic bases indicate to the system that is being intervened and that it must now, from this moment on, produce completely different materials from the previous ones.

[25] Understanding that the system has the four causes as proposed by Aristotle: materialistic and mechanistic evidenced in the physical symptoms, while the formal and final (or better of sense and meaning) is related to the associated psychological and memory contents.

9. Lacan J. The symbolic, the imaginary, and the real [Internet]. Conference held at the Amphitheater of the Sainte-Anne Psychiatric Hospital, Paris; 1953. Available at: lacanterafreudiana.com.ar/2.5.1.4%20%20%20LO%20SIMB,%20LO%20IMAG%20Y%20LO%20REAL,%201953.pdf
10. Nardone G, Portelli C. Knowing through change. Barcelona: Herder; 2006. 248pp.
11. Andrade E. Darwin's demons: semiotics and thermodynamics of biological evolution. Bogotá: Universidad Nacional; 2003.
12. Pinheiro R, Luz M. Effective practices x ideal models: action and thought in the construction of comprehensiveness. In: Pinheiro RA, editor. Construction of comprehensiveness: everyday life, knowledge, and practices in health. Rio de Janeiro: IMS/UERJ-CEPESC-ABRASCO; 2007.
13. Schrödinger E. What is life and mind and matter. New York: Cambridge University Press; 1967. 188pp.
14. Bykov K, Konradi G. Fundamental concepts of physiology. In: Bykov KM, editor. Text-book of physiology. Moscow: Foreign Languages Publishing House; 1960. p. 15–45.
15. Toscano De La Torre F, Pinilla Bonilla LB. The principles of neural therapy from the foundations of nervism to current neuroscience. Salud UIS. 2012;44(2):57–65. Available at: https://revistas.uis.edu.co/index.php/revistasaluduis/article/view/2591
16. Pavlov IP. Conditioned reflexes: lessons on the function of great hemispheres. 3rd ed. Madrid: Ediciones Morata; 2021. p. 433.
17. Sudakov KV. Theory of functional systems: a keystone of integrative biology. In: Nadin M, editor. Anticipation: learning from the past. The Russian/soviet contributions to the science of anticipation. Cognitive systems monographs. Vol. 25. New York: Springer; 2015. p. 153–73. Available at: https://doi.org/10.1007/978-3-319-19446-2_9.
18. Pinilla-Bonilla LB. Critical analysis of the theoretical-methodological procedures of A. D. Speransky's research that support neural therapy from the Peircean logic. Master's thesis. Bogotá: Universidad Nacional de Colombia; 2010. 119p. Available at: https://repositorio.unal.edu.co/handle/unal/6873
19. Pinilla-Bonilla LB. Application of the Peircean research method to Speransky's work. In: Oostra A, Zalamea F, editors. Cuadernos de sistemática Peirceana. Bogotá: Editorial Nomos; 2012. p. 93–114. Available at: https://www.unav.es/gep/bibliopeirceana.html.
20. Bykov KM, Kurtsin IT. Cortico-visceral pathology. 2nd ed. Madrid: Atlante; 1968. p. 849.
21. Kurismaa A. From integrative biology to the nerve impulse: rethinking neural information and semiotics in the functional systems perspective. Adapt Behav. 2023;31(1):87–101. https://doi.org/10.1177/10597123221089557.
22. O'Connor J, Seymour J. Introduction to NLP. Barcelona: Urano; 2007.
23. Shapiro F. Eye movement desensitization and reprocessing—EMDR. Mexico City: Pax; 2004.
24. Adamec RE, Stark-Adamec C, Saint-Hilaire JM, Livingston KE. Basic science and clinical aspects of procaine HCl as a limbic system excitant. Prog Neuro-Psychopharmacol Biol Psychiatry. 1985;9(2):109–19. Available at: https://doi.org/10.1016/0278-5846(85)90073-9.
25. Ketter TA, Andreason PJ, George MS, Lee C, Gill DS, Parekh PI, Willis MW, Herscovitch P, Post RM. Anterior paralimbic mediation of procaine-induced emotional and psychosensory experiences. Arch Gen Psychiatry. 1996;53(1):59–69. https://doi.org/10.1001/archpsyc.1996.01830010061009.
26. Adinoff B, Devous MD, Best SE, Alexander D, Kelly Payne J, Williams M. Dose-response measures of rCBF and subjective changes following procaine in healthy female volunteers. Psychiatry Res. 2002;114(3):123–35. https://doi.org/10.1016/s0925-4927(02)00008-2.
27. Matulewicz P, Orzeł-Gryglewska J, Braszka Ł, Zawistowski P, Jurkowlaniec E. Hippocampal theta rhythm after local administration of procaine or amphetamine into the ventral tegmental area in fear conditioned rats. Neurosci Lett. 2015;589:132–7. Available at: https://doi.org/10.1016/j.neulet.2015.01.049. Epub 2015 Jan 21.
28. Løvtrup S. Ontogeny and phylogeny from an epigenetic point of view. Hum Dev. 1984;27(5/6):249–61. Available at: http://www.jstor.org/stable/26764458

29. Feil R, Fraga M. Epigenetics and the environment: emerging patterns and implications. Nat Rev Genet. 2012;13:97–109. Available at: https://doi.org/10.1038/nrg3142.
30. Peedicayil J. Genome-environment interactions and psychiatric disorders. Biomedicines. 2023;11(4):1209. https://doi.org/10.3390/biomedicines11041209. PMID: 37189827; PMCID: PMC10136093.
31. Labra-Spröhnle F. Human, all too human: Euclidean and multifractal analysis in an experimental diagrammatic model of thinking. In: Nadin M, editor. Anticipation across disciplines. Cognitive systems monographs. Vol. 29. New York: Springer, Cham; 2016. p. 105–33. Available from: https://doi.org/10.1007/978-3-319-22599-9_9.
32. Klefbeck J, Dabas E. Network therapy: a treatment method in crisis situations. Family Syst & Health. 2000:47–63.
33. Walsh F. Family resilience (2nd ed): strategies for strengthening it. Madrid: Amorrortu editors; 2012.
34. Morales L. A proposal for integrating psychotherapy into biographical history: management of adult patients with homeopathy. Master's thesis. Bogotá: Universidad Luis G. Páez; 2015.
35. Bronfenbrenner U. The ecology of human development: experiments in natural and designed environments. Barcelona: Paidós; 1987.
36. Ceberio M, Watzlawick P. The construction of the universe. Buenos Aires: Herder; 2006.
37. Gergen K, McNamee S, Kaye J, Hoffman L, Goolishian H, Andersen T, Cecchin G. Therapy as social construction. Buenos Aires: Paidos; 1996.
38. Téllez A. Clinical hypnosis, an Ericksonian approach. Mexico City: Trillas; 2020.
39. Paul-Cavallier F. Hypnosis according to Erickson. Madrid: Bernett-Danilo; 1995.
40. Grinder J, Bandler R. Frogs into princes: transcription of the seminar by the creators of NLP. Madrid: Gaia; 2001.
41. Shapiro F. EMDR, eye movement desensitization and reprocessing therapy, basic principles, protocols, and procedures. Mexico City: EMDR Library; 2019.
42. Berne E. Games people play: psychology of human relationships. Mexico City: Dana; 1966.
43. Saéz-Alonso R. Psychological games according to transactional analysis, two do not play unless they want to. Madrid: CCS; 2001.
44. Cyrulnik B. From gesture to word: the ethology of communication in living beings. Barcelona: Gedisa; 2004.
45. Freud S. 17th conference. The meaning of symptoms. In: Freud S. Complete works. Amorrortu editors: Buenos Aires; 1993.

Chapter 23
Paraclinical Strategies in Neuraltherapeutic Medicine

Eduardo Humberto Beltrán Dussán

1 Introduction

One of the most important objectives in Neuraltherapeutic Medicine is the appropriate localization of the interfering fields to precisely define the application of stimuli with local anesthetics and thus achieve the best results in patients [1].

Life history and a thorough physical examination are essential to establish circumstantial and temporal correlations associated with the clinical manifestations that are part of the various reasons for consultation, and thus try to locate possible interfering fields [2].

In the life of each patient, organ systems are subject to continuous modifications, many of them originating in accidental traumatic, inflammatory or infectious processes, surgical interventions, or other types of circumstances. Interfering fields are not always structured immediately after the action of the factors that give rise to them, and almost always require a variable time during which the organism can maintain the ability to communicate in a compensated way, until clinical manifestations secondary to interference in communication systems gradually appear [3, 4].

2 Identification of Interfering Fields

There are several strategies that allow the existence of interferences in biological communication systems to be evidenced, when they are not easily identifiable clinically. One of these strategies is the use of diagnostic imaging, through which

E. H. Beltrán Dussán (✉)
Faculty of Medicine, Universidad Nacional de Colombia, Bogotá, Colombia
e-mail: ehbeltrand@unal.edu.co

L. B. Pinilla Bonilla et al. (eds.), *Neuraltherapeutic Medicine*,
https://doi.org/10.1007/978-3-032-03257-7_23

anatomical, traumatic, therapeutic, or other circumstances that have occurred in the past and that may have been structured as interfering fields can be established [5].

Factors that generate interfering fields such as various prosthetic materials, osteosynthesis, foreign bodies, abnormal growths, or alterations in biological structures, among others, can at some point begin to generate interference in the communication systems, causing a complex of symptoms in patients. The use of current diagnostic images ranging from X-rays, ultrasound, nuclear medicine studies, various CT modalities, magnetic resonance imaging, or integration strategies of various images, according to the latest advances in technology, allows the identification of these circumstances [6–9].

One of the most widely used has been images of the oral cavity [10, 11] through which it is possible to identify interfering fields that guide management that must be carried out in coordination with dentists and their specialties, taking into account the concepts of neurofocal dentistry [12–14].

Another way to locate interfering fields is the identification of local temperature variations, which can be established by careful physical examination or with the use of thermography systems, such as infrared thermography by which it is possible to identify temperature variations at sites corresponding to biological interference compared to neighboring tissues, allowing for more precise localization [15].

When there are interfering fields, variations in sensitivity may also occur in the surrounding areas, which can be identified clinically or through algometry systems, [16] which allow the most sensitive areas on the body surface to be objectively identified and thus be able to locate the most appropriate sites for neural therapy medicine interventions.

Interfering fields can also manifest themselves through variations in surface or deep circulation, identifiable through careful observation or using Doppler technology, which allows variations in the circulation of the examined terrain to be objectively established through images that are quite precise in their location [17, 18].

Skin turgor in the areas surrounding the interfering fields can be identified by clinical examination by analysis by manually rolling the folds and moving them, identifying areas with irregularities [19], or identifying variations in the skin's electrical conductivity by electrophysiology-based electronic methods [20].

To identify variations in sweating, new iodine-impregnated paper techniques have been developed, which have been standardized by computer to identify the activation of sweating in place of the old iodine and starch test, which was performed by applying an iodine solution to the area, allowing it to dry and then applying starch powder to evaluate the change in iodine color as an indicator of excessive sweating [21].

Within the conceptualization of Neuraltherapeutic Medicine, it is considered that many interfering fields can be centralized in specific areas of the brain and begin to command interfering activities from the central nervous system. The identification of this phenomenon could be documented by brain mapping techniques in order to obtain a more objective appreciation of corticalization phenomena and also be used as reference points for the evaluation of therapeutic responses [22, 23].

The possibility of identifying interfering fields through measurements with the methodology of Voll's Electroacupuncture has been described, being able to have information on some body areas of their location or identify changes in electrical activity in the path of the scars to specifically locate the altered areas. [24].

All these technologies, which provide safety for the interventions to be performed, should continue to be analyzed with a research-based evaluation to consolidate their usefulness in the practice of Neuraltherapeutic Medicine.

References

1. Dosch P, Dosch M. The interference field and its elimination by means of lightning reaction. In: Dosch P, Dosch M, editors. Manual of neural therapy according to Huneke. 2nd ed. Stuttgart: Thieme; 2007. p. 78–118.
2. Fisher L. Anamnesis and examination. In: Fisher L. Neural therapy according to Huneke: Mexico. Spanish Version of the Publication by Hipocrates Verlag, Stuttgart. 2012. p. 76–84.
3. Kidd R. Interference fields. In: Kidd R, editor. Neural therapy applied neurophysiology and other topics. Renfrew: Custom Printers of Renfrew Ltd.; 2005. p. 24–40.
4. Barop H. The interference field. In: Barop H. Atlas of neural therapy: Mexico. Spanish Version of the Publication by Hipocrates Verlag, Stuttgart. 2003. p. 14–16.
5. Ford B, Dore M, Moullet P. Diagnostic imaging: appropriate and safe use. Am Fam Physician. 2021;103(1):42–50.
6. Davatzikos C, Sotiras A, Fan Y, Habes M, Erus G, Rathore S, Bakas S, Chitalia R, Gastounioti A, Kontos D. Precision diagnostics based on machine learning-derived imaging signatures. Magn Reson Imaging. 2019;64:49–61. https://doi.org/10.1016/j.mri.2019.04.012. Epub 2019 May 6. PMID: 31071473; PMCID: PMC6832825.
7. Hosny A, Parmar C, Quackenbush J, Schwartz LH, Aerts HJWL. Artificial intelligence in radiology. Nat Rev Cancer. 2018;18(8):500–10. https://doi.org/10.1038/s41568-018-0016-5. PMID: 29777175; PMCID: PMC6268174.
8. Lundström C, Lindvall M. Mapping the landscape of care providers' quality assurance approaches for AI in diagnostic imaging. J Digit Imaging. 2023;36(2):379–87. https://doi.org/10.1007/s10278-022-00731-7. Epub 2022 Nov 9. PMID: 36352164; PMCID: PMC10039170.
9. Velazquez-Albino AC, Imhoff ED, Rinaldi-Ramos CM. Advances in engineering nanoparticles for magnetic particle imaging (MPI). Sci Adv. 2025;11(2):eado7356. https://doi.org/10.1126/sciadv.ado7356. Epub 2025 Jan 8. PMID: 39772674; PMCID: PMC11708890.
10. van der Stelt PF. From pixel to image analysis. Dentomaxillofac Radiol. 2021;50(2):20200305. https://doi.org/10.1259/dmfr.20200305. Epub 2020 Nov 11. PMID: 33119990; PMCID: PMC7860954.
11. Majanga V, Viriri S. Dental images' segmentation using threshold connected component analysis. Comput Intell Neurosci. 2021;2021:2921508. https://doi.org/10.1155/2021/2921508. PMID: 34950198; PMCID: PMC8691977.
12. Barciela Calderón J, de la Torre Roses M, Cabrera Carballo N, Barrios Rosdríguez MA. Neurofocal dentistry as part of neural therapy. Revista Archivo Médico de Camagüey. 2002;6(6):661–8. Retrieved on October 14, 2024, from http://scielo.sld.cu/scielo.php?script=sci_arttext&pid=S1025-02552002000600014&lng=es&tlng=es
13. Kidd R. Dental aspects of neural therapy. In: Kidd R, editor. Neural therapy applied neurophysiology and other topics. Renfrew: Custom Printers of Renfrew Ltd.; 2005. p. 72–84.
14. Dosch P, Dosch M. The dental interference field. In: Dosch P, Dosch M, editors. Manual of neural therapy according to Huneke. 2nd ed. Stuttgart: Thieme; 2007. p. 91–9.

15. Kesztyüs D, Brucher S, Wilson C, Kesztyüs T. Use of infrared thermography in medical diagnosis, screening, and disease monitoring: a scoping review. Medicina (Kaunas). 2023;59(12):2139. https://doi.org/10.3390/medicina59122139. PMID: 38138242; PMCID: PMC10744680.
16. Castien RF, Coppieters MW, Durge TSC, Scholten-Peeters GGM. High concurrent validity between digital and analogue algometers to measure pressure pain thresholds in healthy participants and people with migraine: a cross-sectional study. J Headache Pain. 2021;22(1):69. https://doi.org/10.1186/s10194-021-01278-8. PMID: 34253164; PMCID: PMC8276500.
17. Chipperfield AJ, Thanaj M, Clough GF. Multiscale, multidomain analysis of microvascular flow dynamics. Exp Physiol. 2020;105(9):1452–8. https://doi.org/10.1113/EP087874. Epub 2020 Feb 7.
18. Kim ES, Sharma AM, Scissons R, Dawson D, Eberhardt RT, Gerhard-Herman M, Hughes JP, Knight S, Marie Kupinski A, Mahe G, Neumyer M, Poe P, Shugart R, Wennberg P, Williams DM, Zierler RE. Interpretation of peripheral arterial and venous Doppler waveforms: a consensus statement from the Society for Vascular Medicine and Society for Vascular Ultrasound. Vasc Med. 2020;25(5):484–506. https://doi.org/10.1177/1358863X20937665. Epub 2020 July 15.
19. Dosch P, Dosch M. Examining the Patient. Skin. In: Dosch P, Dosch M, editors. Manual of neural therapy according to Huneke. 2nd ed. Stuttgart, Thieme; 2007. p. 68–71.
20. Abe Y, Nishizawa M. Electrical aspects of skin as a pathway to engineering skin devices. APL Bioeng. 2021;5(4):041509. https://doi.org/10.1063/5.0064529. PMID: 34849444; PMCID: PMC8604566.
21. Gagnon D, Ganio MS, Lucas RA, Pearson J, Crandall CG, Kenny GP. Modified iodine-paper technique for the standardized determination of sweat gland activation. J Appl Physiol (1985). 2012;112(8):1419–25. https://doi.org/10.1152/japplphysiol.01508.2011. Epub 2012 Feb 9. PMID: 22323650; PMCID: PMC3331585.
22. Markello RD, Hansen JY, Liu ZQ, Bazinet V, Shafiei G, Suárez LE, Blostein N, Seidlitz J, Baillet S, Satterthwaite TD, Chakravarty MM, Raznahan A, Misic B. Neuromaps: structural and functional interpretation of brain maps. Nat Methods. 2022;19(11):1472–9. https://doi.org/10.1038/s41592-022-01625-w. Epub 2022 Oct 6. PMID: 36203018; PMCID: PMC9636018.
23. Alexander-Bloch AF, Shou H, Liu S, Satterthwaite TD, Glahn DC, Shinohara RT, Vandekar SN, Raznahan A. On testing for spatial correspondence between maps of human brain structure and function. NeuroImage. 2018;178:540–51. https://doi.org/10.1016/j.neuroimage.2018.05.070. Epub 2018 Jun 1. PMID: 29860082; PMCID: PMC6095687.
24. Dosch P, Dosch M. Equipment-based methods. In: Dosch P, Dosch M, editors. Manual of neural therapy according to Huneke. 2nd ed. Stuttgart: Thieme; 2007. p. 118–20.

Chapter 24
The Diagnosis in Neuraltherapeutic Medicine

Laura Bibiana Pinilla Bonilla and Jazmín Ariza-Tarazona

1 The History of the Concept of Diagnosis and Its Limitations

The concept of diagnosis can be traced back to Hippocratic physicians, such as Alcmaeon of Crotona. In Homeric times, the verb "diagignoskein", a Greek word that means to distinguish or discern, was used. To be more precise, day means "through" and gignoskein means "to know," a concept that was also known as he diagnostike tekhne (the art of distinguishing or identifying diseases) [1, 2]. In other words, this expression means:

> To know technically an individual disease (…) to know how to discern it precisely among all the others and to penetrate visually into what is not seen of it through what is apparent in it. [1]

In some ancient texts, the term skeptomani (meaning to observe carefully or examine in detail) had been used as an equivalent of diagignoskein, since the act of diagnosing "concerns not only the external and apparent, but also the internal and essential" [1].

L. B. Pinilla Bonilla (✉)
Faculty of Medicine, Master in Alternative Medicine, Neural Therapy Area, Universidad Nacional de Colombia, Bogotá, Colombia

Integrated Health Services Subnetwork of the South, Research and Innovation Center, Bogotá, Colombia
e-mail: lbpnillab@unal.edu.co

J. Ariza-Tarazona
Master in Alternative Medicine, Neural Therapy Area, Faculty of Medicine, Universidad Nacional de Colombia, Bogotá, Colombia

L. B. Pinilla Bonilla et al. (eds.), *Neuraltherapeutic Medicine*,
https://doi.org/10.1007/978-3-032-03257-7_24

Until this point in history, the diagnostic exercise was assumed as an act of research and observation to not only identify cases of disease but also to unravel its causes. However, with the arrival of the modern age, under a classificatory scheme and based on analysis, an exercise of describing the "ways of getting sick" was introduced, which was called nosography. With the work of Thomas Sydenham in the seventeenth century, the concepts of "clinical picture and morbid species" were introduced with the intention of reducing diseases to species in a similar way to how botanists do in their phytologies [3].

According to Laín Entralgo [4], in the modern age three notions of disease began to be introduced, which, according to some authors, constituted the biological conception of disease. The first of these notions is the anatomoclinical configuration configured since Galen and which assumes the disease as a visible and verifiable lesion. The second notion is the pathophysiological one, which understands that the disease is a process that begins before the pathological injury or change in structure. And, finally, the etiopathological notion that was born with the microbial theory of diseases, which, in turn, opened the door so that not only microorganisms were considered as the only agents capable of causing disease, but also this possibility was extended to physical and chemical agents that can also invade the organism altering it [5].

The entry of this biological conception into medicine led to the conception of disease as an "entity" capable of incorporating, landing, and developing in the body. That is to say, the disease is objectified [3] by considering itself as something external to the organism, which must be fought at all costs and must be "separated" from the person. By separating the disease from the person they had as prey, then this human being could return to their previous self and return to "normality." This conception of normality, which comes from statistics, presents the difficulty that it ignores the individual processes of getting sick [6, 7]. These and other limitations of this conception are expanded upon in Chap. 19 of this book.

From the perspective of Neuraltherapeutic medicine, the processes of illness and their corresponding diagnoses are read through another lens. These processes are intertwined with multiple internal and external factors in the life of each being and make the dispositions to get sick absolutely unique and dependent on each biography [6, 7]. Chapter 19 delves into various elements that lead to a reinterpretation of the concept of illness for neuraltherapeutic medicine; in Chap. 20, emphasis is placed on the life history and the influence of sociocultural aspects in the interpretation of both their body and what it means to get sick for that being; and in Chap. 46, it delves into how environmental, social, historical and cultural aspects are integrated in a diagnostic exercise applied to the community and primary health care environment.

In the following section, the foundations and implications that this new conception has for the diagnostic field in neuraltherapeutic medicine will be presented.

2 Fundamentals of the Diagnostic Approach in Neural therapeutic Medicine

The vision of diagnosis within the practice of Neuraltherapeutic medicine, together with the health-disease conception, underwent a transformation throughout history in the Colombian territory (see Chaps. 3 and 18).

As mentioned in other chapters of this book, Neuraltherapeutic medicine was nourished by different sources, such as neural therapy according to Huneke from Germany, synthetic physiology from Russia (Chap. 13), conceptions from British nervism (see Chap. 14), complexity sciences (Chap. 7), among others.

As far as diagnosis is concerned, Neuraltherapeutic medicine borrowed from the German school elements of the diagnostic scheme that at the same time guide therapy [8, 9]. From synthetic physiology, he took Pavlov's concept of corticalization, Ukhtomsky's conception of the dominant focus [10] and the non-linear and integrative conception of the nervous system that determines a specific course or development of pathologies or neurodystrophies within the organism according to Speransky [11]. From British nerves, especially from the neurologist Henry Head, it takes elements concerning the extent of irritations in the organism and the factors that facilitate their generalization [12, 13]. Finally, it draws on different theories of the complexity sciences, especially the applications of the theory of nonlinear dynamic systems and chaos theory to the concept of health, disease [14–16] and applications to the conception of the functioning of the nervous system as a whole where nonlinear and creative phenomena occur constantly [17] and where communication and information management processes also occur that can be understood from a quantum perspective [18, 19] (See Table 24.1).

Table 24.1 Conceptual elements from different fields and theories that contributed to the structuration of a new diagnostic approach in NTM

Elements for a new diagnostic conception in NTM	
NT school according to Huneke [8, 9]	Pathological alterations are due to irritations located at the following levels: 1. Local 2. Segmental 3. Interfering field (remote location)
Synthetic physiology or Russian nervism [10, 11]	1. Neurodystrophies (pathologies) could have the next stages: (a) Segmental distribution (included the symmetric and contiguous distribution) (b) Extension beyond the segment (c) Generalization or corticalization 2. Physical changes are interwoven with emotional and behavioral changes (monistic perspective) 3. After an organism interacts with environmental agents, the organism is never the same again. Therefore, a new organism is being created at every moment by its interactions with the environment 4. In the brain, dominant centers are permanently created and destroyed both at a physiological and pathological level, in a non-local manner, given the temporary associative nature (conditioned reflex) of the NS

(continued)

Table 24.1 (continued)

Elements for a new diagnostic conception in NTM	
British nervism [12, 13]	1. The rules for generalization are the next: (a) Segmental distribution (including the symmetric and contiguous distribution) (b) Extension to lower resistance areas (remote extension) (c) Complete generalization 2. Visceral diseases have a semiological expression, whether in superficial or deep tissues 3. Mental changes are related to visceral disease (monistic perspective)
Complexity sciences [14–19]	From the perspective of complexity sciences, biological systems are considered to have the following characteristics: 1. They experience constant processes of exchanging matter, energy and information with the environment as open systems which behave far from equilibrium. When their dynamics are close to the equilibrium, the systems are getting closer to the thermodynamic death 2. Experience non-local phenomena thanks to the non-linear interrelationship between their parts and due to the quantum behaviors in nature 3. Their processes are constantly changing, irreversible, and therefore evolutionary. So, there are homodynamic process more than homeostatic ones 4. They experience self-organization processes where new creative patterns emerge constantly within their structure

Source: Own elaboration

3 Diagnostic Approach in Neural therapeutic Medicine

As mentioned in the previous section, Neuraltherapeutic medicine integrated and synthesized various elements from the previously mentioned schools and theories to build its own notion of diagnostic practice. When applying these concepts and elements to the theory and practice of Neuraltherapeutic medicine, the following consequences are derived for the diagnostic conception:

1. *Diagnosis as a dynamic and open process:* Diagnosis is not a "state," but a "process" that the individual goes through and that tends to change with each internal and external factor that is related to his or her biography. Diagnosis, therefore, is only an interpretation or a temporary reading of dynamic and adaptive processes that have been developing in the patient. There can be no room for definitive or static diagnoses. Every time the same patient comes to our office for a check-up, it is really a new organism since it is a thermodynamically open system.
2. *The problem of nosographic classifications*: Speransky [11] demonstrated through his research that the tendency of medicine to classify diseases according to their differences is a mistake. This author, on the contrary, invites us to unite the different pathologies according to their similarities in order to arrive at a synthetic and unified theory in medicine. Therefore, a diagnostic scheme for Neuraltherapeutic medicine aligned with the principles of synthetic physiology

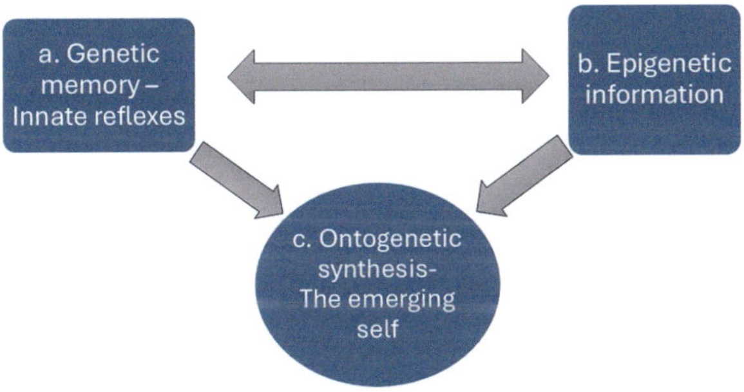

Fig. 24.1 The figure illustrates how ontogeny is a process of synthesis from which "being" constantly emerges, and which is determined by both genetic/innate reflexes and by epigenetic factors involving extrinsic and intrinsic variables. Genetic and epigenetic factors can influence each other during this ontogeny. (Source: Authors)

moves away from the nosographic classificatory proposals of biomedicine, as will be seen later.

3. *The individuality of the diagnosis*: As mentioned in Chap. 22, ontogenetic development involves a series of transformations that take place in living beings, involving their genetic and epigenetic memories, which in turn are based on innate and conditioned reflexes, respectively (See Fig. 24.1).

The information from the environment that has the capacity to modify the epigenetic aspect of organisms, together with the information from individual experiences and experiences, causes unique interpretative synthesis processes to be generated within each organism, constantly changing in each being.

Disease and health from this framework are part of a process of interpretation and assignment of meaning that each being experiences within its becoming.

Considering that, according to synthetic physiology, the conditioned or acquired reflexes that develop in ontogeny are the vast majority of the physiological reflexes of organisms [10], this supports the claim that no two or more identical physiological dynamics can exist. Each organism builds its own temporal associations that determine unique physiological or pathological pathways. Therefore, the nosographic classification system that implies a series of symptoms and signs and a natural development or course of the disease would not have validity from this perspective, since it ignores the individual dynamics and reflexes acquired during the life history of each being.

As an example, two women of the same age, from the same socioeconomic strata, may have developed a series of signs and symptoms that from biomedicine have been labeled as migraine, but in one woman this process may have an irritative origin within the maxillomandibular terrain, while in the other woman it may come from a pathological reflex established in her gynecological area. Interwoven with stories of emotional trauma during their gestations. Obviously, the treatment in each case is absolutely different: in the first case, the diagnosis must lead to treatment and a thorough examination of the oral cavity with diagnostic support and perhaps an assessment by a neurofocal dentist; while, in the second case, the patient could benefit from an infiltration in the uterovaginal plexus in addition to a therapeutic approach to her emotional traumas.

4 Diagnosis as a Dynamic Process in Neuraltherapeutic Medicine

Inspired by the diagnostic schemes developed by the school of Neural Therapy according to Huneke [8, 13], pathophysiological dynamics can be identified that present qualitative differences according to their location, temporality, and dominant expression.

4.1 Pathophysiological (or Irritative) Dynamics According to their Location

1. *Local irritation*: It corresponds to a pathological manifestation that is still circumscribed in the direct area of the first injury. It does not present manifestations or alterations of the other components of the embryologically related segment. There is no symmetrization of clinical manifestations, and there are no signs of generalization or corticalization.
2. *Segmental irritation*: corresponds to a reflex involvement of the other elements derived from embryological metameres, such as dermatomes, myotomes, sclerotomes, or viscerotomas related to the site of the initial lesion. Originally, embryological reflexes are innate or unconditioned, which means that these reflexes tend to be the least variable between different individuals, presenting slightly more predictable dynamics. However, like any innate reflex, they cannot escape the possibility of associating with other information within the nervous system, constituting conditioned reflexes.

   Within life history, it is therefore important to carry out a review of all the systems based on their embryological connections, which allows for the rapid evaluation of all the components of the same segment. As an example, if a person consults for pain in the lower limbs, e.g., located in the leg, ankle and foot, it is important to ask about the other structures that are embryologically linked to these. The affectation in this case is located in the territory of L4-S3. Therefore, it is essential to also check how the genitourinary system and the rectus sigmoid, which receive the same innervation, are located, as well as to check how the other components of the lumbosacral plexus are located (see Chap. 14).
3. *Metasegmental irritation or beyond the segment:* This type of irritation has been classically called the "interfering field" phenomenon since the German school and, more recently, "neuromodulatory trigger" [20]. Its foundation from synthetic physiology is based on the phenomena of temporal associations that occur within the natu-

ral function of cortical coupling of the nervous system [10]. This phenomenon of temporal association is what allows the generation of conditioned reflexes, which are characterized by being dynamic and non-linear. Within the life history, for this reason it is important to carry out an inquiry of all the events organized chronologically, in order to be able to identify previously affected places of the organism and their temporal associations (regardless of their apparent anatomical distance) with other incoming information or afferents that the organism registered at the same time. According to synthetic physiology, a first stimulus/information that reaches the organism can modify its internal dynamics and can become a dominant focus or center. This dominant focus ends up attracting other incoming information to this neuronetwork at the same time in that nervous system, leaving two (different) neuronetworks linked thanks to their simultaneous activation (see Chap. 13).

4. *Generalization and corticalization*: A state of generalization corresponds to an affectation of more than three segmental levels. Henry Head [12] described factors that facilitated generalization that consisted of fever, anemia, mental shock, and menstruation in women. However, a pathology that has been developing for a long time without treatment (chronic) tends to extend by contiguity to other metamers or nearby segments, extends by symmetry, and toward sites of least resistance (or previously affected in the life history), generating an increasing commitment of other segmental levels until reaching a complete generalization. When these processes occur, the inhibitory mechanisms of that organism are generally altered, which can be evidenced by general sensitization phenomena (lowering the pain threshold), mental alterations or irritability, as well as affecting the sleep pattern (as an indicator of natural inhibitory mechanisms).

   On the other hand, although the concept of corticalization is more related to the visceral reflexes that underwent a conditioning process in the cerebral cortex, in daily practice, it has been acquiring a wider use, which is applied when the physical examination finds reflex involvement in the area of the head with increased sensitivity located in each of the specific regions for each of the viscera of the trunk according to Head.

4.2 Pathophysiological (or Irritative) Dynamics According to Their Temporality

1. *Acute process*: it is the one that usually develops in the 3 days following an injury or event experienced by the patient. The symptoms can be perceived as intense and affect the performance of daily tasks. Generally, it is circumscribed to an area or segment.
2. *Subacute process*: It is that pathophysiological dynamic that tends toward stability in the system, manifesting symptoms cyclically and repetitively, and that are sustained for a period of 1–8 weeks.
3. *Chronic process*: it is that neurodystrophic process that tends to remain stable within the body, manifesting symptoms in a cyclical and repetitive way for more than 8 weeks.

4.3 Pathophysiological (or Irritative) Dynamics According to Their Dominant Expression

Although, according to the monistic position of Neuraltherapeutic medicine it cannot be considered that the psyche is in any way separate from the physical dimension of the being, it is possible that, at certain moments, there is a dominant expression in one of the two spheres. To expand on this matter, it is worth quoting an analogy with the dual nature of the phenomenon of light, which, depending on various circumstances, can behave as a particle (physical) or as a wave (mental).

1. *In the physical sphere:* At a certain time, the patient who attends the consultation manifests mostly symptoms in the physical area, orienting the therapeutic management towards this area.
2. *In the mental and emotional sphere*: At a certain time, the patient may have a manifestation of emotional or mental predominance, orienting therapeutic management towards an approach to their traumatic or non-adaptive memories.

4.4 Diagnostic Tools

In the preceding chapter (Chap 23), paraclinical strategies are addressed.

5 The Importance of Integration Within the Diagnostic Approach of the Dominant Foci or Centers: An Illustrative Case

As discussed in Chap. 13, a dominant center is a focus of excitation in the nervous system that modifies the activity of other nerve centers or nerve networks, thus attracting incoming impulses simultaneously. These centers have increased excitability, taking the lead that generates a disposition or a certain pattern of reactions in the nerve centers [21].

The dominant foci can influence the functional dynamics of the other centers to which the irritative process extends or they can also inhibit their normal functioning. Additionally, its influence can reach sites distant from the initial or dominant focus; i.e., a non-local dynamic.

The following is a hypothetical illustrative case of a female patient who presents as an initial pathological alteration a neurodystrophy or inflammatory disorder of the female genital organs, i.e., in the language of biomedicine, an inflammatory pelvic disease. This inflammatory process begins after a dystotic delivery that was complicated by postpartum endometritis.

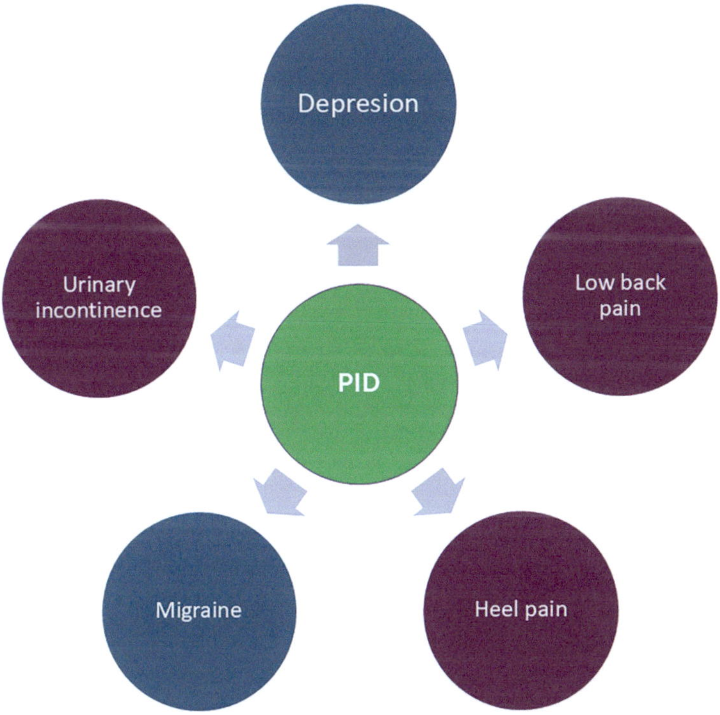

Fig. 24.2 It shows a case of a dominant center located in the gynecological area, which originated other disturbances in the embryological parts related to it and temporarily associated with this first area. (*Source:* Own elaboration)

Its inflammatory condition of the genital area is prolonged over time, so that it begins to affect other structures (see Fig. 24.2) of the same segment that are embryologically related, which are found in violet color: urinary incontinence, heel pain, and low back pain. But additionally, this initial focus takes on so much strength that it ends up generating distant effects, generating irritation in the head area, and finally generating mental changes such as depression. In this case, the genital focus is an example of a dominant focus or center that has both embryological expressions based on innate reflexes and also non-local or remote expressions, supported by temporal associations (conditioned reflexes).

Performing this type of diagnosis can allow that, with an intervention, in this case directed towards the genital terrain, a therapeutic benefit can be obtained by modulating inflammation and improving the trophism of the tissues associated with embryologically, (in this case bladder, heel, and lumbar region), as well as generating an improvement of remote manifestations such as migraine and depression.

References

1. Lain EP. The origins of medical diagnosis. Dynamis Acta Hispanica ad Medicinae Scientiarumque Historiam Illustrandam. 1981;1(1):3–15.
2. Coronado H. Medical diagnosis. Biociencias. 2016;11(1):69–73. Available from: https://revistas.unilibre.edu.co/index.php/biociencias/article/view/2872
3. Niño ED. Becoming ill as semiosis. Contribution to a logical-semiotic critique of medical practice. Thesis. Bogotá: Universidad Nacional de Colombia; 2000. 140p.
4. Laín Entralgo P. Universal history of medicine. Barcelona: Salvat; 1974.
5. Quevedo E. The health-disease process: toward a non-positivist clinic and epidemiology. Permanent seminar on health and administration. Bogotá: Pontificia Universidad Javeriana; 1990.
6. Cardozo AM, Pinilla LB, Andrade LE. Rethinking the concept of illness from evolution and emergence. In: Beltrán E, Vega J, editors. Neural therapeutic medicine: an approach from complex medical systems. Bogotá: Universidad Nacional de Colombia; 2013. p. 73–102.
7. Payán JC. Vital disobedience. Buenos Aires: Salbe Ediciones; 2005.
8. Dosch P, Dosch M. Manual of neural therapy according to Huneke. 2nd ed. Stuttgart: Thieme; 2007.
9. Fisher L. In: Niño Ibarra MC, editor. Neural therapy according to Huneke; neurophysiology, therapeutic injection techniques, vol. 1. 3rd ed. Mexico: Unknown editorial; 2012. p. 1–261.
10. Konradi G. Activity of the nervous system. In: Bykov KM, editor. Text-book of physiology. Moscow: Foreign Languages Publishing House; 1960. p. 516–670.
11. Fisher L. Neural therapy: neurophysiology, therapeutic injection techniques. 5th edition. Stuttgart: Georg Thieme Verlag; 2019. p. 208.
12. Navarro K, Pinilla L. Henry Head's contributions to the neuroanatomical and physiological foundations of segment therapy. Med UIS. 2013;26(2):33–44.
13. Head H. On disturbances of sensation with especial reference to the pain of visceral disease. Brain. 1893;16(1–2):1–133.
14. Boubaker O. Chaos in physiological control systems: health or disease? Chaos Theory Appl. 2024;6(1):1–12. Available from: https://dergipark.org.tr/en/pub/chaos/issue/83761/1413955
15. Goldberger AL. Non-linear dynamics for clinicians: chaos theory, fractals, and complexity at the bedside. Lancet. 1996;347(9011):1312–4. https://doi.org/10.1016/s0140-6736(96)90948-4.
16. Goldberger AL, Amaral LA, Hausdorff JM, Ivanov PC, Peng CK, Stanley HE. Fractal dynamics in physiology: alterations with disease and aging. Proc Natl Acad Sci USA. 2002;99(Suppl 1):2466–72. https://doi.org/10.1073/pnas.012579499.
17. Freeman WJ. The physiology of perception. Sci Am. 1991;264(2):78–87. Available from: http://www.jstor.org/stable/24936793
18. Jibu M, Hagan S, Hameroff SR, Pribram KH, Yasue K. Quantum optical coherence in cytoskeletal microtubules: implications for brain function. Biosystems. 1994;32(3):195–209. https://doi.org/10.1016/0303-2647(94)90043-4.
19. Freeman W, Vitiello G. Matter and mind are entangled in two streams of images guiding behavior and informing the subject through awareness. Mind Matter. 2016;14(1):7–24. Available from: https://www.ingentaconnect.com/contentone/imp/mm/2016/00000014/00000001/art00002
20. Engel R, Barop H, Giebel J, Ludin SM, Fischer L. The influence of modern neurophysiology on the previous definitions of "segment" and "interference field" in neural therapy. Complement Med Res. 2022;29(3):257–67. https://doi.org/10.1159/000522391.
21. Zueva EY, Zuev KB. The concept of dominance by A.A. Ukhtomsky and anticipation. In: Nadin M, editor. Anticipation: learning from the past. The Russian/Soviet contributions to the science of anticipation, Cogn Syst Monogr, vol. 25. New York: Springer; 2015. p. 13–35. https://doi.org/10.1007/978-3-319-19446-2_2.

Part VII
Therapeutic System in Neuraltherapeutic Medicine

Chapter 25
Therapeutic Approach in Neuraltherapeutic Medicine

Laura Bibiana Pinilla Bonilla and Jazmín Ariza-Tarazona

1 General Therapeutic Guidelines

The therapeutic approach in Neuraltherapeutic medicine involves several aspects, such as the injection of procaine, lifestyle adjustments (Chap. 27), dietary adjustments, identifying and avoiding exposure to environmental (Chap. 28) and electromagnetic (Chap. 17) toxins, and recognizing the sociocultural and environmental environment that characterizes the person's habitat and may be a determining factor of their health.

Cases that require special attention to emotional traumas should be considered (see Chap. 41), as well as cases that require referral and assessment by other specialties or other health professionals, such as neurofocal dentists (chap. 43) or psychologists, or even other medical-surgical specialties, when the state of dystrophies exceeds the scope of neural therapeutic intervention.

On the other hand, when performing the intervention with procaine, it is important to keep in mind the principles set out by Pavlov in the framework of synthetic physiology and apply them to the therapeutic field. According to what has been discussed in Chaps. 13 and 22, interventions with procaine are weak irritant stimuli that can easily act in a modulatory manner [1]. Other chapters of this textbook also show that these interventions can act as inhibitory and desensitizing agents (Chap.

L. B. Pinilla Bonilla (✉)
Faculty of Medicine, Master in Alternative Medicine, Neural Therapy Area, Universidad Nacional de Colombia, Bogotá, Colombia

Integrated Health Services Subnetwork of the South, Research and Innovation Center, Bogotá, Colombia
e-mail: lbpnillab@unal.edu.co

J. Ariza-Tarazona
Master in Alternative Medicine, Neural Therapy Area, Faculty of Medicine, Universidad Nacional de Colombia, Bogotá, Colombia

L. B. Pinilla Bonilla et al. (eds.), *Neuraltherapeutic Medicine*,
https://doi.org/10.1007/978-3-032-03257-7_25

41). It is important to note that the process of inhibition or desensitization of pathological irritation takes time and requires reinforcement [2]. When a therapeutic intervention has had a positive effect on the modulation of inflammation and on the improvement of the trophism of that organism, but has not been able to achieve a complete disappearance of the signs and symptoms of that patient, it is advisable to reinforce the previously established therapy.

2 Therapeutic Guidelines for the Approach to Pathophysiological (or Irritative) Dynamics According to Their Location

Prior to any therapeutic approach, the anamnesis, the system review, the chronological description of the history (Chap. 20), the physical examination (Chap. 21), and the intervention after the pertinent analysis must be carried out.

Usually, the intervention starts with a more local and segmental approach. If the therapeutic response to superficial interventions is still only partial after several reinforcements, deep approaches in nodes and plexuses are chosen. An example will be taken as a patient who comes to the clinic for asthma that is difficult to manage with the therapy established by pneumology. Within the life history and evaluation carried out, the neuraltherapist considers that the irritation is at a segmental level and decides to start treatment in the Head's zone of the lungs. After several reinforcements (two or three), the patient manifests an improvement of no more than 50% or indicates a transient improvement that does not last more than 30 days, and the pathological or dystrophic condition is restored. In these cases, the doctor may make the determination to perform a deep approach, for example, through the performance of a stellate ganglion technique. On this occasion, after the intervention in this ganglion, it was possible to obtain a remission of symptoms of almost 100%, which only reappears slightly when there is seasonal flu.

In accordance with the classification of types of irritation set out in Chap. 24, the approach will depend on the neuraltherapeutic diagnostic exercise:

(a) *Local irritation*: Following a physical examination, the treatment for this type of irritation takes place directly at the pathological manifestation site. This treatment could be made through the application of injections in the superficial tissues or in deeper tissues as appropriate. An example of a local approach may be the application of papules or periarticular injections near the external malleolus in the case of an ankle sprain.
(b) *Segmental irritation*: The management strategy for this type of irritation should be derived from the specific management of segmental therapy, which is presented in Chap. 30. This, in turn, is based on Chap. 15 on segmental physiology. After carrying out an evaluation of surface sensitivity and deep tissues, such as fascia, muscle, and osteoarticular tissues, and following the embryological distribution, the intervention is performed according to the respective findings. Depending on the signs found on physical examination, the level of depth and

the level of technique to be used are determined, whether it is the application of papules, injections into scars, injections into subcutaneous tissues, fascia, muscle, pre-periosteal, or joint injections.

(c) *Metasegmental irritation by dominant focus*: once a dominant focus in the nervous system has been identified by life history and physical examination, the treatment is carried out. Subsequently, the professional may evaluate the therapeutic effect in its areas of influence. For instance, if a patient comes in for help with a lung problem that caused bronchial hyperreactivity for the first time during pregnancy, the doctor may decide to do an approach to the uterovaginal plexus as a treatment. After the plexus is performed, the response in the lung organ is evaluated in the next consultation.

(d) *Generalization or corticalization*: this type of case must be evaluated in a very detailed way to identify the focus of dominance in the same way. A very common generalization example is found in cases diagnosed by conventional medicine as fibromyalgia. The life history in these cases, must be aimed at finding the origin of when the symptoms began localized in some anatomical region, which progressed until they reached a generalization. Ideally, this treatment should be directed toward the anatomical places where everything originated. Similarly, if it is a case where an emotional trauma is identified as a trigger, as shown in Chap. 41, emotional traumas also have sites of body anchorage, and these would constitute a therapeutic objective.

3 Therapeutic Guidelines for the Approach to Pathophysiological (or Irritative) Dynamics According to Their Temporality

The classification of dystrophy or pathology (acute, subacute, or chronic) will determine the time to carry out the interview and initial approach.

(a) *Acute pathology*:

Whether in an outpatient or inpatient setting, if the patient presents with acute and very severe pain (with a VAS > 8/10), it may be necessary to first address the patient's desperate pain. Clinical experience in neural therapy has indicated that it has a significant impact on pain management (see Chap. 42, on clinical applications). Therefore, from a humanistic perspective, in these cases it is advisable to first focus on alleviating human suffering. Then, delve deeper into the search for the cause of the dystrophy. Occasionally, the patient's condition and their relationship with the physician allow for rapid identification of the interfering field or focus of dominance from that initial consultation or interconsultation, allowing for intervention. It is important to be vigilant and conduct follow-up to rule out possible urgent surgical pathologies.

Not only are painful pathologies treatment objectives in these acute cases. For example, it is also possible to treat mental and emotional disorders in acute cases, which may correspond to cortico-visceral pathologies, through minimally invasive approaches and with excellent results [3].

(b) *Subacute or acute non-painful pathology*: If the patient is attending for acute non-painful or subacute diseases, such as vertigo, respiratory diseases (otitis, bronchitis, pharyngotonsillitis, laryngitis, pneumonia), gastroenteritis, colitis, genital and urinary tract infections, facial paralysis, eye infections, acute sinusitis, or exacerbated rhinitis, among others, the approach should be more focused on the acute and subacute condition. This approach must be made by the evaluation of all systems and directed life history. The need for a referral to the emergency department needs to be assessed.

(c) *Chronic pathology*: If the patient attends for chronic diseases, the approach allows for a much more extensive review by systems and the description of the history in the timelines to make an intervention that favors, preferably, an approach to the interfering field or focus of pathological dominance, as the case may be.

4 Technical Guidance

It is beyond the scope of this textbook to comprehensively cover each of the techniques mentioned below, because they have already been described extensively in various sources throughout history, some of them included in Techniques Atlases [4] and others in textbooks [5–9]. Instead, this textbook will include in Part VIII some techniques, with a special focus on innovative developments and new proposals.

To perform the techniques, the puncture site, needle direction, and intervention depth must be considered.

Depending on the stage of the district (see Chap. 24), one or more of the following techniques will be required[1] [5, 7]:

- Papule: a technique that performs a wheal on the epidermis, leaving an appearance of orange peel skin with a change in coloration (whitish and raised skin) where the branches of the spinal nerve in the dermatome are intervened. This procedure is generally more painful than deeper procedures due to the greater number of nociceptors located in the dermis. Papules have very favorable effects, from changes in the extracellular matrix to the spinal nerve associated with your dermatome.
- Scars: These are considered frequent fields of irritation. The intervention must extend from the epidermis and dermis to the deepest tissue. Please keep in mind that some scars are much smaller in the epidermis than in deep tissues.

[1] If more information on superficial or deep techniques is required, the reader is suggested to consult the different atlases of neural therapy that are published by different authors in Germany [4–8] or Turkey [9].

- Subcutaneous tissue and fascia injection: It is a deeper injection into the dermis and subcutaneous cellular tissue, including superficial fascia and trigger points.
- Injection into muscle tissues: A technique that directly injects muscle mass or its tendons, including trigger points.
- Pre-periosteal injection: This injection infiltrates the tissues near the periosteum, which is adjacent to the bone.
- Intra-articular injections: Injection that intervenes directly into the joint cavity. Remember that this type of infiltration requires adequate training and, as a requirement, disinfection.
- Perivasal or intravasal injections: Injections made into surrounding tissue and the nerve network surrounding or within blood vessels.
- Injection around organs (thyroid, tonsils, prostate, periodontal tissue).
- Injections into plexuses, ganglia, sympathetic chains, cranial nerves, and nerves presented below under a topographical scheme:

  1. *Head*: supraorbital nerve (V1), infraorbital nerve (V2), nasociliar nerve, upper maxillary nerve (V2), nasopalatine nerve (V2), infratrochlear nerve, atriculotemporal and greater auricular nerve, lower maxillary nerve (V3), inferior dental nerve (V3), mental nerve (V3), facial nerve (VII), vagus nerve (X) , glossopharyngeal nerve (IX), greater and lesser occipital nerve, and ganglia such as the ciliary, otic, pterygopalatine, Gasser's ganglion, or cervical sympathetic chain.
  2. *Neck*: phrenic nerve, spinal or accessory nerve, superficial cervical plexus, retrostyloid technique (or technique to access the vicinity of the superior cervical ganglion, facial nerve, glossopharyngeal nerve, vagus nerve, spinal nerve, and internal carotid plexus), stellate ganglion, thyroid gland, superior and inferior laryngeal nerve.
  3. *Trunk*: intercostal nerves, solar plexus, celiac plexus, lumbar sympathetic chain.
  4. *Pelvis and genitals*: sacral roots, cauda equina, uterovaginal plexus by vaginal way and suprapubically, prostatic gland perineally and suprapubicly, pudendal nerve perineally and para-ischiatic.
  5. *Extremities*: axillary nerve or plexus, radial nerve, ulnar, median, interdigital nerves, sciatic nerve, cluneal nerves, femoral nerve, geniculate nerves, common peroneal nerve, superficial peroneal nerve, deep peroneal nerve, posterior tibial nerve, sural nerve, and saphenous nerve.

5 Medical Supplies and Devices in Neuraltherapeutic Medicine

To talk about therapeutics, the elements and supplies that will be described below must be considered. These supplies and devices, their denominations, and characteristics may vary according to the availability and legislation of each country.

The medical office or clinic should be equipped with the standards of each country and generally include the basic equipment for a general or specialized medical consultation.

The basic supplies for the performance of neural therapeutic intervention are the following:

- Disposable syringes.
- Disposable needles.
- Procaine 1–2% (or available depending on the country); if failing that, use lidocaine.
- Disposable gloves.
- Antisepsis elements (gauze, alcohol, chlorhexidine, and hydrogen peroxide).
- Tongue depressor.
- Lantern.
- Gynecological table.
- Mechanical algometer.
- Specula.
- Intravenous infusion equipment (macrodrip/microdrip IV set, intravenous catheter, 0.9% saline, sodium bicarbonate).

Regarding syringes, 1 mL, 3 mL, 5 mL, and 10 mL can be used, which will be chosen according to the volume required in the procedure. In dentistry, carpule syringes are also used.

The needles are classified according to gauge and length in inches. In Colombia, 30G and 27G gauge needles are available, with sizes that can vary from half an inch, one inch, or one and a half inches. In other countries, 25G is also used.

With regard to the longest and largest diameter needles, the following references are generally used:

- G23—6 cm × 0.6 mm
- G23—8 cm × 0.6 mm
- G21—12 cm × 0.8 mm.

Regarding the therapeutic neural agent, procaine is the anesthetic of choice due to its low toxicity due to its rapid metabolism by plasma esterases (see Chap. 26). In case of absence of procaine, a second option for its use is lidocaine, but it should be taken into account that its metabolism is hepatic and that it has a longer half-life. The usual concentrations of the commercial forms of procaine and lidocaine are 1% and 2%, although they may vary by country. In some cases, considering the principle of applying a mild and nonspecific neural stimulus, procaine can be diluted with saline solution to obtain concentrations of 0.75%, 0.5% or 0.25%, especially in older patients or in people with strong responses or exacerbations.

On the other hand, if a history of irritative reactions is found within the life history due to the administration of local anesthetics, for example, in the use of dental interventions, the application should be done with caution. Although the possibility of procaine type 1 allergy is extremely rare [10], the neural therapist should evaluate this possibility and perform susceptibility tests using procaine concentrations below 0.5%.

5.1 *Other Forms of Use of Local Anesthetics*

Within neural therapeutic medicine, it is possible to use the therapeutic neural agent (procaine or lidocaine) in other ways, namely:

(a) Topicals and patches.
(b) Irrigation of areas such as nasal, ocular, otic, pharyngeal, vaginal, urethral, rectal.
(c) Oral use in capsule form, available in some European countries.
(d) Systemic application by infusion, usually intravenous (see Chap. 40).

6 The Art of Reducing Loads

The authors of this chapter refer to the art of reducing loads, such as the process of prior analysis of the life history and the physical examination of the patient to identify, in advance, the possible dominant or irritative foci that may be markedly exacerbated in patients, if they have not been previously managed. This strategy was created from the occurrence of real cases of patients in whom the exacerbation presented could have been avoided through an adequate prior analysis and initial management of local irritative foci. This strategy emphasizes an exhaustive anamnesis of all previous foci that can be identified in the life history (pathological, surgical, traumatic, dental, gynecological, among others).

Below are two real cases of which the academy was aware. In the first case, a stellate ganglion technique was applied as the first neuraltherapeutic intervention, due to severe and refractory migraine, in a patient without prior exhaustive assessment of the maxillomandibular terrain. The patient had an impacted wisdom tooth on the ipsilateral side of the pain. After the application of the technique, the patient had extreme pain that led her to hospitalization for refractory pain without achieving control, until a panoramic x-ray was performed, where this situation was identified. Once the dental extraction was performed, the patient was asymptomatic.

The second case involved a patient who underwent a first neuraltherapeutic technique on the upper cervical ganglion due to a headache. Subsequently, the patient experienced paralysis of the third cranial nerve, which required approximately 1–2 months to recover. When reviewing the life history of the case, the patient had undergone an intraocular lens insertion, a focus that had not been managed neuraltherapeutically through a local approach in the ocular area.

From these cases, and many others that are not mentioned in this space, it was concluded and learned that local irritations should be treated initially and later segmentally, before performing deeper approaches such as nodes or plexuses. This to reduce unwanted exacerbation reactions for the patient or the therapist. From the authors' experience, if this "reduction of loads" is carried out through the early treatment of local and segmental irritations in this order, this facilitates that patients have more favorable evolutions, and that they do not even require management with deep interventions.

From the theory of nervism (see Chap. 13), these exacerbations can be explained by the fact that in the nervous system, there are dominant excitation foci and dominated or secondary excitation foci. When the focus is dominant, it generates both inhibition and excitation processes on other minority foci. If the focus to be treated in the Neuraltherapeutic intervention is not the dominant or primary focus, but a focus associated with it is intervened, the stimulation that is carried out through the Neuraltherapeutic impulse generates that the dominant center attracts this incoming impulse to itself, generating greater excitation of it. Whereas when the dominant focus is addressed directly, an inhibitory phenomenon is generated on it [11, 12]. Within the history of neural therapy, there is a case that can clearly illustrate this physiological phenomenon. This is the case of the first phenomenon in seconds that occurred in a patient who was injected in the shoulder, but that a few days later generated an activation of a focus that was apparently silent from an old osteomyelitis scar (see Chap. 2). The osteomyelitis scar was the dominant focus, and the shoulder was dominated by it.

6.1 Factors That Facilitate Exacerbations

Within the practice of Neuraltherapeutic medicine, there are several factors that can facilitate the generation of exacerbations, such as:

(a) *Starting treatment ignoring conditions of vulnerability*: sometimes patients with multiple comorbidities, especially the elderly, may come to the Neuraltherapeutic medicine consultation. Since pain is the most frequent consultation in Neuraltherapeutic medicine, it is important that the doctor, before starting a treatment aimed at reducing pain, evaluates conditions of vulnerability, such as:

   (i) History of coronary heart disease.
   (ii) History of chronic obstructive pulmonary disease.
   (iii) History of kidney disease.
   (iv) History of epilepsy or central nerve injuries.
   (v) History of some other disease that has had significant consequences (hospitalizations) and is currently apparently inactive.

   In these cases, it is of utmost importance that, prior to treatment with Neuraltherapeutic medicine in a somatic region to improve pain, these active or silent foci are identified, and priority management is given the high risk of exacerbation.

(b) *Irritating and high-acid-load foods*: Foods that are traditionally known to be "irritants" in popular knowledge should be avoided as much as possible, such as pork or other foods that have a high acid load, promoting a state of low-grade metabolic acidosis. In the specific case of pork meat, it has been found that this irritant effect can be attributed to high concentrations of histamine [13].

On the other hand, some research has been emerging that evaluates the ability of foods to produce acidic or basic precursors under the concept of potential renal acid load (PRAL). In general, high-protein foods, such as meat, cheeses, eggs, and the like, have been found to increase PRAL, while fruits and vegetables decrease it. Foods with a high PRAL have been associated with the development of metabolic alterations, arterial hypertension, renal, bone and muscle alterations due to the state of low-grade metabolic acidosis [14, 15]. Therefore, it is advisable to invite the patient to migrate to more balanced eating habits that avoid chronic low-grade inflammation.

(c) *Abrupt discontinuation of medications*: When patients begin treatment with Neuraltherapeutic medicine and begin to show significant improvement, it is common for them to express the desire to discontinue some or all of the medications due to their adverse effects, mainly. When this happens, the doctor must be cautious not to proceed with an abrupt suspension of the drugs, and preferably, this process should be agreed upon with the specialist who formulated the medication. Generally, this suspension is not performed during the first session but after a series of minimal sessions with a sustained improvement over time that is observable and verifiable, including by diagnostic imaging or laboratories. If the final decision is to suspend medications, it is advisable that this be done gradually so as not to generate rebound effects.

(d) *Initiation of deep or intravascular techniques without reducing loads*: as already mentioned in the previous section, the first Neuraltherapeutic treatments must be aimed at reducing irritative loads at a local and segmental level.

7 Post-therapeutic Reactions

Typical reactions following neuraltherapeutic medicine interventions usually occur within the first 48 h and consist of a group of symptoms that tend to be common among individuals. The most frequent symptoms tend to be local discomfort at the puncture site, such as erythema, heat, pruritus, and ecchymosis. These expected reactions tend to improve with hot physical means.

On the other hand, there are slightly more general reactions that are less frequent, such as fever, dizziness, headache, asthenia, adynamia, and the transient increase in pain or discomfort that was the reason for consultation. While these reactions last, the patient should drink plenty of fluids, try not to consume irritating foods during this period, and not have a high acid load. The medicines that are prescribed during this time depend on what the doctor thinks is best, such as whether painkillers are needed to help with symptoms or homeopathic, phytotherapeutic, or homotoxicological medicines are chosen.

Characteristically, reactions do not tend to last more than 72 h after the procedure. If there are any symptoms that persist over time after 72 h, the doctor should evaluate whether it is rather an exacerbation of an irritative focus previously established in the patient's nervous system, and that should be treated.

8 Types of Response to Neural therapeutic Stimulus

After the neuraltherapeutic intervention, several types of responses can occur according to the type of nervous system of each patient. Pavlov described different types of nervous systems according to three basic properties that he called strength, balance, and mobility [11]. The first of these relates to the limit of the working capacity of cortical nerve cells in relation to the excitation processes that are triggered in them. The second talks about the relationship between excitation and inhibition, and whether or not both processes are equally active in the cerebral cortex. And the last one talks about the ease and speed that the cortex has to generate changes between one state and another.

Pavlov, in fact, described four types of nervous systems that he defined as choleric, sanguine, melancholic, and phlegmatic. Strong reactions are usually generated in sanguine and choleric types. Balanced reactions are usually triggered in the sanguine and phlegmatic types. Unbalanced reactions are generally triggered between melancholic and choleric and, finally, weak reactions, between melancholic and phlegmatic types.

Understanding the types of the nervous system can guide the doctor on the possible reactions that can be expected after a neuraltherapeutic intervention. However, Pavlov himself also mentioned that these types of nervous systems or personalities are not fixed during ontogeny. That is, they are susceptible to being modified according to the experience to which the individual is exposed.

With this in mind, three types of response can be identified after neuraltherapeutic intervention:

1. *Immediate or rapid responders*: these are types of nervous system whose response may manifest itself in the following hours or immediately in the doctor's office after NTM intervention. Now, depending on whether it's a balanced or unbalanced type, the reaction may tend toward transient exacerbation or simply resolution, respectively.
2. *Intermediate responders*: these are types of nervous systems that tend to respond in a period of between 24 and 72 h with different types of nuances.
3. *Late or slow responders*: these are types of nervous systems that tend to exhibit delayed reactions, that is, after 72 h. In general, in this type of responder, the reactions are not as intense and can also be slow with respect to the change that occurs in the organisms.

It is also important to keep in mind that the nervous system of an individual with a certain personality will not always have the tendency to be same. Reactions can also change depending on the tone of the nervous system at the time. For example, a nervous system that is very acutely irritated, with intense pain or a serious illness, when receiving a weak stimulus, is very likely to generate a transmarginal inhibition. Transmarginal inhibition develops when the intensity of a stimulus exceeds a certain limit and the result is not intensification, but weakening or total inhibition of the reflex [11].

These types of responses may also depend on previous emotional states or previous foods or the amount of irritation to which that organism has been exposed prior to the neuraltherapeutic intervention. All these factors can be elements that the neuraltherapist can identify when monitoring this type of reactions and responses in patients, and it also helps to define the plan and periodicity of successive interventions that are required.

References

1. Vishnevsky A. The Novocain blockade and balsamic oil antiseptics as a pathogenic therapeutic form. Cartago: Buenos Aires; 1958.
2. Pavlov IP. Conditioned reflexes: lessons on the function of the great hemispheres. 3rd ed. Madrid: Ediciones Morata. 2021, 433pp. [Spanish].
3. Ruiz-Mejía AF, Beltrán-Dussán EH, Morales-Hernandez LA, Pinilla-Bonilla LB. Neural therapy approach in a hospitalized patient with acute stress disorder. Case Rep. 2020;6(1):25–32. Available from: http://www.scielo.org.co/scielo.php?script=sci_arttext&pid=S2462-85222020000100025&lng=en
4. Dosch M. Atlas of neural therapy: with local anesthetics. 3rd ed. Stuttgart: Thieme. 2012. 224p.
5. Dosch P, Dosch M. Manual of neural therapy according to Huneke. 2nd ed. Stuttgart: Thieme; 2007.
6. Barop H. Textbook and atlas of neural therapy. Diagnosis and therapy with local anesthetics. New York: Thieme; 2017. Available at: https://thieme.co.uk/9783132410497/textbook-and-atlas-of-neural-therapy/
7. Fisher L. Neural therapy: neurophysiology, therapeutic injection techniques. 5th edition. Stuttgart: Georg Thieme Verlag; 2019. p. 208.
8. Weinschenk S. Handbook of neural therapy: diagnostics and therapy with local Anesthetics. 1st ed. Munich: Elsevier, Urban & Fischer; 2010. [German].
9. Nazlikul H. Neural therapy textbook. Istanbul: Nobel Kitabevi; 2010. [Turkish]
10. Weinschenk S, Mergenthaler C, Armstrong C, Göllner R, Hollmann MW, Strowitzki T. Local anesthetics, procaine, lidocaine, and mepivacaine show vasodilation but no type 1 allergy: a double-blind, placebo-controlled study. Biomed Res Int. 2017;2017:9804693. https://doi.org/10.1155/2017/9804693. Epub 2017 Dec 11. PMID: 30035116; PMCID: PMC6049527.
11. Konradi G. Activity of the nervous system. In: Bykov KM, editor. Textbook of physiology. Moscow: Foreign Languages Publishing House; 1960. p. 516–670.
12. Zueva EY, Zuev KB. The concept of dominance by A.A. Ukhtomsky and anticipation. In: Nadin M, editor. Anticipation: learning from the past. The Russian/Soviet contributions to the science of anticipation, Cognitive systems monographs, vol. 25. New York: Springer; 2015. p. 13–35. https://doi.org/10.1007/978-3-319-19446-2_2.

13. Chung BY, Park SY, Byun YS, Son JH, Choi YW, Cho YS, Kim HO, Park CW. Effect of different cooking methods on histamine levels in selected foods. Ann Dermatol. 2017;29(6):706–14. https://doi.org/10.5021/ad.2017.29.6.706.
14. DiNicolantonio JJ, O'Keefe J. Low-grade metabolic acidosis as a driver of chronic disease: a 21st century public health crisis. Open Heart. 2021;8(2):E001730. https://doi.org/10.1136/openhrt-2021-001730. PMID: 34702776; PMCID: PMC8549658.
15. Osuna-Padilla IA, Leal-Escobar G, Garza-García CA, Rodríguez-Castellanos FE. Dietary acid load: mechanisms and evidence of its health repercussions. Nephrology. 2019;39:343–54. https://doi.org/10.1016/j.nefroe.2019.08.001.

Chapter 26
Local Anesthetics in Neuraltherapeutic Medicine

Margarita Santamaría and Guillermo Ospino

1 Introduction: History Was Born in Latin America

The inhabitants of the Andean region during the pre-Columbian era used the leaf of a small shrub called coca (*Erythroxylum coca*) for both maintenance and ritual purposes. Early Spanish writings noted its properties as a substance that reduced hunger and fatigue among the natives of America. According to legend, the coca leaf was given to the Inca people by Manco Capac, son of the sun [1–3].

The narrative continues with the introduction of coca leaves into Europe and their subsequent examination by naturalists, particularly Thomas Moreno y Maíz [4]. In his 1868 monograph titled *Recherches quimiques et physiologiques sur l'erithroxylum coca du Perou et la cocaine,* naturalist Moreno y Maíz details the properties of both the plant and its traditional preparations, as well as the characteristics and applications of its extract, cocaine.

In 1859, the Italian Paolo Mantegazza declared the coca leaf as a new and exciting weapon against diseases [5]. Despite its millenary use in America and its introduction in Europe, history attributes to Albert Niemann, a German chemist, the isolation of the alkaloid, cocaine, and the binding of it with hydrochloride salts for possible therapeutic use [1, 6].

The rise of modern medicine in the first half of the twentieth century generated a growing need to optimize surgical procedures, among which pain management during interventions stood out. It was the German ophthalmologist Karl Koller (1857–1944) who, when observing the anesthetic properties of cocaine in eye

M. Santamaría (✉)
Faculty of Medicine, Universidad Nacional de Colombia, Bogotá, Colombia
e-mail: sesantam@unal.edu.co

G. Ospino
Department of Surgery, Hospital Universitario Nacional, Bogotá, Colombia
e-mail: geospinor@unal.edu.co

L. B. Pinilla Bonilla et al. (eds.), *Neuraltherapeutic Medicine*,
https://doi.org/10.1007/978-3-032-03257-7_26

surgery, divulged the characteristics of this substance. His study not only focused on its anesthetic effects, but also on the consequences that would eventually lead to addiction, a fact he shared with his friend, the celebrated psychoanalyst Sigmund Freud (1856–1939) [1, 7, 8].

The adverse effects associated with cocaine prompted pharmacologists in the late nineteenth century to seek new compounds that demonstrated anesthetic properties without the accompanying side effects. Consequently, in 1904, the German chemist Alfred Einhorn (1856–1917) synthesized novocaine, a compound exhibiting anesthetic properties like those of cocaine. Novocaine could be used in larger quantities without the primary issues presented by cocaine, such as toxicity, short duration of anesthesia, inability to sterilize the solution, and high cost, among other concerns [1, 2].

Novocaine, renamed procaine in North America during World War I, prompted the development of local anesthesia as a crucial component in surgical procedures in addition to the early identification of its anti-inflammatory and organism-regulating properties. During the first half of the twentieth century, its widespread use was evidenced, being used by Vishnevsky and Speransky in Russia; Huneke in Germany; Leriche, Dos Ghali, and Hazard in France; and Danielopolu and Parhon in Romania. Exhibiting not only local anesthetic properties but also non-systemic anesthetics, procaine contributed significantly to improving the evolution of patients by reducing the incidence of infections, improving the body's trophic functions, and positively influencing the rehabilitation process [9–11].

While novocaine blockades were being developed in Europe, Russia, and North America in 1929 an alkaloid was discovered on a pest-resistant barley farm. This discovery led Holger Erdtman (1902–1989) to investigate the compound, called gramine. Later, Nils Löfgren (1913–1967) and Bengt Lundqvist (1922–1953) working with a isogramine derivative, developed in 1948 a substance with a longer anesthetic duration than procaine, which would be marketed as lidocaine [12].

2 Chemical Structure of Local Anesthetics

Local anesthetics are molecules that are made up of three parts (Fig. 26.1) [13]:

- Lipophilic end which is composed of an aromatic ring.
- Hydrophilic end with an amino terminal group.
- Intermediate chain, with an ester or amide-type bond that allows them to be divided into two large groups: amino esters, such as procaine and amino amides, such as lidocaine.

Ester-type local anesthetics are rapidly metabolized by plasma esterases within 4 to 8 min, producing para-aminobenzoic acid (potentially allergenic) and diethylaminoethanol [14].

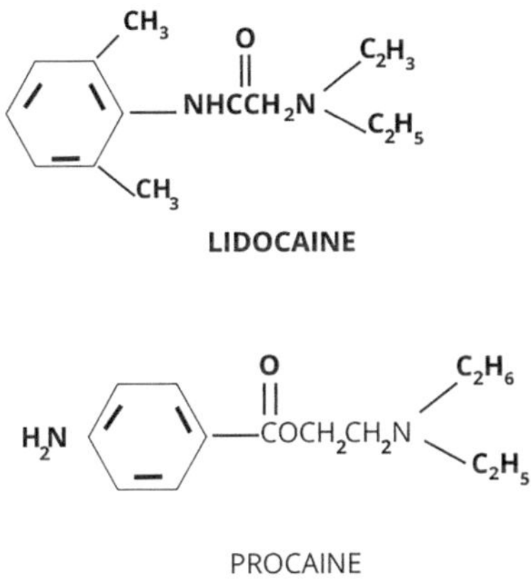

Fig. 26.1 Chemical structure of the local anesthetics: procaine and lidocaine (*Source*: Own elaboration)

Local anesthetics are weak bases, and in aqueous solution the protonated cationic form (due to the affinity of the amine end) and the neutral fat-soluble form are in equilibrium. The proportion of the two forms determines the pKa, or dissociation constant at the pH of the surrounding medium; that is, each local anesthetic has an ionized percentage at pH 7.4; the higher the pKa, the greater the ionized fraction there will be in the solution. Since local anesthetics act within the cell, the ratio of the pKa of the drug to the pH of the tissue in which it is applied determines how quickly the effect is achieved; the higher the non-ionized (fat-soluble) fraction, the faster it will enter the cell. This is why anesthetics with lower pKa have shorter action latencies. The pKa of procaine is 8.9, and that of lidocaine is 7.9 [15, 16].

3 Physiology of Nerve Conduction

Neurons can get electrically excited because they have ion channels in their cell membranes. An action potential is made when these channels, mostly sodium channels, open. In the resting state, neuronal membranes have a negative charge of between −60 and −90 mV (resting membrane potential). Any stimulus that reduces the negative potential to the threshold of −55 mV causes an action potential that allows massive sodium ions to enter the cell and potassium to exit through voltage-gated ion channels, until the electrical potential reaches +40 mV, which is known as depolarization. Subsequently, the sodium channels are inactivated, and the flow of potassium ions allows repolarization to the resting state, the restoration of the membrane potential is achieved through the Na/K ATPase pumps, with the consequent energy consumption [15].

4 Mechanism of Action

Local anesthetics operate primarily by reversibly blocking the activity of sodium channels. Additionally, they have activity on potassium channels, nicotinic receptors, NMDA receptors, and G proteins. The main clinical effect of local anesthetics is on the voltage-dependent sodium channel; once inside the cell, the local anesthetic reaches a new state of equilibrium (ionized and non-ionized form) determined by the intracellular pH. The ionized form acts on the channel when it is open and inactive. Once bound, the local anesthetic prevents neuronal transmission, and nerve block depends on its concentration. The clinical effect ends when the drug diffuses from the cell interior to the extracellular space and the systemic circulation [16].

5 Pharmacokinetics

The plasma concentration of local anesthetics is determined by their absorption, metabolism, and excretion.

Absorption: The rate and extent of systemic absorption of local anesthetics depends on multiple factors such as: injection site, dose, physicochemical properties of local anesthetics, and addition of vasoconstrictors. Injection into highly vascularized tissue results in high plasma concentrations of local anesthetics in a short time [17]. Systemic absorption according to the application site is:

1. Intravenous
2. Intercostal
3. Caudal
4. Epidural
5. Plexo braquial
6. Sciatic
7. Subcutaneous injections.

Metabolism: Ester-type anesthetics such as procaine have metabolism through plasma esterases, except for cocaine which is metabolized in the liver by carboxylesterases. Amide-type anesthetics have their metabolism under hepatic biotransformation through the cytochrome p450 system. The metabolites of amide-type anesthetics are excreted by the kidneys [15, 18].

6 Toxicity

Local anesthetics are safe when administered correctly. However, it has been documented that toxicities can occur due to unintentional intravascular, intrathecal, or intraneural injections, or by systemic absorption if the maximum recommended doses are not respected [16].

LAST (Local Anesthetic System Toxicity): Its incidence increases with a relative overdose of local anesthetics. The main manifestations are first observed in the central nervous system, followed by cardiovascular involvement. Other scenarios include intravascular injection of local anesthetics, which can cause cardiovascular collapse. Injections in the cervical region present the risk of inadvertently entering the cerebral circulation or even the subarachnoid space, which can cause seizures or depression of the central nervous system. The initial symptoms vary according to the plasma concentration of the local anesthetic and patient-specific factors, such as acidosis and protein binding, and can present a wide range of manifestations [16, 19].

Central nervous system toxicity: Anxiety, dizziness, perioral numbness, fainting, and tinnitus, which are caused by blockage of the brain's inhibitory pathways. Other signs observable in possible local anesthetic poisoning are chills, muscle spasms, tremors, and, finally, generalized tonic-clonic seizures [16].

Cardiovascular system toxicity presents with plasma concentrations higher than those required for CNS toxicity; there is no pattern or arrhythmia typical of local anesthetic poisoning. It manifests itself with hypotension, arrhythmias, myocardial depression, cardiovascular collapse, and complete heart block, with life commitment [15, 20].

Prevention is the key to avoiding toxicity from local anesthetics. Systemic absorption depends on the blood supply in the area of administration. It is essential to know the anatomy of the site, respect the maximum doses, aspirate before injecting to avoid intravascular punctures, and administer the dose slowly while maintaining verbal contact with the patient.

The maximum recommended dose for lidocaine is 3 mg/kg patient weight; the addition of epinephrine increases the maximum recommended dose of lidocaine to 7 mg/kg body weight. The maximum total dose of procaine in adults is 1000 mg in 24 h. Since dilutions of procaine used in Neuraltherapeutic medicine range from 0.25% (i.e., solutions with 2.5 mg of procaine per mL) to 0.5% (5 mg of procaine per mL), the probability of reaching these maximum doses during interventions is low [13, 21].

Treatment: being alert to the presentation of signs or symptoms of toxicity is the first step of treatment; if suspected, it is necessary to suspend the administration of the medication, request help, ensure adequate ventilation, and prepare for possible management of the patient's airway, since hypoxia, hypercarbia, and acidosis worsen management. In the case of the presence of seizures, benzodiazepines are the preferred agents for their control; however, any other hypnotic medication can be used.

The management of cardiovascular compromise should follow the guidelines of advanced life support, with the following considerations: The use of epinephrine should be prudent, since doses greater than 1 mcg/kg can induce malignant arrhythmias. The use of vasopressin, calcium channel blockers, and beta-blockers should be avoided, as these can aggravate the prognosis by their interaction with ion channels. Arrhythmias should be treated with amiodarone. It is crucial to start lipid solution treatment as soon as possible [15].

7 Other Properties of Local Anesthetics

This effect on the limbic system is shown by a rise in cerebral blood flow following intravenous administration of procaine. This rise lasts for up to 90 minutes after administration, which could explain how it affects patients' mood [14, 15]. Other parts of this book talk about the effects of procaine on the body (Chap. 40) and on patients' mental health (Chap. 41). This chapter only talks about some of its other effects besides stopping nerve impulses and being useful for pain management.

- Anti-inflammatory: Local anesthetics, through the activation and adhesion of leukocytes, suppress the release of pro-inflammatory cytokines such as interleukin 6, interleukin 8, and C-reactive protein [22].
- Antiarrhythmics: They reduce automatism, especially of ectopic foci, and increase the absolute refractory period, reducing the phenomenon of reentry. (The doses at which cardiac toxicity occurs from procaine are 3 to 5 times higher than those produced by antiarrhythmics.) [14].
- Antineoplastic: Its possible antineoplastic effects are explained by the generation of apoptosis, reduction of neoplastic cell migration, and favoring immunocompetence. Research has demonstrated that procaine epigenetically reduces DNA methylation, thereby halting the growth of gastric and breast cancer cells [22–24].
- Antithrombotic: by inhibition of platelet aggregation [22].
- Antimicrobials with action on the growth of mycobacteria, gram-positive, gram-negative, fungi, and influenza A viruses [22, 25–27].

8 Conclusions

Local anesthetics are drugs that transformed medical practice by eliminating discomfort associated with medical-surgical operations. Currently, they have not been supplanted by any alternative pharmacological agents, and their characteristics are continually being examined in response to the escalating demands of a society increasingly susceptible to oncological diseases and the implications of aging.

They are a crucial instrument in Neuraltherapeutic medicine, considering the impulses produced through their administration, following careful clinical assessment, yield outcomes unattainable with alternative medications.

References

1. Arthur GR, Courtney KR, Covino BG, Garfield JM, Gintant AI, Gissen AJ, et al. Handbook of experimental pharmacology. Local Anesthetics. [Internet]. Strichartz GR, editor. Berlin, Heidelberg: Springer; 1987. 292p. (Handbook of experimental pharmacology; vol. 81). Available from: http://link.springer.com/10.1007/978-3-642-71110-7
2. Ruetsch YA, Boni T, Borgeat A. From cocaine to ropivacaine: the history of local Anesthetic drugs. Curr Top Med Chem [Internet]. 2005;1(3):175–82. [Cited 2025 Jan 10]. Available from: https://www.eurekaselect.com/article/26557
3. Stolberg VB. The use of coca: prehistory, history, and ethnography. J Ethn Subst Abuse [Internet]. 2011;10(2):126–46. [Cited 2025 Jan 10]. Available from: https://www.tandfonline.com/doi/abs/10.1080/15332640.2011.573310
4. Moreno y Maíz T. Chemical and physiological research on Erythroxylum Coca from Peru and cocaine [Internet]. Paris: Louis Leclerc Libraire-éditeur; 1868. [Cited 2025 Jan 10]. Available from: https://bibliotecadigital.bnp.gob.pe/bitstreams/87cbc9ef-3c24-4632-9e5b-f8292be3c50e/download
5. Redman M. Cocaine: what is the crack? A brief history of the use of cocaine as an anesthetic. Anesth Pain Med. 2011;1(2):95–7.
6. Calatayud J, González Á. History of the development and evolution of local anesthesia since the coca leaf. Anesthesiology. 2003;98(6):1503–8.
7. Markel H. About coca: Sigmund Freud, Carl Koller, and cocaine. JAMA [Internet]. 2011;305(13):1360–1. [Cited 2024 Dec 26]. Available from: https://jamanetwork.com/journals/jama/fullarticle/896143
8. Markel H. An anatomy of addiction: Sigmund Freud, William Halsted, and the miracle drug cocaine. New York: Pantheon Books. 2011. 314pp.
9. Gradinaru D, Ungurianu A, Margina D, Moreno-Villanueva M, Bürkle A. Procaine – the controversial geroprotector candidate: new insights regarding its molecular and cellular effects. Oxid Med Cell Longev [Internet]. 2021;2021:3617042. [Cited 2025 Jan 24]. Available from: https://onlinelibrary.wiley.com/doi/full/10.1155/2021/3617042
10. Leriche R. Treatment of embolism and thrombosis of the cerebral vessels. Br Med J [Internet]. 1952;1(4752):231–5. [Cited 2025 Jan 24]. Available from: https://www.bmj.com/content/1/4752/231
11. Speransky AD. A basis for the theory of medicine. New York: International Publishers; 1943.
12. Warner DS, Gordh T, Gordh TE, Lindqvist K. Lidocaine: the origin of a modern local anesthetic. Anesthesiology [Internet]. 2010;113(6):1433–40. [Cited 2024 Dec 27]. Available from: http://links.lww.com//ALN/A649
13. Heavner JE. Local Anesthetics. Curr Opin Anaesthesiol [Internet]. 2007;20(4):336–42. [Cited 2025 Jan 24]. Available from: https://journals.lww.com/co-anesthesiology/fulltext/2007/08000/local_anesthetics.11.aspx
14. Gomez L, Gianchino L. Intravenous procaine: past or future of anesthesiology? In: Aldrete J, Paladino M, editors. Pharmacology for anesthesiologists, intensivists, emergency physicians, and pain medicine. Rosario: Corpus; 2006. p. 255–61.
15. Paladino M, Marelli D. Pharmacology of local Anesthetics. In: Aldrete J, Paladino M, editors. Pharmacology for anesthesiologists, intensivists, emergency physicians, and pain medicine. Rosario: Corpus; 2006. p. 263–71.

16. Taylor A, McLeod G. Basic pharmacology of local anaesthetics. BJA Educ [Internet]. 2020;20(2):34–41. [Cited 2025 Jan 24]. Available from: http://www.bjaed.org/article/S2058534919301520/fulltext
17. Suzuki S, Gerner P, Lirk P. Local anesthetics. In: Hemmings HC, Egan T, editors. Pharmacology and physiology for anesthesia: foundations and clinical application. 2nd ed. New York: Elsevier; 2019. p. 390–411.
18. Bill TJ, Clayman MA, Morgan RF, Gampper TJ. Lidocaine metabolism: pathophysiology, drug interactions, and surgical implications. Aesthet Surg J [Internet] 2004;24(4):307–11. [Cited 2025 Jan 24]. Available from: https://doi.org/10.1016/j.asj.2004.05.001.
19. El-Boghdadly K, Pawa A, Chin KJ. Local anesthetic systemic toxicity: current perspectives. Local Reg Anesth [Internet]. 2018;11:35. [Cited 2025 Jan 19]. Available from: https://pmc.ncbi.nlm.nih.gov/articles/PMC6087022/
20. Mather LE, Copeland SE, Ladd LA. Acute toxicity of local Anesthetics: underlying pharmacokinetic and pharmacodynamic concepts. Reg Anesth Pain Med [Internet]. 2005;30(6):553–66. [Cited 2025 Jan 24]. Available from: https://rapm.bmj.com/content/30/6/553
21. Qiao W, Lin Y. Local anesthetics. In: Barash P, Cullen B, Stoelting R, Cahalan M, Stock C, editors. Clinical anesthesia. 9th ed. Philadelphia: Wolters Kluwer Health; 2023. p. 529.
22. Mahendru K, Sarma R. World Federation of Societies of Anesthesiologists. Perioperative lignocaine. [Internet]. 2024. [Cited 2025 Jan 24]. Available from: https://resources.wfsahq.org/atotw/perioperative-lignocaine/
23. Li YC, Wang Y, Li DD, Zhang Y, Zhao TC, Li CF. Procaine is a specific DNA methylation inhibitor with anti-tumor effect for human gastric cancer. J Cell Biochem [Internet]. 2018;119(2):2440–9. [Cited 2025 Jan 24]. Available from: https://pubmed.ncbi.nlm.nih.gov/28926119/s
24. Villar-Garea A, Fraga M, Espada J, Esteller M. Procaine is a DNA-demethylating agent with growth-inhibitory effects in human cancer cells. Cancer Res. 2003;63(16):4984–9.
25. Razavi BM, Fazly Bazzaz BS. A review and new insights to antimicrobial action of local anesthetics. Eur J Clin Microbiol Infect Dis [Internet]. 2019;38(6):991–1002. [Cited 2025 Jan 19]. Available from: https://pubmed.ncbi.nlm.nih.gov/30680564/
26. Johnson SM, Saint John BE, Dine AP. Local anesthetics as antimicrobial agents: a review. Surg Infect (Larchmt) [Internet]. 2008;9(2):205–13. [Cited 2025 Jan 19]. Available from: https://pubmed.ncbi.nlm.nih.gov/18426354/
27. Callahan ZM, Roberts AL, Christopher AN, Gadomski SP, Kuchta KM, Costanzo CM, et al. The effect of commonly used local anesthetic on bacterial growth. J Surg Res [Internet]. 2022;274:16–22. [Cited 2025 Jan 19]. Available from: https://pubmed.ncbi.nlm.nih.gov/35114483/

Chapter 27
Neuraltherapeutic Medicine and Lifestyle

Eduardo Humberto Beltrán Dussán

1 Introduction

Lifestyle is the way in which the human being relates to the different levels of his existence both physically, emotionally, and mentally, in interaction with the spiritual and also with the social. It has been shown that a good lifestyle is a fundamental factor so that the best conditions are always maintained [1–3].

In Neuraltherapeutic Medicine and in all conceptions of Medicine, a healthy lifestyle has been considered one of the best strategies to ensure the best quality health and the best results in therapeutic interventions [4, 5].

2 Structure of the Human Being

At the moment of conception, the new being acquires information for its physical, emotional, and mental structure and a biological program that directs the processes of growth, development and self-maintenance with a determination of how it will be physically, how it will feel and how it will think [6]. From that moment on, he begins to interact with physical, emotional and mental factors that are in the environment and will generate modifications in his development [7–9].

The physical or material level has to do with the body structure, the emotional level corresponds to feelings and the mental level is made up of thoughts. Factors such as food, physical exercise, sleep, breathing, the environment, body hygiene habits, hygiene of feelings, and hygiene of thoughts are essential to stay in the best possible condition and achieve the happiness that is the goal of life [10, 11].

E. H. Beltrán Dussán (✉)
Faculty of Medicine, Universidad Nacional de Colombia, Bogotá, Colombia
e-mail: ehbeltrand@unal.edu.co

L. B. Pinilla Bonilla et al. (eds.), *Neuraltherapeutic Medicine*,
https://doi.org/10.1007/978-3-032-03257-7_27

The individual is the product of his structure acquired from the moment of conception, of his biological program of self-maintenance, and of the interactions with the different physical, emotional, and mental factors with which he is related [12].

3 Food

Food is the process by which living beings incorporate the nutrients essential to maintain all their structures. In human beings, this process has developed throughout the history of humanity, and it can be identified how food was initially acquired from natural sources in the environment and how the process was transformed until the current industrialization and commercialization of food [13].

One of the greatest difficulties, at present, is to get people to maintain good eating habits, since industrialization has led to the consumption of foods that have been processed through chemical strategies in order to prolong the shelf life, changes in their appearance, taste, smell, coloration, etc., using additives, preservatives, flavorings, and other artificial methods, which force the body to be under the influence of these elements that overload the organic systems and little by little could deconfigure biological information. In addition, the industrialization of agriculture, livestock, poultry, fish farming, and almost all food sources using chemical inducers deteriorate the quality and purity of food [14–16].

For a long time, there has been an attempt to identify the ideal diet for human beings, but according to the research carried out, it has been possible to establish the existence of very important differences in each individual or groups of individuals that make it impossible for there to be a single diet that is the most suitable for everyone. Advances in biological research on human beings have identified genetic and molecular characteristics of each person that have made it possible to establish more appropriate dietary orientations [17, 18].

The genetic and molecular differences of each person command the interaction with the different components of the diet, therefore, current recommendations on the type of diet must be based on individuality, taking into account the foods that generate the best compatibilities to consume them and those that can cause discomfort and recurrent interference to avoid them [19, 20].

The most important thing is to try to consume foods that are pleasant, that have been produced in a biological way, in the most natural way possible, and that cover the requirements of carbohydrates, proteins, fats, vitamins and minerals, and all nutritional requirements, taking into account genetic and molecular individuality [21].

Fasting has been recognized as a lifestyle strategy and as an adjuvant therapy, and it is advisable to do it totally or partially as long as you have medical guidance and supervision [22].

4 Physical Exercise

Physical exercise is the way to maintain the body structures in the best possible way, functional and active, favoring the processes of blood circulation, elasticity and consistency of tissues and its positive impact on the emotional and mental spheres and on all organic systems, being considered as a strategy that must be implemented daily to maintain vital functions in an optimal way [23–27].

The most important thing is to perform the minimum daily exercises required to maintain the most appropriate physical conditions. At home, in any area with good ventilation, a routine can be carried out that should begin with breathing exercises, followed by a gentle jog that should be increased, and then continue with active movements of all body segments from head to toe, integrating breathing exercises. It can be started with periods of 15 minutes that should be progressively increased [28–32].

Sports do not replace the minimum daily routine and should be performed according to individual satisfaction, taking into account the age group to which one belongs and the differences that have currently been established from the genetic and molecular point of view to choose, according to the individual characteristics of each person, the various sports that have been classified as light, moderate or high competition [33–35].

5 The Dream

Sleep is the biological process of recovering body energy through rest and the release of the physical or material components of emotional and mental processes [36, 37].

It is important to take into account several aspects related to sleep such as the site, which must be free of electromagnetic fields and other stimuli that can be perceived by the sense organs for the recovery process to be effective, which is achieved by turning off and disconnecting from the electrical network all the electronic devices that are in the bedroom. The elements on which the body structures rest must be as comfortable and natural as possible, as well as the sleeping clothes. Body orientation with the head directed, as far as possible, toward the north or failing that towards the south. The relationships with the circadian cycles of light lead to the recommendation to be asleep before midnight so that in this way the relationship of the epiphysis with melatonin and its regulation on the various regulation systems occur in a coordinated way. Sleep times should be a minimum of 5 h and a maximum of 8 h and preferably during the night for restful sleep. When lying down to sleep, people should try to eliminate persistent thoughts and accumulated anxieties, which can be achieved through breathing processes [38–40].

When you wake up in the morning, the first thing you should do is be thankful for sleep and for life and prepare for exercise.

6 Breathing

Respiration, from the physiological point of view, is the automatic, self-maintained and self-regulated process by which the organism has the possibility of exchanging gaseous elements by entering the oxygen necessary for the performance of all the biological processes of the different cells that constitute the organs and in the same way to be able to eliminate metabolic waste processes to prevent their accumulation within the organism [41–43].

Breathing is not only a process of gas exchange, it is a biological circuit integrated with different systems at the physical, emotional, and mental level that coordinates the behavior of different organic functions [44–46].

That is why it is important to be aware of this tool for the exchange and mobilization of body energies and to learn its proper realization, managing the inspiratory and expiratory times with abdominal breathing, making pauses in inspiration and exhalation. There are recommendations regarding the duration of these times, which vary between 4 and 8 s in each period, but it is possibly best to do them at a time that best suits each individual [47]. In addition, breathing exercise has been recommended to eliminate pathological processes and strengthen the organ systems, which is achieved by visualizing the areas in conflict in one breath and expelling them to the outside in an expiratory phase and in the next breath, taking in inspiration the force of the universe and internalizing it in the expiratory phase. These benefits of breathing have been confirmed and described in scientific publications [48, 49].

7 The Environment

The environment is the around with which one is in permanent contact and is made up of physical, emotional, and mental factors. All these components are part of the integrity of the human being and therefore affect the quality of life of individuals. A good lifestyle has to do with the environment in all aspects, so you should always be in contact with an environment rich in pure air, sun, and all-natural components, away from all possible pollutants [50–52].

8 Hygiene Habits

Hygiene habits have to do with two fundamental concepts: cleanliness and care. Cleanliness refers to the maintenance of structures free of contamination and dirt, and care refers to the maintenance and development of the integrity of structures [53].

As individuals perform on the physical, emotional, mental, spiritual, and social levels, hygiene must be maintained at all these levels. Hygiene at the material level refers to the cleanliness and care of all body structures, clothing and all the elements with which one is in contact on a daily basis. Emotional hygiene refers to maintaining the best feelings in relation to oneself and in relation to others. Mental hygiene is related to maintaining positive and optimistic thoughts [54].

9 Happiness

Happiness is the goal of life and refers to living in constant harmony with all the events that arise. To achieve this, it must be understood that all circumstances, including adversity, are things that must occur in order to always obtain a benefit. When circumstances arise, they must be analyzed and interpreted positively to find the reason for being and be grateful for the learning that is obtained [55].

Do not assume non-existent situations and especially those that generate negative or pessimistic thoughts, which cause a great consumption of energy and unnecessary anguish [56].

Always maintain positive thoughts about the circumstances that occur or will occur. For no reason, think about negative or disastrous situations, because the power of the mind or the word can cause these situations to materialize and occur in some way [57].

Before any thought, always look for the positive aspects and think in the direction of the good things that may happen to try to materialize. No matter how negative any situation may seem, there are always positive circumstances that should be detected, analyzed, learned, and thanked [58, 59]. These strategies should be implemented and practiced within the family union [60].

The past is the experiences that have been had and that can no longer be modified. Adverse situations should be accepted and never considered as punishment for the decisions made, as they generate feelings of guilt that harm personal integrity. The ideal is to learn to observe experiences, understanding that the things that have happened are circumstances that necessarily had to be present to always generate a positive result. The future is the circumstances that will come according to what has been built, and even though it is good to analyze it, it should not be a cause for unnecessary anguish and worries [61].

We must be measured with the enthusiasm generated by positive circumstances, taking into account that they are the reward of efforts and decisions so as not to fall into inappropriate celebrations.

References

1. Phillips EM, Frates EP, Park DJ. Lifestyle medicine. Phys Med Rehabil Clin N Am. 2020;31(4):515–26. https://doi.org/10.1016/j.pmr.2020.07.006. Epub 2020 Sept 9. PMID: 32981575.
2. Alonso-Stuyck P. Parenting and healthy teenage lifestyles. Int J Environ Res Public Health. 2020;17(15):5428. https://doi.org/10.3390/ijerph17155428. PMID: 32731468; PMCID: PMC7432849.
3. China Kadoorie Biobank Collaborative Group. Healthy lifestyle and life expectancy free of major chronic diseases at age 40 in China. Nat Hum Behav. 2023;7(9):1542–50. https://doi.org/10.1038/s41562-023-01624-7. Epub 2023 July 10. PMID: 37430072; PMCID: PMC7615116.
4. Parkinson MD, Stout R, Dysinger W. Lifestyle medicine: prevention, treatment, and reversal of disease. Med Clin North Am. 2023;107(6):1109–20. https://doi.org/10.1016/j.mcna.2023.06.007. Epub 2023 Jul 16. PMID: 37806726.
5. Brennan J, Phelps K, McGrady A, Schultz P. Introducing lifestyle medicine into family medicine: theory and applications. Int J Psychiatry Med. 2024;59(4):415–23. https://doi.org/10.1177/00912174231215917. Epub 2023 Nov 17. PMID: 37975426.
6. Berresi M, Gilbert S. Developmental biology. 13th ed. Sunderland: Sinaur Associates Inc; 2023.
7. Fouqueau L, Polechová J. Eco-evolutionary dynamics in changing environments: integrating theory with data. J Evol Biol. 2024;37(6):579–87. https://doi.org/10.1093/jeb/voae067. PMID: 38941551.
8. Zhang Y, Koene M, Chen C, Wagenaar C, Reijneveld SA. Associations between the built environment and physical activity in children, adults and older people: a narrative review of reviews. Prev Med. 2024;180:107856. https://doi.org/10.1016/j.ypmed.2024.107856. Epub 2024 Jan 12. PMID: 38220061.
9. Smith JW. Immersive virtual environment technology to supplement environmental perception, preference and behavior research: a review with applications. Int J Environ Res Public Health. 2015;12(9):11486–505. https://doi.org/10.3390/ijerph120911486. PMID: 26378565; PMCID: PMC4586687.
10. Jiao H, Kalsbeek A, Yi CX. Microglia, circadian rhythm and lifestyle factors. Neuropharmacology. 2024;257:110029. https://doi.org/10.1016/j.neuropharm.2024.110029. Epub 2024 Jun 7. PMID: 38852838.
11. Sharma H, Keith Wallace R. Ayurveda and epigenetics. Medicina (Kaunas). 2020;56(12):687. https://doi.org/10.3390/medicina56120687. PMID: 33322263; PMCID: PMC7763202.
12. Donelan SC, Hellmann JK, Bell AM, Luttbeg B, Orrock JL, Sheriff MJ, Sih A. Transgenerational plasticity in human-altered environments. Trends Ecol Evol. 2020;35(2):115–24. https://doi.org/10.1016/j.tree.2019.09.003. Epub 2019 Nov 6. PMID: 31706627; PMCID: PMC9440440.
13. Alt KW, Al-Ahmad A, Woelber JP. Nutrition and health in human evolution-past to present. Nutrients. 2022;14(17):3594. https://doi.org/10.3390/nu14173594. PMID: 36079850; PMCID: PMC9460423.
14. Alsaffar AA. Sustainable diets: the interaction between food industry, nutrition, health and the environment. Food Sci Technol Int. 2016;22(2):102–11. https://doi.org/10.1177/1082013215572029. Epub 2015 Feb 13. PMID: 25680370.
15. van Ruth SM, van der Veeken J, Dekker P, Luning PA, Huisman W. Feeding fiction: fraud vulnerability in the food service industry. Food Res Int. 2020;133:109158. https://doi.org/10.1016/j.foodres.2020.109158. Epub 2020 Mar 9. PMID: 32466937.
16. Lane MM, Gamage E, Du S, Ashtree DN, McGuinness AJ, Gauci S, Baker P, Lawrence M, Rebholz CM, Srour B, Touvier M, Jacka FN, O'Neil A, Segasby T, Marx W. Ultra-processed food exposure and adverse health outcomes: umbrella review of epidemiological meta-analyses. BMJ. 2024;384:e077310. https://doi.org/10.1136/bmj-2023-077310. PMID: 38418082; PMCID: PMC10899807.

17. Kiani AK, Bonetti G, Donato K, Kaftalli J, Herbst KL, Stuppia L, Fioretti F, Nodari S, Perrone M, Chiurazzi P, Bellinato F, Gisondi P, Bertelli M. Polymorphisms, diet and nutrigenomics. J Prev Med Hyg. 2022;63(2 Suppl 3):E125–41. https://doi.org/10.15167/2421-4248/jpmh2022.63.2S3.2754. PMID: 36479483; PMCID: PMC9710387.
18. Carlberg C. Nutrigenomics in the context of evolution. Redox Biol. 2023;62:102656. https://doi.org/10.1016/j.redox.2023.102656. Epub 2023 Mar 11. PMID: 36933390; PMCID: PMC10036735.
19. Ordovas JM, Ferguson LR, Tai ES, Mathers JC. Personalised nutrition and health. BMJ. 2018;361:bmj.k2173. https://doi.org/10.1136/bmj.k2173. PMID: 29898881; PMCID: PMC6081996.
20. Agrawal P, Kaur J, Singh J, Rasane P, Sharma K, Bhadariya V, Kaur S, Kumar V. Genetics, nutrition, and health: a new frontier in disease prevention. J Am Nutr Assoc. 2024;43(4):326–38. https://doi.org/10.1080/27697061.2023.2284997. Epub 2023 Nov 28. PMID: 38015713.
21. Bogard JR, Downs S, Casey E, Farrell P, Gupta A, Miachon L, Naughton S, Staromiejska W, Reeve E. Convenience as a dimension of food environments: a systematic scoping review of its definition and measurement. Appetite. 2024;194:107198. https://doi.org/10.1016/j.appet.2023.107198. Epub 2024 Jan 2. PMID: 38176442.
22. Tang D, Tang Q, Huang W, Zhang Y, Tian Y, Fu X. Fasting: from physiology to pathology. Adv Sci (Weinh). 2023;10(9):e2204487. https://doi.org/10.1002/advs.202204487. Epub 2023 Feb 3. PMID: 36737846; PMCID: PMC10037992.
23. Matei D, Trofin D, Iordan DA, Onu I, Condurache I, Ionite C, Buculei I. The endocannabinoid system and physical exercise. Int J Mol Sci. 2023;24(3):1989. https://doi.org/10.3390/ijms24031989. PMID: 36768332; PMCID: PMC9916354.
24. Gao L, Zhu L, Hu L, Hu H, Wang S, Bezerianos A, Li Y, Li C, Sun Y. Mid-task physical exercise keeps your mind vigilant: evidences from behavioral performance and EEG functional connectivity. IEEE Trans Neural Syst Rehabil Eng. 2021;29:31–40. https://doi.org/10.1109/TNSRE.2020.3030106. Epub 2021 Feb 25. PMID: 33052846.
25. Guan Y, Yan Z. Molecular mechanisms of exercise and Healthspan. Cells. 2022;11(5):872. https://doi.org/10.3390/cells11050872. PMID: 35269492; PMCID: PMC8909156.
26. Szychowska A, Drygas W. Physical activity as a determinant of successful aging: a narrative review article. Aging Clin Exp Res. 2022;34(6):1209–14. https://doi.org/10.1007/s40520-021-02037-0. Epub 2021 Dec 7. PMID: 34873677; PMCID: PMC9151514.
27. Zhang L, Liu Y, Wang X, Zhang X. Physical exercise and diet: regulation of gut microbiota to prevent and treat metabolic disorders to maintain health. Nutrients. 2023;15(6):1539. https://doi.org/10.3390/nu15061539. PMID: 36986268; PMCID: PMC10054346.
28. Messonnier LA. Physical exercise or activity and energy balance or metabolism in the context of health and diseases. Nutrients. 2023;15(23):4909. https://doi.org/10.3390/nu15234909. PMID: 38068767; PMCID: PMC10708250.
29. Pettigrew S, Jongenelis MI, Talati Z, Myers G, Sapountsis N. Dimensions of the diet-exercise relationship in later life: a qualitative study. Aust N Z J Public Health. 2023;47(5):100090. https://doi.org/10.1016/j.anzjph.2023.100090. Epub 2023 Sept 30. PMID: 37783034.
30. Piercy KL, Troiano RP, Ballard RM, Carlson SA, Fulton JE, Galuska DA, George SM, Olson RD. The physical activity guidelines for Americans. JAMA. 2018;320:2020–8.
31. Huang A, Wang E, Sanger S, Papaioannou A, Rodrigues IB. Comparison of national and international sedentary behaviour and physical activity guidelines for older adults: a systematic review and quality appraisal with AGREE II. PLoS One. 2023;18(11):e0294784. https://doi.org/10.1371/journal.pone.0294784. PMID: 38011139; PMCID: PMC10681178.
32. Hu D, Zhou S, Crowley-McHattan ZJ, Liu Z. A comparative study of the physical activity guidelines for children and adolescents from five countries and WHO. Front Public Health. 2024;12:1421843. https://doi.org/10.3389/fpubh.2024.1421843. PMID: 39071153; PMCID: PMC11272551.

33. Egan B, Sharples AP. Molecular responses to acute exercise and their relevance for adaptations in skeletal muscle to exercise training. Physiol Rev. 2023;103(3):2057–170. https://doi.org/10.1152/physrev.00054.2021. Epub 2022 Nov 17. PMID: 36395350.
34. Furrer R, Handschin C. Molecular aspects of the exercise response and training adaptation in skeletal muscle. Free Radic Biol Med. 2024;223:53–68. https://doi.org/10.1016/j.freeradbiomed.2024.07.026. Epub 2024 July 24. PMID: 39059515.
35. Noone J, Mucinski JM, DeLany JP, Sparks LM, Goodpaster BH. Understanding the variation in exercise responses to guide personalized physical activity prescriptions. Cell Metab. 2024;36(4):702–24. https://doi.org/10.1016/j.cmet.2023.12.025. Epub 2024 Jan 22. PMID: 38262420.
36. Baranwal N, Yu PK, Siegel NS. Sleep physiology, pathophysiology, and sleep hygiene. Prog Cardiovasc Dis. 2023;77:59–69. https://doi.org/10.1016/j.pcad.2023.02.005. Epub 2023 Feb 24. PMID: 36841492.
37. Xu Y, Schneider A, Wessel R, Hengen KB. Sleep restores an optimal computational regime in cortical networks. Nat Neurosci. 2024;27(2):328–38. https://doi.org/10.1038/s41593-023-01536-9. Epub 2024 Jan 5. PMID: 38182837; PMCID: PMC11272063.
38. De Pasquale C, El Kazzi M, Sutherland K, Shriane AE, Vincent GE, Cistulli PA, Bin YS. Sleep hygiene – what do we mean? A bibliographic review. Sleep Med Rev. 2024;75:101930. https://doi.org/10.1016/j.smrv.2024.101930. Epub 2024 Apr 16. PMID: 38761649.
39. Grandner MA, Fernandez FX. The translational neuroscience of sleep: a contextual framework. Science. 2021;374(6567):568–73. https://doi.org/10.1126/science.abj8188. Epub 2021 Oct 28. PMID: 34709899; PMCID: PMC8761057.
40. Zisapel N. New perspectives on the role of melatonin in human sleep, circadian rhythms and their regulation. Br J Pharmacol. 2018;175(16):3190–9. https://doi.org/10.1111/bph.14116. Epub 2018 Jan 15. PMID: 29318587; PMCID: PMC6057895.
41. Krohn F, Novello M, van der Giessen RS, De Zeeuw CI, Pel JJM, Bosman LWJ. The integrated brain network that controls respiration. elife. 2023;12:e83654. https://doi.org/10.7554/eLife.83654. PMID: 36884287; PMCID: PMC9995121.
42. Guyenet PG, Bayliss DA. Central respiratory chemoreception. Handb Clin Neurol. 2022;188:37–72. https://doi.org/10.1016/B978-0-323-91534-2.00007-2. PMID: 35965033; PMCID: PMC10557475.
43. Gargaglioni LH, Marques DA, Patrone LGA. Sex differences in breathing. Comp Biochem Physiol A Mol Integr Physiol. 2019;238:110543. https://doi.org/10.1016/j.cbpa.2019.110543. Epub 2019 Aug 22. PMID: 31445081.
44. Del Negro CA, Funk GD, Feldman JL. Breathing matters. Nat Rev Neurosci. 2018;19(6):351–67. https://doi.org/10.1038/s41583-018-0003-6. PMID: 29740175; PMCID: PMC6636643.
45. Olschweiller S, Sauer JF. Respiration-driven brain oscillations in emotional cognition. Front Neural Circuits. 2021;15:761812. https://doi.org/10.3389/fncir.2021.761812. PMID: 34790100; PMCID: PMC8592085.
46. Homma I, Masaoka Y. Breathing rhythms and emotions. Exp Physiol. 2008;93(9):1011–21. https://doi.org/10.1113/expphysiol.2008.042424. Epub 2008 May 16. PMID: 18487316.
47. Ashhad S, Kam K, Del Negro CA, Feldman JL. Breathing rhythm and pattern and their influence on emotion. Annu Rev Neurosci. 2022;45:223–47. https://doi.org/10.1146/annurev-neuro-090121-014424. Epub 2022 Mar 8. PMID: 35259917; PMCID: PMC9840384.
48. Saoji AA, Raghavendra BR, Manjunath NK. Effects of yogic breath regulation: a narrative review of scientific evidence. J Ayurveda Integr Med. 2019;10(1):50–8. https://doi.org/10.1016/j.jaim.2017.07.008. Epub 2018 Feb 1. PMID: 29395894; PMCID: PMC6470305.
49. Korkmaz A, Bernhardsen GP, Cirit B, Koprucu Suzer G, Kayan H, Biçmen H, Tahra M, Suner A, Lehto SM, Sag D, Saatcioglu F. Sudarshan Kriya yoga breathing and a meditation program for burnout among physicians: a randomized clinical trial. JAMA Netw Open. 2024;7(1):e2353978. https://doi.org/10.1001/jamanetworkopen.2023.53978. PMID: 38294813; PMCID: PMC10831575.

50. Lauriola P, Crabbe H, Behbod B, Yip F, Medina S, Semenza JC, Vardoulakis S, Kass D, Zeka A, Khonelidze I, Ashworth M, de Hoogh K, Shi X, Staatsen B, Knudsen LE, Fletcher T, Houthuijs D, Leonardi GS. Advancing global health through environmental and public health tracking. Int J Environ Res Public Health. 2020;17(6):1976. https://doi.org/10.3390/ijerph17061976. Erratum in: Int J Environ Res Public Health 2020;17(22):E8568. https://doi.org/10.3390/ijerph17228568. PMID: 32192215; PMCID: PMC7142667.
51. Evans GW. The built environment and mental health. J Urban Health. 2003;80(4):536–55. https://doi.org/10.1093/jurban/jtg063. PMID: 14709704; PMCID: PMC3456225.
52. Macia L, Galy O, Nanan RKH. Editorial: modern lifestyle and health: how changes in the environment impacts immune function and physiology. Front Immunol. 2021;12:762166. https://doi.org/10.3389/fimmu.2021.762166. PMID: 34764963; PMCID: PMC8576351.
53. Curtis V, Schmidt W, Luby S, Florez R, Touré O, Biran A. Hygiene: new hopes, new horizons. Lancet Infect Dis. 2011;11(4):312–21. https://doi.org/10.1016/S1473-3099(10)70224-3. PMID: 21453872; PMCID: PMC7106354.
54. Pérez Alonso-Geta PM, Moreno MCB. Hygiene and eating healthy habits and practices in Spanish families with children aged 6 to 14. Int J Environ Res Public Health. 2020;17(22):8671. https://doi.org/10.3390/ijerph17228671. PMID: 33266434; PMCID: PMC7700584.
55. Singh S, Kshtriya S, Valk R. Health, hope, and harmony: a systematic review of the determinants of Happiness across cultures and countries. Int J Environ Res Public Health. 2023;20(4):3306. https://doi.org/10.3390/ijerph20043306. PMID: 36834001; PMCID: PMC9963575.
56. Carrero G, Makin J, Malinowski P. A mathematical model for the dynamics of happiness. Math Biosci Eng. 2022;19(2):2002–29. https://doi.org/10.3934/mbe.2022094. Epub 2021 Dec 24. PMID: 35135239.
57. Steptoe A. Investing in happiness: the gerontological perspective. Gerontology. 2019;65(6):634–9. https://doi.org/10.1159/000501124. Epub 2019 Sept 10. PMID: 31505514; PMCID: PMC6878748.
58. Alexander R, Aragón OR, Bookwala J, Cherbuin N, Gatt JM, Kahrilas IJ, Kästner N, Lawrence A, Lowe L, Morrison RG, Mueller SC, Nusslock R, Papadelis C, Polnaszek KL, Helene Richter S, Silton RL, Styliadis C. The neuroscience of positive emotions and affect: implications for cultivating happiness and wellbeing. Neurosci Biobehav Rev. 2021;121:220–49. https://doi.org/10.1016/j.neubiorev.2020.12.002. Epub 2020 Dec 8. PMID: 33307046.
59. Dilman I. Happiness. J Med Ethics. 1982;8(4):199–202. https://doi.org/10.1136/jme.8.4.199. PMID: 7154036; PMCID: PMC1059427.
60. Izzo F, Baiocco R, Pistella J. Children's and adolescents' happiness and family functioning: a systematic literature review. Int J Environ Res Public Health. 2022;19(24):16593. https://doi.org/10.3390/ijerph192416593. PMID: 36554474; PMCID: PMC9778774.
61. Sharma H. Ayurveda: science of life, genetics, and epigenetics. Ayu. 2016;37(2):87–91. https://doi.org/10.4103/ayu.AYU_220_16. PMID: 29200745; PMCID: PMC5688840.

Chapter 28
There Is No Human Health If There Is No Environmental Health

Esperanza Cerón-Villaquirán

1 Introduction: We Are Gaia

> Life defines and maintains the material conditions necessary for its survival, and the entire planet reflects the behaviour of a single organism, even a single living creature. (Lovelock, GAIA)

> The world is not made of objects but of relationships. (Jordi Pigem)

Gaia is no longer a theory; it is not for a place where quantum physics, biology, and chemistry, which were never separated in life, have met again in complex thinking. It is painting now a biocentric path that hopefully will move us away from anthropocentrism [1].

We are connected in every sense of the word: we inter-be with other species in DNA, in the basic morphology of vertebrates, in the common composition of photopigments in the eyes of any species, in the similarities of breathing through the alveoli or through the stomata. In the spiral shapes that are repeated in the constellations, in sunflowers or in snails. We are interbeing because every year 98% of our atoms are exchanged with the environment, although we are still the same being.

In 2012, thirteen neuroscientist gathered in Cambridge, accompanied by Stephen Hawking, declared in what constitutes a true manifesto that animals, even in the absence of a neocortex, are aware of themselves and the world around them, being capable of intentional and even ethical behaviors with different species. The scientists presented evidence that animals share the same neurological substrates as humans, such as neuroanatomical, neurochemical, and neurophysiological ones [2].

Plant neurobiology [3] provides new evidence every day about the intelligence and problem-solving capacity of plants, which learn from experience, keep memories, and even act collectively and take care of the weakest [4].

E. Cerón-Villaquirán (✉)
Faculty of Medicine, Universidad Nacional de Colombia, Bogotá, Colombia
e-mail: esperania@gmail.com

L. B. Pinilla Bonilla et al. (eds.), *Neuraltherapeutic Medicine*,
https://doi.org/10.1007/978-3-032-03257-7_28

At the intracellular level, reality surpasses fantasy: beings capable of living autonomously, or cooperating with those who are different, to make endosymbiosis and first produce nucleated beings, incorporate others (mitochondria, for example), and gradually grow in complexity towards multicellular beings [5]. They invented sexual reproduction and death at the same time: two pieces of information from beings of different sexes come together to form a single totipotential cell that, when reproduced, becomes pluripotent to differentiate into specialized organs. One of these organs will produce the cells of reproduction because the being to which it belongs, at some point, will reach thermodynamic equilibrium, that is, death. All this happens, but not before, probably, finding another half that, with new information, maintains and increases complexity in and with new learning processes [6].

The microbiome, of which we still know little, is teaching us that we must consider it as another tissue of the human body due to its indispensability to guarantee the proper functioning of the digestive system and the entire body [7].

Our knowledge of what we call junk DNA has come to show us that here there are embedded ancestral viruses, a kind of fossil that seems to bring back from time immemorial information that at any given time can play a role in favor or against the health of the individual [8].

At this point, there is no doubt that life operates in a network not only within each kingdom of nature but between all of them, with the planet and the solar system co-evolving away from equilibrium, co-learning in self-organization/autopoiesis in a process of emergences between the living, the inert, and cultures. Each being and everyone interdepend and interrelate in one way or another; it happens both in the intracellular field and within the entire biosphere.

A team from the *Université Libre de Bruxelles* trying to understand a small group of interactions inside a cell, ended up concluding that complexity increases exponentially: any attempt at representation gives a "horror graph" because "everything does everything to everything" [9].

Co-evolution is a process of mutual adaptation-co-learning, metamorphosis, where collaboration, symbiosis, and other forms of co-adaptation *in, on, and with* the environment prevail; where the past, present, and future seem to maintain a permanent dialogue. Recognizing that we belong to Gaia is an important step in understanding environmental health as well as human health [10]. The new biology is showing us about diverse intelligence in all living beings, or as the philosopher Hans Jonas says, "The organic in its simplest forms involves the mind; and the mind, even in its most complex forms, involves the organic."

The present chapter seeks to situate itself in a dialogue between complex thinking, critical epidemiology developed by the Latin American public health perspective of the social/environmental determination of health, and a neuraltherapeutic perspective. It is, therefore, an essay that we hope to enrich with and from other disciplines that work on the health of any living being in any kingdom of nature and from any perspective. We do not intend more than to stimulate a debate and, in our case, to ground it in the neuraltherapeutic exercise.

2 The Problem and Its Origins

> (…) Objective reality has evaporated and what we observe is not nature itself but nature exposed to our method of interrogation. (Heisenberg, Nobel Prize in Physics 1932)

We live in the Anthropocene-an era in which anthropocentrism as an episteme, as a hegemonic paradigm, sustains a model of development in the hands of a minority that monopolizes and benefits from globally assembling a reality in which the nature that we are is a "thing" that is there for the supposed benefit of all. This model, without a doubt, is leading us to the sixth extinction of so many forms of life that will undoubtedly also reach the human species.

The academic and political constitution of this reality in our current world depends on such a paradigm, which in turn is based, as Heisenberg said, on a "method of interrogation." A science that "beyond its technical projections, and like any other scientific discipline, is part of the symbolic power, which is the power to constitute" what is called reality from myth, language, art or science [11]. Precisely what Heisenberg and Bordieu are alluding to is that "nature itself" and "life itself," have so far been outside a scientific position that puts life above any consideration or idea of progress based on infinite growth on a finite planet.

This same paradigm has marked the paths of the hegemonic disciplines of human health since we do not consider the interdependencies with the environment:[1] we think about health from the perspective of the disease of "individual bodies," fragmented into parts, enzymes, and chemical substances extracted from a single static process. Health seeks all the "anti": anti-fever, antibodies, antibiotic, anti-diarrheal, antiparasitic, anti-cancer. Moreover, health also uses the language of war: to fight disease, viruses, etc.; that is, the symbolic language that a "certain medicine" has created for us, not for health, but harmonious with that Cartesian way of understanding science and human development. And the worst part is that it develops increasingly expensive technologies to which is attributed to the character of science and on which it places all answers. Health is taught and exercised, as if it were a matter of doctors, devices, technologies, and medicines, managed by transnational corporations in which profit prevails over the common good.

At this point, a new paradigm is beginning to make its way, since the evidence of the climate crisis has brought to the forefront of the debate the interdependence and interrelation (interbeing) of everything that makes up planet Earth and sustains life. There is a new look at human and environmental health from the approach of social and environmental determination of health, criticizing the Cartesian view. This view reduces everything to the cause-and-effect phenomena of the disease and to the identification of risk factors to which people individually are considered exposed, ignoring the living conditions in which they move. The difference with the WHO's Determinants of Health approach is that:

[1] We do not develop it here, but there is a way of interpreting epigenetics that is equally anthropocentric, which remains for debate.

"... it cannot explain the relationship between the social system, ways of living and health; nor understand the class-based distribution of the forms and intensities of human exposure to dangerous processes, nor the differential vulnerability of groups situated in distinct social insertions; nor deeply comprehend the society-nature metabolism and its social impact. And finally, with this model, it is impossible ´to know society to transform it´ toward a deeper health that would be the pillar not only of a new public health but also of the construction of a new healthy civilizational model". [12]

Therefore, speaking of the problem and its origins, we have so far assumed as "scientific" only that which is quantifiable. Therefore, in addition to shifting from a positivist to a biocentric paradigm, we also require a new symbolism that is consistent across myth, language, art, and science. As Einstein said, "*We cannot solve our problems with the same thinking we used when we created them.*"

3 What Is Environmental Health?

Bringing biology to life and building a biology that is worthy of life. (Brian Goodwin)

According to the WHO, it is an area of study that analyzes environmental factors that affect human health. Specifically, it defines it as "that discipline that includes those aspects of human health, including quality of life and social well-being, that are determined by physical, chemical, biological, social, and psycho-social environmental factors" [13].

This definition falls short in that environmental health, more than an area of study, is an inherence, a complex emergence resulting from that dialogue between everything when it is alive on the planet (what we today call inert) and cultures.

It is a technical definition that fragments the development of the subject in specific studies on air quality, water, toxics and ends up focusing on healthy environments as a matter of individual responsibilities, remaining far from the complex approach that weaves these interrelationships beyond anthropocentrism, that recognizes the interdependencies, and that in particular does not avoid talking about the predatory model of development.

Environmental health is that complex set of autopoietic emergencies that keep the planet away from the state of equilibrium thanks to life as Lovelock postulated in the books already cited.

The complexity of the matter lies in the network of interdependent interrelations. As in the aforementioned study by Pigem, conducted by the Free University of Brussels, this network would mathematically produce a "horror graph" because, within the cell they examined, "everything is related to everything else and vice versa". This extraordinarily complex network, extending even beyond the exosphere, is posited to have sustained life—generically conceived—in a state of autopoiesis marked by ever-increasing complexity.

In an interconnected world, it is not scientific to address separately the different factors that have led the planet today in what has come to be called extinction, caused by a way of life of 1% of humanity that accumulates wealth increasingly at the cost of the destruction of the biosphere. Environmental health is, at the same time, the health of ecosystems, including water and air, it is the health of soils, of coexistence relationships, of interrelations with the solar system, of what we think and feel, falling short in this enunciation.

4 To Talk About Environmental Health in Neuraltherapeutic Practice

We must return to the interdependent interconnection of everything with everything. Only for positivist academic purposes do we speak of the outside and the inside, of above and below, of heaven and earth. Until now, we have been taught ecology as something that is always outside our bodies, "there," in that strange nature, and lately we are learning about the microbiota as "that other" strange and added. We learned medicine, veterinary medicine, dentistry and botany, broken down into their parts.

From our disconnected mind, we think in the soil, on the one hand, and the chemical that must be "added" because we forgot with our science that it is alive. Furthermore, some agrochemical multinationals, even more disconnected and with conflicts of interest, provide us with a generic product to "avoid" us from experimenting.

Consider a human or non-human animal body with a hepatic disease, with liver tests confirming it. Along comes a multinational pharmaceutical company, whose primary interest is economic profit. The industry already possesses the necessary resources to treat it. This allows us to maintain our comfort zone, as an authority outside our consultant's relationship knows what resources to provide.

Due to obvious limitations, we will speak without talking about air, water, soil and the complex "internal" ecology of living in the singular. We will talk without any claim to exhaust and with the intention of expanding the dialogue about anthropogenic chemical contamination of food and pharmaceuticals.

As food was the first thing that any living being sought on Earth and we continue to do so, we agree with the phrase of the German philosopher Ludwig Feuerbach: "We are what we eat"; and with Hippocrates: "Let your medicine be your food and your food be your medicine."

But what do we eat today? The vast majority of the planet's inhabitants consume, in one way or another, what has been touched for decades by agrochemical multinationals, whose industrial origin comes from the residual stocks of toxins that remained after the so-called world wars and that pharmaceutical companies decided to take advantage of both in agriculture and in the food industry—not nourishments—because there is a difference between eating and nourishing [14].

These multinationals whose products can be found in any department store or sidewalk store and in all the languages of the world are the ones that now, thanks to researchers such as Dr. Carlos Monteiro of Brazil, among others, and adopted by the WHO, are technically called *ultra-processed foods*, and in many countries, they are beginning to be given consumer warning seals [15].

Ultra-processed foods are defined by the WHO/PAHO as "industrial formulations that are sold ready to eat or drink." They contain many ingredients (colorants, flavorings, perfumes, foaming agents, stabilizers, flavor enhancers, preservatives, stabilizers, antibiotics, antifungals, coagulants, anticoagulants, microplastics, heavy metals, synthetic hormones, as well as salt, sugars and industrial fats, etc.), which make them highly palatable and addictive. Its caloric value is high in contrast to its poor nutritional and polluting value.

All these foods—not nourishments—are characterized by being made in the laboratory with chemical substances, many of them toxic, inflammatory, carcinogenic, obesogenic, which affect fertility and hormonal development (endocrine disruptors), cognition, mental health, etc., and with which we have not co-evolved on the planet. Their daily consumption several times a day and from birth fed with artificial formulas, end up altering our "internal" ecology, our microbiota, and the health of the entire GAIA. In living beings, we are seeing the symptoms and signs of morbidity and mortality, qualitative and quantitative evidence that we are asked to ignore because the industry does not deal with or care about the risks involved in bio-impregnation, nor the effects of mixtures and recombinations of the more than 50 million chemical substances that the Chemical Abstracts Service recognized as being used in ultra-processed foods in 2010 [16].

To be brief: at breakfast, we eat branded cereal and margarine. At lunch and dinner, we consume sausages, transgenic corn, drinks with added sugars, and fruits and vegetables from monocultures with a high content of agrotoxins and less nutritional content, meats from monofarms, all of them ultra-processed.

The fact is that the business is so good, and it is concentrated in just 10 brands, which control the world market, bankrupt and absorb local enterprises, and influence the health and agri-food public policies of all countries. The worst part is that they are supported by global and omnipresent advertising apparatuses that convince the average citizen that they are nutritious, time-saving, delicious (no doubt because they are loaded with glutamate and other flavor enhancers), give spark to life, are energetic, etc. A path by which they discourage the immense culinary and biodiverse wealth of the peoples [17].

According to a report by the WHO's European Office on Child Health, it was recognized that European children were born with more than 300 synthetic chemicals that did not exist in their grandparents' bodies [18], we cannot imagine with the global pollution of soil, air and water how these figures have been able to grow exponentially in the world.

In the scenario of our professional practice, we tend to overlook these possible factors of interrelation with the environment. Hence, the life history of the patient must include these elements related to daily food, modes and means of cooking, and the water and drinks he/she consumes. Also, the elements that he/she uses for personal hygiene from mouth to body, the products that he/she uses to make up, the indoor and outdoor environment of his/her home, exposure to other pollutants such as electromagnetic radiation, the effects described in the literature, and the medications that he/she is taking, etc. [19].

Health cannot be reduced to a fragmented biomedical approach that views it as merely the absence of disease and responds with "anti" strategies and treatments. Such a view ignores the web of interdependences in which life unfolds, and it is precisely this web that sustains and makes life possible. A paradigm shift is urgently needed from a positivist and anthropocentric science to a biocentric science, one that recognizes the multiplicity of intelligences in all living beings , the co-evolutionary processes of cooperation and symbiosis , and the systemic interrelations that define health at every scale. Whoever controls our food and medicines controls our freedom. This is why, in the deepest sense, the struggle for environmental health is inseparable from the struggle for human health, dignity and autonomy. For all this reason, human health cannot exist without environmental health, and vice versa and is not a merely a slogan, but a reality that must guide science, medicine, public health and civilization itself.

References

1. Lovelock J, Bateson G, Margulis L, Atlan H, Varela F, et al. Gaia, implications of the new biology. Barcelona: Kairos; 1987.
2. Low P. The Cambridge Declaration on Consciousness. Proceedings of the Francis Crick Memorial Conference, Churchill College, Cambridge University, July 7. 2012. p. 1–2.
3. Mancuso S. The nation of plants. Paradela LD, translator. Barcelona: Galaxia Gutenberg; 2020.
4. Fox Keller E. Seduced by the living. Barcelona: Fontalba; 1983.
5. Margulis L, Sagan D. The origins of life. Valencia: PUV; 2019.
6. Margulis L, Sagan D, Garcia. What is sex? Barcelona: Tusquets; 1998.
7. Prieto PA. Fundamentals of the microbiota and the microbiome. Advances in research on the human gut microbiome. Rev Med (Bogotá). 2023;141(45):229–46.
8. De la Rosa S, et al. Endogenous retroviruses shape pluripotency specification in mouse embryos. Sci Adv. 2024;10(4):eadk9394.
9. Pigem J. Vital intelligence. Barcelona: Kairos; 2015.
10. Lovelock J. We belong to Gaia. Barcelona: Editorial Gg; 2021.
11. Bourdieu P. Intellectuals, politics, and power. Buenos Aires: UBA/Eudeba; 2000.
12. Breilh J. The social determination of health as a tool for transformation towards a new public health (collective health). Rev Fac Nac Salud Pública. 2013;31:13–27.
13. World Health Organization. Environmental Health [Internet]. Available at: https://www.who.int/health-topics/environmental-health#tab=tab_1
14. Cabeza MD. The globalized agro-food system: food empires and social and ecological degradation. Rev Econ Crítica. 2010;10:32–61.
15. Parra DC, da Costa-Louzada ML, Moubarac JC, Bertazzi-Levy R, Khandpur N, Cedi. Association between the consumption of ultra-processed foods and the nutritional profile of the diet of Colombians in 2005. Salud Publica Mex. 2019;61(2):147–54.
16. Ravi N, Bhabananda B, Ian R, Cribb J, Kuar B, Paul C, et al. Chemical pollution: a growing danger and potential catastrophic risk to humanity. Environ Int. 2021;156:106616.

17. Montagut X. Globalized foods: food sovereignty and fair trade. Barcelona: Icaria Editorial; 2006.
18. World Health Organization, European Union, European Environment Office. Children's health and environment. Copenhagen: WHO; 2002. Available at: https://iris.who.int/bitstream/handle/10665/107856/9789289072977-eng.pdf?isAllowed=y&sequence=1
19. Vivas E. The hidden face of the global agro-food system. Peasant struggles. Proposals, networks, and alliances. Barcelona: Grupo ETC; 2008.

Chapter 29
Precautions and Risks in Neuraltherapeutic Medicine

Eduardo Humberto Beltrán Dussán

1 Introduction

To practice medicine in a responsible and ethical way, it is necessary to consider the precautions and risks within your practice. These circumstances can be classified into variables that are related to: the medications to be used, the elements of application, the techniques used in therapeutic practice, and the patients and the therapists.

2 Precautions and Risks in Relation to Medicines

In neuraltherapeutic medicine (NTM), short-acting local anesthetics are used in microdoses, taking into account that the objective of their application is not the anesthetic result but other actions described in their mechanisms of action such as the stabilizing capacity of membranes, among others [1]. For this reason, the use of Procaine [2] or Lidocaine [3] is recommended in concentrations that do not exceed 1% as far as possible.

Some hypersensitivity reactions to these drugs have been described in the literature, which are not frequent; and occasional adverse reactions on the cardiovascular system, respiratory, nervous system, and liver function, more related to the use of high doses [4]. The recommendation for responsible practice of NTM is to have clear knowledge about the concentrations, doses, pharmacological aspects, toxicity, and adverse effects of these therapeutic agents, in order to try to avoid all possible risks [5–7].

E. H. Beltrán Dussán (✉)
Faculty of Medicine, Universidad Nacional de Colombia, Bogotá, Colombia
e-mail: ehbeltrand@unal.edu.co

L. B. Pinilla Bonilla et al. (eds.), *Neuraltherapeutic Medicine*,
https://doi.org/10.1007/978-3-032-03257-7_29

Other medications should not be mixed with local anesthetics when performing NTM interventions in order to be objective in the evaluation of outcomes.

Hypersensitivity and allergic reactions to the drug can be established prior to the interventions, by skin tests or by evaluating the conjunctival response that has been validated by artificial intelligence methods [8].

In some publications, the addition of bicarbonate has been suggested to reduce pain at the time of application, especially in the papule modality, which has been based on the experience of the use of this buffer strategy in other medical and dental specialties [9–11]. As it is not a standardized practice in all cases, if it is performed, all aseptic conditions must be met.

3 Precautions and Risks in Relation to the Application Elements

All the elements to be used in the practice of NTM such as needles and syringes and local anesthetic containers must be disposable, and intradermal injectors must guarantee their total sterilization [12].

4 Precautions and Risks in Relation to Techniques

The application of local anesthetics in NTM can be classified as superficial and deep. Superficial applications, which usually correspond to papules, are found under direct vision, and for this reason, practically no accidents are described by their application. Deep blood cells, on the other hand, are not under direct vision and could generate lesions of vascular and anatomical structures that could result in secondary complications, so it is very important to remember the anatomy of the areas to be operated on, always aspirate with the syringe before application to avoid intravascular applications and observe patients after deep applications [13, 14].

Taking into account these circumstances, the possibility of using methods such as ultrasound in the in-depth applications of NTM is considered, which will allow, as a safety measure, a direct view at the time of the intervention. This strategy has already been applied in some conventional medicine procedures with excellent results [15, 16].

All areas to be operated on with NTM should be disinfected beforehand, and when an infected or potentially infected area is affected, the application equipment should be changed, if other interventions are to be performed at other sites [12].

5 Precautions and Risks in Relation to the Patient

The conditions of each patient must be analyzed exhaustively. Precautions should be taken in patients on anticoagulation or with hemorrhagic pathologies, especially in deep applications that are difficult to control [17, 18]. If the use of NTM is considered essential, the special characteristics of each patient should be taken into account, and in anticoagulated patients, anticoagulants should be discontinued according to their pharmacological characteristics, with an adequate time before application [19, 20].

In cancer patients undergoing treatment, avoid NTM interventions during periods of immunosuppression generated by medications, and do them when patients are outside the risk period [21].

In immunosuppressed patients, those who are systemically compromised or in critical conditions, try to do as few interventions as possible [22].

6 Precautions and Risks in Relation to the Therapist

Before the application of NTM procedures, adequate hand washing and sterile gloves should be used in the application of deep techniques, recommendations that arise from the consensus on health care safety existing in the literature [23]. Colombian legislation considers that interventions are carried out by health professionals in the specific field of their profession, with postgraduate training in NTM [24].

References

1. Vinyes D, Muñoz-Sellart M, Fischer L. Therapeutic use of low dose local anesthetics in pain, inflammation, and other clinical conditions: a systematic scoping review. J Clin Med. 2023;12(23):7221. https://doi.org/10.3390/jcm12237221. PMID: 38068272; PMCID: PMC10707454.
2. Gradinaru D, Ungurianu A, Margina D, Moreno-Villanueva M, Bürkle A. Procaine – the controversial geroprotector candidate: new insights regarding its molecular and cellular effects. Oxidative Med Cell Longev. 2021;2021:3617042. https://doi.org/10.1155/2021/3617042. PMID: 34373764; PMCID: PMC8349289.
3. Bahar E, Yoon H. Lidocaine: a local anesthetic, its adverse effects, and management. Medicina (Kaunas). 2021;57(8):782. https://doi.org/10.3390/medicina57080782. PMID: 34440986; PMCID: PMC8399637.
4. Brunton LL, Knollmann BC. Goodman & Gilman's the pharmacological basis of therapeutics. 14th ed. New York: McGraw Hill; 2023.
5. Becker DE, Reed KL. Local anesthetics: review of pharmacological considerations. Anesth Prog 2012;59(2):90–101; quiz 102–3. https://doi.org/10.2344/0003-3006-59.2.90. PMID: 22822998; PMCID: PMC3403589.

6. Sheikh NK, Dua A. Procaine. 2023. In: StatPearls [Internet]. Treasure Island (FL): StatPearls Publishing; 2024.
7. Torp KD, Metheny E, Simon LV. Lidocaine toxicity. 2022. In: StatPearls [Internet]. Treasure Island (FL): StatPearls Publishing; 2024.
8. Yarin Y, Kalaitzidou A, Bodrova K, Mösges R, Kalaidzidis Y. Validation of AI-based software for objectification of conjunctival provocation test. J Allergy Clin Immunol Glob. 2023;2(3):100121. https://doi.org/10.1016/j.jacig.2023.100121. PMID: 37779521; PMCID: PMC10509841.
9. Hockett D, Kress L, Mac Donald R, Krenzischek DA, Maheshwari A. Effectiveness of buffered lidocaine for local anesthesia during liver biopsy. Gastroenterol Nurs. 2021;44(3):172–6. https://doi.org/10.1097/SGA.0000000000000542. PMID: 33927155; PMCID: PMC8162227.
10. Hyttönen M, Nietosvaara Y, Reito A, Sirola J, Heikkinen N, Savolainen A, Räisänen MP. Protocol for a double-blinded randomised controlled trial investigating the use of adjunct bicarbonate in carpal tunnel release: a single-centre study. BMJ Open. 2023;13(9):e071488. https://doi.org/10.1136/bmjopen-2022-071488. PMID: 37723109; PMCID: PMC10510898.
11. Gorrela H, Srujana T, Arthi S. Buffered versus non-buffered local anaesthesia in minor oral surgery – a comparative study. Ann Maxillofac Surg. 2024;14(1):15–20. https://doi.org/10.4103/ams.ams_168_21.
12. Beltrán EH, Urrego DZ. A medical system called neural therapeutic medicine. In: Beltrán EH, Vega JA, editors. Neural therapeutic medicine: an approach from complex medical systems. Bogotá D.C.: Universidad Nacional de Colombia; 2013. p. 29–49.
13. Dosch P. Dosch M. The technics of neural therapy. In: Dosch P., Dosch M. Manual of neural therapy according to Huneke. 2nd Ed. Stuttgart. Thieme. 2007: 261–288.
14. Rathmell JP. Complications in Pain Medicine. In: Cousins MJ, Horlocker TT, Brindenbaugh PO, Carr DB, editors. Neural blockade in clinical anesthesia and pain medicine. 4th ed. Philadelphia: Lippincott Williams & Wilkin; 2009. p. 1223–67.
15. Xiong X, Xiong Y, Liu G. Systematic review and meta-analysis: safety of ultrasound-guided peripheral venipuncture and catheterization. Ann Palliat Med. 2021;10(11):11721–32. https://doi.org/10.21037/apm-21-3163.
16. Huang C, Li J, Guo Y, Zhang Y, Luo W, Diedrich DA, Zhang T, Huang W, Xiao Y. Ultrasound-assisted lumbar puncture with a horizontal and perpendicular Paramedian approach based on positioning in patients with abnormal spinal anatomy: a case report and technical description. BMC Anesthesiol. 2023;23(1):410. https://doi.org/10.1186/s12871-023-02368-7.
17. van Baarle FEHP, van de Weerdt EK, Suurmond B, Müller MCA, Vlaar APJ, Biemond BJ. Bleeding assessment and bleeding severity in thrombocytopenic patients undergoing invasive procedures. Transfusion. 2020;60(3):637–49. https://doi.org/10.1111/trf.15670. Epub 2020 Jan 31. PMID: 32003910; PMCID: PMC7079124.
18. McCulloch M, Nachat A, Schwartz J, Casella-Gordon V, Cook J. Acupuncture safety in patients receiving anticoagulants: a systematic review. Perm J. 2015;19(1):68–73. https://doi.org/10.7812/TPP/14-057. Epub 2014 Nov 24. PMID: 25432001; PMCID: PMC4315381.
19. Mehic D, Neubauer G, Janig F, Kaider A, Ay C, Pabinger I, Gebhart J. Risk factors for future bleeding in patients with mild bleeding disorders: longitudinal data from the Vienna bleeding biobank. J Thromb Haemost. 2023;21(7):1757–68. https://doi.org/10.1016/j.jtha.2023.03.006. Epub 2023 Mar 15.
20. Dhakal P, Rayamajhi S, Verma V, Gundabolu K, Bhatt VR. Reversal of anticoagulation and management of Bleeding in patients on anticoagulants. Clin Appl Thromb Hemost. 2017;23(5):410–5. https://doi.org/10.1177/1076029616675970. Epub 2016 Oct 26.
21. Sparreboom A, Baker SD. Pharmacokinetics and pharmacodynamics of anticancer drugs. In: De Vita VT, Lawrence TS, Rosenberg SA, editors. Cancer: principles and practice of oncology. 12th ed. Philadelphia: Wolters Kluwer; 2023. p. 231–8.
22. Dosch P, Dosch M. Procaine hypersensitive and accidents. Countermeasures in accidents. Important rules for practical applications. In: Dosch P, Dosch M, editors. Manual of neural therapy according to Huneke. 2nd ed. Stuttgart: Thieme; 2007. p. 277–88.

23. Yilma M, Taye G, Abebe W. Magnitude of standard precautions practices among healthcare workers in health facilities of low and middle income countries: a systematic review and meta-analysis. PLoS One. 2024;19(4):e0302282. https://doi.org/10.1371/journal.pone.0302282. PMID: 38687766; PMCID: PMC11060540.
24. Congreso de la República de Colombia. Law 1164 of 2007 "by which provisions are made regarding human talent in health." Article 19. Available at: https://www.minsalud.gov.co/normatividad_nuevo/ley%201164%20de%202007.pdf. Consulted on 8 Feb 2025.

Part VIII
Some Techniques and New Trends in Neuraltherapeutic Medicine

Chapter 30
A New Approach to Segmental Therapy

Jazmín Ariza-Tarazona and Laura Bibiana Pinilla Bonilla

1 Introduction

The knowledge of the embryology of the nervous system, together with the extensive enrichment of the semiology proposed by Dr. Head [1] and Dr. Mackenzie [2], as well as other authors of segmental anatomy and physiology [3], allows for more precise diagnosis and segmental therapy, with a special focus on visceral diseases.

The first step in this approach is to perform a complete physical examination (Chap. 21), using a mechanical algesimeter or algometer to assess surface sensitivity. Evaluation with this instrument provides information on the specific sensitivity of a dermatomic level and is considered positive if the patient presents sensitivity with a pressure of 4 kg/cm^2, which is approximately the pressure needed to whiten the nail bed of the thumb [4]. In this way, a visceral pathology or disease can be identified early, even long before the patient presents any symptoms or changes can be found in the laboratories [3].

The most remarkable aspect of this new approach to therapeutics is the individualization of segmental therapy. The classic schemes of neural therapy, such as the "crown of thorns," the "pulmonary vest," or "abdomen segment," among others [5],

J. Ariza-Tarazona
Master in Alternative Medicine, Neural Therapy Area, Faculty of Medicine, Universidad Nacional de Colombia, Bogotá, Colombia

L. B. Pinilla Bonilla (✉)
Faculty of Medicine, Master in Alternative Medicine, Neural Therapy Area, Universidad Nacional de Colombia, Bogotá, Colombia

Integrated Health Services Subnetwork of the South, Research and Innovation Center, Bogotá, Colombia
e-mail: lbpnillab@unal.edu.co

L. B. Pinilla Bonilla et al. (eds.), *Neuraltherapeutic Medicine*, https://doi.org/10.1007/978-3-032-03257-7_30

which have been widely disseminated and used, are protocol schemes[1] that, in addition, ignores important aspects of embryological knowledge. From the approach of Neuraltherapeutic medicine, protocols deny any possibility of respecting individualization.

Additionally, the knowledge of segmental anatomy allows us to understand that the segments described as classic do not completely encompass the reflex metameric area. As an example, a pulmonary or cardiac pathology can extend in its clinical manifestations to the head, neck, or upper extremity area, in addition to the chest.

Likewise, frequently occurring pathologies, such as plantar fasciitis or talalgia, are derived from irritation in the lower hypogastric segment (due to pelvic viscera pathologies), which in turn depends on the lumbosacral plexus.

In the following section, a new individualized segmental approach scheme presented by the authors is proposed.

2 Individualized Segmental Approach

Before performing the procedure, the first step is to make a complete life history (Chap. 20), a detailed physical examination (Chap. 21), and an analysis to arrive at the neural therapy diagnosis (Chap. 24).

Chapter 15 provides detailed information on segmental physiology based on the Head and Mackenzie zones [1, 2, 6] that should be taken into account for therapy. The areas of each of the organs of the head, neck, trunk, and pelvis are described. The therapeutic approach of this new segmental approach is outlined below:

1. Define the segmental area that requires intervention. Examples: segmental area of the liver, segmental area of the bladder, and segmental area of the eye.
2. According to the physical examination and life history, define the metameric level to be operated on (dermatome, fasciotome, myotome, sclerotome, or all).
   (a) *In case of dermatome intervention*: after evaluation with a mechanical algesimeter, perform an intradermal or subdermal infiltration with the local anesthetic in the patient's positive points. For this, short-length, smaller-gauge needles (1/2 or 1 in. (2.54 cm) × 30 G) are usually required, with a papule application volume of 0.1 cc. Later on, we will indicate how to apply the application in the zones according to the Head.

[1] Here the term "protocol" refers to the fixed and invariable scheme of application of a treatment in pre-established sites that do not depend on a sensitivity test. In the example of the crown of thorns, it is a scheme of applying subdermal papules to the scalp in an arrangement similar to having a crown of thorns on the head. In the case of the "pulmonary vest," it refers to the application of anteroposterior parasternal papules in the manner of a vest. In the case of some other segment, such as the abdomen, it refers to the application of papules applied equidistantly and distributed over a specific surface of the skin. All these applications, under the classic scheme, did not depend on any skin sensitivity test to explore the "individual" points of each patient.

(b) *In case of fasciotome intervention*: perform subdermal and subcutaneous cellular tissue infiltration with the local anesthetic in the sites where fascia alterations are found in the physical examination. For this purpose, use a 1 in. × 30 G needle, with a volume per application of approximately 0.5 cc.
(c) *In case of myotome intervention*: intramuscular infiltration is performed with the local anesthetic in the places where trigger points, contractures, or muscle hyperalgesia are found. The needle varies according to the depth at which the muscle is located; it can range from 1 in. to 1 1/2 in. × 27G with an approximate volume of 1 cc.
(d) *In case of sclerotomy intervention*: a pre-periosteal infiltration with the local anesthetic is performed in the places where a trophic lesion or periosteal scar is suspected. The needle varies according to the depth at which the bone structure is located. This can vary between 0.5 and 1.5 in. × 27 or 30 G with an approximate volume of 1 cc.

    Caution: In case of approaching the thoracic area, in myotoma or sclerotoma, you should act with caution regarding the depth due to the risk of pleural injury. In the anterior, lateral and posterolateral areas, preferably do not go deeper than 1 cm in the intercostal spaces of thin people.

3. Treatment of Head's zones: This intervention depends on the physical examination with the mechanical algometer. The vast majority of patients will manifest superficial skin sensitivity to a greater or lesser extent in the areas described by Henry Head in cases of visceral disease, including the teeth. However, some patients express it earlier or later, depending on their sensitivity threshold and their type of nervous system. Some patients, presenting with diseases of the trunk viscera, may not show superficial sensitivity in the chest, abdomen, or pelvis, but they do in the corresponding reflex Head's zone. Mackenzie also described that in "rare" cases where there is no hypersensitivity of the skin when examined with the blunt-tipped instrument (equivalent to the algesimeter), it is generally found that the deeper tissues (muscles, fascia, periosteum and joints) can exhibit sensitivity [7].

    The intervention in the dermatome and Head's zones is performed directly on the identified points of hypersensitivity with the mechanical algesimeter. In the event that a patient exhibits a large number of hypersensitivity points, it is advisable to initiate the intervention at the maximum pain points (MP) according to Head [1, 6] shown in Chap. 15. Performing the intervention on the MP frequently causes the sensitivity of the remaining points in the same area to decrease or disappear.

    Monitoring through MP also allows for the evaluation of the effect of the intervention carried out, serving as indicators of the trophic status of the viscera.

3 From Deep to Superficial Techniques

During the Forum of Neural Therapy held in Vienna in 2019, Pinilla[2] presented a conference in which some experiences and research with the new segmental approach were shared.

One of these studies was carried out by Estévez [8], within the framework of a master's thesis in the area of neural therapy of alternative medicine at the National University of Colombia. The medical records of patients treated by the specialty in Neuraltherapeutic medicine at the El Tunal hospital in southern Bogotá between 2015 and 2018 were retrospectively reviewed.

A sample of 80 patients who consulted for different types of musculoskeletal pain was taken. Patients reported having between 2 and 8 painful musculoskeletal symptoms in different locations. When comparing the differences in VAS between the start and end of treatment (8 sessions), a statistically significant reduction was found. The average number of sessions required to achieve complete pain elimination was 3.72 sessions.

Surprisingly, 93.21% of the interventions needed to reduce pain were superficial, while only 7.8% needed deep procedures in the plexus or ganglia.

In the Forum in Vienna, Pinilla concluded that in Colombia, the inclusion of this knowledge derived from Head and Mackenzie has allowed effective treatment in Neural Therapy practice in less time than before with the minimum requirement of making deep injections and, in consequence, minimizing the risk of adverse effects.

4 Illustrative Clinical Cases

Next, two clinical cases will be presented; one of them is a theoretical case, and the second case is a patient of the private consultation, who duly agreed and signed the informed consent.

4.1 Clinical Case: Pelvic Pathology

A 25-year-old female patient presented with plantar pain of 3 years' duration. She had consulted orthopedics, where they diagnosed plantar fasciitis and bilateral calcaneal spurs, giving conventional management with physical therapy without pain control. In search of different alternatives, she consults the Neuraltherapeutic medicine service, where it is found that, in the patient's life history, the pain begins at the age of 22, the pain is daily, it is exacerbated by periods of prolonged standing. The

[2] Pinilla Bonilla L. B. From Deep to Superficial Techniques. International Forum of Neural Therapy. Vienna, 2019. Information available at: https://ignh.de/forum-neural-therapy-international/

VAS is 6/10 and can reach VAS 8/10. Her menstrual cycle further intensifies the pain. Due to its characteristics, pain affects the sole, back, and sometimes the neck of the foot. When she is in an ovulatory cycle, the patient reports that the pain rises to the area of the calf muscles.

On the review by systems, the patient indicated that she had dyspareunia and dysmenorrhea of VAS 4 to 8/10 in each menstrual period, irregular cycles since menarche, with heavy bleeding and expulsion of clots. These symptoms began at the age of 21 when she began IUD planning (intrauterine device: copper T), which was removed at 6 months due to non-tolerance. She currently uses birth control methods with a barrier method (condom), and despite this change, bleeding has continued with the same characteristics since the placement of the intrauterine device. In the important history, the patient reported the presence of a urinary tract infection at the age of 23 and of repeated vaginal infections due to candida.

On physical examination, the following signs have found: normal vital signs, hypersensitivity in the occipital area of the scalp with the mechanical algesimeter, coldness in the infraumbilical abdomen and pelvis area (T10 to L1), sensitivity to examination with the algesimeter in the same dermatomes, sensitivity in the L1 dermatome in the anterior thigh, pain on palpation of the pubic symphysis, positive Mackenzie's sign in the sacral area (pain on palpation of the spinous processes from S1 to S4), tenderness in the area of insertion of fascia lata at the level of the left knee, pain on palpation of the bilateral internal and external malleoli and pain on palpation of the calcaneus (See Fig. 30.1).

The following diagram is presented for verification of symptomatic areas.

It is evident that the patient has clear genitourinary symptoms with involvement from T10 to S4 that is reflected in both the pelvic, sacral, and lower limb areas. When the intervention is performed, with the first approach to the points of skin

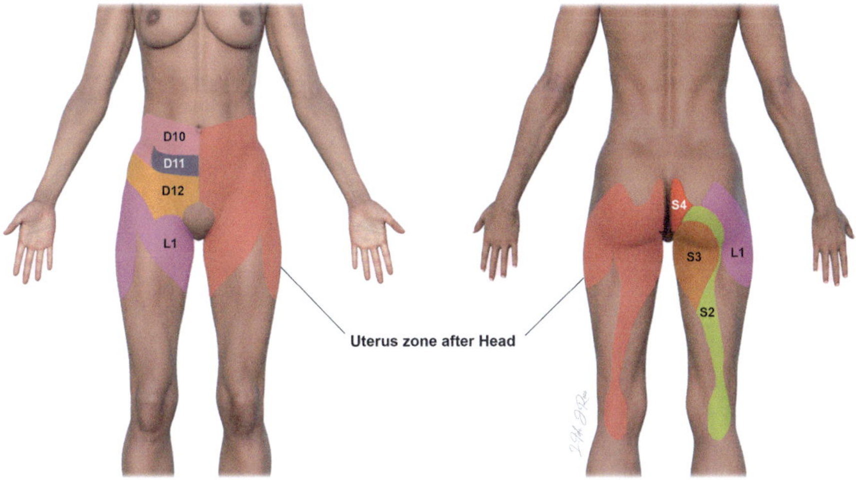

Fig. 30.1 Diagram of the head zone of the uterus

hypersensitivity located in the Head's zone of the anteroposterior uterus, the patient improves plantar pain by 80%, decreases the volume of menstrual bleeding and symptoms in the lower limbs, and decreases sensitivity in the scalp. It should also be remembered, as explained above, that visceral pathology can be reflected in the head when there is already a possible case of corticalization, and that it is reflected in the Head's zones of the head, according to each viscera [7].

4.2 Clinical Case: Cardiac Pathology

We describe a case of a 65-year-old male patient who has a herpes zoster rash on his right arm, causing a VAS 8/10 burning pain. He went to the emergency department, where they prescribed oral antivirals, NSAIDs, and topical local lidocaine gel. Despite medical management, the pain does not improve. In Neuraltherapeutic medicine consultation, symptoms of mild dyspnea have been found for 2 months in ambulation. He denies any other type of symptomatology. Important background: mixed dyslipidemia in control with lipid-lowering management.

During the physical examination, we found that the vital signs were within normal limits. A herpetiform rash is evident in the right upper limb that involves the ulnar area at the level of the fingers of the hand (fourth finger external lateral aspect and fifth finger) and the axillary area, with active vesicles (See Fig. 30.2).

In addition to the distribution of the lesions, there are points of sensitivity in the area of the left anterior thorax (Head's zone of heart). Intervention was performed on the points of maximum pain in the area of the head of the heart from C7 to T1 and T4 to T6, but the patient was sent for a cardiology study (although the patient did not have clear symptoms of cardiac pathology, the symptom of dyspnea and the distribution of the rash indicate possible irritation in the cardiac area).

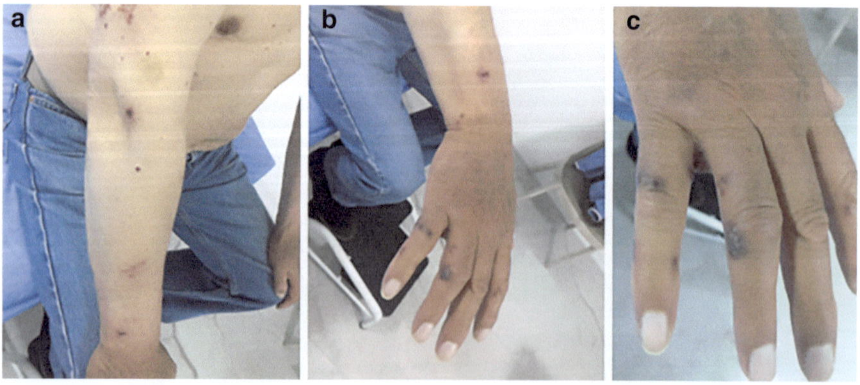

Fig. 30.2 Photographs of Head's zone of heart in patient with Herpes Zoster. Photograph **a**, shows the involvement of the ulnar area of the arm and forearm; photograph **b** and **c**, show the involvement of the ulnar area in the forearm and hand. (Photograph supplied by Jazmín S. Ariza)

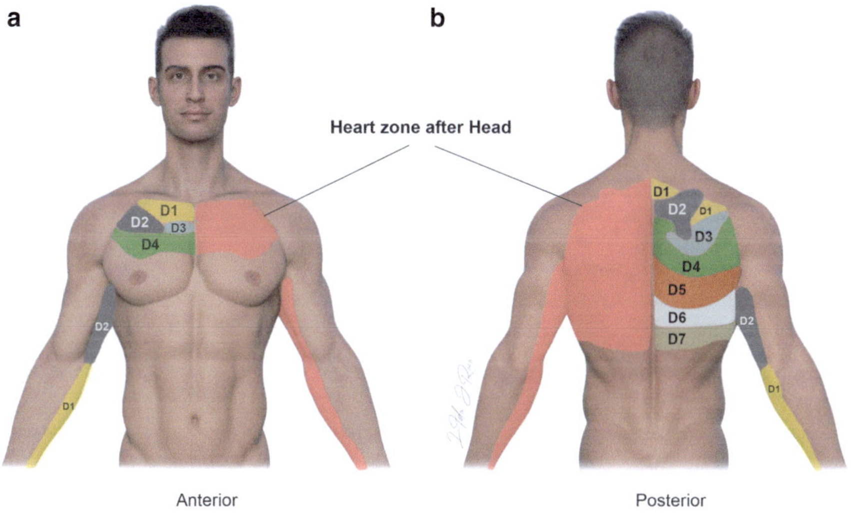

Fig. 30.3 Cardiac head zone diagram

Fig. 30.3 is presented for verification of symptomatic areas.

Pain was controlled in the patient with Neuraltherapeutic medicine and subsequent studies showed that there was an obstruction of more than 80% in the descending coronary artery, which was managed with stenting.

This last case demonstrates that the information provided by the Head's zones is also evident before the patient shows clear signs and symptoms. Regarding laterality, it should not always be expected homolaterally in a single viscera but should be guided by the area described.

References

1. Head H. On disturbances of sensation with special reference to the pain of visceral disease. Brain. 1893;16(1–2):1–133.
2. Mackenzie J. The meaning and mechanism of visceral pain as shown by the study of visceral and other sympathetic (autonomic) reflexes. Br Med J. 1906;30:1523–8.
3. Wancura-Kampik I. Segmental anatomy. 1st ed. Munchen: Elsevier Urban & Fisher Verlag; 2009.
4. Okifuji A, Turk DC, Sinclair JD, et al. A standardized manual tender point survey. I. Development and determination of a threshold point for the identification of positive tender points in fibromyalgia syndrome. J Rheumatol. 1997;24(2):377–83.
5. Dosch P, Dosch M. Manual of neural therapy according to Huneke. 2nd ed. Stuttgart: Thieme; 2007.
6. Head H. On disturbances of sensation with special reference to the pain of visceral disease: part II. Head and neck. Brain. 1894;17(3):339–480.
7. Mackenzie J. Some points bearing on the Association of Sensory Disorders and Visceral Disease. Brain. 1983;16:321–53. https://doi.org/10.1093/brain/16.3.321.
8. Estevez E. Contribution of neuraltherapeutic medicine to the management of patients with osteo-muscular pathologies. Master's thesis. Bogotá: Universidad Nacional de Colombia; 2020. 46p.

Chapter 31
New Technique of Vagus Nerve

Laura Bibiana Pinilla Bonilla, Jazmín Ariza-Tarazona, Luz Amparo Arias-López, and Juliana Henao

1 Anatomy and Path of the Vagus Nerve

The tenth cranial nerve, vagus nerve (from the Latin nervus vagus), named for its wandering path (See Fig. 31.1), has its apparent origin in the retroolivar sulcus, emerging between the glossopharyngeal nerve and the spinal nerve [2].

He was called the wandering protector (because of his long journey in various viscera). Nowadays, it is a therapeutic target because it establishes several relationships with the immune system, has analgesic properties, influences the relationships between appetite and obesity, and is related to memory, among other functions [3].

L. B. Pinilla Bonilla (✉)
Faculty of Medicine, Master in Alternative Medicine, Neural Therapy Area,
Universidad Nacional de Colombia, Bogotá, Colombia

Integrated Health Services Subnetwork of the South, Research and Innovation Center,
Bogotá, Colombia
e-mail: lbpnillab@unal.edu.co

J. Ariza-Tarazona
Master in Alternative Medicine, Neural Therapy Area, Faculty of Medicine,
Universidad Nacional de Colombia, Bogotá, Colombia
e-mail: jsarizatarazona@gmail.com

L. A. Arias-López
Faculty of Medicine, Morphology Department, Master in Human Morphology,
Universidad Nacional de Colombia,
Bogotá, Colombia
e-mail: luaariaslo@unal.edu.co

J. Henao
Private Practice, Medellín, Colombia
e-mail: juhenaoa@unal.edu.co

L. B. Pinilla Bonilla et al. (eds.), *Neuraltherapeutic Medicine*,
https://doi.org/10.1007/978-3-032-03257-7_31

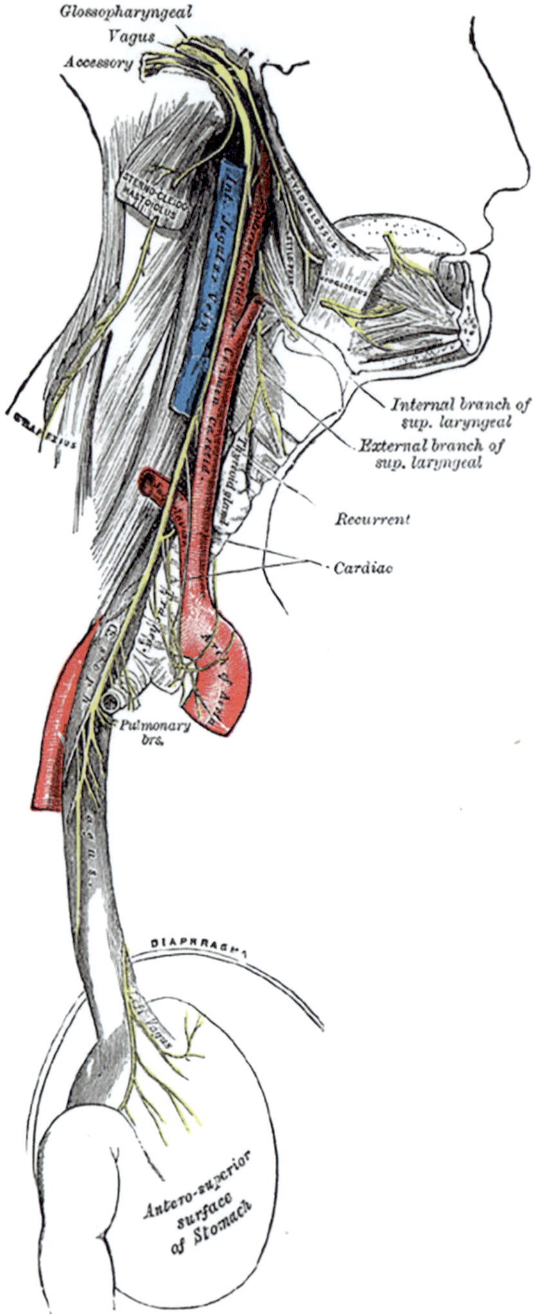

Fig. 31.1 The vagus nerve and its path are shown. (Taken from Gray [1])

Table 31.1 Functions of the vagus nerve

No.	Sensitivity	Sensory	Motor
1.	The mucosa of the epiglottic vallecula, the epiglottis and the portion of the larynx that is close to the glottic branch and inferior to the vocal cords [2]. This innervation is given by one of the branches of the NC X called the internal branch of the superior laryngeal nerve [3]	Taste of the vallecula and the epiglottis [2]. And part of the root of the tongue; soft palate and oropharynx	Skeletal striated muscles of the larynx. This innervation is given by one of the branches of the X NPC called the inferior or recurrent laryngeal nerve [3]. As well as the cricothyroid muscles and the inferior constrictor muscle of the pharynx
2.	The carotid body [2]		Gastric and hepatic secretor
3.	The esophagus, lower respiratory tract, heart, thymus, aorta, gastrointestinal tract, liver, gallbladder, and portal vein [5]		Parasympathetic innervation of the heart, airway, lungs, kidneys—Via vagosympathetic splenic reflex—[6]
4.	Spleen [6]		Vasodilation
5.			Gastric peristalsis, duodenal, jejunal, ileal, cecum, appendix, ascending colon and 2/3 right of the transverse colon

Source: Taken and modified from Henao [2]

It supplies nerves to the pharynx, esophagus, larynx, trachea, bronchi, heart, stomach, pancreas, liver, and organs supplied by the superior mesenteric artery. This is done through small networks of nerves that connect to the myenteric or Auerbach plexuses, where the parasympathetic postsynaptic fibers are found [3]. Acetylcholine (Ach) of neuronal and non-neuronal origin (T lymphocytes) is its neurotransmitter [4].

It has three components that are related to sensitivity, sensory, and motor functions [2] (See Table 31.1).

2 Central and Peripheral Connections and Anastomosis with Other Structures

In the central nervous system, the collection of neuronal cells is known as the nucleus. In the peripheral nervous system, it is known as the ganglion. Thus, the sensory fibers of the vagus nerve possess their neuronal body in the nucleus of the solitary tract, the motor fibers are located in the nucleus ambiguus, and the parasympathetic fibers in the dorsal nucleus of the vagus nerve [2].

The vagus nerve is part of the group called cranial parasympathetic, along with the common ocular motor nerve (NC III), the facial nerve (NC VII) and the glossopharyngeal nerve (NC IX). In addition to the parasympathetic function of the NC X, it has somatomotor, somatosensory, visceromotor, and viscerosensory functions. The somatomotor function corresponds to the innervation of the pharynx (swallowing movement) and gives the motor innervation of the muscles of the larynx to contribute to phonation. With regard to somatosensory function, it innervates part of the lingual root, the pharyngeal and laryngeal mucosa [2].

The visceromotor function is given by the peristalsis of the digestive tract, from the esophagus to the transverse colon; secretor of the gastric glands; and negative chronotropic. Finally, the viscerosensitivity function is defined by the nerve connections in the lungs and gastrointestinal tract mentioned earlier [1]. In fact, the vagus nerve is considered a mixed nerve given the multiple functions and examples cited above [2].

The vagus nerve, once it originates in the retroolivar sulcus, descends through the jugular foramen, where its first ganglion, called the jugular ganglion [7] or superior, is located.

It is centrally connected to the nucleus of the solitary tract with taste fibers from the facial (VII) and glossopharyngeal (IX) cranial nerves. This serves as a relay for taste. In addition, it is related to the V cranial or trigeminal nerve in the spinal nucleus of the latter, where sensory information is collected from the outer portion of the tympanic membrane, the external auditory canal, the outer ear, and the regional meninges [7].

The three nuclei of the vagus nerve are: main motor, formed by the ambiguous nucleus, with corticonuclear afferent fibers from both hemispheres and with its efferent fibers, which innervate constrictor muscles of the pharynx and intrinsic muscles of the larynx. The parasympathetic or dorsal nucleus of the vagus, with afferent fibers from the hypothalamus, and its efferent fibers are distributed through the thoraco-abdominal viscera to the distal third of the transverse colon. The sensory nucleus, which is the lower part of the solitary tract nucleus, is related to afferent information that terminates in the spinal nucleus of the trigeminal nerve, forming multiple connections [2].

Anastomosis of the vagus nerve with the following cranial nerve has been described, depending on the site of the anastomosis, namely:

(a) Anastomosis with XI in the jugular node.
(b) Anastomosis with IX in the jugular node.
(c) Anastomosis with VII in the auricular branch of the vagus; the posterior auricular nerve; the posterior aspect of the pinna and the posteroinferior aspect of the external auditory canal.
(d) Anastomosis with XII in the plexiform node.

Additionally, the vagus nerve is anastomosed with the great sympathetic and with C1–C2 in the plexiform ganglion. The latter anastomosis has been described as inconstant.

3 Functions of the Vagus Nerve

3.1 Classic

Traditionally, it has been known that the vagus nerve carries fibers mainly from the parasympathetic subdivision of the autonomic nervous system, which are responsible for arteriole dilation, pupillary miosis, cardiac and airway innervation, stimulation of gastric and hepatic secretion, and gastrointestinal peristalsis. In addition, it has a sensory function in the epiglottis and larynx, a motor function in the larynx and pharynx where it collaborates with phonation and swallowing, respectively. And a sensory function providing the taste information of the vallecula, epiglottis, part of the root of the tongue, soft palate, and oropharynx [2].

3.2 Non-classical

Within the non-classical pathway, there is the function that the vagus nerve plays in inflammation. Kevin Tracey's approach to the theory of inflammation in the early 2000s was thought to have been the first to describe these uses. Nonetheless, since the 1880s transcutaneous electrical stimulation of the vagus nerve and cervical sympathetic stimulation have been described as being used for seizures [4]. In the 1930s, Vishnevsky surgeons used interventional techniques that they called cervical sympathetic vagus block for therapeutic purposes for patients with thoracic trauma, with excellent results in infection prevention, shock, and pain control [8].

Tracey proposed that cholinergic neurons can modulate acute inflammatory responses through the nervous system, that acts as a reflex, modulating several systems such as the immune and endocrine [9].

Two pathways are known within the inflammatory response. One pathway, called the diffusible pathway, in which the circulatory system intervenes, and the second pathway is the so-called neural pathway. When DAMP or PAMP (Damage-Associated Molecular Patterns or Pathogen-Associated Molecular Patterns) are present in the local tissue, inflammation-causing substances such as IL-1 (interleukin 1) or TNF (tumor necrosis factor) are produced. These substances stimulate neutrophils and lymphocytes. The information is transported through the circulation to initiate the production of ACh (acetylcholine). This, in turn, stimulates the production of glucocorticoids and, therefore, of anti-inflammatory substances such as IL 10 (interleukin-10), glucocorticoids and spermine, among others. This pathway is slow and depends on the concentration of the gradients of the substances involved [9].

The second pathway is neural, where macrophages are also involved. When these are stimulated by local proinflammatory substances, the information travels through sensory afferents from the vagus nerve to the nucleus of the solitary tract in the hypothalamus. This results in an efferent response (through the motor fibers of the vagus) which involves the production of ACh that, when binding to the receptor in the macrophage, decreases the production of TNF. It is considered a neural reflex pathway, where information from a specific stimulus enters through the afferent route, generating an efferent response. This pathway is rapid, integrated into the nervous system, and its response is in the form of a reflex arc.

Other receptors that are stimulated on macrophages, such as substance P receptors, when activated, increase TNF production. This correlates to a pathway that sustains pain, and through sympathetic pathways, this production can be increased or decreased by stimulating adrenaline/noradrenaline receptors [9]. This pathway is mainly found in the reticuloendothelial tissues of organs such as the liver, spleen, kidney, and gastrointestinal system.

The importance of vagus nerve stimulation today lies in the wide pathology in which it can have a therapeutic action through measures such as external stimulation. There are invasive and non-invasive vagus stimulation devices. In the first cases, side effects such as dysphonia, paresthesia's, Horner's syndrome, dyspnea, vocal cord paralysis, dyspepsia, neuropathic pain around the stimulator, bradycardia, asystole, hematoma or infection have been described. In the second cases, local discomfort, skin irritation and muscle pain can occur. If the cost and frequency of application are added to this, it could be an option with several disadvantages for the patient [10].

4 Intervention/Stimulation Techniques on the Vagus Nerve

In the context of neural therapy and the Russian school, the following techniques have been described:

4.1 Sympathetic Vague Block According to the Vishnevsky

In their work "Novocaine Blocks and Oleobalsamic Antiseptics as a Special Form of Pathogenic Therapeutics" [8], Soviet surgeons named Vischnevsky detail a technique to reach the vagus nerve, which they call vagossympathetic block, and describe it as a physiological technique of crawling infiltrate. To achieve this, the patient must lie supine on a table with the head displaced to the opposite side of the doctor. A roll is placed under the shoulders and the shoulder is lowered from the side to be treated, moving the arm downwards.

Next, the focus is on the anatomical repair needed. Apply strong pressure with the index finger on the back part of the sternocleidomastoid muscle "above the point where it joins the external jugular vein," directing pressure toward the middle of the structures in this area. A wheal is made in this place, the needle is inserted inwards and slightly upwards, facing the anterior surface of the spine. For this procedure, they recommend injecting a volume of 30 to 50 cc of 0.25% novocaine (procaine) solution, in small quantities of 2 to 3 cc, which will permeate the vasculonervous sheath where perineural contact produces its action without causing effects on the patient [8].

The Vischnevsky considered this technique quite safe for the protection of the cervical vascular bundle, since by moving the sternocleidomastoid muscle towards the midline, the vessels that run on the anterior surface of the spine are separated. According to the description of the technique, the needle will pass through the aponeurosis of the sternocleidomastoid, guiding the solution behind the middle sheet of the neck aponeurosis [8].

In addition, they mention other techniques without going into the details of their application:

- Alexandrin proposed injecting the novocaine solution through the open mouth at the level of the soft palate, between the posterior and lateral wall of the pharynx, directing the needle horizontally.
- Ajutin described another technique following the anterior border of the sternomastoid muscle in the direction of the vasculonervous bundle.

However, these techniques were not used by the Vishnevskys. On the contrary, the sympathetic vagus block was used even bilaterally by the Vishnevskys in the prophylaxis and therapy of pleuropulmonary shock (rib cage trauma during the war), by interrupting irritation through the truncal nerves of the neck, not only affecting the vagus nerve, but also the sympathetic system [8].

4.2 *Vagus Nerve Injection According to Peter Dosch*

The technique described by the Germans addresses both cranial nerve nerves, the glossopharyngeal nerve (NC IX) and the vagus nerve (NC X). They recommend the injection of 2 to 3 cc of procaine with a needle of 0.8 mm in diameter and 50–60 mm in length. The needle is inserted at right angles to the skin, between the tip of the mastoid and the angle of the jaw, until it makes contact with bone in the styloid process. The anesthetic is put in at the front and to a depth of 30—40 mm if the glossopharyngeal is to be reached, and in a dorsal direction if the vagus nerve is to be addressed. After the intervention, there may be a sensation of "lump" in the throat, dysphagia and loss of sensation in the pharyngeal mucosa, which indicates blockage of the glossopharyngeal nerve. Both vagus and glossopharyngeal nerves on the same side are frequently blocked, but the authors do not recommend performing this technique bilaterally due to the risk of bilateral recurrent nerve paresis [11].

5 New Technique for Approaching the Vagus Nerve by Transpharyngeal Route

The technique proposed in this chapter arose from the observation and research question posed by Pinilla L: Considering how close the posterolateral wall of the pharynx is to the carotid sheath, through which the vagus nerve passes, would a transpharyngeal approach be a feasible and easy way to intervene on this nerve? Would it be possible to intervene on the vagus nerve by using the same access site to infiltrate the tonsils and just by changing the depth of the injection?

An experimental design in cadavers was then proposed, for which it was accompanied by professors Ariza and Arias, and the support of the Department of Morphology of the National University of Colombia.

5.1 *Investigation on Cadavers*

The first step was to recreate the most common access in neural therapy, which is via the retrostyloid pathway in a cross-section at the level of the mastoid. Figure 31.2 shows that a 1.5-in. needle enters through the retrostyloid access and must travel at least 4 cm to reach the carotid sheath. By this route, the needle is also very close to the exit of the facial nerve.

When compared with the second route, which is the new transpharyngeal route, it is observed that the needle should only enter 2 cm from the anterior pillar of the tonsils. In this way, the facial nerve is avoided (Fig. 31.3).

The second phase consisted of carrying out a study on cadavers, in which tests were carried out by injecting methylene blue in two cases (vagus nerve stained with blue, positive test):

1. In cadaver with an unaltered carotid sheath to check the staining status of the superficial fascias close to it:

The needle was inserted with a syringe loaded with methylene blue into a cadaver with an undamaged carotid sheath. 1 cc was applied, entering through the lower pole of the platoglossal arch with a needle 30 degrees to the right with respect to the midline (Fig. 31.4). 5–10 min later, a submandibular window and dissection were performed to verify the status of the carotid sheath, which was indeed stained.

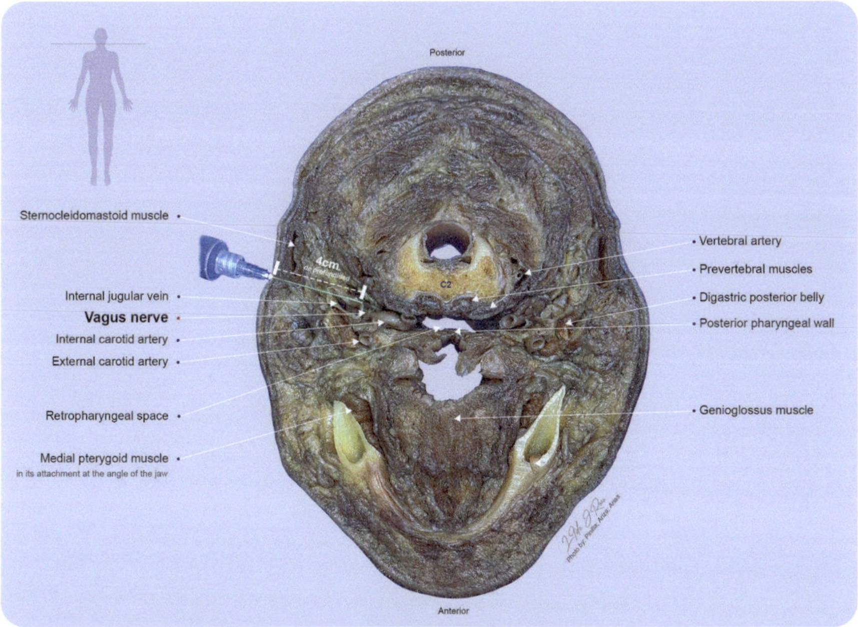

Fig. 31.2 Cross-section: top view at the level of the mastoid, where the needle is observed entering through the retrostyloid space. The vagus nerve and its relationship to blood vessels are shown. (Source: Photograph taken by the authors, edited by Luis F. Jaimes, with the support of the Department of Morphology of the National University of Colombia)

2. In the dissected carotid sheath to check the staining status of the vagus nerve directly.

For this second part, the corresponding dissection of the carotid sheath was first performed at the submandibular level. Subsequently, the needle was introduced with a syringe loaded with methylene blue, and 1 cc was applied, entering through the lower pole of the palatoglossal arc at a needle 30° to the right with respect to the midline (Fig. 31.5). After 5–10 min, the staining check on the vagus nerve is performed directly in this case.

3. Diffusion through the fasciae.

In the cadaver, it was evident that the stain covered a large part of the lateral cervical fascia. The cervical fascias acquire a relevant function due to its continuity and contiguity through their fibers with elements of the cranial cavity. The pretracheal fascia, which is part of the deep cervical fascia, is continued with the oropharyngeal fascia at the back and top and fuses with the carotid sheath laterally. On the other hand, the prevertebral fascia forms an extension sheath for the

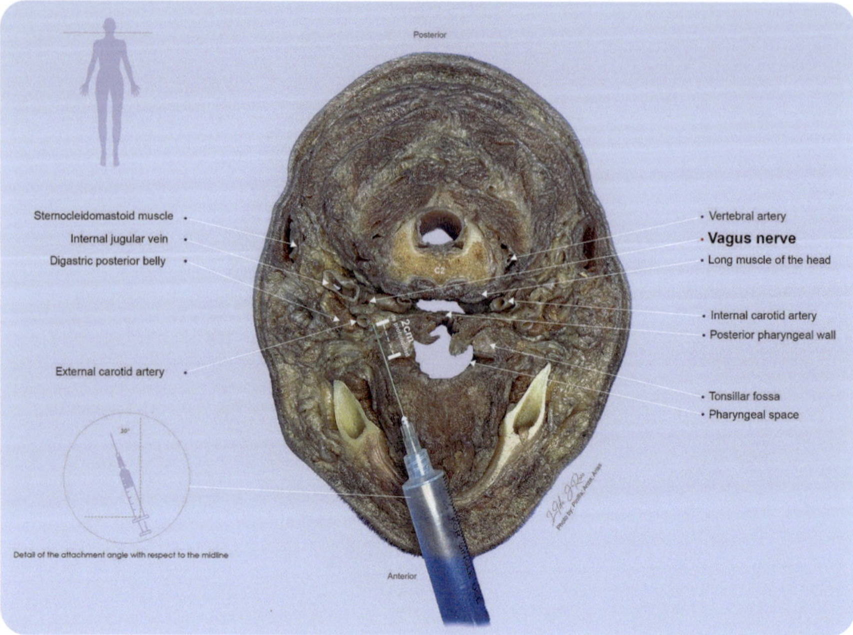

Fig. 31.3 Cross-section and upper view at mastoid level. Transpharyngeal entry to the vicinity of the carotid sheath is observed. (Source: Photograph taken by the authors, edited by Luis F. Jaimes, with the support of the Department of Morphology of the National University of Colombia)

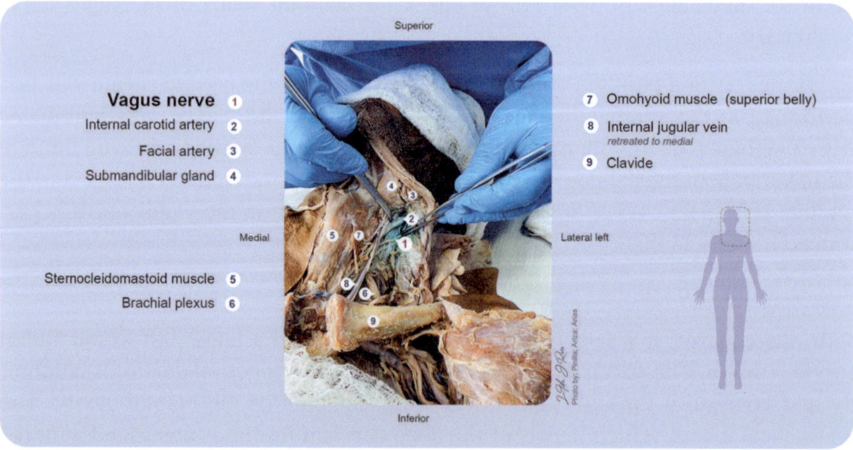

Fig. 31.4 The submandibular window with a positive test after methylene blue infiltration in the palatoglossal arch is shown. (Source: Photograph taken by the authors, edited by Luis F. Jaimes, with the support of the Department of Morphology of the National University of Colombia)

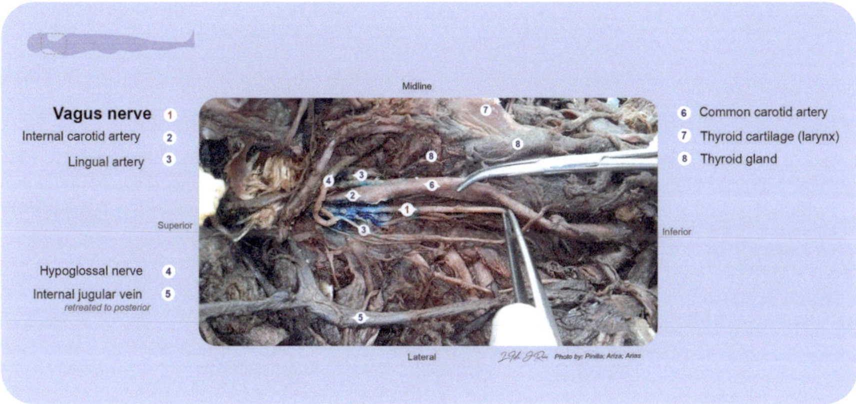

Fig. 31.5 A left submandibular and anterolateral view is shown, where the components of the carotid sheath after dissection are observed. The vagus nerve is marked with positive staining with methylene blue. (Source: Photograph taken by the authors, edited by Luis F Jaimes, with the support of the Department of Morphology of the National University of Colombia)

spine that anchors to the base of the skull at the top and fuses with the carotid sheath anteriorly. The carotid sheath involves important neurovascular structures such as the common carotid artery, the internal jugular vein, and the vagus nerve [12].

From the above, it can be deduced that there is a relationship between the cervical fascia and the dura mater directly and with the other meninges indirectly. The main connection is given by the continuity of the periosteal spinal dura mater with the deep cervical fascia of the neck. Likewise, the carotid sheath contains structures that are in proximity to the meninges, more specifically to the dura mater, especially at the base of the skull, where the dura mater is continuous with the meningeal layers that surround the brain. In the neck, the spinal dura mater is in contact with the prevertebral layer of the deep cervical fascia, which provides support and stability to the spinal cord in this region. In the same way, this connection could also be supported by the embryological origin shared by the fascial system and the dura mater [13].

5.2 Description of the Technique

(a) *Materials*: 3 or 5 mL syringe with 30 G × 1 in. needle.
(b) *Application of procaine*: 1–1.5 mL of procaine at 0.5% or 1%.
(c) *Patient position and anatomical repairs*: The patient may be seated or supine or in a supine position. To make this decision, the patient is asked to open their mouth, and an observation of the uvula, soft palate, and palatal pillars is made to determine a classification according to the Mallampati score. If it is a type 1

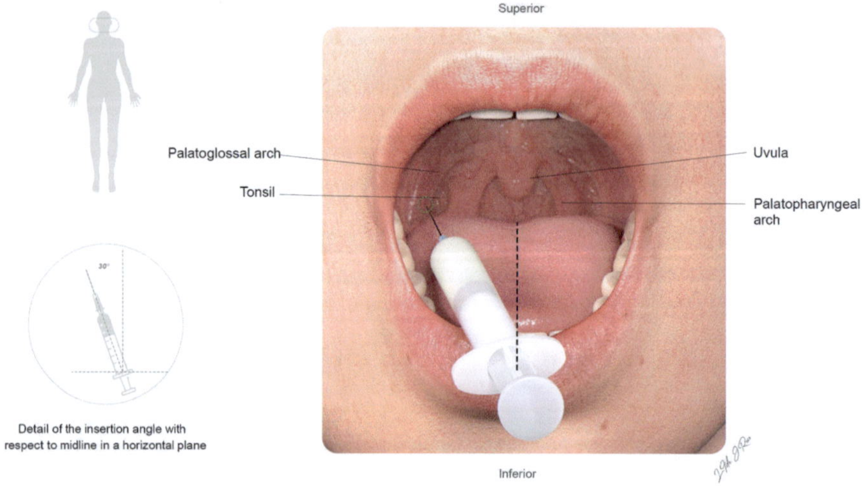

Fig. 31.6 A patient's oral cavity and anatomical repairs are shown. The needle is oriented at 30° from the midline, and its entry point at the lower pole of the anterior palatal pillar is shown. (Source: Authors. Illustrations by Luis F. Jaimes)

or 2, the technique can be performed in a supine position. If it is a type 3 or 4, it is advisable to perform the technique sitting down and preferably with a headrest. To perform the technique, one must be able to visualize the lower pole of the palatoglossal arc, which will be the point of insertion of the needle. To do this, use a tongue depressor.

(d) *Technique*: As can be seen in Fig. 31.6, the needle must be inserted oriented 30° to the side with respect to the midline of the body. Through the lower pole of the palatoglossal arc, make the direct insertion (without prior papule) of the needle about 2 cm deep in the direction indicated, applying the procaine in the vicinity of the carotid sheath. It may be advisable to perform aspiration to verify that the application is not intravascular. However, the small amount of procaine application, the concentration used, and the suggested gauge of the needle, make this application a safe technique. It is important to understand that the mechanism by which vagus nerve stimulation is achieved is thanks to a principle of diffusion through the cervical fascia.

5.3 Indications and Precautions

(a) *Indications*

(i) *Segmental treatment:* This technique can be used as a segmental treatment, in the case that several superficial interventions have already been attempted in the segment with partial or transient improvement. The pathologies for which it could be indicated are based on its primary connections and anastomoses described above, such as dystrophies of the tongue, larynx, pharynx, respiratory system, heart and some large vessels, gastrointestinal system including the portal vein, and kidney through the vagossympathetic reflex of the spleen.

(ii) *Treatment in case of pathological dominance*: Likewise, it can be indicated when a pathological dominance is suspected, the effects of which can be evidenced by affecting other organs and systems at a distance.

(iii) *Complementary treatment in inflammatory pathologies:* Based on Kevin Tracey's research, the modulating role of vagus nerve inflammation in different inflammatory pathologies has been evidenced. However, it is not recommended that the treatment of these pathologies be limited to the stimulation of the vagus nerve, but that it be carried out in addition to the treatment of the affected segment or the pathological dominances of this organism, according to its life history.

(b) *Precautions*:

This technique is generally safe to use. The authors have made an approximate number of 450 applications during 7 years of observation, with no mention of complication, even during bilateral applications carried out during the pandemic. However, it is preferable to make unilateral applications, since this would prevent more intense post-infiltration reactions.

(i) *Reduction of previous loads*: Preferably, only perform this technique once irritative loads have been reduced (see Chap. 25 on the therapeutic approach in Neuraltherapeutic medicine). Furthermore, one could perform this technique in combination with a treatment aimed at the foci of dominance or irritative foci active in the patient at the time of consultation. For instance, if an organism has had irritations in other areas (for example, the heart or lungs, a history of arrhythmias, coronary heart disease, colitis, diverticulosis, or surgeries), it is very important to address these sources of irritation as soon as possible, even before doing a stimulation of the vagus.

(ii) *Coagulation disorders*: Take due precautions in cases of coagulation disorders. If necessary, request a hematology concept. In case the patient is taking anticoagulants, evaluate the possibility that the patient discontinues, 3 days before the procedure, the use of them.

(iii) *Hypotension or bradycardia*: No "vasovagal" effects have been observed so far after the application of this technique, such as syncope, bradycardia or hypotension. However, be sure to take your blood pressure and heart rate before the procedure. Avoid performing this technique if you find hypotension or bradycardia.

5.4 Immediate Post-infiltration Reactions

Given that the site where the Neuraltherapeutic nerve is injected is an area through which the glossopharyngeal nerve also runs and the cervical sympathetic chain is also located a few centimeters behind the carotid sheath, it is possible to observe some of the following immediate reactions after performing this technique, but with a transitory nature (usually lasting 2–5 min).

- Difficulty swallowing (due to intervention on the glossopharyngeal nerve).
- Open rhinolalia (due to momentary hypomobility of the soft palate).
- Dysphonia (by the superior laryngeal branch).
- Cough (from stimulation of the vagus).
- Horner's syndrome (by the proximity of the cervical sympathetic chain, via cervical fascia).

Before performing the technique, make sure that you have explained to the patient the expected reactions, which can reduce the anxiety that some patients may have about the procedure.

Acknowledgements We would like to express our deepest gratitude to Professor Luis Enrique Caro Henao of the Department of Morphology at the National University of Colombia, who granted us access to the Anatomical Dissection Laboratory during the pandemic to test the vagus nerve access technique and also supported us in cadaver dissections.

References

1. Gray H. Anatomy of the human body. Plate 793. Philadelphia: Lea & Febiger; 1918. [Public Domain]. Available at: https://archive.org/details/anatomyofhumanbo1918gray/page/908/mode/2up
2. Henao J. Approach to the vagus nerve in Neuraltherapeutic medicine. Master thesis. Bogotá: Universidad Nacional de Colombia, Faculty of Medicine; 2021.
3. Yuan H, Silberstein SD. Vagus nerve and vagus nerve stimulation, a comprehensive review: part I. Headache. 2016;56(1):71–8. https://doi.org/10.1111/head.12647.
4. Tracey KJ. The inflammatory reflex. Nature. 2002;420(6917):853–9. https://doi.org/10.1038/nature01321.
5. Berthoud HR, Neuhuber WL. Functional and chemical anatomy of the afferent vagal system. Auton Neurosci. 2000;85(1–3):1–17. https://doi.org/10.1016/S1566-0702(00)00215-0. PMID: 11189015.
6. Tanaka S, Abe C, Abbott SBG, Zheng S, Yamaoka Y, Lipsey JE, Skrypnyk NI, Yao J, Inoue T, Nash WT, Stornetta DS, Rosin DL, Stornetta RL, Guyenet PG, Okusa MD. Vagus nerve stimulation activates two distinct neuroimmune circuits converging in the spleen to protect mice from kidney injury. Proc Natl Acad Sci USA. 2021;118(12):e2021758118. https://doi.org/10.1073/pnas.2021758118.
7. Latarjet M, Ruiz-Liard A. Human anatomy. 5th ed. Buenos Aires: Editorial Médica Panamericana, S.A.; 2019. 823 p.
8. Lanska DJ. J.L. Corning and vagal nerve stimulation for seizures in the 1880s. Neurology 2002;58(3):452–459. doi:https://doi.org/10.1212/wnl.58.3.452.

9. Vishnevsky A. Novocain blockade and oleo balsamic antiseptics as a pathogenic therapeutic method. Buenos Aires: Cartago; 1958.
10. Wang L, Wang Y, Wang Y, Wang F, Zhang J, Li S, et al. Transcutaneous auricular vagus nerve stimulators: a review of past, present, and future devices. Expert Rev Med Devices. 2022;19(1):43–61. https://doi.org/10.1080/17434440.2022.2020095.
11. Dosch P, Dosch M. Manual of neural therapy according to Huneke. 2nd ed. Stuttgart: Thieme; 2007.
12. Moore KL, Dalley AF, Agur AMR. Clinically oriented anatomy. 7th ed. Philadelphia: Wolters Kluwer; 2013. 988p.
13. Ünal M, Sezgin AB. Dura mater: anatomy and clinical implication. J Behav Brain Sci. 2021;11:239–47. https://doi.org/10.4236/jbbs.2021.1110019.

Chapter 32
New Technique for Accessing Gasser's Ganglion Through the Pterygopalatine Fossa

Laura Bibiana Pinilla Bonilla, Jazmín Ariza-Tarazona, and Luz Amparo Arias-López

1 Introduction

The purpose of this chapter is to introduce the reader to the new technique of access to Gasser's ganglion through the pterygopalatine fossa. To this end, a general review of the anatomy and route of the trigeminal nerve, the location of Gasser's ganglion, as well as its relationship with the pterygopalatine fossa, will be carried out. Similarly, some pathologies related to the trigeminal nerve for which this technique would be indicated will be reviewed.

It also includes a general review of the techniques described in the field of neural therapy and anesthesia for direct access to Gasser's ganglion, reviewing their limitations and scope. The description of Gasser's new approach technique will include the presentation of research carried out on cadavers in the dissection theater of the Faculty of Medicine of the National University of Colombia. At the end of the chapter, the reader will find a detailed description of the technique and its indications and precautions.

L. B. Pinilla Bonilla (✉)
Faculty of Medicine, Master in Alternative Medicine, Neural Therapy Area, Universidad Nacional de Colombia, Bogotá, Colombia

Integrated Health Services Subnetwork of the South, Research and Innovation Center, Bogotá, Colombia
e-mail: lbpinillab@unal.edu.co

J. Ariza-Tarazona
Master in Alternative Medicine, Neural Therapy Area, Faculty of Medicine, Universidad Nacional de Colombia, Bogotá, Colombia

L. A. Arias-López
Faculty of Medicine, Morphology Department, Master in Human Morphology, Universidad Nacional de Colombia, Bogotá, Colombia

L. B. Pinilla Bonilla et al. (eds.), *Neuraltherapeutic Medicine*,
https://doi.org/10.1007/978-3-032-03257-7_32

2 Anatomy of the Trigeminal Nerve, the Gasser Ganglion, and the Pterygopalatine Fossa

2.1 The Trigeminal Nerve

The trigeminal nerve is a cranial nerve that has a sensory portion that primarily innervates the face and an efferent portion that innervates the chewing muscles. The trigeminal motor pathway originates in the cerebral motor cortex by synapsing in the trigeminal motor nucleus of the pons; from there, the second neuron synapses directly into the chewing muscles. While the bodies of sensory neurons are located in the trigeminal ganglion [1].

The Gasser's ganglion, or trigeminal ganglion, which is the largest of the ganglia of the cranial nerves, is a crescent-like structure located in the cavity of Meckel in the middle cranial fossa at the petrous vertex of the temporal bone, near the carotid canal, in a dural recess (where the meningeal and the periosteal layers of dura mater fold) [2]. This contains the neural bodies of the 3 main branches that will then be distributed in the ophthalmic nerve (V1), maxillary nerve (V2), and mandibular nerve (V3). These branches pass from the skull to the face through three different holes: V1 passes through the sphenoid cleft, V2 passes through the foramen rotundum, and V3 passes through the foramen ovale (see Fig. 32.1) [1].

The trigeminal nerve has nerve ganglia associated with each of its sensory branches: The ophthalmic nerve is related to the ciliary ganglion, the maxillary nerve is related to the pterygopalatine ganglion, and the mandibular nerve is related to the otic ganglion [1]. Each of its roots innervates different structures, among others [4]:

- Ophthalmic (V1): forehead, nose, eyelid, pupil, sclera, ethmoid, lacrimal, tentorium and sickle sensitivity of the brain, and anastomosis with occipital nerve.
- Maxilla (V2): eyelid, nose, cheeks, superior alveolar roots, nasal cavity, maxillary sinus, connection with facial and pterygopalatine ganglion, connection with internal carotid plexus, dura innervation.
- Mandibular (V3): buccal, facial nerve connection, lingual nerve, anastomosis of the atriculotemporal root with branches of the facial nerve and otic ganglion, helix and tragus skin, external otic meatus, branches to TMJ, parotid, dental, duramater innervation.

Among the main functions of the trigeminal nerve, widely recognized, among the most important are [4]:

(a) Sensitive information about the face and scalp.
(b) It innervates mastication muscles and the tensor tympani.
(c) Innervates the temporal muscle.
(d) Proprioceptive information of the teeth.
(e) Multiple connections and reflexes.

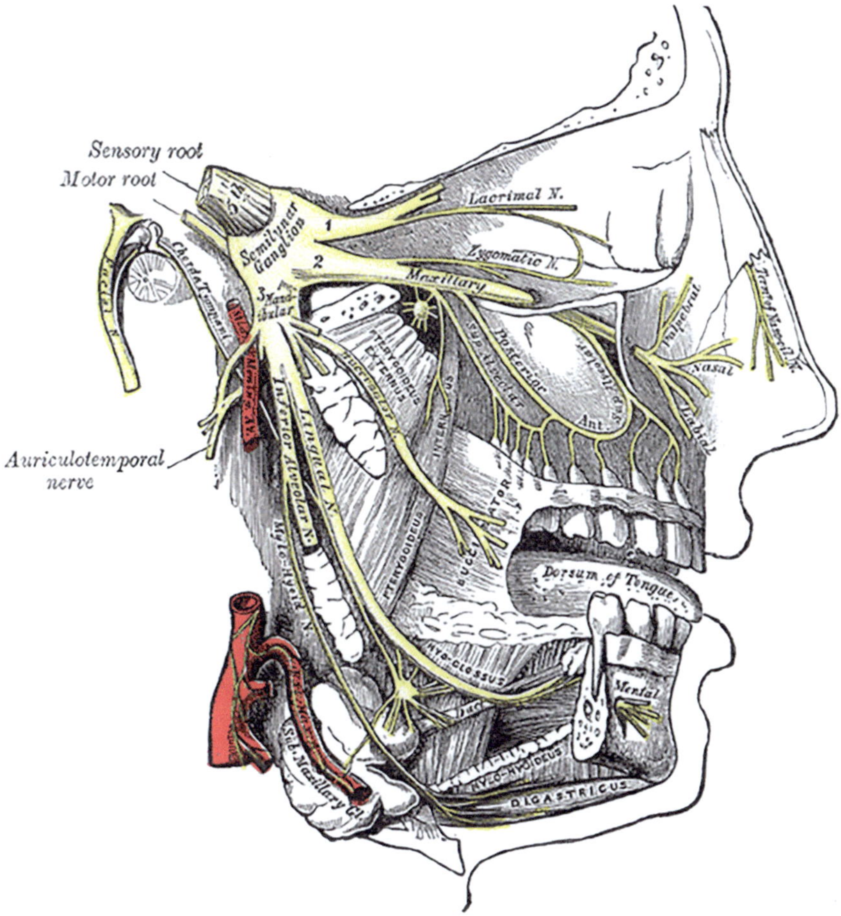

Fig. 32.1 A diagram of the crescent-like ganglion of Gasser and its distribution in the 3 branches is shown. (Take from Gray [3])

Within this last point "e", it is important to mention the participation of the trigeminal nerve in the cornea, blinking, tearing, mandibular, and trigeminal-cardiac reflexes [4]. However, of greater interest to mention are the multiple connections and anastomoses that the trigeminal nerve presents, some of them peripheral and others central.

Among the peripheral connections of interest is its anastomosis with the facial nerve, or VII cranial nerve. In a review of the literature conducted by Hwang et al., it was found that the trigeminal nerve has a wide communication with the facial nerve. Analyzing the scientific literature that refers to cadaver dissection, it was found that the maxillary ramus has the highest frequency of communication with the facial nerve of 95%, the mandibular ramus of 76.7%, and the ophthalmic branch with the lowest frequency of communication of 33.8% [5]. This connection has been clinically evidenced, especially in cases of facial paralysis that have occurred after dental procedures, direct trigeminal lesions, dental lesions, and bone infections [6].

Within the framework of the central connections, many are of interest; however, some of them stand out, such as [4]:

- Connections with the nucleus of the solitary tract that is related to information from the cardiovascular, respiratory, and intestinal systems.
- With cranial nerves IX and X, whose neural projections synapse in the nucleus of the trigeminal spinal tract.
- Third-order connections, which are projections towards the somatosensory cortex, cerebellum, reticular formation, and cingulate cortex, among others.

The trigeminal nerve also forms the trigeminal-cervical complex, which runs from the caudal nucleus of the trigeminal to the C2-C3 segments, also called the paratrigeminal nucleus. This complex has made it possible to understand the very frequent clinical findings of patients with pathologies of the craniofacial organs and structures that present with pain in the structures innervated by the cervical nerve roots [7, 8]. Likewise, it has been experimentally verified that motor neurons can even be activated in the neck thanks to the stimulation of the V pair in humans and animals [9, 10].

2.2 *Pterygopalatine Fossa*

This fossa borders anteriorly with the posterior aspect of the maxillary bone, posteriorly with the pterygoid process of the sphenoid bone, medially with the vertical lamina of the palatine bone, superiorly with the greater wing of the sphenoid bone, and inferiorly with the pyramidal process of the palatine bone. This fossa maintains important anatomical communications, namely, the middle cranial fossa through the foramen rotundum, the orbital cavity through the inferior orbital fissure, the nasal cavity through the sphenopalatine foramen, and the infratemporal fossa through the pterygomaxillary fissure. This fossa contains several anatomical structures such as the maxillary nerve, the pterygopalatine ganglion, the pterygoid duct nerve, and the third portion of the internal maxillary artery [1] [2].

Because it is a place of communication with the middle cranial fossa through the foramen rotundum, through which the V2 root emerges, and because it also contains the pterygopalatine ganglion, this fossa is of special interest when it is desired to therapeutically address the Gasser's ganglion directly (see Fig. 32.2).

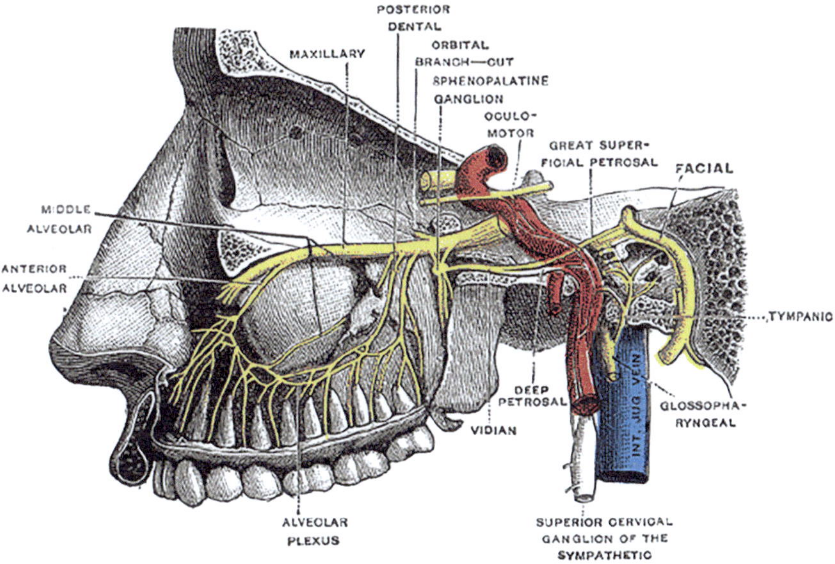

Fig. 32.2 The pterygopalatine fossa is shown containing the pterygopalatine ganglion and the maxillary root or V2. (Taken from Gray [11])

3 Pathologies Related to the Trigeminal Nerve

Among the most common pathologies related to the trigeminal are clearly trigeminal neuralgia and migraine [1]. However, within the framework of the new conceptions of synthetic physiology (See Chap. 13), it is considered that one of the functions of the nervous system that is ubiquitous is the trophic function according to Speransky [12]. From this new framework, taking into account the peripheral and central connections previously described, especially the anastomosis with the facial nerve, among the pathological alterations in the area of the face that can be secondary to a trigeminal dystrophy, are the following, many of them described by Speransky:

(a) Inflammatory disorders of the eye: xerophthalmia, keratitis, conjunctivitis, styes, among others.
(b) Inflammatory disorders of the middle ear: Otitis media, tinnitus.
(c) Inflammatory disorders of the nose: rhinitis and epistaxis.
(d) Sinus disorders: acute and chronic sinusitis.
(e) Disorders of the oral cavity: xerostomia, gingivitis or stomatitis, caries, pulp necrosis, periodontitis, periapical abscesses.
(f) Skin disorders: keratosis, acne, and pigmentation changes.

Taking into account the embryological (see Chap. 14) and central connection with the cervical plexus (trigeminal-cervical complex) mentioned above, the following pathological manifestations can be found:

(a) Neck pain and muscle contractures.
(b) Musculoskeletal alterations in the joints of the upper limbs, including alterations of the rotator cuff muscles.
(c) Vascular alterations such as sympathetic dystrophy.
(d) Alterations of the organs of the neck: larynx, thyroid, parathyroid.

4 Techniques Described

In the field of neural therapy, the approach to the mandibular nerve or the otic ganglion has been described as the one that reaches the vicinity of the Gasser's ganglion. The patient should be seated with the head resting or lying on a table. The needle should be inserted about 30 mm in front of the tragus, in the mandibular notch that forms under the zygomatic arch while the patient's mouth is open. For this technique, a 6 cm by 0.6 mm diameter needle is used, applying about 2–3 mL of procaine. The needle is guided transversely to the opposite side and inserted at a depth of 4 cm until it reaches the pterygoid process. The needle is then removed slightly and carefully brought to the dorsal direction about 5–10 mm until it is about 5 cm deep. Once the place near the foramen ovale has been reached, the patient may report paresthesia. There, it must be aspirated to make sure it has not entered a blood vessel, and then procaine is injected [13, 14]. Among the disadvantages of this technique are the pain generated by the injection due to the diameter of the needle, as well as the possibility of generating a hematoma due to injury to the internal maxillary artery or its branches in the infratemporal fossa.

In the context of anesthesiology, there is another procedure described for access or block of the Gasser's ganglion or trigeminal ganglion. It is usually a procedure that requires a peripheral IV line, sedation, and basic monitoring with electrocardiogram, blood pressure, and pulse oximetry. The patient is placed supine in a position where the head is at maximum extension in order to facilitate vision through the fluoroscope. In this technique, the skin and subcutaneous tissues are anesthetized with 1% lidocaine using a 27 g needle, entering approximately 2.5 cm laterally and 1 cm below the angle of the ipsilateral mouth, directing the needle towards the foramen ovale. A 10 cm needle with fluoroscopy guidance is then advanced until the foramen is reached [15]. Among the disadvantages of this technique, the discomfort that patients may experience is described, along with the injury to the accessory meningeal artery or the dura mater of the floor of the middle cranial fossa.

5 New Technique for Approaching Gasser's Ganglion by Pterygopalatine Fossa

5.1 Research on Cadavers

The technique proposed in this chapter arose from the observation and research question posed by Pinilla L: Is it possible that when infiltrating directly into the pterygopalatine fossa, procaine diffuses through the foramen rotundum towards Gasser's ganglion?

An experimental design was proposed in cadavers, for which it was accompanied by professors Ariza and Arias, and the support of the Department of Morphology of the National University of Colombia.

The different techniques described in the field of neural therapy for pterygopalatine ganglion intervention were evaluated, since these techniques are supposed to enter the fossa. For this access, extraoral and intraoral techniques have been described:

(a) *Extraoral access:* Within extraoral access to the fossa, entry above the zygomatic arch has been described at the midpoint between the external canthus of the eye and the ear [13]. This technique has the disadvantage of being more painful and having the risk of hematoma when punctured due to injury to the internal maxillary artery or its branches in the infratemporal fossa. On the other hand, based on the observation of different skulls, it is observed that when entering extraorally, there would be no guarantee that it would effectively enter through the pterygopalatine fossa, since, in some patients, the size of this fossa may be smaller, making it more likely to knock against the pterygoid process and not enter the fossa.

(b) Intraoral access: it is entered through the greater palatal foramen. This technique could be considered very accurate, since, if the needle enters the palatine canal, it means entering the pterygopalatine fossa [13]. However, apart from being a painful intervention, the authors have observed the presence of hematomas on the palate due to the puncture of the vein or palatine artery. Also, anatomical variations can make it difficult to enter the canal due to narrowness and, in very rare cases, absence of it.

Therefore, the possibility of a different intraoral admission was raised, based on the study of the anatomy, after the last molar directed towards the pterygopalatine fossa, at the end of the palatine bone.[1] For this access to be facilitated in real life, it is necessary to make a bend in the needle of about 45 degrees with respect to a perpendicular midline that passes through the axis of the syringe (see Fig. 32.3a, b).

[1] In patients who have their denture complete up to the wisdom tooth, the posterior edge of the palatal bone is about 1–2 mm behind this tooth. However, in edentulous patients it can also be easily identified by palpating the end of the hard palate and drawing an imaginary line that passes through this posterior edge and projects laterally until it reaches the vestibule.

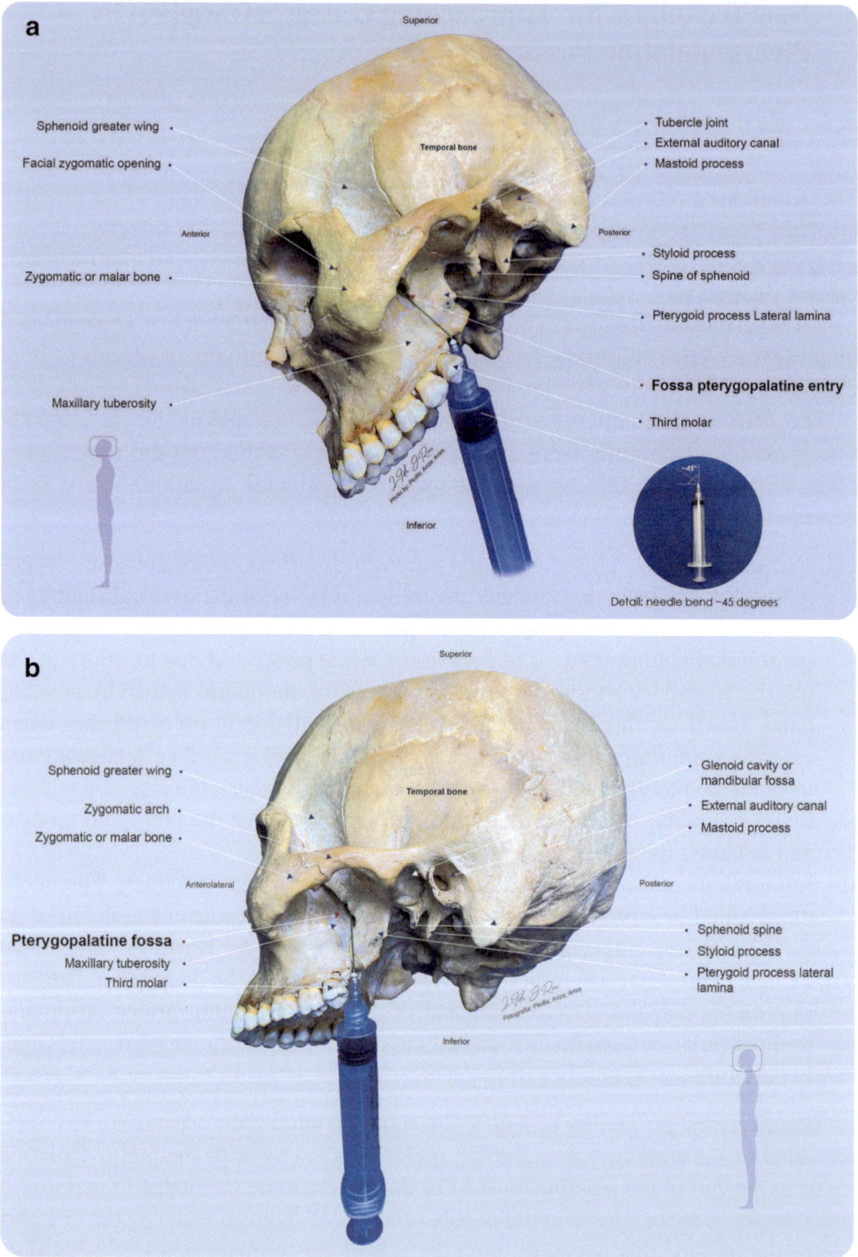

Fig. 32.3 (**a**) Insertion of the needle into the pterygopalatine fossa, lateral view. (**b**) Insertion of the needle into the pterygopalatine fossa, posterolateral view. (Source: Photograph taken by the authors, edited by Luis F. Jaimes, with the support of the Department of Morphology of the National University of Colombia)

When exploring this form of entry into the pterygopalatine fossa in complete skulls, with a 1 1/2 inch needle of 27 G, it could be observed that the needle not only entered completely into the pterygopalatine fossa, but even reached the vicinity of the posterior floor of the orbit, very close to the ciliary ganglion (see Fig. 32.4a, b).

After defining the entry site and the angulation of the needle, a methylene blue test was performed. Thus, a needle was inserted into the corpse with this angulation and posterior to the palatal bone (see Fig. 32.5). To show whether methylene blue could stain the Gasser's ganglion, this test was performed on a cadaver whose brain had been removed, preserving the dura mater so that the middle cranial fossa could be observed. The test was performed on two cadavers, finding a positive test in both, i.e., Gasser's ganglion was indeed stained with methylene blue (Fig. 32.6).

5.2 *Description of the Technique*

(a) *Materials*: 5 cc syringe (for bilateral applications) or 3 cc syringe for unilateral application. 27G × 1.5 inch needle.
(b) *Application of procaine.*
   (i) Unilateral application: 2–2.5 cc of 1% procaine.
   (ii) *Bilateral application*: 1–2 cc of 0.5% procaine on each side.[2]
(c) *Patient position and anatomical repairs*: With the patient in the supine position, anatomical repairs are previously identified to identify the site of needle entry into the pterygopalatine fossa. Clearly identify the end or back edge of the hard palate and draw an imaginary horizontal line over this edge that extends laterally until reaching the vestibule. On this imaginary line at the level of the vestibule is the end of the palatine bone posterior to the third molar. On this point of the mucosa, on the vestibular side, the needle is inserted.
(d) *Technique*: The first step is establishing an angulation of the needle from the base of 45 degrees, always leaving the bevel in the direction of the acute angle (see Fig. 32.3). In other words, when the needle is inserted, the bevel should point toward the patient's midline or nose. During insertion, the needle must move cranially and medially to enter the pterygopalatine fossa. The needle should enter completely as shown in Fig. 32.3 and no resistance should be perceived. Should it encounter resistance, it may be knocking against the palatine rather than entering it. In this case, change the needle, reperform the anatomical repairs, and insert the needle again. Given the low amount and concentration of procaine for this technique, it is not necessary to perform aspiration; however,

[2] The reason why a lower concentration and quantity are injected in the bilateral application is a recommendation of the authors. In sensitive people, it is possible that the sensation of total anesthesia of the face may be uncomfortable or generate anxiety. Additionally, the tone of the chewing muscles can be lost, generating difficulty speaking for a few minutes. It has been observed that this reaction can be avoided with lower concentration and less quantity.

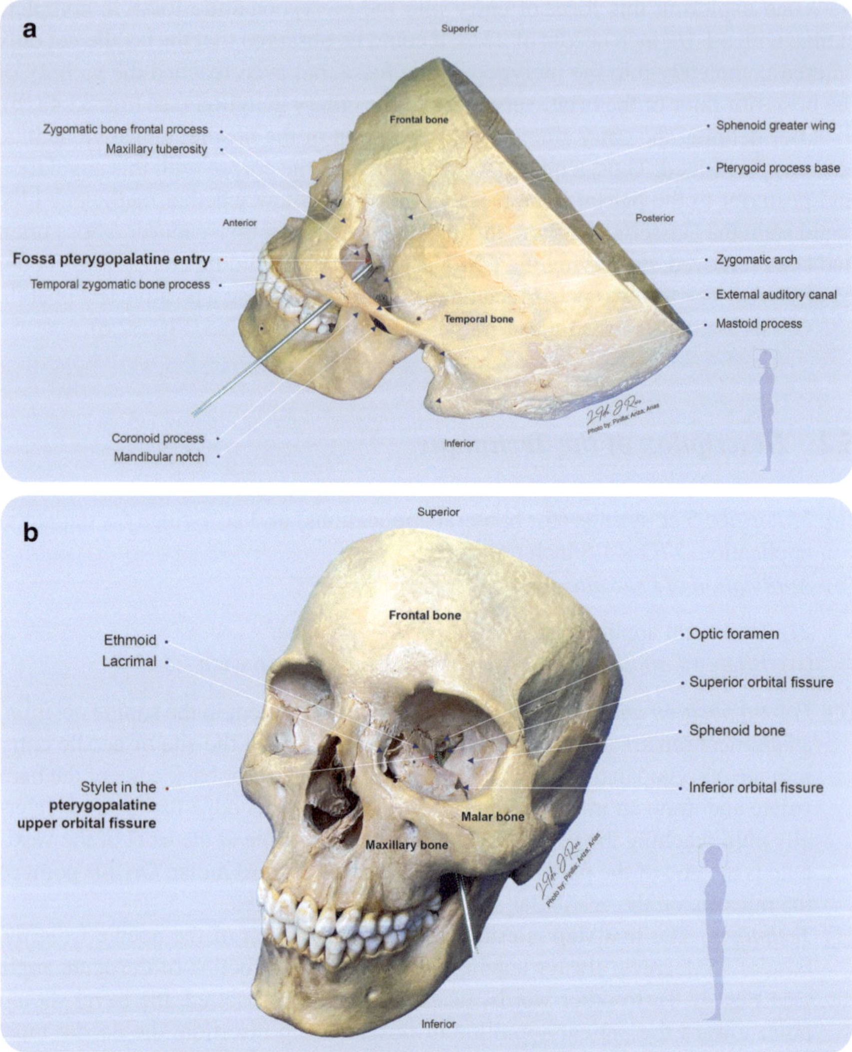

Fig. 32.4 (**a**) A metal stylet is inserted into the pterygopalatine fossa through the anatomical repair site under study. Lateral view. (**b**) Anterolateral view of the metal stylet inserted into the pterygopalatine fossa, finding that, upon entering approximately 3.5 cm deep, the anatomical proximity of the ciliary ganglion on the floor of the orbit is reached. (Source: Photograph taken by the authors, edited by Luis F. Jaimes, with the support of the Department of Morphology of the National University of Colombia)

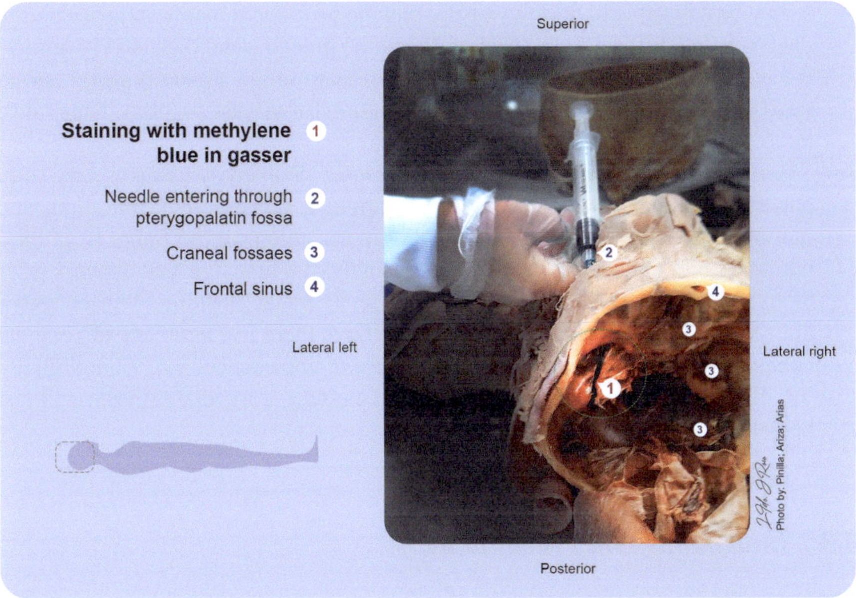

Fig. 32.5 A test was done in the dissection theater with the insertion of the needle angled at 45 degrees toward the posterior edge of the palatal bone, injecting methylene blue approximately 1 cc. superior view. (Source: Photograph taken by the authors, edited by Luis F Jaimes, with the support of the Department of Morphology of the National University of Colombia)

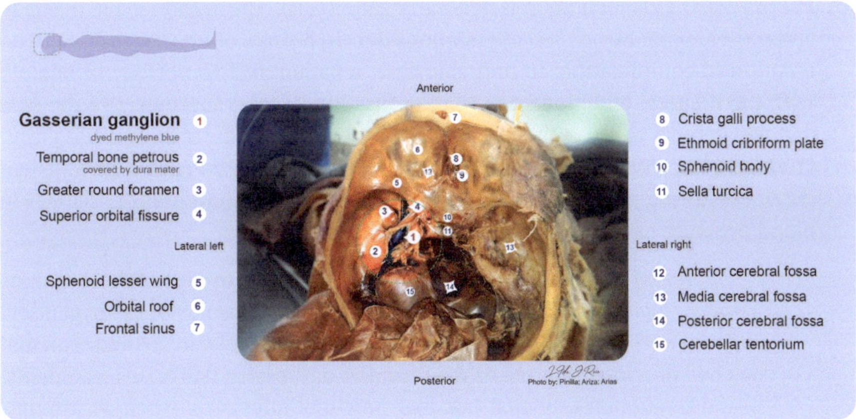

Fig. 32.6 An image showing the middle cranial fossa, where the coloration of the Gasser's ganglion with methylene blue is shown on the left side. (Source: Photograph taken by the authors, edited by Luis F Jaimes, with the support of the Department of Morphology of the National University of Colombia)

it may be advisable to do so to ensure that the procaine remains extravascular in the fossa and diffuses to the Gasser. Inject the procaine and then slowly remove the needle. At the end, ask the patient to remain in the supine position and to raise the chin slightly, maintaining this position for at least 2–3 min. Then move on to sensitivity assessment.

(e) *Sensitivity assessment for verification purposes*: Sensitivity changes vary from patient to patient based on the amount applied, procaine concentration, and individual sensitivity threshold. Changes in sensation can be found from mild paresthesia to almost total anesthesia. Usually, the first sign that appears prior to hypoesthesia/anesthesia is the presence of malar flushing. Subsequently, after the sensitivity test on the skin of the face, there is a tendency to generate changes in sensitivity in the following order of appearance: V2, V3 and finally V1. If the anesthetic used was procaine, the effect of hypo/anesthesia will last between 5 and 10 min.

5.3 *Indications and Precautions*

(a) *Indications*: This technique can be used as a segmental treatment, in case several superficial interventions have already been attempted in the segment with partial or transient improvement. The pathologies for which this technique could be indicated are mentioned in the third section of this chapter. Likewise, it can be indicated when a pathological dominance is suspected, but with the precautions indicated below.

(b) *Precautions*: This technique is generally safe to use. The authors have made an approximate number of 500 applications during 8 years of observation, with no mention of complication. In only one case, a patient had an episode of anxiety with the bilateral technique due to the sensation of total anesthesia of the face and the inability to move the jaw due to the relaxation of the masseter and pterygoid muscles, which lasted about 10 min. Other mild reactions include transient dizziness lasting no more than 5 min. No heart rhythm alterations or changes in blood pressure have been detected so far in any patient.

   (i) *Reduction of previous loads*: Preferably, only perform this technique once irritative loads have decreased in the superficial branches of the trigeminal or facial nerve (due to their anastomosis). For example, in an organism that has had previous injuries to the face and oral cavity (surgeries, accidents, dental treatments), or that has had previous infections (such as mumps, conjunctivitis, styes, sinusitis, periapical abscesses, among others), it is important to perform the respective interventions. In the oral cavity, these may include infiltration of dental foci such as implant sites, root canals, extractions, or other periapical or periodontal inflammations. In other contexts, infiltration of the supraorbital nerve, infraorbital nerve, mental nerve, ciliary ganglion, atriculotemporal nerve, nasopalatine nerve, maxillary nerve, lower dentary, among others, may be required.

(ii) *Coagulation disorders*: take appropriate precautions in cases of bleeding disorders. If necessary, request a hematology consult. In case the patient is taking anticoagulants, evaluate the possibility that the patient suspends, 3 days before the procedure, the use of them.
(iii) *Trismus*: In case of trismus secondary to severe trigeminal neuralgia or some other similar disorder, it is usually beneficial to first perform a bilateral infiltration of the masseterine nerve that crosses the mandibular notch and provides the motor innervation to obtain a relaxation of the same muscle. In this way, the patient will be able to perform the oral opening and will facilitate the performance of this technique.

References

1. Martínez-Lozano A. Anatomical review and introduction of concepts in pterygopalatine fossa techniques in neuraltherapeutic medicine, for the management of related pathologies. Master's thesis. Bogotá: Universidad Nacional de Colombia; 2022. p. 52. Available at: https://repositorio.unal.edu.co/handle/unal/82028
2. Yu M, Jozsa F, Donohoe C. Neuroanatomy, Lunate Ganglion. [Updated 2023 Mar 20]. In: StatPearls [Internet]. Treasure Island (FL): StatPearls Publishing; 2025. Available from: https://www.ncbi.nlm.nih.gov/books/NBK556085/
3. Gray H. Anatomy of the Human Body. Plate 778. Philadelphia: Lea & Febiger; 1918, p. 890. [Public Domain]. Available at: https://archive.org/details/anatomyofhumanbo1918gray/page/890/mode/2up
4. López G, Salazar JI, Osuna E. Anatomical, physiological, and embryological description of the trigeminal nerve in the conceptual framework of neural therapy as a frequent interfering field substrate. NOVA Magazine. 2012;10:83–100. [Spanish]. Available at: https://revistas.unicolmayor.edu.co/index.php/nova/article/view/194
5. Hwang K, Yang SC, Song JS. Communications between the trigeminal nerve and the facial nerve in the face: a systematic review. J Craniofac Surg. 2015;26(5):1643–6. https://doi.org/10.1097/SCS.0000000000001810.
6. Kawano-Hokama M, Shiratori-Tusita LN, Pinilla-Bonilla LB, Cruz-Rodríguez Y. The potential role of trigeminal nerve irritation in the pathophysiology of bell's palsy. A case report from a neural therapy perspective. Case Rep. 2022;8(2):1. https://doi.org/10.15446/cr.v8n2.93840.
7. Bartsch T, Goadsby PJ. The trigeminocervical complex and migraine: current concepts and synthesis. Curr Sci Inc. 2003;7:371–6. https://doi.org/10.1007/s11916-003-0036-y.
8. Shiratori Tusita LN, Fischer L. Chronic therapy-resistant neck pain in a fifty-year-old man: the role of partially impacted third molars – case report and new pathophysiological insights. Complement Med Res. 2023;30(3):270–4. https://doi.org/10.1159/000529293.
9. Leandri M, Gottlieb A, Cruccu G. Head extensor reflex evoked by trigeminal stimulation in humans. Clin Neurophysiol. 2001;112(10):1828–32. https://doi.org/10.1016/s1388-2457(01)00648-4.
10. Zeredo JL, Toda K, Soma K. Nature of neck motor unit activities evoked by different trigeminal inputs in rats. J Dent Res. 2003;82(5):402–5. https://doi.org/10.1177/154405910308200515.
11. Gray H. Anatomy of the Human Body. Plate 779. Philadelphia: Lea & Febiger; 1918, p. 891. [Public Domain]. Available at: https://archive.org/details/anatomyofhumanbo1918gray/page/890/mode/2up
12. Speransky AD. A basis for the theory of medicine. New York: International Publishers; 1943.
13. Dosch M. Atlas of neural therapy: with local anesthetics. 3rd ed. Stuttgart: Thieme; 2012. p. 224.

14. Fisher L. In: Niño Ibarra MC, editor. Neural therapy according to Huneke; neurophysiology, therapeutic injection techniques, vol. 1. 3rd ed. Mexico: unknown editorial; 2012. p. 1–261.
15. Chaturvedi A, Dorado F, Shanthanna H, et al. How I do it: gasserian ganglion block for trigeminal neuralgia. ASRA Pain Medicine News. 2023;48 https://doi.org/10.52211/asra050123.011.

Chapter 33
Facial Nerve Technique

Luis Fernando Córdoba-Llanos, Edna Cecilia Garzón-Fuentes, and Francisco Echandía-Bocanegra

1 Introduction

The facial nerve is the seventh cranial nerve, and for its study, it is usually divided into four segments as follows [1]:

- The core and tracts.
- The cisternal segment that runs through the internal ear canal.
- The intratemporal segment that passes through the bony canal of the facial nerve.
- The peripheral segment that begins at the stylomastoid foramen.

Other authors classify the intracranial segment into five sections: cisternal, canalicular, labyrinthine, tympanic, and mastoid [2].

The facial nerve is associated with four brainstem nuclei: the facial motor nucleus, the superior salivatory nucleus, the spinal nucleus of the trigeminal nerve, and the nucleus of the solitary tract. This nerve carries branchial motor (special visceral efferent), visceral motor (parasympathetic), special sensory (taste), and

Luis Fernando Córdoba-Llanos died before publication of this work was completed.

L. F. Córdoba-Llanos (Deceased)
Faculty of Medicine, Universidad del Cauca, Popayán, Colombia

E. C. Garzón-Fuentes (✉) · F. Echandía-Bocanegra
Master in Alternative Medicine, Neural therapy Area, Faculty of Medicine, Universidad Nacional de Colombia, Bogotá, Colombia
e-mail: ecgarzonf@unal.edu.co; fechandia@unal.edu.co

L. B. Pinilla Bonilla et al. (eds.), *Neuraltherapeutic Medicine*,
https://doi.org/10.1007/978-3-032-03257-7_33

general sensory fibers. It plays a central role in both voluntary and emotional facial expression: voluntary facial movements are mediated peripherally through the facial nerve, which serves as the final common pathway for cortical motor commands to the muscles of facial expression [1]. Motor neurons that go to the upper part of the face are partially decussated, while those on the lower face do so completely.

The branchial motor function includes the innervation of the posterior belly of the digastric, the stylohyoid, and the stapedius muscle of the stapes, which participates in the motor reflexes of the middle ear. The facial nerve carries special sensory (gustatory) fibers that convey taste sensation from the anterior two-thirds of the tongue to the nucleus of the solitary tract, and general afferent fibers that transmit cutaneus sensation from the posterior region of the auricule to the spinal nucleus of the trigeminal nerve.

The visceral motor (parasympathetic) function of the facial nerve arises from the superior salivatory nucleus and provides secretomotor control to the lacrimal, nasal, and palatine glands via the greater petrosal nerve (through the pterygopalatine ganglion), as well as to the sublingual and submandibular glands via the chorda tympani nerve. The greater petrosal nerve joins sympathetic fibers from the carotid plexus—carried by the deep petrosal nerve—to form the nerve of the pterygoid canal (Vidian nerve).

The facial nerve emerges from the pontomedullary sulcus, near the cerebellopontine angle, and courses together with the eighth cranial nerve (vestibulocochlear) within a common sheath in its cisternal segment before entering the internal acoustic meatus. It then proceeds through the bony facial canal (Fallopian canal), reaching its intratemporal portion, which is divided into three segments: labyrinthine, tympanic, and mastoid. Before exiting through the stylomastoid foramen, the nerve passes through the geniculate ganglion, where it joins the intermediate nerve of Wrisberg, which carries special sensory (taste) afferent fibers and preganglionic secretomotor fibers destined for the lacrimal gland. From this point, it continues as the greater superficial petrosal nerve, which conveys secretomotor fibers to the lacrimal and nasal glands [1].

In the longest intratemporal, segment—the mastoid portion—two important branches arise: the nerve to the stapedius muscle, and the chorda tympani nerve which exits the temporal bone through the petrotympanic fissure to join the lingual nerve. Along this pathway, its carries special sensory (taste) afferent fibers from the anterior two-thirds of the tongue, as well parasympathetic efferent fibers to the submandibular ganglion.

After leaving the skull through the styloimastoid foramen, the facial nerve runs anteriorly between the styloid process and the posterior belly of the digastric muscle, passing behind the stylohyoid muscle, until it reaches the parotid gland (Figs. 33.1 and 33.2).

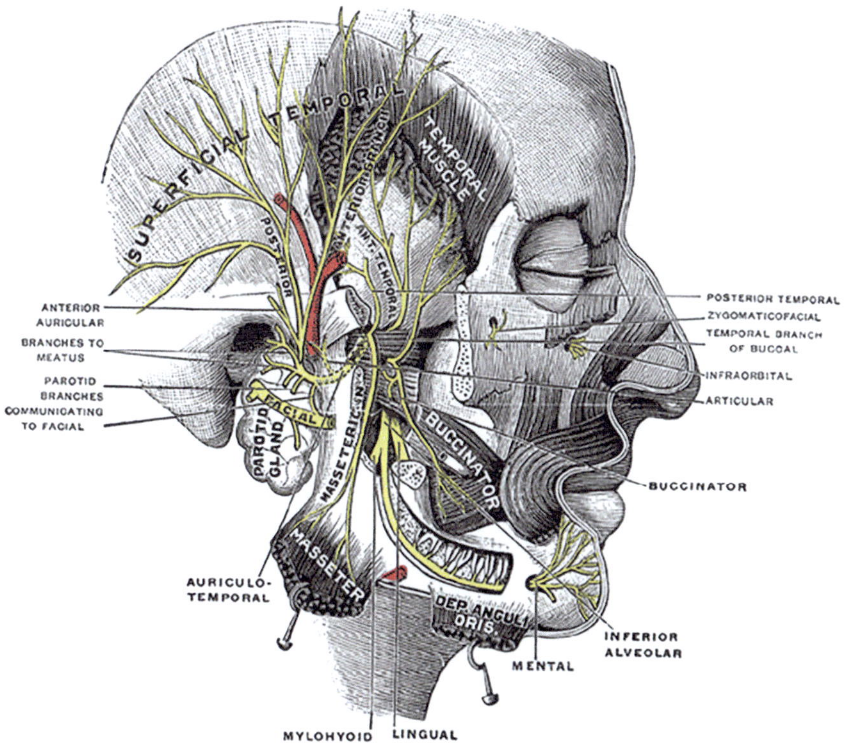

Fig. 33.1 Diagram of the peripheral section of the facial nerve. (*Source*: Taken from [3])

Before entering the gland, it gives off three branches: the posterior auricular branch (supplying the occipital and posterior auricular muscles), the branch to the posterior belly of the digastric muscle, and the branch to the stylohyoid muscle. Within the parotid gland, the facial nerve divides into two main trunks—the temporofacial (upper) and cervicofacial (lower)—which further branch into five terminal divisions: temporal, zygomatic, buccal, marginal mandibular, and cervical, forming the parotid plexus. This plexus fans out over the masseter muscle and communicates with branches of the trigeminal nerve, mainly the auriculotemporal and buccal nerves. Along this course, the facial nerve maintains a close relationship with the retromandibular vein and the external carotid artery (and its maxillary and superficial temporal branches), which is clinically significant for its identification during surgical and therapeutic procedures and interventions.

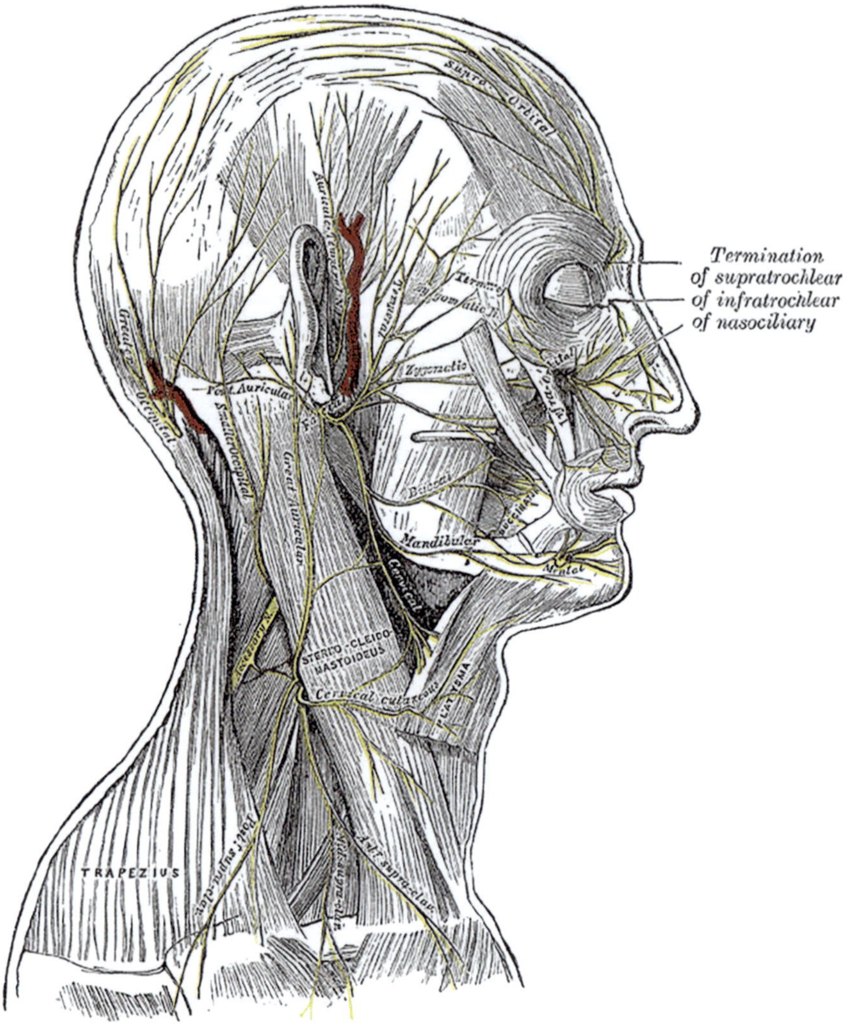

Fig. 33.2 Peripheral section of the facial nerve. (*Source*: Taken from [4])

2 Anatomical and Functional Relationships

Whit technological advances in morphological studies and in paraclinical imaging such as CT and MRI [2], knowledge of functional anatomy of the cranial nerves has been greatly enriched. These advances have revealed numerous anastomotic connections between pairs of cranial nerves, related both to topographical proximity and to functional interactions, and have highlighted the considerable anatomical variability among individuals. In particular, the facial nerve has been shown to establish connections with the trigeminal nerve, including branches of the auriculotemporal, buccal, mental, lingual, infraorbital, zygomatic, and ophthalmic nerves. Additionally, it forms connections with branches of the vestibulocochlear, glossopharyngeal and vagus nerve, as well as with branches of the cervical plexus, such as the great auricular nerve (C2–C3), the greater and lesser occipital nerves (C2), and the transverse cervical nerve (C2–C3) [5–11].

3 Clinical Conditions Related to the Facial Nerve

A wide range of signs and symptoms may lead clinicians to consider its involvement for therapeutic intervention, always taking into account that each decision must be framed within the patient's own life history (see Chaps. 18, 20, and 24).

Among the symptoms involving the facial nerve are the following: impairment of the muscles of facial expression (eye closure, smiling, frowning, puckering of the lips, etc.); loss of taste perception in the anterior two-thirds of the tongue; altered sensation in the retroauricular region and external auditory canal; superficial sensory disturbances of the auricle and mastoid region; dysfunction of the lacrimal, submandibular, and sublingual glands; symptoms of auditory hypersensitivity related to the stapedial reflex; and altered secretory function of the mucosa of the nasal cavity, hard and soft palate, and peri-uvular region.

As discussed throughout this book, biomedical diagnoses do not, in themselves, determine treatment in Neuraltherapeutic Medicine (Chaps. 18, 20, and 24). Nevertheless, recognizing the pathologies that may affect each segment of the facial nerve can help guide clinical and therapeutic decision-making [1]. The facial nerve can be affected at different levels:

- *Supranuclear lesions:* involving the motor cortex (precentral and postcentral gyri), including ischemic or neoplastic lesions of the central nervous system.
- *Nucleus and fascicular lesions:* Affecting the facial nucleus or its tracts, including pathologies of the cerebellopontine angle and the internal auditory canal.
- *Intratemporal segment:* tumors of the internal auditory canal, schwannomas, or other lesions.
- *Peripheral segment* including congenital conditios such as Eagle's syndrome (elongated styloid process) [12].
- *Inflammatory diseases:* acute or subacute viral Bell's palsy and inflammatory diseases of the perigeniculate area. Herpes zoster otic syndrome, or Ramsay-Hunt syndrome. Basilar meningitis, such as tuberculosis or sarcoidosis. Inflammatory or infectious disease of the middle ear, petrosal apex, or skull base may also involve the nerve
- *Vascular conditions:* hemifacial spasm due to compression at the root entry zone or cisternal segment by vascular malformations, hemangiomas, or aneurysms in the distal vertebral, basilar, or smaller posterior circulation arteries, such as the anteroinferior cerebellar artery (AICA) or the posteroinferior cerebellar artery (PICA).

- *Neoplastic conditions*: primary facial nerve schwannoma, facial nerve hemangioma, and head or neck tumors involving the petrous or parotid region, such as adenoid cystic carcinoma.
- *Traumatic lesions:* craniofacial trauma, particularly fractures of the temporal bone, or petrosal apex, due to the vulnerability of the perigeniculate and labyrinthine regions.

4 Described Techniques for Accessing the Facial Nerve

From a functional point of view, the numerous anastomotic connections among the cranial nerves highlight the integrated operation of the nervous system as a whole. Likewise, they enrich the diagnostic and therapeutic possibilities in patients, particularly for Neuraltherapeutic Medicine that recognizes the postulates of nervism and its dystrophies. These dystrophies may result from an irritation component near the affected segment or reflect a distant disturbance or irritation process.

In Neuraltherapeutic Medicine, a technique know as *Supreme* has been used to access the facial nerve and the upper cervical sympathetic chain in the neck region. This technique involves accesing a common anatomical area that is shared by the facial, glossopharyngeal, vagus, accessory, hypoglossal, and upper cervical ganglia nerves, as well as the proximity of important vascular structures such as the internal carotid artery and the internal jugular vein. This technique is highly non-specific and may entail an increased risk, due to its proximity to the stylomastoid and jugular foramina.

Mathias Dosch, in the context of Neural Therapy, described the *Supreme* technique as a unified one for injection in the immediate vicinity of the upper cervical ganglion and the retrostyloid region. The needle insertion point for the technique is located at the intersection point of two auxiliary lines. A vertical line that descends along the anterior edge of the mastoid process and a horizontal line, at a distance of one finger, above the mandibular angle. A 5–6 cm needle is used, inserted perpendicular to the skin. The application of 3–5 cc of neuralterapeutic solution is indicated at a depth of 3–4 cm, using the styloid process as the anatomical landmark [13, 14].

However, the most common and safest technique for the application of Neural Therapy in the specific territory of the facial nerve is through a more direct approach to the retrostyloid region, in the vicinity of the stylomastoid foramen, where the facial nerve of the skull emerges. This technique is derived from the classic anesthesiology technique of Dr. O'Brien, modified by Nadbath and Rehman, and later, by Spaeth [15, 16].

In this classic technique described in anesthesiology, the reference point for the application is located immediately below the external auditory meatus between the anterosuperior border of the mastoid process and the posterior border of the mandibular ramus. Locating the injection site can be facilitated by asking the patient to open and close their mouth. Using a short (12 mm) 25-gauge needle, a papule is made into the skin, followed by insertion of the needle to its maximum depth. Aspiration is performed before administering 3 mL of local anesthetic, followed by a recommendation for local massage to dissipate the local anesthetic [17].

Precaution: When performing this technique, it is important to remember the close proximity of the stylomastoid foramen to the jugular foramen, where the glossopharyngeal (IX), vagus (X), and accessory (XI) nerves emerge [17], as well as the nearby internal carotid artery and internal jugular vein.

In Neural Therapy texts, a specific application is described for the facial nerve, approaching approximately 10 mm medially and cranially from the tip of the mastoid process, directed toward the stylomastoid foramen. This application is complemented by a fan-shaped infiltration along the course of the facial nerve anterior to the ear, beginning from a point just anterior to the attachment of the earlobe [14, 18].

Figures 33.3 and 33.4 show two computerized axial tomography images where these anatomical relationships and the injection site in the stylomastoid space can be seen.

An anatomical review conducted in India reported that, although significant racial variations exist in the position of the stylomastoid foramen relative to the mastoid process, in 83.51% of 100 skulls examined (both male and female), the stylomastoid foramen was located anterior to the line passing through the superior margin of the anterior border of the mastoid process. The mean distance from the center of the stylomastoid foramen to the mastoid tip was 15.26 ± 1.4 mm on the right and 14.32 ± 1.8 mm on the left [19]. Accordingly, when performing an anesthetic or

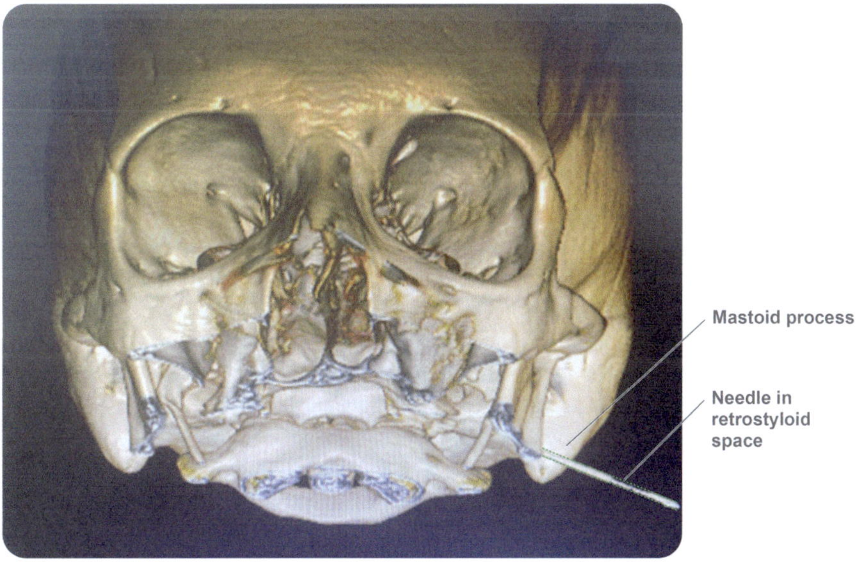

Fig. 33.3 CT image showing a needle entering the stylomastoid space, previous view. (*Source*: Luis Fernando Córdoba personal archive. *Edited*: Luis Fernando Jaimes)

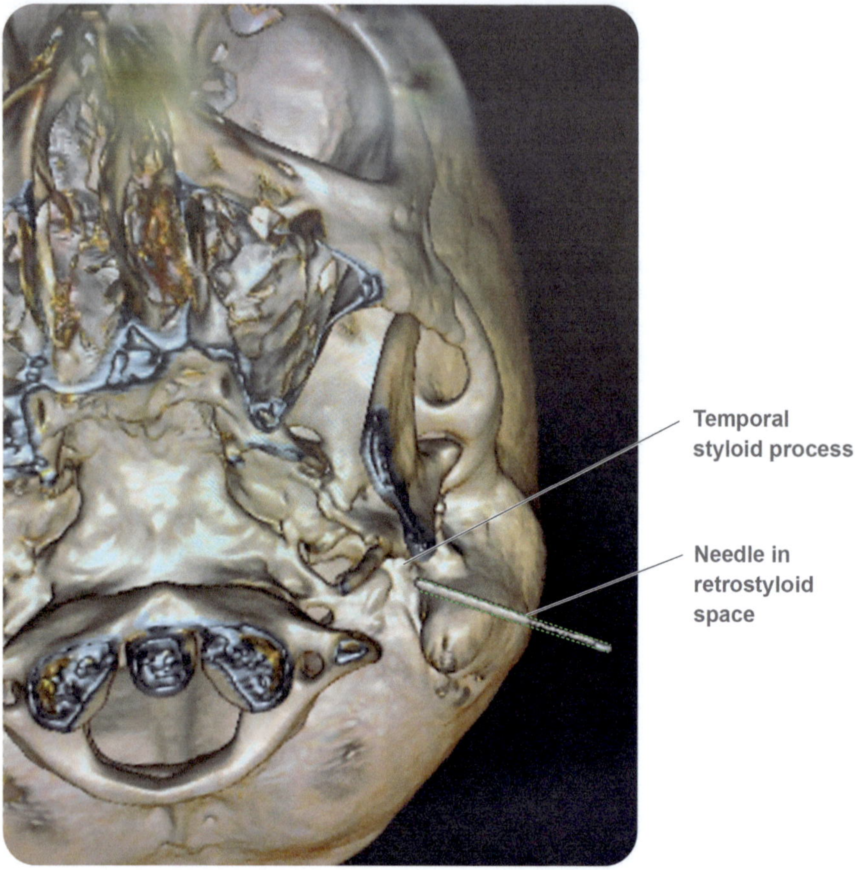

Fig. 33.4 CT image showing the needle entering the stylomastoid space, anterior and inferior view. (*Source*: Luis Fernando Córdoba personal archive. *Edited*: Luis Fernando Jaimes)

neuraltherapeutic application near the stylomastoid foramen: when the needle is inserted along the anterior border of the mastoid process, to reach this region it should be directed slightly anteriorly and medially. If the needle is inserted from the tip of the mastoid process, it should be directed slightly upward (superiorly), anteriorly, and medially [19].

In the morphological study of the retrostyloid space conducted by Franco and Santamaría at the National University of Colombia in 2014, it was evident how in that area there is proximity of very easy access to cranial pairs VII, IX, X, XI, and XII, together with the superior cervical ganglion, depending on the direction of the needle and the depth of insertion, reaching the facial nerve first at approximately 2,1 centimeters away (Figs. 33.5 and 33.6) [20].

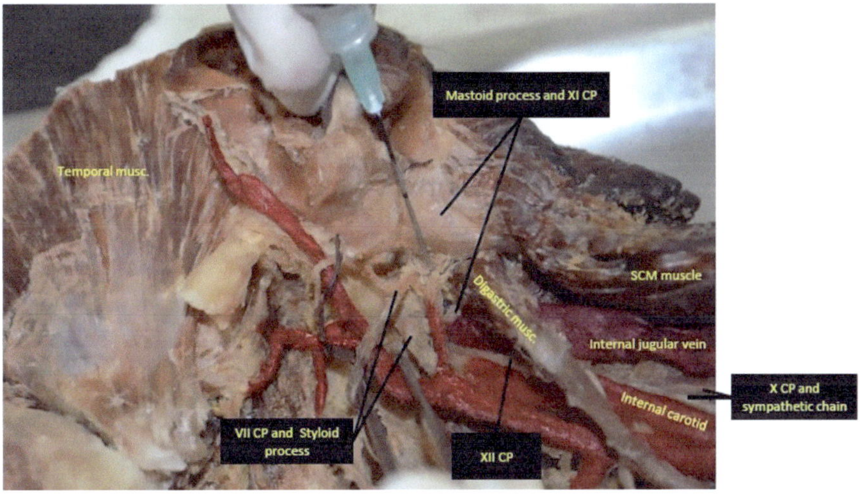

Fig. 33.5 Morphological study image showing the location and depth of the facial nerve in the retrostyloid space. The image provides a lateral and inferior view. (*Source*: Taken from [20])

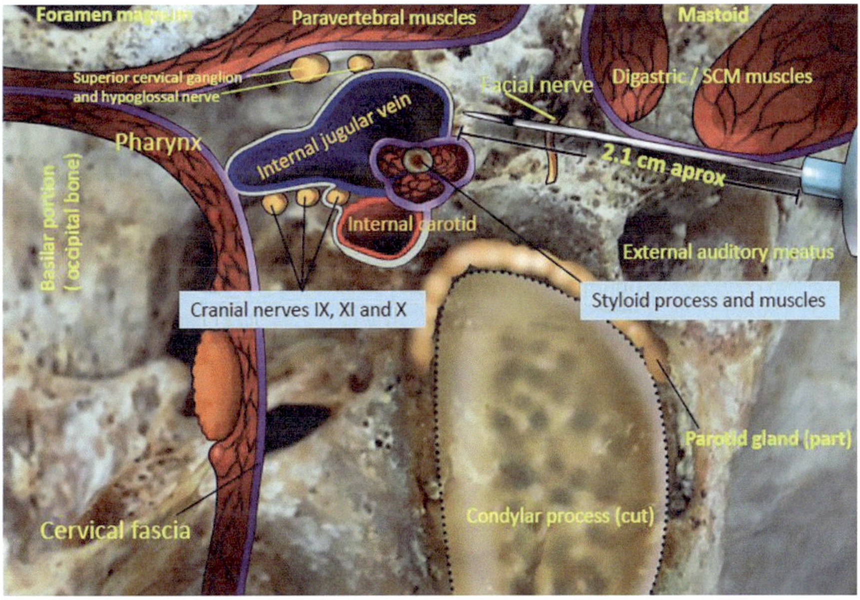

Fig. 33.6 Scheme of a transverse section illustrating the relationships in the retrostyloid space of cranial nerves VII, IX, X, XI, and XII, and the superior cervical ganglion. (*Source*: Taken from [20])

5 Technique for Accessing the Facial Nerve in Neuraltherapeutic Medicine

The most commonly used technique in Neuraltherapeutic Medicine takes the mastoid process and the mandibular ramus as a reference and is described below:

(a) *Materials*: 2.5 or 4 cm needle (1–1.5 in.), 3–5 mL syringe.
(b) *Application of procaine*: 2.5–4 mL of 0.5% procaine.
(c) *Patient position and anatomical landmarks:* The patient must be in a supine position with the head turned to the opposite side from where the application will be made. Locate the mandibular ramus, mastoid process, and ear canal.
(d) *Technique:* At the midpoint between the posterior border of the mandibular ramus and the anterior border of the mastoid process, and immediately below the external auditory canal, the needle is inserted perpendicular to the skin, toward the anterior part of the mastoid process. Once in contact with the anterior border of the mastoid, the needle is redirected slightly forward, 5 to 10 degrees (Fig. 33.7), advancing approximately 1 cm beyond the bone contact described, positioning itself near the stylomastoid foramen. In total, approximately 2 to 2.5 cm should be penetrated from the plane of the skin.
(e) In some cases, injections targeting the peripheral branches of the facial nerve are indicated. For this purpose, techniques described in anesthesiology, may be used. Van Lint block: the anesthetic is injected to block the peripheral terminal branches supplying the orbicularis oculi. The injection is place just above the eyebrow and below the inferior orbital margin through a point approximately 2 cm posterior to the lateral orbital rim, at the level of the lateral cantus. The O'Brien block, also known as a facial trunk block, is performed at the level of the mandibular neck, near the condylar process, to block the proximal trunk of the facial nerve. In the modified O'Brien block approach places the injection at the dorsal rim of the mandible near the tragus of the ear. Atkinson block: targets the superior or temporofacial branch of the facial nerve accessed from the inferior margin of the zygomatic bone. A subcutaneous injection is made along the midpoint of the line between the inferior border of the zygoma and the temporomandibular joint; 2–5 mL of anesthetic solution are injected along this line in both directions [19, 21].

    Although local anesthetics are not used for anesthetic purposes in Neuraltherapeutic Medicine/Neural Therapy, these standard anestesiology techniques provide practical approaches that may be adapted to neuraltherapeutic applications depending on the specific clinical context.

Indications:

- As treatment for interference fields or dominant pathological foci, based on the patient's life history and physical findings (see Chap. 24).
- For secondary disorders due to trophic alteration of the innervation of the facial nerve or its anastomoses.
- As segmental therapeutic support for the pathologies described in Sect. 3, whose clinical presentation primarily affects the facial region.

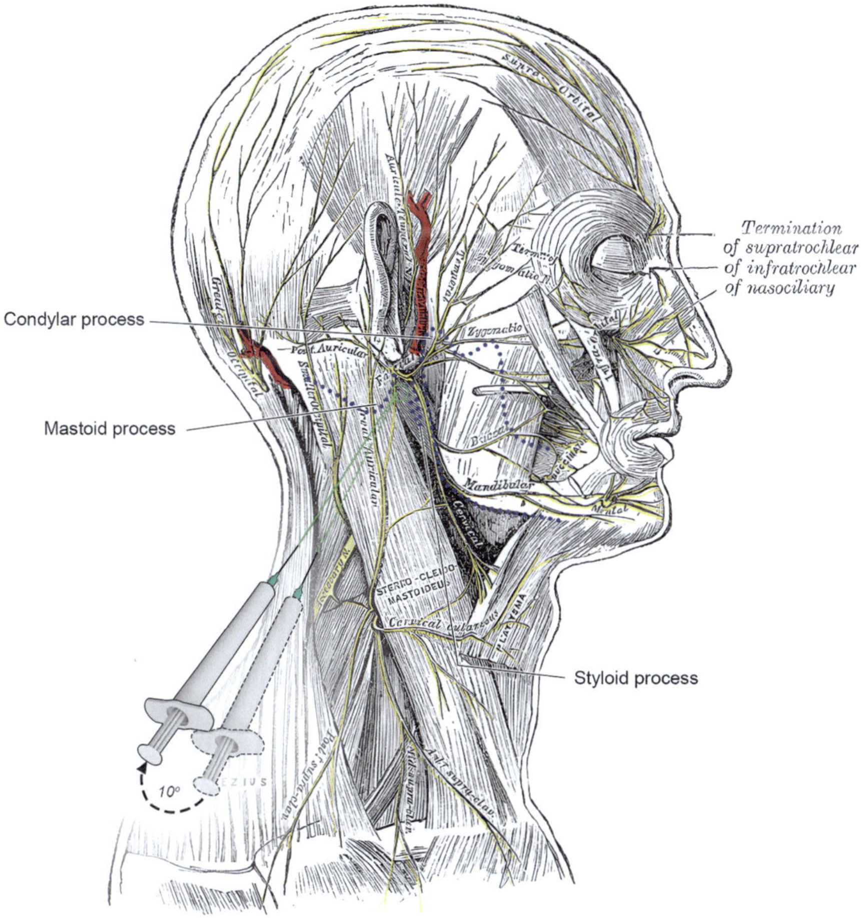

Fig. 33.7 Diagram of access to the peripheral trunk of the facial nerve in the retrostyloid space. (*Source*: Taken and modified from [4])

6 Post-infiltration Reactions and Recommendations

- Depending on the level of intervention, transient paresthesias or partial/complete hemifacial and cervical paresis may occur on the ipsilateral side for about 10–15 minutes. These effects can be uncomfortable, so the patient should be informed and reassured in advance.
- According to the type of infiltration, hematomas, including a parotid hematoma, may occur. Injections should be performed slowly, after aspiration, using non-traumatic needles (27G × 2.5 to 4 cm), depending on the patient's build.
- A transient sensation of vertigo is also possible due to the connections with the vestibular cochlear nerve.

- Ipsilateral Horner may manifest for a brief period as a result of the vagal and upper cervical plexus connections, particularly when the needle is advanced deeper than indicated.

References

1. Phillips D, Bubash LA. The facial nerve: anatomy and common pathology. Semin Ultrasound CT MR. 2002;23(3):202–17. Available from: https://pubmed.ncbi.nlm.nih.gov/12168997/
2. Ottaiano AC, Gómez GD. Lourenção Freddi TdA. The facial nerve: anatomy and pathology. Ultrasound Semin CT MRI. 2023;44(2):71–80. https://doi.org/10.1053/j.sult.2022.11.005. Available from: https://pubmed.ncbi.nlm.nih.gov/37055142/
3. Gray H. Anatomy of the human body, plate 781. Philadelphia: Lea & Febiger; 1918. p. 894. Available from: https://archive.org/details/anatomyofhumanbo1918gray/page/894/mode/2up
4. Gray H. Anatomy of the human body, plate 790. Philadelphia: Lea & Febiger; 1918. p. 904. Available from: https://archive.org/details/anatomyofhumanbo1918gray/page/894/mode/2up
5. Mahajan R, Jain K, Kalsotra P, Bloria S. Transient facial nerve paralysis in two patients following zygomaticotemporal nerve block: case studies. Indian J Anaesth. 2023;67(7):664–6. https://doi.org/10.4103/ija.ija_985_22. Available from: https://pubmed.ncbi.nlm.nih.gov/37601948/
6. Cobo JL, Solé-Magdalena A, Menéndez I, de Vicente JC, Vega JA. Connections between the facial and trigeminal nerves: anatomical basis for facial muscle proprioception. JPRAS Open. 2017;12:9–18.
7. Shoja MM, Oyesiku NM, Griessenauer CJ, Radcliff V, Loukas M, Chern JJ, et al. Anastomoses between lower cranial and upper cervical nerves: a comprehensive review with potential significance during skull base and neck operations. Part I: trigeminal, facial, and vestibulocochlear nerves. Clin Anat. 2014;27(1):118–30.
8. Diamond M, Wartmann CT, Tubbs RS, Shoja MM, Cohen-Gadol AA, Loukas M. Peripheral facial nerve communications and their clinical implications. Clin Anat. 2011;24(1):10–8.
9. Baumel JJ. Trigeminal-facial nerve communications: their function in facial muscle innervation and reinnervation. Arch Otolaryngol. 1974;99(1):34–44.
10. Yang HM, Won SY, Kim HJ, Hu KS. Sihler staining study of anastomosis between the facial and trigeminal nerves in the ocular area and its clinical implications. Muscle Nerve. 2013;48(4):545–50.
11. Velasco I, Salinas F, Aguilar L, Gallego A, Pastrián J, Fariña R, et al. Anatomical considerations in parotidectomy: literature review based on a case. Int J Morphol. 2013;31(1):231–8.
12. González-García N, Porta-Etessam J, García-Azorín D. Eagle's syndrome: towards a clinical definition. Neurologia. 2021;36(6):412–7. https://doi.org/10.1016/j.nrleng.2018.03.007. Available from: https://pubmed.ncbi.nlm.nih.gov/34238523/
13. Dosch M. Illustrative atlas of neural therapy techniques with local anesthetics. 1st ed. Mexico: Latinoamericana Publishing; 2016. 155p.
14. Dosch P, Dosch M. Manual of neural therapy according to Huneke. 2nd ed. Stuttgart; New York: Thieme; 2007. 416p.
15. Hessemer V. Peribulbar anesthesia versus retrobulbar anesthesia with facial block: techniques, local anesthetics and additives, akinesia and sensory blockade, complications. Klin Monbl Augenheilkd [Internet]. 1994;204(2):75–89. [Cited 2025 Mar 9]. Available from: http://www.thieme-connect.com/products/ejournals/html/10.1055/s-2008-1035503
16. Atkinson WS. Facial nerve block. Am J Ophthalmol [Internet]. 1964;57(1):144–5. [Cited 2025 Mar 9]. Available from: https://www.ajo.com/action/showFullText?pii=0002939464920501
17. Herlich A. Focused local anesthesia and analgesia for head and neck surgery. Int Anesthesiol Clin. 2012;50(1):13–25. Available from:. https://doi.org/10.1097/AIA.0b013e318218f6ee.

18. Fisher L. Neural therapy according to Huneke: neurophysiology, therapeutic injection techniques. 3rd ed. In: Niño Ibarra MC, editor. Mexico: Unknown publisher; 2012. 261p.
19. Sharma N, Varshney R. Morphometry of stylomastoid foramen and its clinical application in facial nerve block. Saudi J Anaesth [Internet]. 2015;9(1):60. [Cited 2025 Mar 9]. Available from: https://pmc.ncbi.nlm.nih.gov/articles/PMC4279352/
20. Franco Castillo JC, Santamaría EM. Retrostyle space, nerve junction: VII, IX, X, XI, XII cranial nerves and the superior cervical sympathetic ganglion. Morfolia [Internet]. 2014;6(2) [Cited April 15, 2025]. Available from: https://revistas.unal.edu.co/index.php/morfolia/article/view/45359
21. Schimek F, Fahle M. Techniques of facial nerve block. Br J Ophthalmol [Internet]. 1995;79(2):166–73. [Cited 2025 Mar 11]. Available from: https://pmc.ncbi.nlm.nih.gov/articles/PMC505050/

Chapter 34
The Cervical Spine

Hüseyin Nazlikul and Fatma Gülçin Ural Nazlikul

1 The Cervical Spine (CS)

The cervical spine is the shortest and most mobile part of the spine, connecting the head to the trunk. It contains the spinal cord and, laterally, the blood vessels that supply and drain the brain. The cervical spine is made up of seven differently shaped vertebrae that are connected to each other, the skull and the thoracic spine. The vertebrae from C3 to C7 are almost identical in their basic structure. However, the first and second cervical vertebrae (C1 and C2) differ significantly in shape, justifying the division of the cervical spine into upper and lower segments. The first two cervical vertebrae, together with the joints at the base of the skull, form the upper cervical spine, formerly known as the "craniovertebral joints."The upper joint between the atlas and the occiput and the lower joint between the atlas and the axis also differ significantly from each other [1–3].

The articular surfaces of the atlas for the atlantooccipital joints are oval and converge medially anteriorly, whereas those for the atlantoaxial joint are round. According to Fryette's principles, the upper cervical spine exhibits contralateral

H. Nazlikul (✉)
International Federation of Medical Associations of Neural Therapy – IFMANT, Schattenhalb, Switzerland

Nazlikul Naturel Foundation for the Development of Healthy Habitats, Istanbul, Turkey

Faculty of Medicine, Department of Biophysics, Istanbul University of Health and Technology, Istanbul, Turkey
e-mail: hnazlikul@web.de

F. G. U. Nazlikul
Faculty of Medicine, Physical Medicine and Rehabilitation, Istanbul Health and Technology University, Istanbul, Turkey
e-mail: fatma.nazlikul@istun.edu.tr

L. B. Pinilla Bonilla et al. (eds.), *Neuraltherapeutic Medicine*,
https://doi.org/10.1007/978-3-032-03257-7_34

coupling of rotation and lateral flexion, while the C2 to C7 region exhibits ipsilateral coupling of these movements [4–6].

Movement between adjacent vertebrae is restricted. The combined movement of many segments results in a significant range of spinal motion. Depending on the location and orientation of the facet joints, the range of motion varies in different planes of the spine. In addition, the rib cage limits the movement of the thoracic spine, while the rotation of the pelvis increases the movement of the trunk. The functional movement of the spine depends on the sum of the different spinal segments and the orientation of the pelvis [7, 8].

1.1 Diagnostic Information

The roots of the sympathetic nervous system are located between segments C8 and L2, but its peripheral distribution is not only segmental. According to the principle of divergence, the sympathetic system branches into many spinal segments [9, 10].

From a neuraltherapeutic point of view, the peripheral distribution of the sympathetic nervous system is of immense importance. Both afferent and efferent sympathetic nerves travel along spinal nerves and vascular structures to reach their innervated areas. This explains why all tissues with spinal innervation and arterial supply also have sympathetic innervation. In addition to the vascular or spinal nerve, other tissues are important for access to the sympathetic nervous system [6, 11, 12].

The afferent branches of the sympathetic system, like other afferent nerves, enter the spinal cord from the dorsal roots. The nerve cells of this system are located in the dorsal root ganglia. At the spinal level, the synaptic connections between afferent and efferent neurons form polysynaptic (indirect) and monosynaptic (direct) reflex arcs via interneurons, independent of the somatic or visceral nervous system [2, 5, 6, 9].

The cervical spine, consisting of seven vertebrae, forms the basis for the connection between the head and the trunk (see Fig. 34.1). In addition to the static function, these vertebrae allow three levels of head movement: forward and backward tilt, rotation, and lateral tilt. For these functions to work properly, the capsule-ligament apparatus and muscles must function smoothly. The static and dynamic function of the cervical spine is primarily controlled by the spinal nervous system through afferent-efferent pathways [4, 5, 13–15].

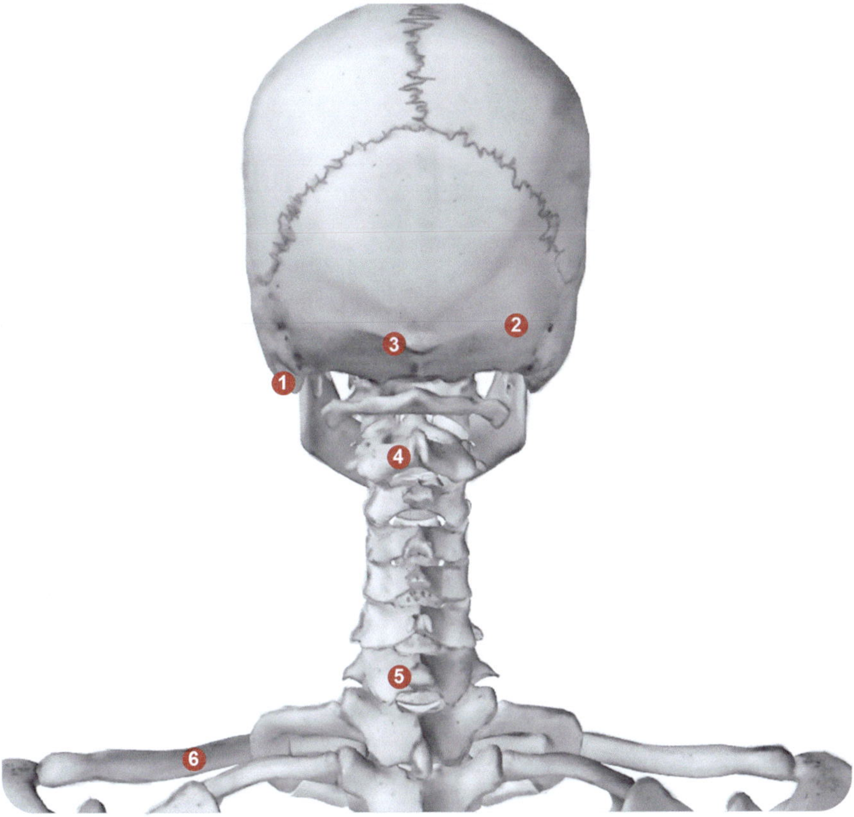

Fig. 34.1 Palpation of Bony Landmarks. Numbers identify the following structures: (1). Processus mastoideus, (2). Linea nuchae superior/inferior, (3). Protuberantia occipitalis externa, (4). The spinous proccss of C2, (5). The spinous process of C7, (6). The superior angle of the scapula. (Source: Own elaboration)

1.2 Important Notes on Spinal Indications

- PRM (physical and rehabilitation medicine), physiotherapy, and orthopedics: Treatment of the spine, joints, ligaments, and muscles is possible through the sympathetic nervous system.
- Extremity diseases can be treated via neuraltherapeutic medicine through joints, ligament capsule structures, vessels, nerves, and muscles.
- Thoracic and abdominal diseases, gynecological, urological, and andrological disorders: Treated through the corresponding segments. Reflexive somatic changes due to organ disease can be clinically evaluated through sympathetic afferent irritation-induced somatic changes in skin, muscle, and spinal function.
- Painful movement restriction in the cervical spine post-trauma.
- Pseudoarticular disorders of the upper extremity and shoulder girdle.
- Root Irritations of the cervical plexus and brachial plexus.

- Myotendinosis of the upper limbs, periarthropathy.
- Spondylodiscitis.
- Interference field-induced disorders [1, 5].

1.3 Cervical Syndrome: Cervical Spine Syndrome (CSS)

Diagnosis is often delayed by factors such as long clinical duration, muscle hypertonia, pain in other parts of the spine, local pain, reflex pain, and basic movement and postural problems. It also requires good history-taking and examination skills, especially when symptoms are caused by weather changes, hormonal imbalances or inflammatory conditions. Manual examination is essential to diagnose functional disorders accurately and promptly [6, 12].

1.3.1 Functional Disorders of the Cervical Spine (May Extend to T5)

- Constipation.
- Hypermobility.
- Muscle dysfunction.
- Interference fields.
- Projection syndromes.

Dysfunctions of the upper cervical spine manifest as neck pain radiating into the head. Disorders originating in the lower cervical spine manifest as neck pain radiating into the arm. Dysfunctions originating in the mid-cervical region may be visceral in origin, related to the phrenic nerve, thyroid gland, or tonsils, and affect internal organs [2, 5, 10].

1.4 Cervico-Trigeminal Convergence (See Fig. 34.2)

- Receptive field of the neck:
  - Explicit nociception and proprioception from suboccipital muscles and joints: Occiput—C3.
- Cervico-trigeminal convergence:
  - Spinal nucleus of the trigeminal nerve (“medullary dorsal horn”).
  - C1–C3, N. V, (N. VII, IX, X, XII).
- Direct projections to the vestibular nuclei:
  - C1–C3.
  - Trigeminal nerve (N.V.)

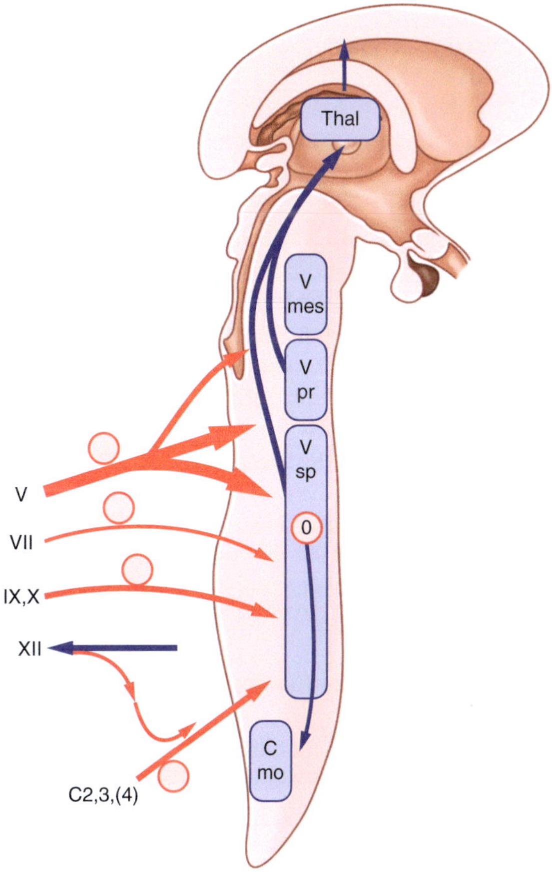

Fig. 34.2 Cervico-trigeminal convergence as a basis for craniovertebral syndrome. This figure shows the nucleus of the spinal trigeminal nerve (V sp) convergence of afferents C1–C3 and N. trig. "trigemino-cervical convergence" VII, IX, X, and XII. (Source: Own elaboration)

1.4.1 Specific Assignments

- C1: N. suboccipitalis.
  - No dermatome—but R. meningeus to the dura.
  - Innervates MM. obliquus capitis superior, rectus capitis minor.
  - Innervates atlas segments of longer neck extensors (e.g., M. splenius) with dorsal branches.
- C2: N. occipitalis major, N. occipitalis minor.
  - Large dermatome occipital and posterior dura mater.
  - Motor (together with C1) to nearly all atlas muscles.
  - Innervation of the atlas musculature: approx. 60% from anterior branches of the upper cervical nerves.

- C3: N. occipitalis tertius.
  - Smaller dermatome occipital and suboccipital.
  - Atlas segments from M. levator scapulae, M. longissimus cervicis with anterior branch.
  - Cervical joints C3 with dorsal branches [5]

1.4.2 Symptoms of Cervicobrachial Syndrome (C3–T4)

- Myofascial pain in the levator scapulae muscle (C3).
- Myofascial pain in the supraspinatus muscle (C4).
- Myofascial pain in the deltoid, biceps muscle (C5).
- Myofascial pain with pronation/supination and flexion/extension of the wrist (C6).
- Myofascial pain in the triceps muscle (C7).
- Myofascial pain in the finger flexors (C8).
- Myofascial pain in the finger extensors (T1).
- Sympathetic reactions (circulation, sweating, heart, respiration) of the upper sympathetic trunk and cervical ganglia (T1–T4).

1.4.3 Mobility of the Cervical Spine

The examination of the mobility of the cervical spine should focus on the active and passive movements that the cervical spine can perform (see Fig. 34.3). Possible movements include:

- Ventral flexion.
- Dorsal flexion.
- Lateral flexion.
- Rotation.

  Nodding movements ventrally and dorsally (maxillary/C1).
  Lateral inclination (maxillary/C1)

- Translation ventrally, dorsally, and laterally.

1.4.4 Cervical Spine Syndrome (CSS Syndrome)

Cervical spine syndrome (CSS syndrome) can be divided into three main categories based on the affected vertebrae:

1. Upper cervical spine syndrome (C1–C3):
   - Neck pain radiating to the head.

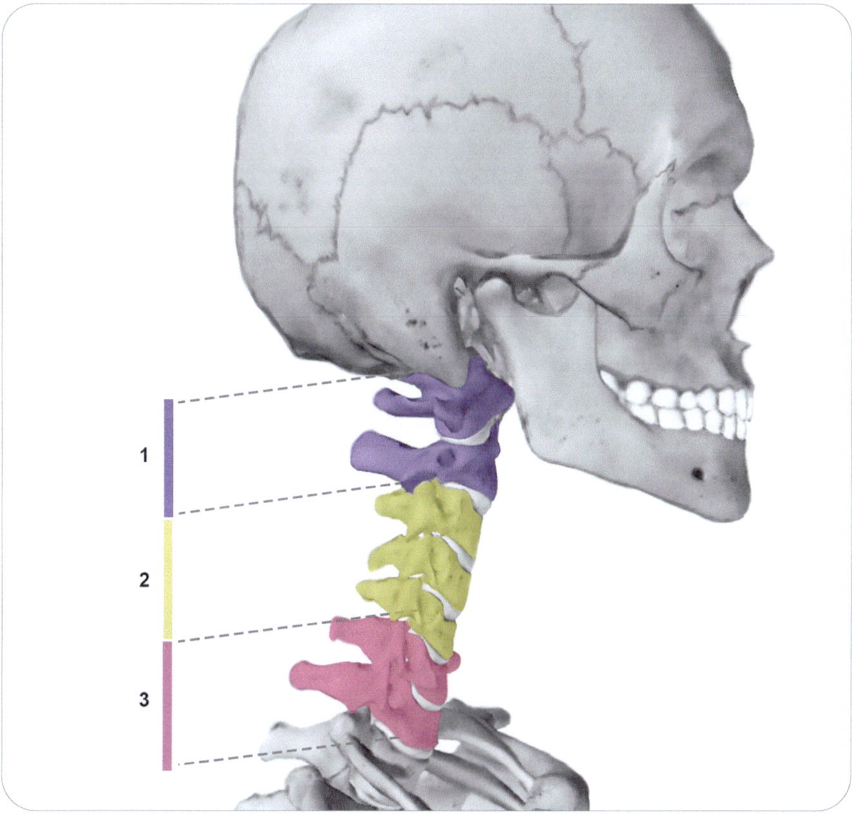

Fig. 34.3 The image depicts a side view of the cervical spine and its relationship with the skull. The cervical spine is divided into three distinct regions: 1. **Upper Cervical Spine**: This area, highlighted in purple, consists of the atlas (C1) and axis (C2) vertebrae. These two vertebrae allow for the majority of the head's rotation and support the skull's weight. 2. **Middle cervical Spine**: Represented in yellow, this region includes the mid-cervical vertebrae (C3 to C5). This section provides support and mobility, allowing for flexion, extension, and lateral flexion of the neck. **Lower Cervical Spine**: Depicted in red, this lower portion consists of the lower cervical vertebrae (C6 to C7). This area is responsible for supporting the neck's stability and bears much of the head's weight, contributing to movements like flexion and extension. The color-coding in the image helps to differentiate these three critical regions of the cervical spine, each playing a unique role in neck mobility, support, and overall function. (Source: Own elaboration)

2. Lower cervical spine syndrome (C4–C7):
   - Neck pain radiating to the arm.

   This categorization helps in better understanding the symptoms and developing targeted treatment approaches. In terms of neuraltherapeutic medicine, a third category is also significant:

3. Middle cervical syndrome (C3–C5):
   - **Pseudoradicular symptoms.**
   - **Pronounced vegetative symptoms**:
     - Palpitations.
     - Tachycardia.
     - Tachyarrhythmia.
     - Diaphragmatic motor disturbances.
     - Gastroesophageal disorders.
     - Liver and gallbladder disorders.
     - Thyroid and tonsillar disorders.
     - All disorders related to the N. phrenicus.
     - Roemheld syndrome [16]

1.5 Examination Procedure

- Pain history.
- Inspection.
- Palpation.
- Functional palpation:
  - Joints.
  - Ligaments.
  - Muscles.
- Additional examinations:
  - Neurology (e.g., electromyography, nerve conduction velocity, evoked potentials, etc.)
  - Imaging (X-ray, CT scanner, MRI, scintigraphy).
  - Possibly laboratory/biochemistry tests.

An accurate diagnosis requires a thorough examination. The following points are clarified through anamnesis and functional examination:

- Location and extent of pain.
- The intensity of pain.
- Nature of pain.
- Sensory disturbances.
- Performance decline.
- Pain during coughing, sneezing, and straining.
- Impact of body posture.
- Effects of heat and cold.
- Pain after inactivity.
- Movement restrictions.

- Dental status.
- Temporomandibular joint.
- Waking up early due to pain (e.g., inflammation, such as ankylosing spondylitis).
- Pain that increases suddenly when walking and immediately disappears when sitting (spinal canal stenosis).
- Increased pain intensity with walking/movement (myofascial disorders).
- Occupation/sports.
- Psychosocial factors.

1.6 Facet Joint Position and Movement of the Cervical Spine (Figs. 34.4 and 34.5)

1.6.1 Facet Joint Position in Neutral

- Positioned at a 45° angle relative to the segment, depending on the region and shape of the cervical spine.

1.6.2 Characteristics of the Cervical Spine

- Movement directions and range vary by segment:
  - Occiput-Atlas:
    - Flexion: 10°.
    - Extension: 25°.
  - Atlas-Axis:
    - Rotation: 90°.
    - Flexion: 5°.
    - Extension: 10°.

1.6.3 Cervical Spine Examination

- Total rotation test: left-to-right comparison over the nose for symmetry.
- Inclination test: minimum of 4 cm (2 finger widths).
- Reclination test: approximately 18 cm (hand span).
- Inclined rotation test: lightly held, about 30–40° for upper cervical spine symmetry.
- Reclined rotation test: around 30° for middle/lower cervical spine symmetry.

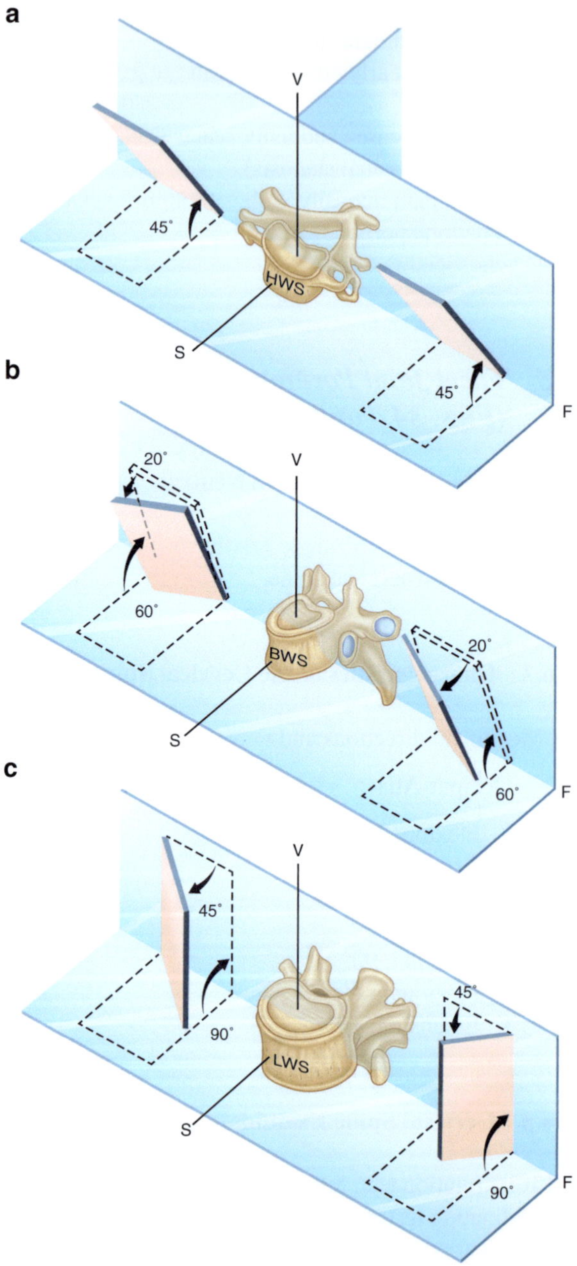

Fig. 34.4 Inclination of facet-joints: CSS: 45°, TSS: 60°, and LSS: 90°. The image shows a schematic representation of the facet joints in the cervical spine (HWS), thoracic spine (BWS), and lumbar spine (LWS). (**a**): The cervical spine (CSS) is depicted with a facet angle of 45°. This angle allows for a high degree of mobility, especially in rotation and flexion/extension. (**b**): The thoracic spine (TSS) shows facet angles of 60° and 20°. The facet joints of the thoracic spine allow for some movement but are mainly restricted to flexion and extension, as the ribs limit rotation and lateral flexion. (**c**): The lumbar spine (LSS) is shown with facet angles of 90° and 45°. This alignment of the facet joints primarily permits flexion and extension while significantly restricting rotation. These illustrations highlight how the orientation of the facet joints affects the mobility and stability of different sections of the spine. Understanding these angles is crucial for grasping the biomechanical properties of the spine and their relevance to diagnostic and therapeutic procedures. (Source: Own elaboration)

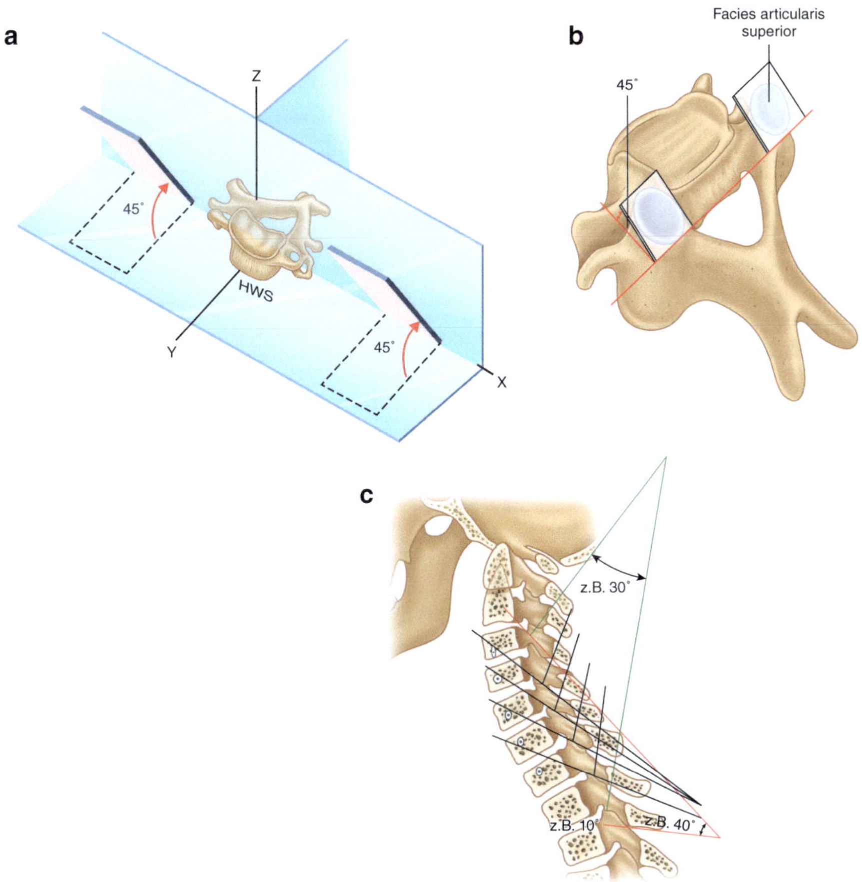

Fig. 34.5 The image shows various views and angles of the cervical spine (HWS) and the facet joints, which are of great importance for diagnosis and treatment. (**a**): This section shows the cervical spine (HWS) in a 3D representation, where the facet joints are shown at a 45-degree angle. This angle is crucial for understanding the alignment and possible directions of movement of the joints, which is necessary for correct diagnosis and therapy. (**b**): Here, an individual facet joint is shown in isolation, also at a 45-degree angle. This representation helps to capture the exact location and angle of the joint surfaces. It is important to note that the joint surfaces are not flat but angled, which affects mobility and load distribution. (**c**): This lateral view of the cervical spine shows various possible angles for diagnostic and therapeutic access, such as 30° and 40°. These angles are essential to ensure the accurate placement of needles or other instruments without endangering adjacent structures. Knowledge of the anatomical structures and correct angles is crucial for accurate diagnosis and the performance of effective treatments, particularly in procedures such as neural therapy or injection therapy at the facet joints. (Source: Own elaboration)

1.6.4 C2–C7 Movement

- Flexion, extension, rotation, and lateral flexion. Each segment shows approximately 10° of flexion, with the greatest flexion between C4–C5 and C5–C6. The greatest extension is also between C4–C5, while lateral flexion mainly occurs between C3–C4 and C4–C5.

1.6.5 Individual Vertebrae

- C1 (Atlas): No body or spinous process, articulates with the odontoid process of C2, and supports the skull.
- C2 (Axis): The most robust cervical vertebra, with the dens serving as the axis for rotation.
- C7: A long spinous process, palpable from the outside, known as the vertebra prominens.

1.6.6 Neuraltherapeutic Approach

- Processus spinosus (PS).
- Local and segmental treatment.
- Injection techniques:
  - Ligaments (ligament injections).
  - Facet joints.
  - Spinal nerves.
  - Sacroiliac joint.
  - Timing points.
  - Ganglion and sacral canal.

1.7 Cervical Spine Injection Techniques

1.7.1 Neck Wheals in the Shoulder Girdle Area

Procedure:

- Location: Initially, paravertebral wheals are placed at the level of the spinous processes of the cervical vertebrae and 2–3 cm away from the spinous processes.
- Injection: Depending on palpation findings, 0.2–0.5 ml of 0.5–1% procaine is injected into local subcutaneous gelosis or hypertonic muscle fibers at the points where the pain is most pronounced upon palpation.

  Technique:

- The spinous processes are the only reliably palpable bony structures in the cervical spine region for injections. The stimulated structure is typically painful on palpation. Injections are administered in the area of the cervical facet joints and spinous processes.

1.7.2 Injection into the Cervical Spine (CS) Facet Joints

Palpation of facet joint-adjacent painful tissue densities: These tissue densities correspond to segmental muscular reflex spasms of the deep paraspinal segmental muscles (medial tract M. erector spinae, Mm. rotatores). They are also known as irritation zones or points [2, 5–7, 9].

Palpation of facet joints on the right: Identify the facet joint line starting from C2/3. Use the right index or middle finger to palpate deeply from the dorsolateral just beside the M. semispinalis capitis. Facilitate the detection of facet joints by gently laterally flexing the CS toward the palpation side with the left hand over the head and aligning the thoracic spine (TS) to avoid cervical hyperextension. Use the opposite-hand arrangement for the left side [2, 5, 6, 9, 10].

Palpation of mobility and end feel: Assess the segmental mobility and end feel of the facet joint from dorsolateral during guided ipsilateral lateral flexion coupled with same-direction rotation, effectively "scanning" the entire CS.

Facet joints characteristics: Facet joints guide the movement of the functional unit through gliding. They consist of synovial tissue and a fibrous capsule, significantly contributing to stability. The orientation of the facet joints varies along the spine, with movement direction dictated by the orientation of their surfaces [5–7, 9, 10].

This procedure, a form of neural therapy, is typically used to manage pain or inflammation associated with cervical facet joint syndrome. The goal is to deliver medication directly to the facet joint to reduce inflammation, alleviate pain, and improve mobility in the cervical spine.

The illustration shows the careful approach required to avoid surrounding structures, such as major blood vessels and nerves, while accurately targeting the facet joint (see Fig. 34.6). The angle of the needle and the positioning of the syringe are critical for the success of this neural therapy procedure, ensuring that the medication is delivered precisely where it is needed.

1.7.3 Injection into Cervical Spine (CS) Facet Joints

Facet joint injection:

- Injection site: 2 cm lateral from the center of the spinous process (PS).
- Injection direction: sagittal.
- Injection depth: 2.5–3.5 cm.

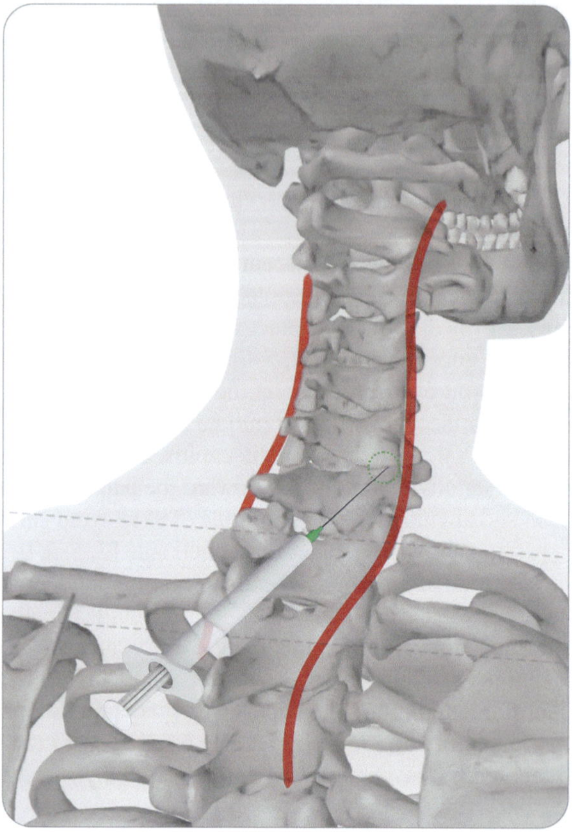

Fig. 34.6 The image depicts a neural therapy procedure where an injection is being administered to the C5 facet joint in the cervical spine. The injection site is clearly marked along the cervical vertebrae, with the needle aimed at the facet joint of the C5 vertebra. The surrounding anatomical structures, including the cervical spine, muscles, and blood vessels, are illustrated to highlight the precise location of the injection. (Source: Own elaboration)

- Materials and local anesthetic (LA): 40 × 0.4 mm needle, 1.5–2 ml of 1% procaine/lidocaine.

Cervical spinal nerve injection: The respective spinal nerve exits the foramen ventrolaterally at the transverse process in the region of the palpable sulcus nervi spinalis (between the anterior and posterior tubercles), where it can be carefully palpated and compared for provocation (see Fig. 34.7).

1.7.4 Cervical Spinal Nerve Injection

Injection technique:

Palpation of the sulcus:

- Procedure: Apply gentle pressure to detect extreme hyperalgesic tenderness indicative of root irritation, which may radiate into the dermatome.

Injection site:

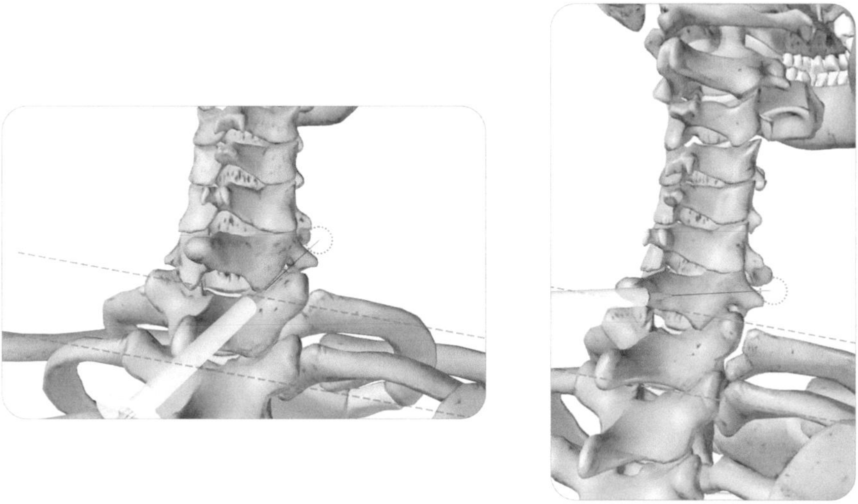

Fig. 34.7 The image shows injections into the cervical nerves, using C5 as an example. (Source: Own elaboration)

- Location: 2 cm lateral to the lower part of the posterior spinous process (SP).
- Direction: Insert sagittally, retract slightly after contacting the facet, then move 1 cm laterally.
- Depth: 3.0–3.5 cm.
- Materials: 40 × 0.4 mm needle.
- Local anesthetic: 3–5 ml of 1% procaine/lidocaine.

Specific technique:

- For cervical spinal nerve injections, the needle is inserted under the spinous process of the vertebra above the targeted nerve. For example, for the C6 spinal nerve, the needle is inserted under the C5 spinous process.

1.7.5 The Importance of the Linea Nuchae in the Diagnosis and Treatment of Cervical Spine Syndrome (CSS) Problems

The Linea Nuchae plays a crucial role in both the diagnosis and treatment of cervical spine (CSS) issues. The cervical vertebrae C2 to C7 project along this line, enabling precise palpatory diagnostics and targeted therapeutic approaches.

Anatomical overview (see Fig. 34.8):

- M. splenius capitis (A/green): This muscle is crucial for the movement and stability of the cervical spine, particularly the segments C4 to C7.
- M. semispinalis capitis (B/orange): This muscle is mainly responsible for the segments C2 and C3 and plays a vital role in the extension and rotation of the cervical spine.

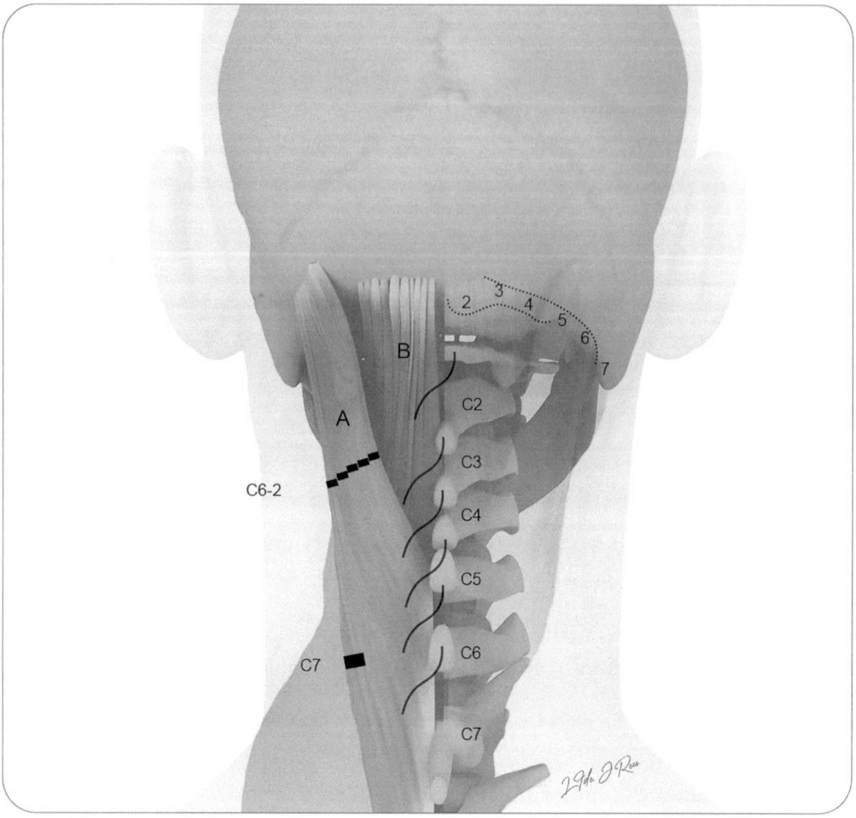

Fig. 34.8 Muscle attachments in the cervical spine and projection of irritation and insertion points. (Source: Own elaboration)

Diagnostic and therapeutic approaches:

1. Palpatory diagnostics:

   - By palpating the points along the Linea Nuchae, sensitive areas can be identified that indicate problems in the corresponding cervical segments (see Fig. 34.9).
   - Particularly, the points corresponding to the muscle attachments of the M. semispinalis capitis (for C2 and C3) and the M. splenius capitis (for C4 to C7) provide valuable diagnostic insights.

2. Therapeutic applications:

   - Muscle relaxation: Targeted massages and manual therapy at the identified points can alleviate muscle tension and improve the mobility of the cervical spine.

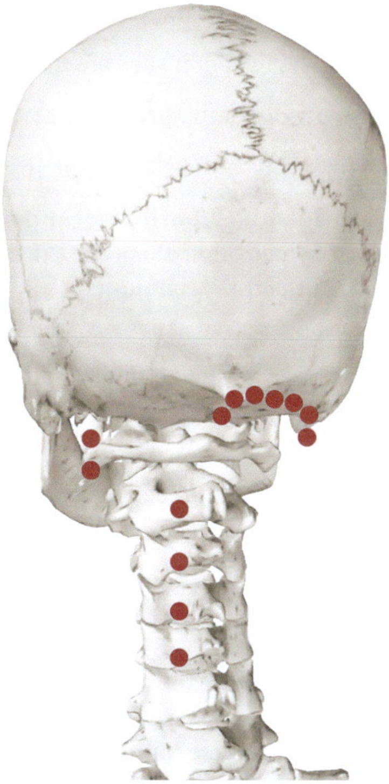

Fig. 34.9 Position of irritation points/ points of cervical insertion. The red dots on the image indicate specific pressure points that are important for cervical dysfunction. These points are crucial for identifying areas of irritation that may be causing or contributing to cervical spine issues. The irritation points can be located either on the linea nuchae or over the musculus multifidus. (Source: Own elaboration)

- Trigger point therapy: Identified trigger points along the Linea Nuchae can be treated with specific pressure techniques and stretching exercises.
- Rotation and extension therapy: Specific exercises to improve the rotation and extension of the cervical spine, considering the muscle attachments of the M. semispinalis capitis and M. splenius capitis.

Neural therapy injections at the linea nuchae and PS points of the cervical spine:

Neural therapy is an essential method for treating pain and functional disorders in the cervical spine (CSS). Specific injection points along the Linea Nuchae and the paravertebral segments (PS) are used to relieve pain and improve the functionality of the cervical spine.

Preparation for Injections:

1. Patient education and consent:
    - The patient is informed about the procedure, goals, and potential risks of the injection.
    - Written informed consent is obtained.
2. Patient positioning:
    - The patient is positioned comfortably, either sitting or lying down, to allow good access to the cervical spine.

3. Hygienic preparation:

   - The injection sites are thoroughly disinfected to prevent infections.

   Injections at the linea nuchae:

1. Injections at sensitive spots (trigger points).

   - **Identification of trigger points**: Sensitive spots (trigger points) are identified by palpation along the Linea Nuchae.
   - **Injection technique**:

     – A thin needle is used to inject the local anesthetic directly into the identified trigger points.
     – Typical local anesthetic: procaine or lidocaine.
     – Dosage: 0.5–1 ml per injection site.

   - **Goal**: The injection reduces muscle tension and alleviates pain by lowering the local threshold of irritation.

   Injections in the paravertebral segments (PS):

1. Injections in the dermatomal and myotomal areas.

   - **Identification of PS points**: The PS points are located along the paravertebral segments of the cervical spine (C2–C7).
   - **Injection technique**:

     – The needle is inserted at an angle of approximately 45 degrees to the skin surface to bring the local anesthetic close to the spinal nerve root.
     – Typical local anesthetic: procaine or lidocaine.
     – Dosage: 1–2 ml per segment.

   - **Goal**: The injection in the PS points aims to influence nerve conduction, thereby achieving pain relief and) improving muscle function.

2. Injections in muscles and ligaments.

   - **Identification of injection sites**: Muscle and ligament structures along the cervical spine are identified by palpation.
   - **Injection technique**:

     – The needle is inserted deeply enough to inject the local anesthetic directly into the affected muscle or ligament structures.
     – Typical local anesthetic: procaine or lidocaine.
     – Dosage: 1–2 ml per injection site.

   - **Goal**: The injection aims to release muscle tension and improve the flexibility and functionality of the ligaments.

   Combination of injection techniques:

- Sequence of injections: The injections typically begin in the dermatomal areas (paravertebral segments) to achieve a systemic effect and then proceed to the specific muscle and ligament injections and trigger points at the Linea Nuchae.
- Mechanism of action: Combining these injection techniques provides comprehensive treatment that addresses both the cause of pain and the muscular and structural problems.

Post-injection care and monitoring:

- Patient monitoring: The patient is monitored for any adverse reactions or side effects after the injections.
- Follow-up: Regular follow-up is essential to evaluate the success of the treatment and adjust further injections if necessary.

Summary
Neural therapy injections at the Linea Nuchae and PS points of the cervical spine are an effective method for treating CSS problems. By targeting local anesthetics at the trigger points, muscle attachments, and paravertebral segments, pain can be alleviated, muscle tension released, and cervical spine functionality improved.

1.7.6 Therapeutic Injections into Ligaments

Neural therapy is a method of complementary medicine where local anesthetics such as procaine or lidocaine are injected to treat chronic pain and functional disorders. This technique can be particularly effective when applied to spinal ligaments to alleviate pain and improve mobility. Below are the basic steps and considerations for performing injections into spinal ligaments (ligamentum flavum and other ligaments of the cervical, thoracic, and lumbar spine):

Anatomical structures (see Fig. 34.10):

- Procc. spinosi.
  - The spinous processes are bony structures that extend backward from the vertebral bodies.
- Lig. supraspinale.
  - This ligament extends along the tips of the spinous processes throughout the spine, connecting them.
- Lig. interspinale.
  - The ligamentum interspinale is located between the spinous processes of adjacent vertebrae, providing additional stability.
- Lig. flavum.
  - The ligamentum flavum is a strong, elastic ligament that extends between the laminae of adjacent vertebrae, closing the vertebral canal posteriorly.

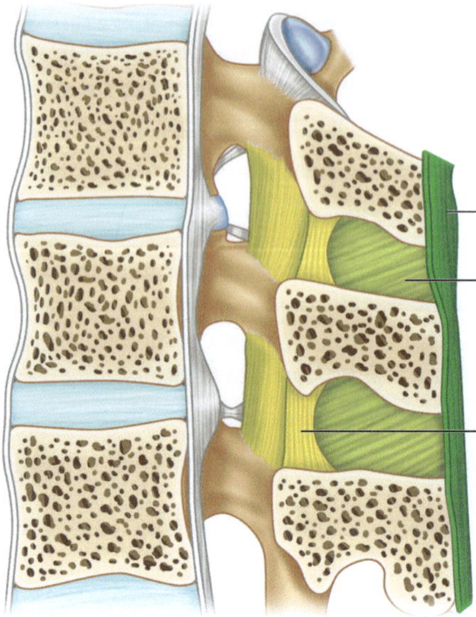

Fig. 34.10 The position of the ligaments along the spine and their relationship to the spinous processes. Injections into these areas are important therapeutic measures for treating various spinal disorders and for pain relief. (Source: Own elaboration)

Injections:

Injections into the spinous processes and ligaments of the spine:

- Injections into the Procc. spinosi.
  - Injections can be administered along the ligamentum supraspinale to reduce inflammation and relieve pain. These injections are often helpful in treating back pain and soft tissue injuries.
- Injections between the spinous processes (interspinous).
  - Injections into the ligamentum interspinale can provide targeted pain relief in the deeper layers of the spine. This technique is frequently used for chronic back pain.
- Injections into the ligamentum flavum.
  - Injections into the ligamentum flavum are typically part of epidural injections used to treat disc herniations and radicular pain. These injections aim to reduce inflammation and swelling that might be pressing on the nerve roots.

Preparation:

- Patient education and consent:
  - The patient should be informed about the procedure and potential risks. Written informed consent is required.
- Sterile conditions:

  - The procedure must be performed under sterile conditions to avoid infections.
- Localization:
  - The exact injection site is determined through clinical examination and, if necessary, imaging techniques (e.g., ultrasound, X-ray).

Procedure:

- Patient positioning:
  - The patient is placed in a position that facilitates access to the desired injection site. This can vary depending on the target region (e.g., prone position for injections into the lumbar spine).
- Disinfection:
  - The skin over the injection site is thoroughly disinfected.
- Local anesthesia:
  - A small amount of local anesthetic is injected subcutaneously to numb the injection site.
- Injection:
  - Under sterile conditions, a fine needle is inserted into the ligament to be treated. The local anesthetic is injected slowly. The amount of anesthetic and the depth of the injection depend on the specific location and individual case.

Aftercare:

- Observation:
  - The patient is monitored for a short period after the procedure to ensure no immediate complications occur.
- Instructions:
  - The patient receives instructions to avoid strenuous activities for a certain period and to monitor for potential side effects.

Specific ligaments:

- Ligamentum flavum:
  - These ligaments connect the laminae of adjacent vertebrae and play an important role in stabilizing the spine. Injections into this ligament require precision to avoid damage to nearby structures.
- Other ligaments of the cervical, thoracic, and lumbar spine:
  - These include the ligamentum longitudinale anterius and posterius, the ligamentum supraspinale, the ligamentum interspinale, and the ligamentum

nuchae (in the cervical spine). Each of these structures has specific anatomical features that must be considered during injection.

Risks and complications

- Infection:
  - One of the most serious complications, which can be minimized by strict sterile techniques.
- Nerve injury:
  - There is a risk of nerve injury, especially with injections near the spine.
- Allergic reactions:
  - Rare, but possible, especially in patients with known allergies to local anesthetics.
- Vascular complications:
  - Accidental injection into a blood vessel can lead to systemic effects of the local anesthetic.

2 Conclusion

Neuraltherapeutic injections into the ligaments of the spine are a specialized technique that should be performed by experienced therapists. A thorough understanding of the anatomy and potential complications is crucial for the safety and effectiveness of the procedure.

Please ensure that all injections are performed by a qualified specialist to minimize risks and complications.

References

1. Frölich E. Manual medicine–medical hand art for diagnosis and therapy. Isny-Neutrauchburg: MWE-Self-Publishing; 2009. Available from: http://www.manuelle-mwe.de
2. Nazlikul H. Textbook of neural therapy. 1st ed. Istanbul: Nobel Kitabevi; 2010.
3. Böhni UW, Lauper M, Locher H. Manual medicine 2. In: Practically applying diagnostic and therapeutic techniques. Stuttgart: Thieme; 2012.
4. Neuhuber WL. Functional neuroanatomy of the Cranio-cervical junction. In: Hülse M, Neuhuber W, Wolff HD, editors. The upper cervical spine. Berlin: Springer; 2005. p. 55–71. https://doi.org/10.1007/3-540-28250-5_6.
5. Nazlikul H. Segmental vertebral dysfunction is a multi-causal event. Manual Med. 2014;52(5):432–6. https://doi.org/10.1007/s00337-014-1141-1.
6. Barop H. Textbook and atlas of neural therapy: diagnosis and therapy with local anesthetics. Stuttgart: Thieme; 2018.

7. Acarkan T, Elmacioglu MA, Nazlikul H. FASET joint syndrome and clinical reflections. J Complement Med Regul Neural Ther. 2019;13(1)
8. Nazlikul H. Neurovegetative, blockades, and manual medicine: autonomic nervous system, blockades, and manual medicine. Manual Med. 2010;6 https://doi.org/10.1007/s00337-010-0805-8.
9. Fischer L. Textbook of neural therapy according to Huneke. 3rd ed. Stuttgart: Hippokrates; 2001. p. 108–11.
10. Weinschenk S. Handbook of neural therapy–therapy with local anesthetics. 2nd ed. Stuttgart: Georg Thieme Verlag; 2020. p. 976.
11. Nazlikul H, Babacan A. The role of neural therapy and injections. In: Babacan A, editor. Pain and injections. Ankara: Türkiye Klinikleri; 2019. p. 110–7.
12. Engel R, Barop H, Gielbel J, Ludin SM, Fischer L. The influence of modern neurophysiology on the previous definitions of "segment" and "interference field" in neural therapy. Complement Med Res. https://doi.org/10.1159/000522391.
13. Dvorák J, Grob D. Cervical spine, diagnostics and therapy. Stuttgart: Thieme; 2010.
14. Bischoff HP, Moll H. Textbook of manual medicine. 6th ed. Balingen: Spitta; 2011.
15. Nazlikul H, Ural FG, Öztürk GT, Öztürk ADT. Evaluation of neural therapy effect in patients with piriformis syndrome. J Back Musculoskelet Rehabil. 2018;31(6):1105–10.
16. Ural FG, Nazlikul H. Diaphragmatic dysfunctions and their treatment: neural therapy and manual medicine as effective approaches. Int Clin Med Case Rep J. 2025;4(1):1–8.

Chapter 35
Techniques of Stellate Ganglion

Sven Soecknick and Guillermo Ospino

1 Introduction

The stellate ganglion block is one of the oldest and most important injections in neural therapy. The reason lies in the widespread linkage of sympathetic nerves to the whole upper part of the body. This means that the sympathetic nervous system supplies the head, neck, shoulder, upper extremities, and chest, along with its internal organs. Consequently, there is a large variety of indications a stellate ganglion block can be used for.

Besides the extraordinary role of the stellate ganglion in segmental neural therapy, the understanding of the autonomic nervous system itself and its influence on immune and inflammatory processes has increased. In this context, the stellate ganglion is also involved in the control of general inflammation processes over feedback loops that come from intestinal vagal or sympathetic signals [1]. Furthermore, autonomic centers in the brain are shown to be under the influence of the stellate ganglion [2].

Due to these findings, the growing interest in stellate ganglion block (hundreds of new publications in the past years) is comprehensible, and the injection is essential in every doctor's neuraltherapeutic practice.

S. Soecknick (✉)
Medical practice Centre for holistic medicine, Lübeck, Germany
e-mail: dr.soecknick@naturmedizin-luebeck.de

G. Ospino
Department of Surgery, Hospital Universitario Nacional, Bogotá, Colombia
e-mail: geospinor@unal.edu.co

L. B. Pinilla Bonilla et al. (eds.), *Neuraltherapeutic Medicine*,
https://doi.org/10.1007/978-3-032-03257-7_35

2 History

In 1936, René Leriche and René Fontaine published the article *L'anesthesie isolee du ganglion etoile: sa technique, ses indications, ses resultats* [3], in which they described the technique used by them during the previous 9 years, treating more than 200 patients for diagnostic and therapeutic purposes. However, the role of the sympathetic nervous system and the interventions that can be made in it for the treatment of multiple conditions began in 1852 with Bernard and Brown-Sequard. At the end of the nineteenth century, resections of the stellate ganglion were performed to treat exophthalmos, glaucoma, and trigeminal neuralgia. Kotzarreff in 1920 reported the use of cervical sympathectomy for the treatment of hyperhidrosis, and in 1921 Jonnesco reported the treatment of angina pectoris with stellate ganglion resection [4].

In 1954, Moore published the book *Stellate Ganglion Block,* in which he described around 20 techniques for performing it, most of them in order to direct the local anesthetic at the level of the transverse process of C7. However, both for ease and for having fewer complications, the approach to the transverse process of C6 has remained the most used technique, whether by anatomical references or with the use of ultrasound [5, 6].

3 Neuroanatomy and Pathophysiology

The sympathetic autonomic nervous system is made up of two ganglion chains that each run anterolateral to the spine, from the base of the skull to the coccyx. On each side there are 3 cervical, 11 or 12 thoracic, 3 or 4 lumbar, and 4 or 5 sacral ganglia, ending in the coccyx with the ganglion impar. Its distribution involves a complex of nerve fibers with interaction in the spinal cord, spinal roots, ganglia, and sympathetic nerves. The cervical sympathetic chain does not receive preganglionic fibers from cervical levels except for the medullary segments C7 to C8 and is made up of three ganglia [4]:

- *Superior ganglion*: located at the level of the vertebral bodies of C2-C3.
- *Middle ganglion*: At the level of the body of C6, the smallest of the cervical chains is inconstant and absent in some individuals.
- *Stellate ganglion*: is mostly a fusion of the inferior ganglion of the cervical sympathetic trunk and the first ganglion of the thoracic sympathetic trunk. It lies embedded by the prevertebral lamina of the cervical fascia, directly anterolateral to the longus colli muscle at the level of the first rib and the transverse process of vertebra seven. In approximately 20%, the two ganglia are not fused, and the inferior cervical ganglion is designated as the stellate ganglion. Anatomical structures of significance around the stellate ganglion are the carotid artery (anteriorly), the subclavian artery (inferiorly), the vertebral artery (anterolaterally), and the esophagus, trachea, and vertebral column (medially) (see Fig. 35.1).

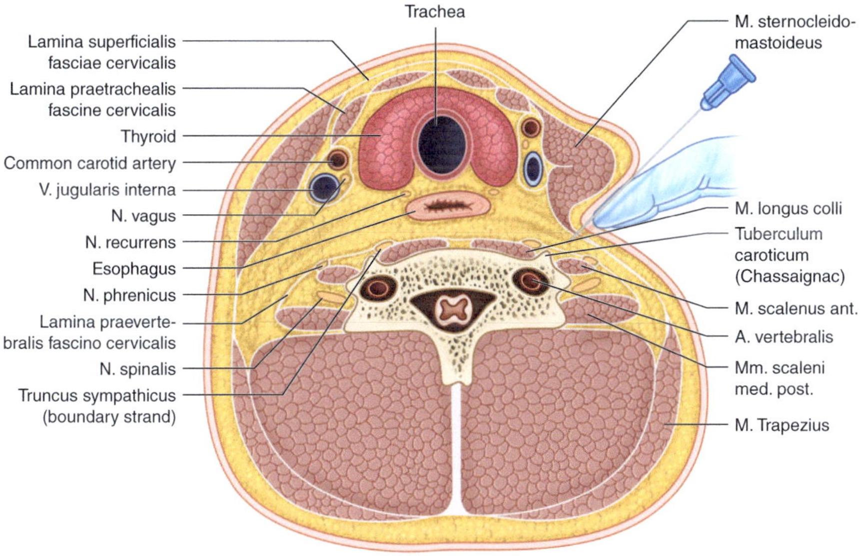

Fig. 35.1 Stellate ganglion block. A cervical cross-section at the level of vertebra C6

The efferent sympathetic input of the stellate ganglion occurs from the intermediolateral nucleus of the spinal segments C7-Th5. As the stellate ganglion switches from the first to the second sympathetic neuron, different diversifications of the phrenic nerve, vagus nerve, laryngeal recurrent nerve, vascular rami, and visceral rami exist. In this way, the stellate ganglion is connected to nearly all structures of the upper half of the body, like the lung, heart, esophagus, thyroid, parathyroid, and thymus. Junctions to the brachial plexus and intercostal nerves ensure the influence on the upper extremity and osteal thorax. The subclavian artery, the vertebral artery, the inferior thyroid artery, and the thoracic internal artery are all affected by treatment of the stellate ganglion through their vascular branches. More peripheral connections over the cardiac plexus also exist to parasympathetic fibers that come from the vagus nerve. In this way, the sympathetic and parasympathetic modulation of the heart is ensured [4].

In the neck, the paravertebral muscles longus capitis, rectus capitis, and longus colli are covered in their anterior part by the prevertebral cervical fascia that extends from the base of the skull to the T4 vertebra. The cervical sympathetic chain then runs along the frontolateral surface of the prevertebral muscles. The fascia and the frontolateral surface of the prevertebral muscles are connected by a space called the interfascial, which lets the local anesthetic that was applied there spread [7].

4 Applications for Stellate Ganglion Block Assorted by Anatomical Region

All named indications can just be examples for the possible treatment of the particular region. According to the basic neuraltherapeutic treatment principles, the success of stellate ganglion block for each indication depends on the individual influences of neuromodulatory triggers in every single patient. After a good clinical assessment and, preferably, after evaluation of dominances, after reduction of irritating loads (see Chap. 25), this could be a treatment to be used in several cases:

1. Disorders of shoulder and arm.
2. Disorders of neck and organs.
3. Disorders of the head.
4. Diseases of thorax and organs.

4.1 Non-segmental

The stellate ganglion is normally used for the neuraltherapeutic influence of the ipsilateral part of the upper body. But modern neurophysiology no longer recognizes segmental boundaries [8]. Therefore, the stellate ganglion plays an increasing role in treating non-segmental diseases. Two of the five most common conditions in which good results have been obtained with this technique are the next [9]:

- Long COVID-19 syndrome [9]
- Breast cancer patients [10]
- Post-perimenopausal symptoms like hot flashes [11]
- Post-traumatic stress disorder (PTBS) [11]
- Chronic fatigue syndrome (CFS).
- Sleep disturbance.
- Hyperinflammation (viral/bacterial) [1]

A bibliometric analysis of stellate ganglion block in the medical literature showed that it is a globally used technique, and the areas of greatest interest are focused on the treatment of arrhythmias, "breast cancer and climacteric medicine, post-traumatic stress disorder, pain management, cerebrovascular diseases, and long COVID syndrome"[12].

5 Contraindications

Anticoagulation (coumarinics, Non-Vitamin K Antagonist Oral Anticoagulants).
Severe heart diseases.

Atrioventricular block 3rd°.
Heart failure NYHA III—IV.
Bradycardia.
Massive lung emphysema due to danger of pneumothorax.
Paresis of the phrenic or laryngeal recurrence nerve at the contralateral side.

6 Injection

Since Leriche and Fontaine described her technique in 1934 [3], different other techniques were described. Reischauer published a dorsal technique at the sixth cervical vertebra. Herget found a technique from the ventral-medial of the sterno-cleidomastoid muscle in 1943 [13]. To reduce complications, in later decades several modifications were made.

The most commonly used approaches that correspond to the lateral technique from Leriche and Fontaine and the paratracheal technique are described. Acquaintance with each technique is crucial for its integration into therapeutic practice. Both approaches, properly performed, are safe and relatively easy to practice.

6.1 Technique According to Leriche and Fontaine

An upright position with a stabilized head is possible; much better is a lying position with a small pillow, if preferred. To get a better feel for Chassaignac's tubercle (the anterior tubercle of the transverse process of the sixth cervical vertebra), the head must be held in a neutral position at first (Fig. 35.2). This position keeps the sternocleidomastoid muscle from tensing up.

To find the correct level of height at the cervical spine, the sternocleidomastoid muscle is divided into three parts. Position the second and third fingers between the lower and middle parts at the dorsal rear edge of the muscle to exert a ventral force. With this maneuver, the neurovascular bundle (common carotid artery, vagus nerve, and internal jugular vein) can be shifted medially away from the injection zone. Now the head is turned about 45° to the contralateral side and slightly hyperextended, while the middle fingers stay constant during the whole palpation and injection process on Chassaignac's tubercle. The point of injection lies one millimeter craniomedial of the middle finger. The direction of injection is 45° medial and dorsal. In 1–2 cm, soft bone contact to Chassaignac's tubercle has to be found. After a double-negative aspiration in two planes for blood and cerebrospinal fluid, a test injection of 0.2 ml is applied. If no negative reactions occur, slowly inject 3–5 mL of 1% procaine [3].

After the injection, the patient should sit up to let the procaine diffuse caudally at the fascia of the longus colli muscle to the stellate ganglion. A mild massage with a swab can accelerate this process.

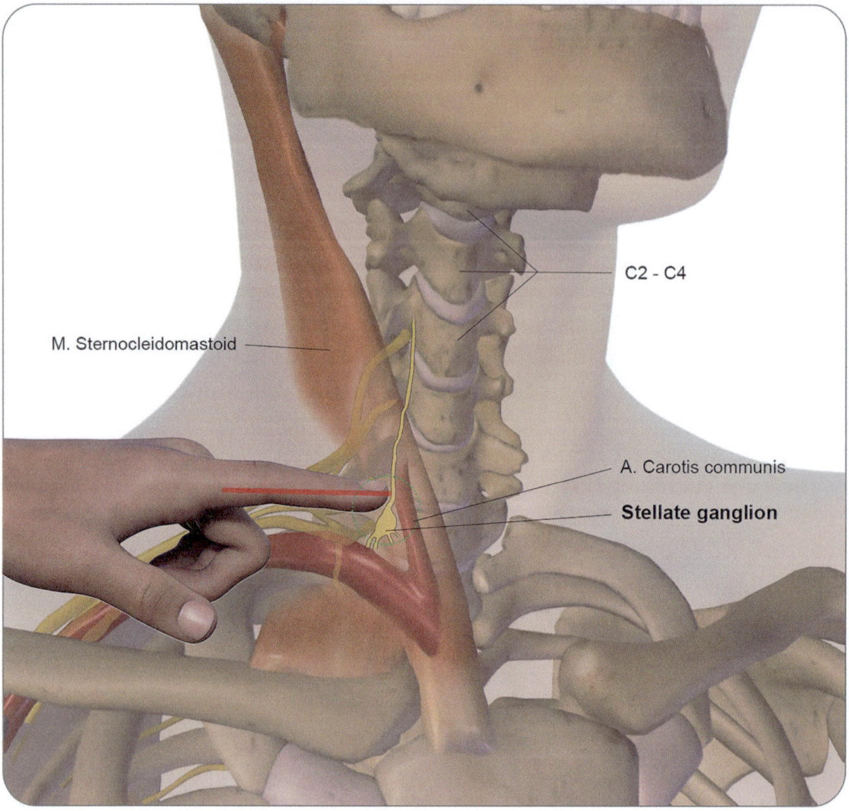

Fig. 35.2 The figure shows the location of the stellate ganglion in the prevertebral area of C6-C7. Furthermore, the figure shows the anatomical relation with other structures such as the sternocleidomastoid muscle, carotid artery, and subclavian artery

6.2 Paratracheal Technique

The advantages described with this technique include greater ease and avoiding making pleural or vertebral artery punctures less likely. Once the patient has been informed of the technique and the side effects, auscultation of the carotid arteries is carried out, and the existence of a carotid murmur contraindicates the procedure.

Place a support under the shoulders and allow the patient in the supine position to slightly extend their neck. Ask the patient to slightly open their mouth, but refrain from swallowing or speaking. With aseptic technique, the cricoid cartilage is located since, at the posterolateral level of the trachea, there will be the transverse process of C6, or the tubercle of Chassaignac. With the non-dominant hand, the carotid pulse is found, and the index finger is used to separate the carotid artery from the internal jugular vein in the middle. To achieve this, use the middle finger to feel the transverse process of C6 as a prominence between the trachea and the blood vessels.

The trachea needs to be slightly separated from the injection site. A needle with a diameter of 27 G and a length of 3–4 cm is introduced perpendicularly into the space created between the two fingers until it contacts the transverse process, and then it is slightly withdrawn to position the tip in the interfascial space (See Fig. 35.3).

Always aspirate at least twice, having rotated the needle 180° to rule out aspiration of blood or cerebrospinal fluid, and proceed to the injection of an aliquot of 0.5 ml of procaine. Thereafter, to really rule out the inadvertent administration of subarachnoid or intravascular, be sure that the patient does not present symptoms, and then the administration of the total dose of procaine (4 to 5 ml at 0.5 or 1%) could be completed. The diffusion of the anesthetic improves with a light massage [6].

Bilateral procedures will not be performed because of the potential for respiratory failure resulting from a block of the phrenic nerve and the recurrent laryngeal nerve.

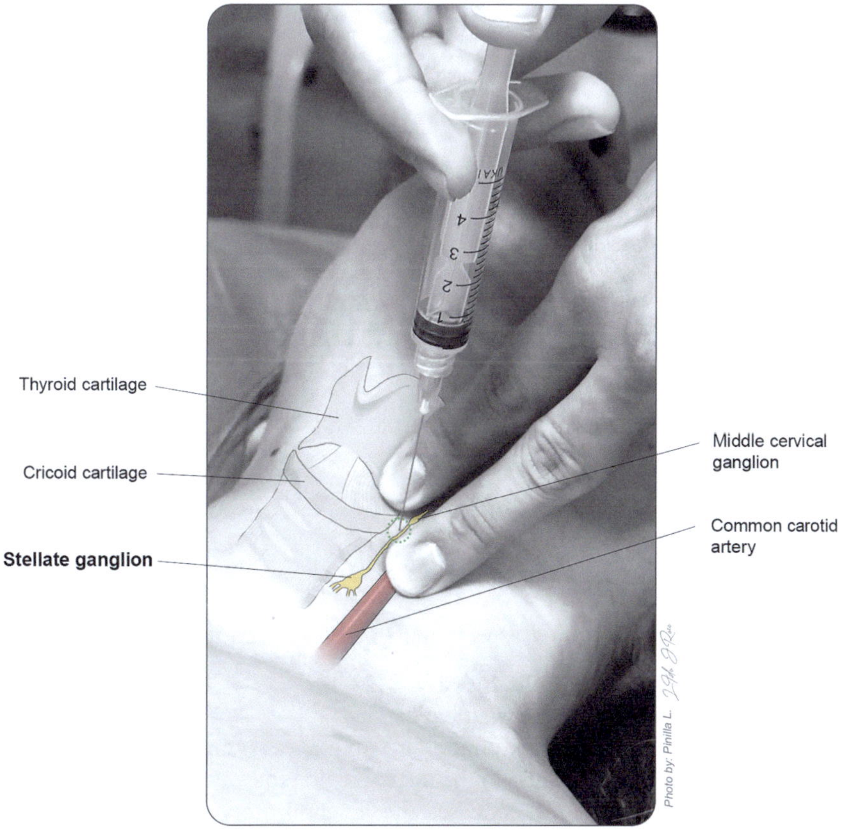

Fig. 35.3 Paratracheal technique to reach the vicinity of the stellate ganglion

6.3 Material

syringe 5 ml,
Needle 0.4 × 20 mm (27G × 1½ inches).
Procaine 1% 3–5 ml.

7 Effects of Stellate Ganglion Block Injection [10, 14]

Horner's Syndrome complex (Miosis, Ptosis, Enophthalmus).
Ipsilateral nostril swelling (Guttman's sign).
Initially mild circulation and pulse depression.
Mild dizziness.
Increasing degree of small conjunctival vessel.
Warmness of ipsilateral Head, arm, or chest.

8 After Injection

Let the patient sit up.
Verbal Monitoring.
Measurement of blood pressure and oxygen saturation.

9 Complications and How to Avoid Them

Among the various complications described by some authors are the following [15]:

- Pneumothorax.
- Total spinal anesthesia.
- Severe hypertension.
- Intrathecal injection.
- Generalized seizures.

Nevertheless, the following aspects must be considered to avoid wrong injections and complications:

- Take enough time for palpation and injection.
- Thoroughly double negative aspiration in two planes (syringe turned in 180°).
- While the carotid artery shifts to the medial region, the vertebral artery remains in close proximity. (In 5–10% of cases, the vertebral artery crosses sixth Cervical vertebra and not seventh Cervical vertebra.)
- Be careful not only of blood but also of liquid aspiration. (No injection!)

- Always do a small test application of 0.2 ml procaine. If any kind of misbehavior, dizziness, or other symptoms happen, do not inject.
- The patient must receive a slow and controlled injection under continual verbal monitoring.
- Too dorsal point of injection and too medialized direction of the needle increase the risk of a cerebrospinal puncture or hitting the intervertebral foramen.
- If too many local anesthetics are used or, in the case of too medial injection, a laryngeal recurrent nerve or phrenic nerve can be reached. Hoarseness or phrenic nerve paralysis may occur for a brief period. Due to the short time of anesthesia of procaine, both effects are harmless, but patients have to be monitored until the end of the anesthetic effect.
- If the point of injection is too caudal or, in the case of extreme lung emphysema, a pneumothorax is possible.

10 Red Flags

Based on some author's experience, with over 3000 documented stellate ganglion blocks and literature [16], the described lateral technique is considered a very safe method. A systematic review, with different techniques and different materials used, found very rare complications such as bleeding, hemorrhagic shock, or convulsion in rates from 1.7/1000 overall [15].

Reasons were identified to be based on the technique itself (blind technique, fluoroscopic technique, ultrasound-guided technique), whereas no technique had any evident advantage.

Other authors, like Hahn Godefroy, found in a retrospective analysis of stellate ganglion block with procaine much lower complication rates from 1/10,000. The much lower fat solubility, the short anesthetic time of procainc, and the use of the lateral technique might be the reasons for the much lower rates of complications in stellate ganglion blocks, as described by other authors.

11 Ultrasound-Guided Technique

For several years, more and more studies with ultrasound-guided stellate ganglion blocks have been published. The description of several different access paths suggests that the correct injection technique may not yet exist [17].

The decision, if ultrasound guidance in stellate ganglion block is a real advantage in neural therapy, is actually in progress. This combined use usually has higher costs due to the learning curve, but suggests more safety and avoidance of complications. Doctors have to be taught ultrasound techniques next to neural therapy; however, ultrasound isn't available at every doctor's practice. These could be reasons for restricted access to sufficient neural therapy. Until studies have not shown safer or more successful evidence in ultrasound technique, the proven procedure should be maintained.

References

1. Fischer L, Barop H, Ludin SM, Schaible HG. Regulation of acute reflectory hyperinflammation in viral and other diseases by means of stellate ganglion block. A conceptual view with a focus on Covid-19. Auton Neurosci. 2022;237:102903.
2. Westerhaus MJ, Loewy AD. Central representation of the sympathetic nervous system in the cerebral cortex. Brain Res. 2001;903(1–2):117–27.
3. Leriche R, Fontaine R. Isolated anesthesia of the stellate ganglion: its technique, indications, and results. Presse Méd. 1934;42(849):200.
4. Acevedo J, Berbeo M, Diaz R, Feo O. Anatomy of the stellate ganglion. Pain. 2007;2(1):1–18.
5. Carron H, Litwiller R. Stellate ganglion block. Anesth Analg. 1975;54(5):567–70.
6. Angel AM. Stellate ganglion block in pain management. Rev Col Anest. 2007;35(3):227–32.
7. Gofeld M, Bhatia A, Abbas S, Ganapathy S, Johnson M. Development and validation of a new technique for ultrasound-guided stellate ganglion block. Reg Anesth Pain Med. 2009;34(5):475–9.
8. Engel R, Barop H, Giebel J, Ludin SM, Fischer L. The influence of modern neurophysiology on the previous definitions of "segment" and "interference field" in neural therapy. Complement Med Res. 2022;29(3):257–67.
9. Duricka D, Liu L. Reduction of long COVID symptoms after stellate ganglion block: a retrospective chart review study. Auton Neurosci. 2024;254:103195.
10. Soecknick S. Stellate ganglion block with procaine in breast cancer survivors with hot flashes and sleep disturbances undergoing endocrine therapy. Medicine (Baltimore). 2024;103(2):e36848.
11. Lipov EG, Lipov S, Joshi JR, Santucci VD, Slavin KV, Vigue SB. Stellate ganglion block may relieve hot flashes by interrupting the sympathetic nervous system. Med Hypotheses. 2007;69(4):758–63.
12. Ren Y, Zhang Z, Li H-P, Zhang P-J, Duo J, Kong H. A comprehensive overview of the stellate ganglion block throughout the past three decades: a bibliometric analysis. Pain Physician. 2024;27:e597–610.
13. Herget R. A simple technique for temporarily blocking the stellate ganglion. Chirurg. 1943;15:680–2.
14. de la Vega Costa KP, Perez MAG, Roqueta C, et al. Effects on hemodynamic variables and echocardiographic parameters after a stellate ganglion block in 15 healthy volunteers. Auton Neurosci. 2016;197:46–55.
15. Goel V, Patwardhan AM, Ibrahim M, Howe CL, Schultz DM, Shankar H. Complications associated with stellate ganglion nerve block: a systematic review. Reg Anesth Pain Med. 2019;44(6):669–78.
16. Hahn-Godeffroy JD. Injection into the stellate ganglion. In: Neural therapy according to Huneke: Freudenstädter lectures, vol. 12; 1988. p. 73–92.
17. Kim H, Song SO, Jung G. A lateral Paracarotid approach for ultrasound-guided stellate ganglion block with a linear probe. J Anesth. 2017;31:458–62.

Chapter 36
The Thoracic Spine

Hüseyin Nazlikul and Fatma Gülçin Ural Nazlikul

1 Injections in the Thoracic Spine

The thoracic spine is the longest section of our spine and consists of 12 similarly shaped vertebrae and the intervertebral discs between them. It serves as the connecting link between the cervical and lumbar spine, making it the longest supporting element of our trunk. In its connection function to the cervical spine, the first 3 to 4 thoracic vertebrae participate in the rotational, flexion, and lateral bending movements of the cervical spine, decreasing from cranial to caudal. We have already referred to the fourth thoracic vertebra as the kinesiological pivot point of the cervical spine (see Fig. 36.1) [1, 3].

1.1 Thoracic Vertebra

It is easily recognized by the rib facets on both sides of the body and the transverse process [1]. The 12 vertebrae that extend from the base of the neck to the last point where the ribs meet the spine are referred to as the thoracic vertebrae. These

H. Nazlikul (✉)
International Federation of Medical Associations of Neural Therapy – IFMANT, Schattenhalb, Switzerland

Nazlikul Naturel Foundation for the Development of Healthy Habitats, Istanbul, Turkey

Faculty of Medicine, Department of Biophysics, Istanbul University of Health and Technology, Istanbul, Turkey
e-mail: hnazlikul@web.de

F. G. U. Nazlikul
Faculty of Medicine, Physical Medicine and Rehabilitation, Istanbul Health and Technology University, Istanbul, Turkey
e-mail: fatma.nazlikul@istun.edu.tr

L. B. Pinilla Bonilla et al. (eds.), *Neuraltherapeutic Medicine*,
https://doi.org/10.1007/978-3-032-03257-7_36

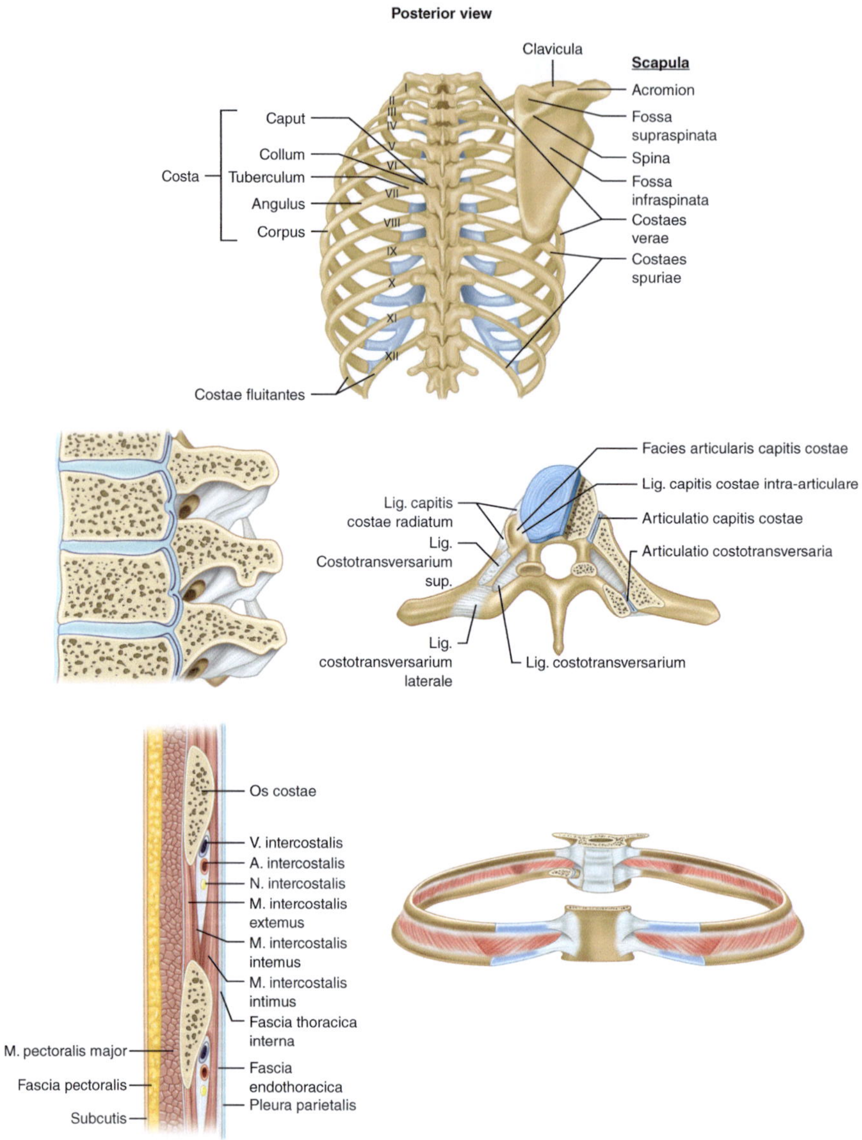

Fig. 36.1 The image illustrates the detailed anatomy of the thoracic region, focusing on the rib cage and its associated structures. Top Section: Shows the posterior view of the rib cage, including the thoracic vertebrae, ribs, and associated landmarks such as the clavicle, scapula, and various parts of the ribs (caput, collum, tuberculum, and angulus). It highlights the articulation of the ribs with the thoracic vertebrae and the structural connections with the scapula and clavicle. Middle Section: Provides a close-up of the thoracic vertebrae, demonstrating the intervertebral discs and the ligaments that stabilize the rib-vertebrae connections, including the ligamentum costotransversarium and ligamentum capitis costae. Bottom Left Section: Highlights the muscles of the thoracic wall, such as the pectoralis major, and the relationship between the ribs and the intercostal muscles.

vertebrae control the motor and sensory innervation of the trunk. When this area is damaged, it can lead to paralysis of the trunk and areas below, resulting in loss of control over the legs, genital organs, and sexual functions, leading to paraplegia [1, 2].

1.2 *Mobility of the Thoracic Spine*

The thoracic spine, with its mobility, serves two different movement systems: first, the trunk as part of the movement apparatus with the shoulder girdle at the cranial end and the pelvic girdle at the caudal end; second, the thorax as the external, mechanically functioning respiratory apparatus. During maximum inspiration, the kyphosis of the thoracic spine is increased, whereas it is flattened during maximum expiration [1].

In its function as part of the musculoskeletal system, the thoracic spine passively participates in the movements of the neighboring sections of the cervical and lumbar spine in its upper and lower regions, respectively, decreasing with increasing distance from these neighboring sections. The 12 thoracic vertebrae differ significantly in structure and function from the other vertebrae.

The caudally oriented spinous processes are located at the level of the next lower thoracic vertebra. This must be considered when examining other vertebral segments and their segmental connections [2]. The articulated connection of the ribs to the vertebrae and spinous processes, as well as the resulting changes in spinal movement, must be taken into account, especially in relation to rotational movements (see Fig. 36.1) [2, 3].

The segmental distribution of the nervous system is most apparent in the thoracic spine. The course of the ribs also includes both afferent-efferent somatic and afferent-efferent sympathetic nerve distributions. The association of the thoracic and abdominal organs with sympathetic innervation to the corresponding thoracic vertebral segments can be utilized for diagnostic and therapeutic purposes (see Figs. 36.2 and 36.3) [3].

Pathological stimuli originating from various regions are reflexively relayed to the axial organ via the ANS. Since this pathway has a bidirectional effect from the center to the periphery and from the periphery to the center, it is possible to interrupt the corresponding pathological stimulus and treat diseases by administering certain injections through the axial organ during treatment [3].

Fig. 36.1 (continued) It also emphasizes the fascial layers, including the fascia endothoracica and pleura parietalis. This comprehensive illustration provides an in-depth view of the structural and functional relationships within the thoracic cage, essential for understanding respiratory mechanics, rib movement, and thoracic stability. Bottom Right Section: Displays a detailed view of the sternocostal joints, where the ribs connect to the sternum. This section also shows the costal cartilages and the surrounding musculature, including the intercostal muscles. (Source: Own elaboration)

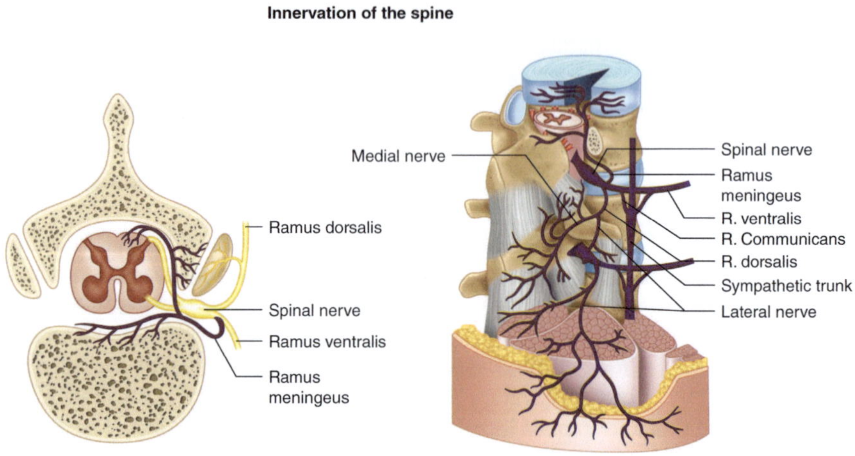

Fig. 36.2 The image illustrates the innervation of the spine and depicts the nerve supply to the vertebral bodies. It shows the various nerve branches emerging from the spinal nerves, including the dorsal ramus, ventral ramus, and meningeal ramus. These nerve branches are responsible for the sensory and motor innervation of the spinal structures. On the left side of the image, there is a cross-section of a vertebra that displays the position of the nerves relative to the spine. On the right side, a more detailed depiction of the nerve pathways along the spine and the adjacent structures, such as the sympathetic trunk and the filamenta, is presented. These anatomical details highlight the functional connections between the nervous system and the spine, which are crucial for movement coordination and sensory perception of the trunk. (Source: Own elaboration)

1.3 Palpation Is Crucial for Diagnosing Thoracic Spine Dysfunctions

1.3.1 Kibler's Skin Fold

Reduced mobility is a possible sign of sympathetic system activation. In cases of chronic dysfunctions, there is increased local skin tension (turgor), with the skin fold becoming thickened and less easily lifted, and local dermographism as an indication of local autonomic dysregulation; this is often accompanied by local hyperalgesia (peripheral sensitization) [4].

1.3.2 Superficial Palpation

Pressure tenderness of the periosteum and ligamentous attachments at the spinous processes, as well as local or regional increases in muscle tone and myofascial trigger points of the paraspinal muscles (e.g., the longissimus system) [4, 5].

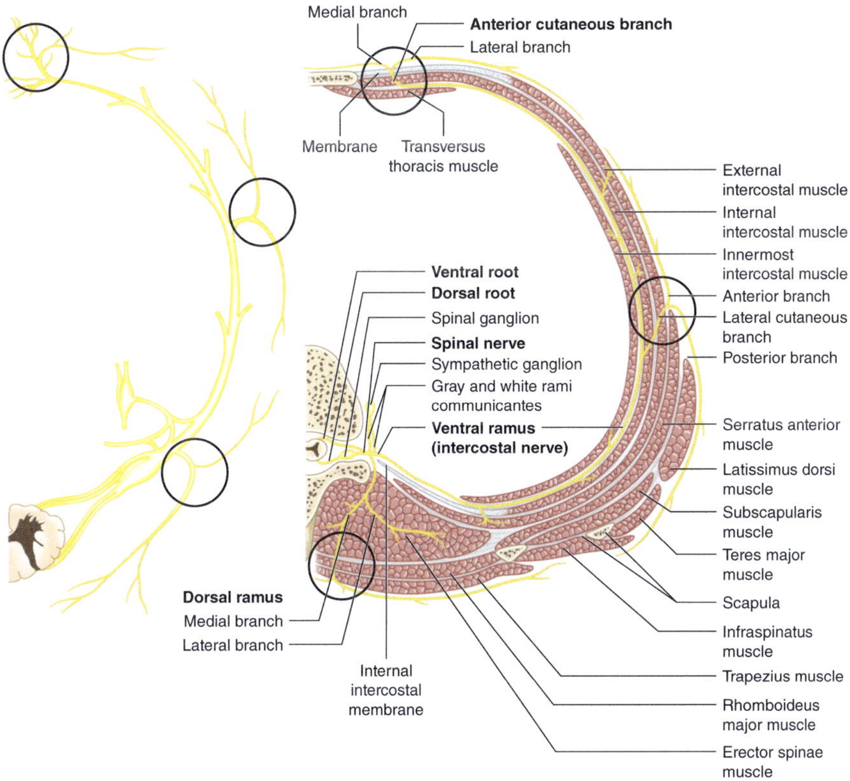

Fig. 36.3 The image presents a schematic depiction of the nerve-vessel bundle entry points along the spine and ribs. These points are located anteriorly, laterally, and sometimes posteriorly on the body and are of diagnostic significance, as they can become hardened and extremely painful in cases of viscerosomatic irritation. Palpation Opportunities: These entry points can be located through palpation, particularly when a hardened, granular texture and tenderness are detected. Palpation of these points can assist in diagnosing viscerosomatic dysfunctions, as the pain often indicates deeper visceral or somatic irritation. Injection Opportunities: For therapeutic purposes, targeted injections can be administered at these points. These injections, often containing local anesthetics or neuraltherapeutic agents, can help alleviate the irritation and restore the function of the affected nerves and tissues. The injections should be precisely administered along the marked entry points to achieve optimal efficacy and symptom relief. (Source: Own elaboration)

1.3.3 Superficial and Deep Palpation

Palpation of paraspinal tissues, bony landmarks, and particularly various muscle tracts and groups to detect regional changes in muscle tone and focal, usually facet joint-adjacent, costotransverse joint-adjacent, and on the costal angle, pressure-sensitive indurations ("irritation zones") (see Fig. 36.4) [4, 5].

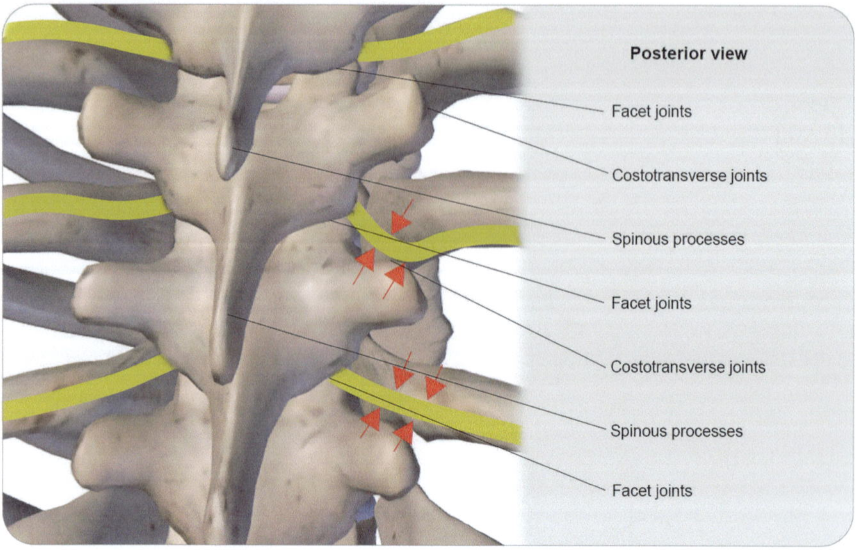

Fig. 36.4 The image provides a schematic representation of the thoracic spine, with a particular focus on the facet joints, costotransverse joints, and the spinous processes of the thoracic vertebrae (T-spine). The red arrows highlight specific points that are significant for diagnosing and treating dysfunctions in these joints. Facet joints are the articulations between the vertebrae that play a crucial role in the mobility of the spine. Costotransverse joints connect the ribs to the transverse processes of the vertebrae, contributing to the stability of the thoracic cage. Spinous processes are bony protrusions that serve as attachment points for muscles and ligaments, playing an important role in the movement and stability of the spine. Identifying and treating these structures is a central aspect of neural therapy, particularly in managing pain and movement restrictions in the thoracic region. (Source: Own elaboration)

1.3.4 Paraspinal Palpation

Directly paraspinal in depth. Focal, facet joint-adjacent, and usually pressure-sensitive increases in tone of the medial deep tract of the erector spinae (rotatores and multifidi muscles). Differentiation between focal muscular irritation due to a movement segment dysfunction and an activated facet joint or another deep-seated pathology is not possible [4, 5].

1.3.5 Palpation of the Transverse Process Region

Coming slightly from the lateral side along the rib, the longissimus system is pushed medially, allowing the palpating finger to reach the dorsal transverse process region. Painful palpation findings are often detected here in cases of dysfunction (see Fig. 36.4).

1.3.6 Palpation of the Costal Angle

In rib joint dysfunction, a local myofascial tone change is found here, which can reflexively be associated with the longissimus and iliocostalis systems with muscle attachments at the costal angle [4, 5].

1.4 Indications [6, 7]

- Painful restriction of movement following cervical spine (CSP), thoracic spine (TSP), and rib trauma.
- Rib fracture.
- Vertebral body fracture.
- Intercostal neuralgia.
- Herpes zoster.
- Thoracic blockade.
- Myotendinosis, spondylodiscitis.
- Reflexive and segmental dysfunctions that occur with the following and adjacent diseases:
  - Stomach (Th6-Th9).
  - Small intestine (Th7-L1).
  - Large intestine (Th7-L1).
  - Kidneys (Th10-L1).
  - Urogenital system (Th10-L2).
  - Heart (Th1-Th5).
  - Bronchi and lungs (Th1-Th4).
  - Pancreas (Th6-Th10).
  - Liver and gallbladder (Th6-Th9).
- In cases where the thorax is considered a disturbance field.

1.5 Neurological Relations: Sympathetic Nervous System [6]

- Th1-Th4: Head + Thorax.
- Th5-Th9: Celiac ganglion (Ggl. coeliacum).
- Th10-Th11: Superior mesenteric ganglion (Ggl. mesentericum sup.)
- Th12-L2: Inferior mesenteric ganglion (Ggl. mesentericum inf.)
- Th2-Th8: Arms.
- Th12-L2: Legs.

2 Injection into Spinous Processes

The tips of the spinous processes are palpated with the upper part of the trunk slightly inclined forward. A 4 cm long needle is advanced perpendicularly to the skin until bone contact is made. After slightly withdrawing the needle and advancing it cranially at a 45° angle, 0.3–0.5 ml of procaine solution is injected. In a depth of 1.5 cm, 1 ml of procaine solution is also infiltrated into the supraspinous ligament and interspinous ligament [6–8].

- *Injection site*: Spinous process.
- Injection direction: After contacting the sagittal plane of the spinous process, the local anesthetic (LA) is injected. The needle is then withdrawn and advanced cranially.
- *Injection depth*: 1–2.5 cm.
- Materials and LA used: 40 × 0.4 mm needle.
- *Amount of local anesthetic* to be used: 0.5–1 ml of 1% procaine/lidocaine.

3 Injection into the Facet Joints of the Thoracic Spine

One finger lateral to the spinous process line, at the level of the midpoint between two adjacent spinous processes, lies the facet joint (see Fig. 36.5) (except in the lower thoracic spine region, where it is located beside the midpoint of the spinous process). Due to individual anatomical variations, these guidelines are only generally indicative [6–8].

4 Injection into the Facet Joints

- *Injection site*: Two posterior spinous processes (PS), 2 cm lateral to the sacroiliac joint (SI).
- Injection direction: Sagittal.
- Injection depth: 2.5–3.5 cm (until bone contact).
- Materials and LA used: 40 × 0.4 mm needle, 0.5 ml of procaine or lidocaine.

5 Injection in the Area of the Costotransverse Joints

The joints are typically located a few millimeters below the intervertebral joints, slightly lateral (2–2½ fingers lateral to the spinous process line). Due to anatomical variations, a completely reliable description is not possible [6–8].

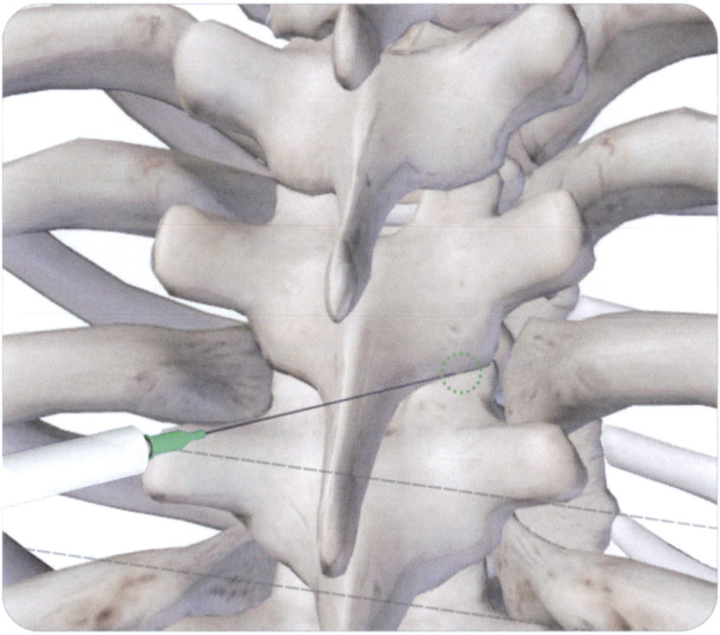

Fig. 36.5 The image depicts an injection technique targeting the facet joints of the spine. The needle is inserted laterally to the spinous process line, directed toward the facet joint. This technique is used to inject local anesthetics into the joint, which helps alleviate pain and improve mobility in cases of facet joint syndrome. (Source: Own elaboration)

The intervertebral joints of the thoracic vertebrae are located approximately 3 cm lateral to the vertical line formed by the spinous processes, aligned with the end of the spinous process of the vertebra above (see Fig. 36.6). The needle insertion is done perpendicular to the skin [9, 10].

- *Injection site*: A few millimeters below the two posterior spinous processes (PS/SP), 3 cm lateral to the sacroiliac joint (SI). Approximately from the SP line to 2 fingers paramedian.
- *Injection direction*: Sagittal only.
- *Injection depth*: 3–3.5 cm (until bone contact). The artery, vein, and costal nerve are located at the cranial edges of the lower rib sections.
- *Materials and LA used*: 40 × 0.4 mm needle, 0.5 ml of procaine or lidocaine.

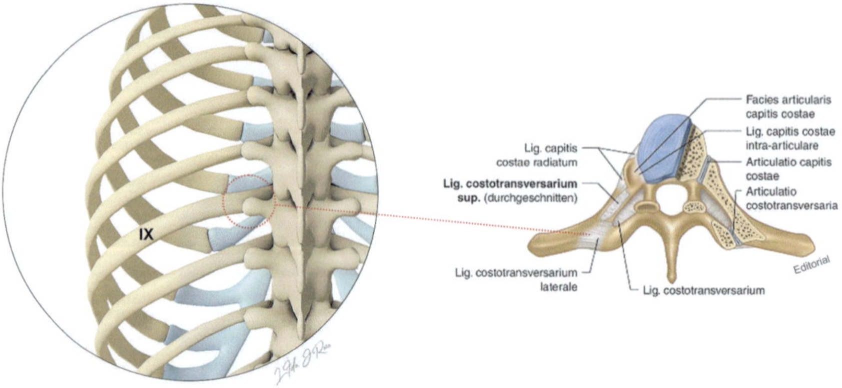

Fig. 36.6 The image provides a schematic representation of the costotransverse joint, which connects the rib to the transverse process of the thoracic vertebra. The arrows indicate the positions for targeted injections into the costotransverse joint, aimed at alleviating pain and improving mobility in this area. (Source: Own elaboration)

6 Injection Around the Intercostal Nerves

6.1 Mobility of the Ribs

During respiratory excursions, the lower ribs follow the upper ones during inspiration, and conversely, the upper ribs follow the lower ones during expiration. It becomes clear that a rib with restricted mobility can create a movement obstruction for the neighboring ribs, thereby potentially causing functional disturbances in entire sections of the thorax.

The tip of the spinous processes is palpated (see Fig. 36.7). The needle is advanced 3–4 cm laterally, perpendicular to the skin, in a slightly cranial direction (approximately 5°). At a depth of 3–3.5 cm (2.5–3 cm in very thin patients), the needle reaches the rib. The needle is then slightly withdrawn, and the tip is slightly lowered, then advanced again to a depth of 0.5 cm. At this point, the lower edge of the rib should be palpated. After two aspiration attempts, 1–2 ml of procaine solution is infiltrated [7, 11].

- *Position*: Lying on the side, with the hand under the head.
- *Injection site*: Angulus costae at the posterior axillary line.
- *Injection direction*: With the arm abducted at a 90-degree angle, insert the needle perpendicular to the rib arch. Once bone contact is felt, slightly withdraw the needle by approximately 1 mm, and push the skin and needle downward. The needle is then advanced perpendicular to the rib until bone contact is felt again. After making contact with the bone, withdraw the needle by about 1 mm, and move the skin with the needle downward toward the lower edge of the rib.
- *Injection depth*: Advance the needle about 3 mm (no deeper due to the risk of pneumothorax), and perform the injection at this point.

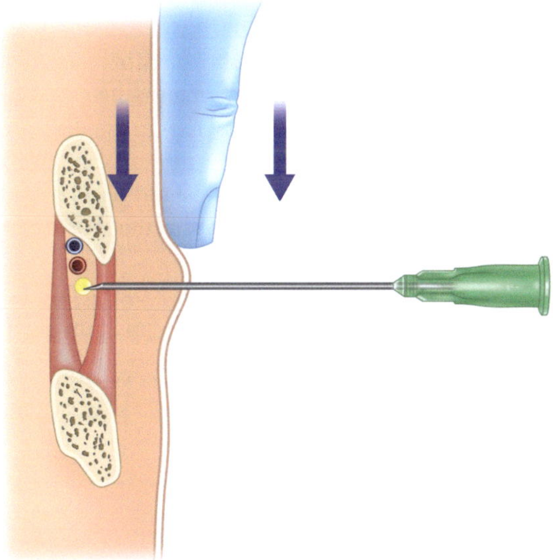

Fig. 36.7 The image illustrates the injection technique targeting the intercostal nerves. The needle is inserted at a specific angle below the rib to reach the intercostal nerve. This technique is used to administer local anesthetics, which can help alleviate pain and improve the function of the affected rib area. (Source: Own elaboration)

- *Materials and LA used*: 40 × 0.4 mm needle, 0.2–0.5 ml of procaine or lidocaine.

Caution—Pneumothorax!: Insert the needle perpendicular to the rib. After making bone contact, withdraw the needle by 1 mm. Press the skin under the rib with your finger. Without changing the direction of the needle, do not insert it more than 3 mm into the skin.

7 Chronic Syndromes Resulting from Thoracic Blockages

The influence of the autonomic nervous system plays a significant role in thoracic blockages. Any restriction in movement during inhalation and exhalation or within the thorax can cause discomfort. All syndromes that worsen while lying down have their origin in the spine. Any stimulus that exceeds the threshold leads to increased tension and heightened sensitivity to additional stimuli in the corresponding segmental musculature.

Chronic syndromes caused by thoracic blockages (first described by the author H. Nazlikul in 2008) can be improved by targeted influence on the autonomic nervous system through neural therapy [12, 13].

Chronic diseases, in particular, are an expression of disrupted self-regulation. Chronicity is a cybernetic problem of irregularly interconnected regulatory circuits. The body operates inefficiently as a whole. Eventually, regulatory capacities become exhausted, and reactivity, in the sense of an adaptation syndrome, weakens according to Selye [13].

Thoracic blockages are areas of irritation that influence the entire organism. A thoracic blockage is characterized by tenderness to pressure, tension, swelling of the connective tissue, and possibly painful restricted mobility [14, 15, 17].

In the case of a prolonged disturbance, hard tension formation occurs. The impact of an irritation of the spinal nerve root in the dermatome, myotome, and sclerotome can be demonstrated particularly through altered sensitivity and motor function. Any stimulus that exceeds the threshold leads to increased tension and heightened sensitivity to additional stimuli in the corresponding segmental musculature [13–16].

As described by H. Nazlikul in his thesis on thoracic blockages [13], Fig. 36.8 centers around the concept of nociception, which arises from joint disorders.

- *Nociception*: Nociception is the process through which pain signals are transmitted to the nervous system, initiating a series of responses.

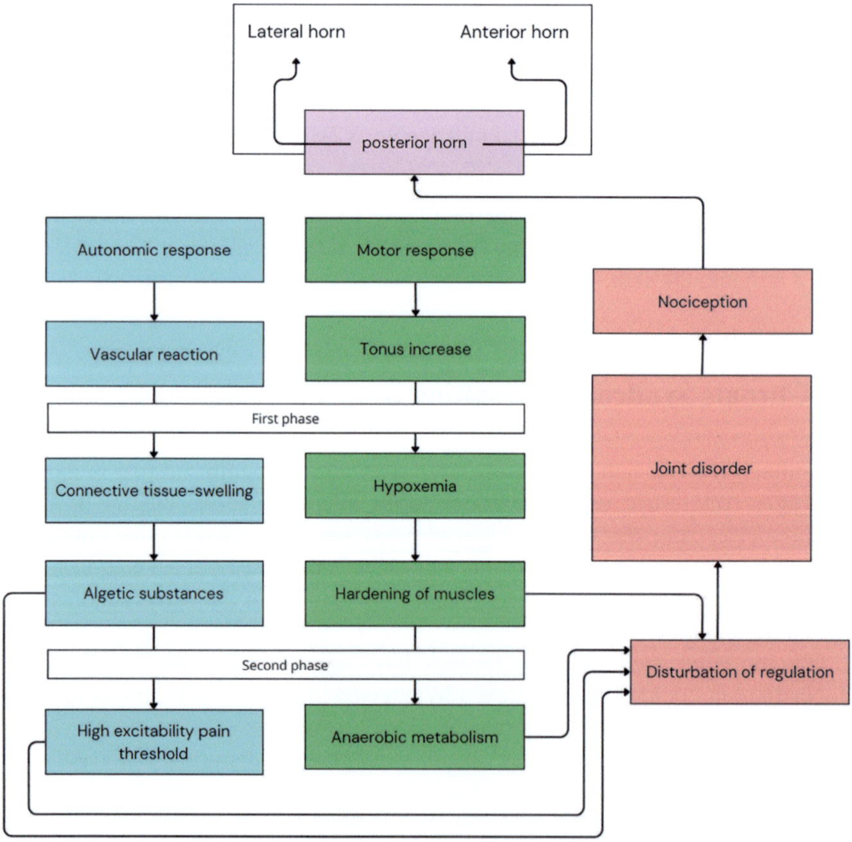

Fig. 36.8 Motor and vegetative nociceptive reactions in joint disorders and the associated progressive regulatory derailment. (Source: Own elaboration)

- *Vegetative response*: On the left side of the diagram, the nociceptive signal is processed through the vegetative (autonomic) nervous system, leading to a vascular reaction. This reaction triggers the first phase, resulting in connective tissue swelling. As this process advances, algogenic substances (pain-producing substances) are released, leading to high excitability and a low pain threshold during the second phase.
- *Motor response*: On the right side, the motor response is activated by the nociceptive signal. This results in increased muscle tone (tonus elevation), initiating the first phase characterized by hypoxemia (low oxygen levels in the tissues). Prolonged hypoxemia leads to hard tension in the muscles, followed by anaerobic metabolism during the second phase.
- *Regulatory derailment*: At the center of the diagram, joint disorder is depicted as the initial cause of regulatory dysfunction. This dysfunction leads to progressive regulatory derailment, affecting both the vegetative and motor responses. The interconnections between these systems create a feedback loop that perpetuates the cycle of pain and dysfunction. This diagram, is used to support the thesis that thoracic blockages contribute significantly to chronic syndromes through complex interactions within the autonomic and motor systems, ultimately leading to widespread regulatory failure.

There is also a connection with unphysiological stress, unfavorable postural patterns, organic injuries or disease consequences, as well as degenerative, inflammatory, or even neoplastic processes. Irritation zones, hereinafter also referred to as interference fields, can focus on a trigger or acupuncture point. These can typically be treated with neural therapy.

Muscles interact with each other and influence motor function in a complex chain reaction. Pathological processes affect the entire chain. The resulting muscular imbalance or irritation disrupts the joint apparatus. The arthromuscular regulatory circuit degenerates in the sense of a regulatory catastrophe, which manifests as an irritation zone.

7.1 Segments Holistically Networked

In his representation of the movement segment, Junghanns demonstrates the diverse and holistic networking of vertebral segments on a cybernetic and regulatory basis (see Fig. 36.9). The static concept of the spine must inevitably give way to the dynamic designation of the axial organ, not least as a subtle body language expression of internal and external posture. The conceptual model "Segmental Reflex Complex" symbolizes the horizontally and vertically oriented reaction linkage of all structures and systems with the movement segment. Treatment of thoracic vertebral blockages directly at the site of occurrence is particularly successful. These blockages are often distributed across the segment. Therefore, a comprehensive

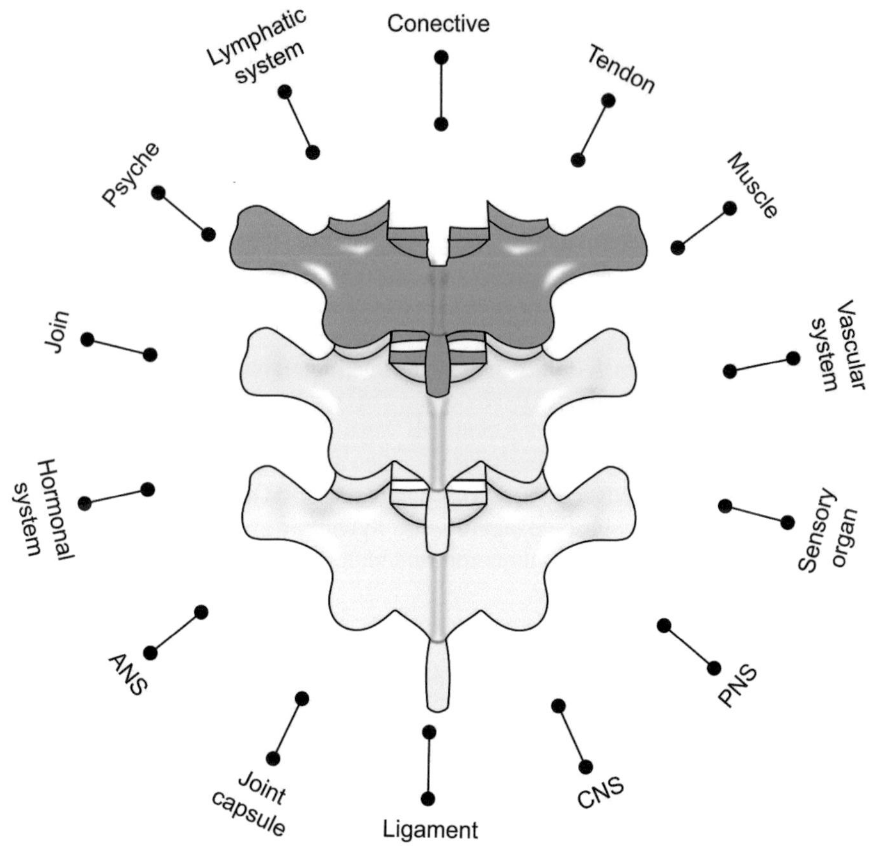

Fig. 36.9 This graphic, adapted from Junghanns' concept of segmental interconnections, illustrates the complex relationships between a vertebral segment and various systems within the body. The graphic emphasizes the segmental reflex complex, demonstrating how the health and function of a vertebral segment can influence and be influenced by these various bodily systems. It serves as a visual representation of the interconnectedness within the body, underscoring the importance of considering these relationships in diagnosis and treatment. (Source: Own elaboration)

examination is essential. It is important in all techniques to treat the patient bilaterally, that is, ventral and dorsal in the same session.

The disturbance of individual systems or the extent to which these processes occur can be verified with experience and appropriate methods. However, due to the complexity of the interconnected structures of the organism, many pathways remain open [13, 17].

Time is a critical dimension in this context. The end stage of the focus of disturbance is degeneration, a rigid regulatory organism, and the chronic stress or irritation syndrome. Irritation zones always represent an additional energy expenditure for the body and a loss of efficiency [13].

7.2 *Functional Definition of Interference Fields*

An interference field is a ubiquitously occurring tissue section with sympathetic innervation, where the afferent fiber component is in a pathological, chronic state of irritation. The oligosymptomatic or asymptomatic nature of the interference field suggests a moderate, rather subthreshold irritation of the sympathetic nervous system [3, 10, 11].

It is more likely that a labile, nonspecific inflammatory situation is present, triggered by organic or inorganic substances or by microorganisms that the organism cannot initially degrade or remove after an injury or illness. In this situation, peptides may be released from nonspecifically functioning inflammatory cells, which themselves constitute the actual substrate of the stimulus for the afferent sympathetic nervous system [13].

Not only organic but also emotional interference fields can, depending on the degree and duration of exposure, lead to excessive reactions in response to additional internal or external stress and thereby cause thoracic blockages.

8 Chronic Syndromes Caused by Thoracic Blockages Can Be Successfully Treated with Neural Therapy

Chronic syndromes caused by thoracic blockages can be improved through targeted influence on the autonomic nervous system with neural therapy [13, 14].

Neural therapy is a holistically oriented form of regulation therapy and can be used either alone or in combination with other conventional therapeutic methods. The targeted injection of small amounts of a local anesthetic (usually 1% procaine or lidocaine solution) is not intended to provide short-term relief from an existing symptom or pain but primarily to eliminate causative factors, thereby creating the conditions for normalization or improvement of function and the body's own regulation. Neural therapy assists the organism in regaining its lost balance by eliminating disturbances. Here, knowledge of the connections between skin areas, vertebral segments, and internal organs is crucial [13, 17].

9 Six Views/Theses on Thoracic Blockages (as Described by the Author Nazlikul) [7, 13]

1. Syndromes that worsen while lying down have their origin in the spine, typically in the thoracic spine (BWS).
2. Chronic diseases mediated through the autonomic nervous system are generally associated with vertebral blockages in the thoracic spine.

3. Chronic non-radicular syndromes of the extremities are mediated by the upper thoracic spine and the sacroiliac joint.
4. Lasting success can only be explained by eliminating interference fields or regulating the autonomic nervous system.
5. A segmental disorder is always identified. The Kibler skin fold technique is an effective method for detecting reflexive signs of disease.
6. Thoracic expansion or inhalation may be restricted.

Regulatory blockages can seriously irritate the autonomic nervous system and impede the effects of therapeutic stimuli. Neural therapy is a method that does not address pain management in the conventional sense but instead eliminates pain-causing factors and creates the conditions for improving function and normalizing regulation.

Neural therapy helps the body regain its lost balance by eliminating disturbances. Knowledge of the connections between skin areas, vertebral segments, and internal organs is crucial in this process.

The key to successful treatment is finding the path to the original source of disturbance. It is not the injection technique or the amount of substance used that is decisive, but rather the understanding of the relationships involved and the targeted injection of small amounts that is critical for success [13, 18].

10 Therapeutic Injections into Ligaments

For injections into ligamentous structures, please consult Chap. 34, subtitle Therapeutic Injections into Ligaments.

References

1. Frisch H. Programmed examination of the musculoskeletal system. Basic examinations of the Thorax (T1 and ribs). 9th ed. Berlin: Springer; 2009. p. 275–310.
2. Dvorák J, Grob D. Thoracic spine: diagnosis and therapy. Stuttgart: Thieme; 2010.
3. Nazlikul H. Segmental vertebral dysfunction is a multi-causal event. Man Med. 2014;52(5):432–6. https://doi.org/10.1007/s00337-014-1141-1.
4. Bischoff HP, Moll H. Textbook of manual medicine. In: Diagnosis and therapy in the thoracic area. 6th ed. Balingen: Spitta; 2011. p. 124–52.
5. Nazlikul H. Neurovegetative system, blockades, and manual medicine. Man Med. 2010;48(6):435–9. https://doi.org/10.1007/s00337-010-0805-8.
6. Nazlikul H. Neural therapy textbook. 1st ed. Istanbul: Nobel Kitabevi; 2010. p. 251–68.
7. Nazlikul H. Neural therapy textbook. In: Thoracic blockades. 1st ed. Istanbul: Nobel Kitabevi; 2010. p. 213–24.
8. Barop H. Textbook and atlas of neural therapy. 2nd ed. Berlin: Haug Verlag; 2015.
9. Nazlikul H, Babacan A. The role of neural therapy and injections. In: Babacan A, editor. Pain and injections. Ankara: Türkiye Klinikleri; 2019. p. 110–7.

10. Barop H. Textbook and atlas of neural therapy. 2nd ed. Stuttgart: Haug Verlag; 2015. p. 196–201.
11. Fischer L. Textbook of neural therapy according to Huneke. 3rd ed. Stuttgart: Hippokrates; 1996. p. 108–11.
12. Böhni UW, Lauper M, Locher H. Manual medicine 2. In: Practical application of diagnostic and therapeutic techniques. Stuttgart: Thieme; 2012.
13. Nazlikul H. Thoracic blockades and the effect of neural therapy in combination with manual therapy. Man Med. 2010;48(5):329–38.
14. Nazlikul H. Neurovegetative system, blockades, and manual medicine: vegetative nervous system, blockades, and manual medicine. Man Med. 2010;6 https://doi.org/10.1007/s00337-010-0805-8.
15. Frölich E. Manual medicine – medical hand skills for diagnosis and therapy. In: Heymann W, editor. Isny-Neutrauchburg: MWE-Self-Publishing; 2009.
16. Bischoff HP, Moll H. Textbook of manual medicine. 6th ed. Balingen: Spitta; 2011.
17. Heymann VW, Locher H, Böhni U, Habring M. Neuroanatomy part 1: facts and hypotheses on afferents and autonomic control. Man Med. 2011;49:473–80.
18. Nazlikul H, Babacan A. The role of neural therapy and injections. In: Babacan A, editor. Pain and injections, vol. 1. Ankara: Türkiye Klinikleri; 2019. p. 110–7.

Chapter 37
Lumbar Spine: Diagnosis and Therapy with Neural Therapy

Fatma Gülçin Ural Nazlikul and Hüseyin Nazlikul

1 Introduction

Following the thoracic vertebrae, the five vertebrae that support the lumbar region are referred to as the lumbar vertebrae. If damage to the lumbar vertebrae compresses the spinal cord, it can result in paraplegia, leading to a loss of control over the legs and the functions of the lower limbs, including genital and sexual abilities.

The lumbar region, comprising five vertebrae, is a common site for chronic and acute conditions. Discs, vertebral joints, ligaments, capsule structures, muscles, vessels, and nerves are all involved in the static and dynamic functions of the lumbar spine (see Figs. 37.1 and 37.2). Due to its topographical location and structure, the lumbar spine is subjected to greater stresses than any other part of the spine, which alone explains the frequency of conditions in this area. A condition in this region rarely affects a single structure, such as an individual vertebral joint. Irritation of one structure acts like a chain reaction, affecting other structures such as vessels, nerves, and muscles, depending on neurophysiological connections [1–3].

F. G. U. Nazlikul
Faculty of Medicine, Physical Medicine and Rehabilitation,
Istanbul Health and Technology University, Istanbul, Turkey
e-mail: fatma.nazlikul@istun.edu.tr

H. Nazlikul (✉)
International Federation of Medical Associations of Neural Therapy – IFMANT,
Schattenhalb, Switzerland

Nazlikul Naturel Foundation for the Development of Healthy Habitats, Istanbul, Turkey

Faculty of Medicine, Department of Biophysics, Istanbul University of Health and Technology, Istanbul, Turkey
e-mail: hnazlikul@web.de

L. B. Pinilla Bonilla et al. (eds.), *Neuraltherapeutic Medicine*,
https://doi.org/10.1007/978-3-032-03257-7_37

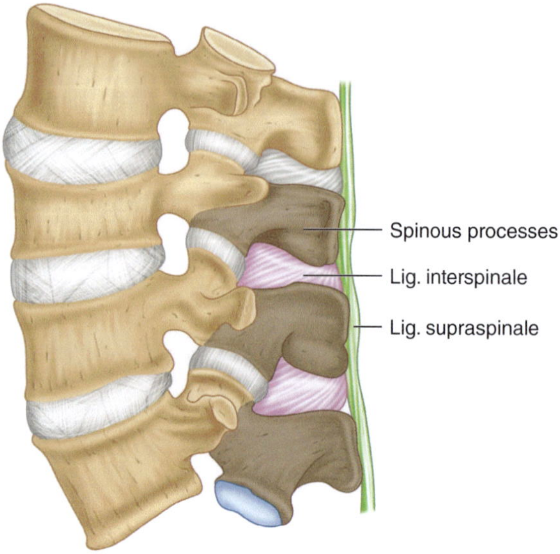

Fig. 37.1 Ligamentary components of the lumbosacral spine. This image shows the anatomical location of the ligaments in the lumbar and lumbosacral spine, specifically the supraspinous ligament and the interspinous ligament. These ligaments connect the spinous processes of the vertebrae and play a crucial role in stabilizing the spine. If these structures are found to be problematic, infiltration may be considered to relieve pain and improve function. (Source: Own elaboration)

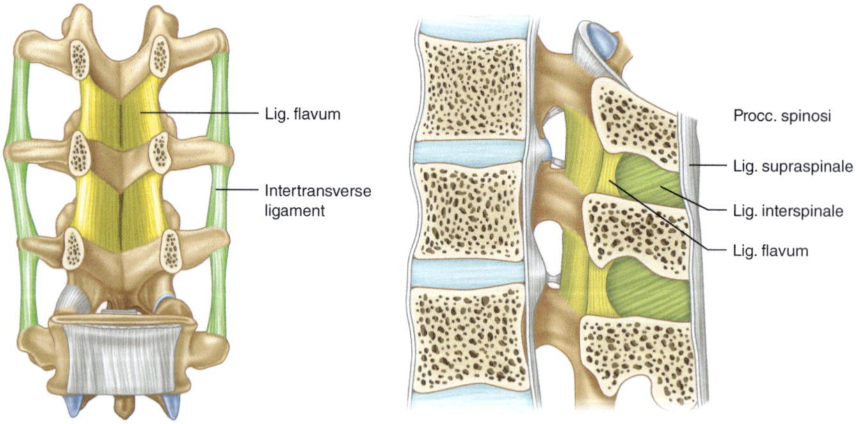

Fig. 37.2 Ligaments of the lumbar and lumbosacral spine play a critical role in spinal stability and are essential targets in neural therapy. (Source: Own elaboration)

1.1 Flexion: Extension

Increases as it descends to the caudal segments, reaching 20° at the lumbosacral level (LS). The LS segment is the most mobile segment for flexion and extension. The lumbar spine provides 60° of spinal flexion, and hip flexion, i.e., pelvic rotation, provides an additional 25° of flexion. Lateral bending: 3° in the LS segment and 6° in the other lumbar segments. Axial rotation: In the LS region, rotation is greater than lateral flexion. It is less in the other regions [2–4].

1.2 Lumbar Spine Mobility

The mobility of the lumbar spine is relatively limited, for example, by the close proximity of the spinous processes, which prevent excessive lordosis. Rotations are possible with only a few degrees in an upright posture; with inclination and divergence of the articular processes, rotational mobility is improved. Nevertheless, the mobility of the lumbar spine and its transition to the sacrum is of great importance for human gait, as physiological shearing forces in the bony pelvis during different standing and walking phases, involving the sacrum, transmit rotational forces to the base of the fifth lumbar vertebra, which then transfers these rotations, decreasing segmentally, to the vertebrae above it [2, 3, 5–7].

In trunk lateral bending, the lumbar spine contributes to the motion, with the stronger lateral bending movements performed in the lower half of the lumbar spine.

In cases of lumbar spine disorders, the hip and sacroiliac joints should always be ruled out. Therefore, differential diagnostic examination of the hip joint, sacroiliac joint, and lumbar spine is crucial, using a sequence of provocation tests in three stages by gradually raising the leg at different fixation points. This approach allows for a quick investigation and identification of the cause.

1.3 Diagnosis of Lumbar Spine Syndrome

The diagnosis of lumbar spine syndrome serves several purposes:

- To uncover the causes of the symptoms, particularly if they require specific or urgent treatment;
- To objectify the symptoms and the resulting functional impairments as a basis for monitoring progress;
- To identify "yellow flags" that may pose a risk for the chronification of the pain syndrome.

Diagnosis of the Lumbar Spine Simple visual inspection, simple examination with the hands and fingers, and anamnesis through spoken word allow us to make 70–80% of the diagnosis and save many X-ray examinations [4, 5, 7, 8].

Conclusion The lumbar spine is highly susceptible to various conditions due to its structural and functional significance. Neural therapy, through its ability to modulate the autonomic nervous system and address interference fields, offers a robust approach to treating lumbar spine-related pain and dysfunctions. Comprehensive diagnostic approaches that include functional and vegetative assessments are essential for the successful application of neural therapy in managing lumbar spine disorders [4, 5, 9–13].

2 Comprehensive Examination Clarifies Functional Connections

This comprehensive examination is essential to clarify the functional relationships within the body, especially in the context of lumbar spine syndrome. The following aspects should be considered:

- *Spinal misalignment*: Are there any spinal misalignments?
- *Chain of functional disorders*: Are there chains of dysfunctions present?
- *Origin from another spinal segment*: Could the problem originate from another level of the spine?
- *Jaw alignment*: How is the alignment of the teeth and jaw?

During the examination, all of the following structures should be considered [2, 4, 6, 14]:

- *Passive structures*: Cartilage, bones, capsules, tendons, and ligaments.
- *Active structures*: Muscles, including their origins, insertions, and trigger points.
- *Supplying structures*: Arteries and nerves.
- *Draining structures:* Veins and lymphatic vessels.
- *Joint and muscle functional chains*: From cranial (head) to caudal (tail end).

2.1 Genesis and Correlations of Lumbar Spine Syndrome

Lumbar spine syndrome can be classified into different types based on the underlying cause [5, 7, 15]:

- *Morphological–anatomical causes*: This includes true lumbago caused by a lumbar prolapse.
- *Blockages*: Particularly sacroiliac joint (SIJ) blockages and symphysis blockages, as well as facet syndrome, which play crucial roles.
- *Structural changes*: Such as scoliosis, fractures, tumors, or pregnancy.
- *Neuropathic pain*: Pain caused by irritation of a nerve, such as lumboischialgia.
- *Degenerative diseases*: Although these account for only a small proportion of the changes.
- *Functional disorders*: These make up the majority of lumbar spine complaints.
- *Vegetatively induced pain*: Often triggered by interference fields, mediated through the autonomic nervous system, and not necessarily related to the lumbar spine itself.
- *Referred pain*: For example, pain originating from the female pelvis that is referred to the sacral region.

2.2 *Specific Lower Back Pain (Approximately 45% of Cases)*

2.2.1 15% of Specific Lower Back Pain Cases [4, 5, 10, 16]:

- Spondylitis.
- Other spinal infections.
- Rheumatoid inflammation of the spine.
- Osteoporosis.
- Tumors, metastases.
- Spondylolisthesis.
- Spinal stenosis.
- Disc herniation.
- Other nerve root compressions.

2.2.2 30% of Specific Lower Back Pain Cases [4, 5, 10, 17, 18]:

- All types of spinal osteoarthritis.
- All other types of degenerative changes in the spine (bones and muscles).

2.2.3 Non-specific Lower Back Pain—55% of Cases [4, 5, 16, 7, 18]

Non-specific lower back pain typically lacks a specific etiology and is often understood within a biopsychosocial framework:

- *Biological causes*: Somatic dysfunction.
- *Psychological causes.*
- *Social causes.*

It is rare to identify a single cause; almost always, it is a combination of multiple factors.

Biological causes [4, 5, 7, 8, 14, 18–20]**:** Functional issues with lumbar muscles, especially:

- *M. multifidus.*
- *M. quadratus lumborum.*
- *M. iliocostalis thoracis.*
- *M. longissimus dorsi.*
  - Functional problems in the thoracolumbar fascia.
  - Segmental intervertebral dysfunction ("blockage").
  - Somatic comorbidity (cervical spine, cranial nerves, including TMJ).

Psychological causes:

- Lack of coping strategies.

- Behavioral problems.
- Anxious, depressive, overwhelmed, or withdrawn personality.
- Psychological comorbidity.

Social causes:

- Dysfunctional family environment.
- Social isolation: lack of friends, unemployment.
- Bullying; heavy and/or monotonous work.
- Lack of compensation for occupational accidents or diseases.

This image illustrates the key ligamentous structures of the lumbar and lumbosacral spine, including the ligamentum flavum, supraspinous ligament, interspinous ligament, and intertransverse ligament. These ligaments connect the vertebrae and contribute significantly to the structural integrity of the spine. In cases where these ligaments are found to be problematic or painful, infiltration through neural therapy can be an effective approach to relieve pain and restore function by addressing disruptions in the autonomic nervous system [1, 6].

3 Functional Examination of the Lumbar Spine

In the lumbar spine region, a functional examination is performed as the first step in a three-step diagnostic process. Initially, the posture and alignment of the lumbar spine are assessed through visual inspection. Observations include any flattening or exaggeration of the lumbar lordosis, the presence of a hyperlordotic kink at the lumbosacral junction, or a dorsolumbar kyphosis, scoliosis, or antalgic posture. A slight scoliosis often manifests only as a more pronounced lumbar bulge on one side, which becomes more apparent during forward bending [2–5, 20] .

Following this, the sequence of spinous processes is palpated and checked for lateral deviations or step formations. In the case of the latter, it is necessary to determine whether it is a true or pseudolisthesis. In true spondylolisthesis, the step formation is found in the spinous process row above the slipping vertebra, while in pseudolisthesis, it is located below the slipping vertebra. This occurs because, in true spondylolisthesis, the spinous process of the slipping vertebra remains stationary due to the split in the interarticular portion [2, 3, 6].

3.1 Assessment of Schober's Sign and Ott's Sign

Schober's Sign: The functional examination includes both general and segment-specific assessments. During forward bending, Schober's sign and the finger-floor distance are initially measured. It is important to note that, in addition to lumbar

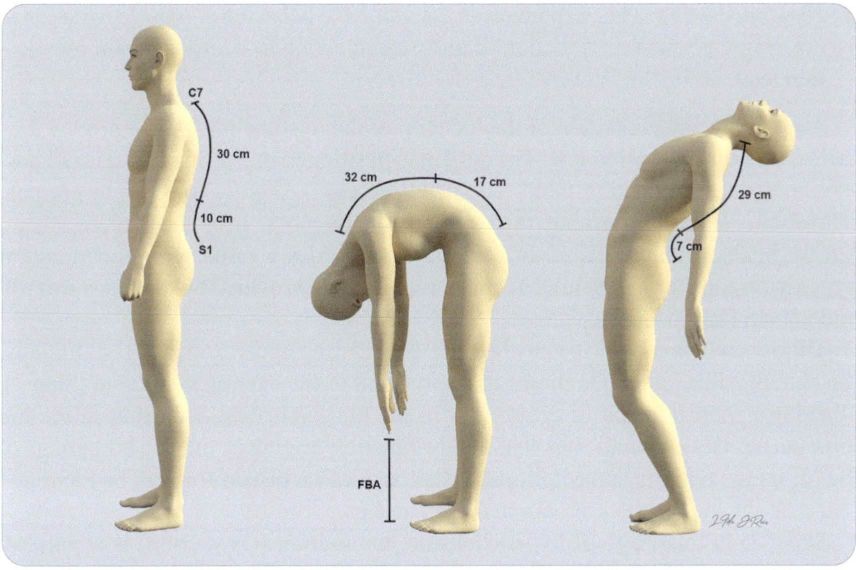

Fig. 37.3 This illustration depicts the assessment of the Otto and Schober signs to evaluate spinal mobility. Measurements are taken in an upright position, during maximum forward flexion, and during backward extension. Normal values for the Schober sign range around 29/30/32–34 cm, indicating the flexibility of the lumbar spine. The graphic demonstrates the method for assessing spinal mobility using the Otto and Schober signs. The first image shows the starting position, where measurement points are marked on the spinous processes of C7 and S1. The second image illustrates forward flexion, where the increase in distance between the marks is measured, indicating the spine's flexibility. The third image shows backward extension, where a decrease in the distance is measured to assess the lumbar spine's mobility. These measurements help identify limitations or deviations in spinal movement. (Source: Own elaboration)

spine mobility, the function of the hip joints (especially) and shortening of the hamstring muscles are also significant factors. The measurement of the mid-distance around L1 can also be included .

Ott's Sign: A point is marked 30 cm distal to the spinous process of C7, and changes in length during maximal forward and backward bending are measured. The normal values are approximately 29/30/32–34 (See Fig. 37.3) [2, 3, 20].

3-Step Hyperextension Test

The 3-step diagnostic approach, introduced by Bischoff (Bischoff & Moll 2011), involves the following procedures [2, 3, 6]:

1. *Assessment of functional mobility*: This step aims to identify relative hypomobility by evaluating the functional range of motion.
2. *Identification of specific irritation*: Using the so-called "irritation point," this step identifies specific irritation in the muscles associated with segmental innervation of the sacroiliac joint (SIJ).

3. *Dynamic testing*: This step involves assessing the behavior of muscle irritation to determine a pain-free direction of movement, acting as a targeted pain provocation test.

A more precise indication of the location of the dysfunction can be provided by the 3-step hyperextension test. The patient is positioned in a prone and relaxed posture on a flat examination table. The head section is slightly lowered to promote relaxation. When performing this differential diagnosis test, the patient should remain in the prone position. In cases of hyperlordosis while lying down and/or hyperextension pain in the lumbar spine, relief can be provided by placing a soft roll underneath [2, 3, 14, 17].

This test was first described by Mennel as the 3-step hyperextension test. Initially, the patient's iliac crest (Os ilium) is firmly fixed to the examination table (Step 1), allowing hyperextension to occur only in the hip joint. Pain occurring in the hip joint during this step indicates that the dysfunction originates there. Shortenings of the M. rectus femoris and M. iliopsoas that also cause discomfort can be identified based on the localization of pain to these muscles.

Stage 2: In this stage of hyperextension, the sacrum (Os sacrum) is stabilized, which now includes the sacroiliac joint (SIJ) in the movement. Any pain occurring in the SIJ region, or pain that is added to the existing hip pain, indicates involvement of the sacroiliac joint (see Fig. 37.4).

Stage 3: A counterforce is applied to the lower lumbar spine, incorporating the lumbosacral junction into the examination. In this stage, only a slight counterforce is applied because it is important not to exclude the cranial sections from the movement and to avoid applying too much force, which could adversely affect both the posterior fibrous ring of the lumbosacral disc and the vertebral joints in this area.

Author's note: The 3-step hyperextension test is performed with the patient in a prone position and provides the examiner with insights into whether the condition involves the hip joint, the sacroiliac joints, or the lumbosacral junction.

Summary

- *Patient position*: Prone on a flat table.
- *Examiner position*: On the opposite side, facing the table.
- *Stage* 1: Fixation of the iliac crest—assesses the hip joint. (Consider hip involvement in cases of pain or restricted movement.)
- *Stage* 2: Fixation of the sacrum—assesses both the hip and SIJ. (Consider SIJ involvement in cases of pain or restricted movement).
- *Stage* 3: Gentle counterforce applied to the lumbosacral junction—assesses all three components. (Consider lumbar spine involvement in cases of pain or restricted movement).
- *Pitfalls*: Insufficient stabilization of the opposing structures in stages 1 and 2.

Indications [4, 5, 7, 9, 16, 18, 21]

- Lower back pain.
- Spondyloarthrosis.
- Spondylopathy.

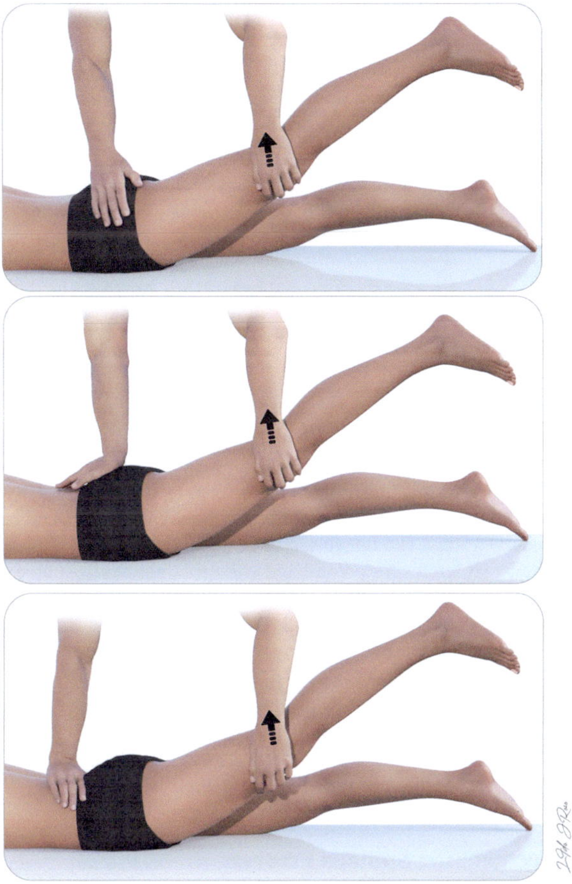

Fig. 37.4 Stages hyperextension test. Three-stage examination to determine dysfunctions in the hip area, sacroiliac joint or lumbar area: Top figure: The patient lies in the supine position, and the leg is lifted with the knee extended. This phase is used to detect possible dysfunctions in the hip joint. Middle figure: The patient lies in a prone position, and the leg is raised again with the knee extended. This phase focuses on the sacroiliac joint and possible dysfunctions in this area. Bottom figure: The patient's leg is raised with the knee bent to test the flexibility and possible dysfunctions in the lumbar area. This examination helps to identify the exact location of a dysfunction in the lower back or pelvic area. (Source: Own elaboration)

- Lumbar disc herniation.
- Spinal canal stenosis.
- Nerve root compression.
- Vertebral fractures (new and old, including osteoporotic compression fractures).
- Tumors and metastases.
- Lumbar spine injuries.
- Scheuermann's disease, degenerative diseases of the lumbar spine.
- Spondylolisthesis.
- Lumbar interference fields.

The stimulation therapy is conducted with a wheal-array over the spinous processes of the lumbar spine and an infiltration into the paravertebral region about 3–4 cm at the same level of the affected segment.

Injection into the Spinous Processes

First of all, Fig. 37.5 describes some anatomical orientation points and anatomical landmarks to consider for the treatment of the lumbosacral spine. Painful spinous

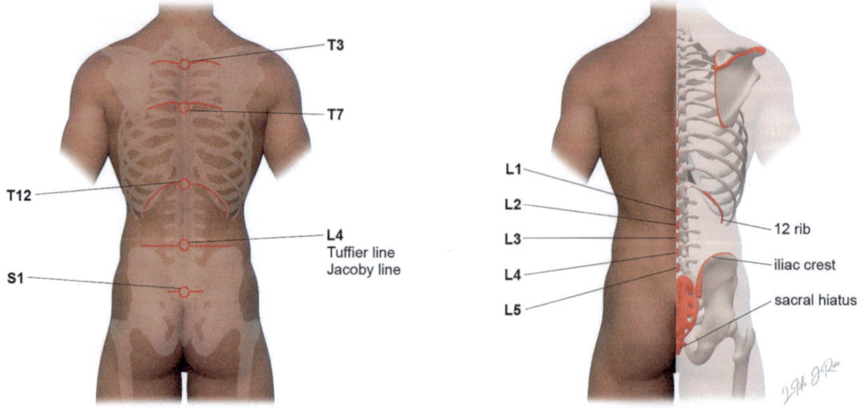

Fig. 37.5 Anatomical orientation points of the lumbar and lumbosacral spine. This illustration highlights key anatomical landmarks, such as the iliac crest, sacral hiatus, and various vertebral levels, which are crucial for ensuring accurate localization and height assessment during therapeutic interventions. The image serves as a guide for identifying the correct vertebral levels and surrounding structures for precise and effective treatment. (Source: Own elaboration)

processes are identified through palpation. After forming a wheal, a 2–3 cm long needle is advanced until it contacts the bone. A 0.5 ml solution of procaine is infiltrated into the supra- and interspinous ligaments, which extend to the superior and inferior spinous *processes*. The needle is withdrawn slightly and redirected approximately 60° cranially and caudally to infiltrate these ligaments. The injection depth is about 2 cm [10–13].

Injection Site: Spinous Process

- *Direction of injection*: Once the sagittal SP (spinous process) is contacted, the local anesthetic (LA) is injected, the needle is withdrawn, and then redirected cranially and caudally to infiltrate the supra- and interspinous ligaments.
- *Depth of injection*: 1–2.5 cm.
- *Equipment used*: 40 × 0.4 mm needle.
- *Amount of local anesthetic used*: 0.5–1 ml of 1% procaine/lidocaine.

Lumbar facet injection:

The facet joints of the lumbar spine are located approximately 4–5 cm deep and 2–2.5 cm lateral to the midline of the spinous process. Painful spinous processes are identified by palpation. With the upper body slightly inclined forward, a 6 cm long needle is inserted about 2–2.5 cm lateral to the midline at the level of the midpoint of the spinous process (see Figs. 37.6 and 37.7). Facet injections are usually not performed at a single level, as the facets are innervated by two dorsal rami nerves. If it is unknown whether the second branch originates from an upper or lower vertebra, three injection levels are recommended: the affected facet, one lower facet, and one upper facet [7, 10–13, 20, 22].

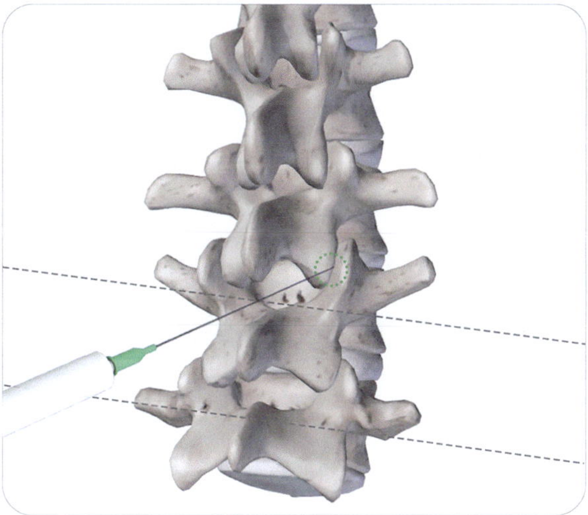

Fig. 37.6 LCS facet injection: This illustration shows the correct positioning of the needle for an injection into the lumbar facet joints. The goal is to place the needle in the lower third of the spinous process to ensure precise delivery of the medication. (Source: Own elaboration)

Injections into the Lumbar Facet Joints (See Fig. 37.8)

- *Injection site*: In the middle third of the lower part of the posterior spinous process (SP), with a 2–2.5 cm paramedian approach.
- *Direction of injection entry*: strictly sagittal.
- *Injector*: 60 × 0.6 mm needle.
- *Injection depth*: 4–5 cm (until bone contact).

Lumbar Sympathetic Chain [10, 11]

- *Injection site*: Middle of the L3 spinous process, 3.5 finger-widths lateral.
- *Injection direction:* 30 degrees medially in the horizontal plane.
- *Needle*: Depending on body size, 60–120 × 0.8 mm.
- *Injection depth*: After approximately 8 cm (reaching the anterior surface of the vertebral body), advance the needle an additional 1–2 cm.

Injections for Spinal Nerves [10–12]

Since they form a functional unit in the diagnosis of diseases affecting the lower extremities, the spinal nerves L1–L4 are examined together.

After exiting the spinal canal, the spinal nerves converge in the lumbar plexus and innervate the ventromedial part of the leg as peripheral nerves. The branches of the spinal nerves are intertwined.

The spinal nerves are grouped into segments and innervate the peripheral nerves (iliohypogastric nerve T12-L1, ilioinguinal nerve T12-L1, genitofemoral nerve L1-L2, lateral femoral cutaneous nerve L2-L3, obturator nerve L2-L4, femoral nerve L2-L4), leading to a segmentally complex innervation of the muscles, so that the failure of one segment results in the loss of function of various muscle segments but not the entire muscle.

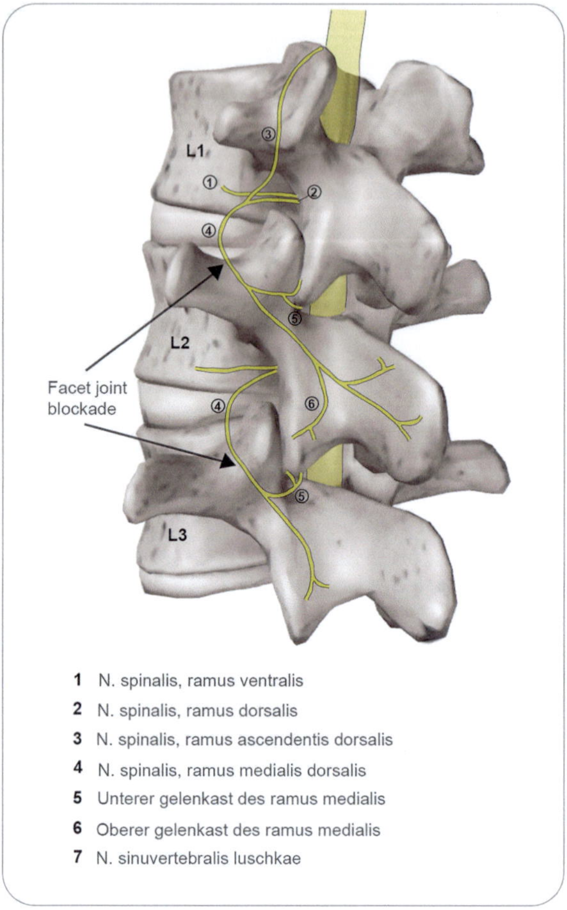

Fig. 37.7 Facet blockade: This image illustrates the anatomical position of the lumbar facet joints and the neural innervation provided by the spinal nerves. Key structures include the ramus ventralis n. spinalis, ramus dorsalis n. spinalis, and various branches such as the ramus medialis, which are involved in the innervation of the facet joints. These nerves are crucial in transmitting pain signals in conditions where facet joint dysfunction occurs, often leading to a facet joint blockade. (Source: Own elaboration)

Indications

- Diseases of the adductor muscles of the thigh and quadriceps muscles.
- Lumbago originating from the L1–L4 segment.
- Nerve compression.
- Groin pain.
- Unspecified groin pain.
- Obturator neuralgia.
- Gonarthropathy (e.g., chondropathia patellae, retropatellar osteoarthritis).

Injections at L1–L4 Spinal Nerves [10–12]

The patient sits with a slight forward inclination of the upper body. The iliac crest line is marked. The spinous process closest to this line corresponds to L4. The spinous process at this level is marked depending on which spinal nerve is involved (see Fig. 37.9).

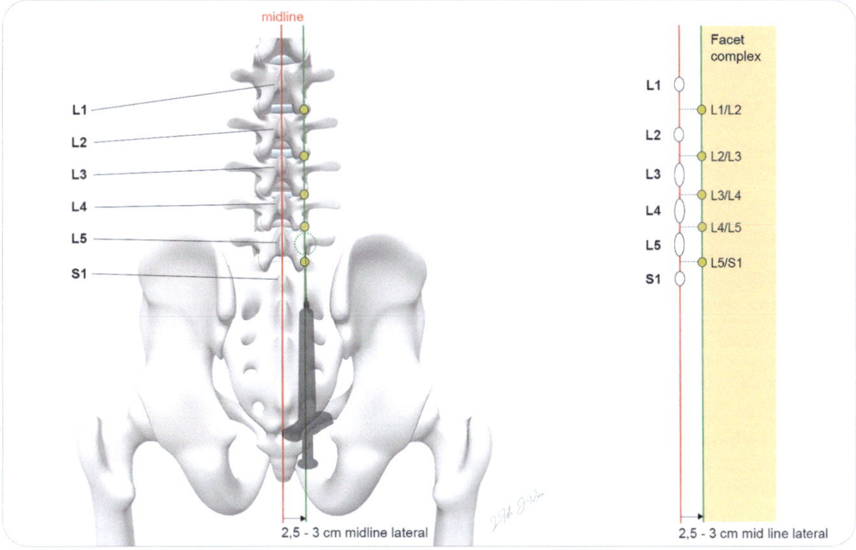

Fig. 37.8 Injections into the lumbar facet joints: This illustration shows the anatomical orientation and correct placement of the needle for injections into the lumbar facet joints. The injection site is located 2.5–3 cm lateral to the midline (PS) at the level of the corresponding vertebral segments. After a perpendicular insertion, once bone contact is made, a fan-shaped pericapsular infiltration is performed to ensure effective treatment of the facet complex. (Source: Own elaboration)

Injection site: In the lower part of the posterior spinous process (SP), 3 cm lateral to the SI (2.5 fingers lateral and 1 finger cranial).
Direction of injection entry: Sagittal approach.
Injector: 60 × 0.60 mm or 80 × 0.60 mm.
Injection depth: 5–7 cm.

Injection around the Spinal Roots L5–S3 [10–12]

The sacral plexus consists of the anterior part of the spinal nerves L5-S3 as well as branches of the R. ventralis originating from L4. An important point for diagnosis and neuraltherapeutic treatment is that in approximately 20% of cases, the segment of the sacral plexus is shifted cranially or caudally (M. Clara). The innervation area includes only the flexion zone of the lower limbs via the r. ventral connection and also the dorsal lumbar and sacral region via the r. dorsales nervi spinales, which do not merge into a plexus. Therefore, during the stimulation of a spinal nerve, a clinical reaction in the lumbar and sacral regions as well as in the lower limbs can be expected.

The simultaneous blockade of somatic nerve components is of secondary importance in neural therapy, unlike in local anesthesia. The goal is to achieve better blood circulation and a short-term reduction of the sympathetic afferent stimulus, which is amplified in the diseased state by reflex effects on the somatic nervous system and all other tissues.

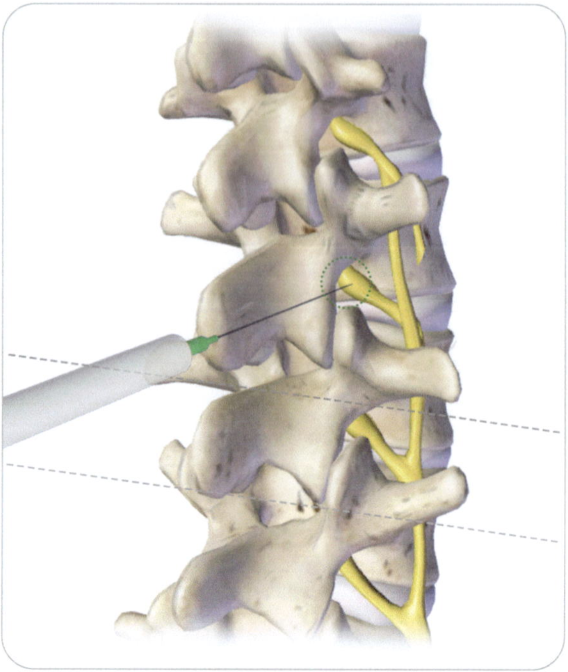

Fig. 37.9 Injections at L1–L4: Injection into spinal nerves in the lumbar spine region: This illustration shows the correct placement of the needle for an injection into the lumbar spinal nerves. The needle is carefully introduced into the perineural space to ensure precise administration of medication near the nerve root. This allows for effective treatment of radicular pain and other neurological symptoms caused by irritation or inflammation of the spinal nerves in the lumbar region. (Source: Own elaboration)

This explains why neural therapy for diseases of the lumbar spine, sacrum, and lower limbs is performed via the spinal roots of the sacral plexus.

Dysfunctions

- Dysfunction of the gluteal muscles.
- Muscles of the thigh flexors.
- Lower leg and foot muscles.
- In circulatory disorders of the lower limbs.
- In interference field problems considered at the L1-L4 levels.
- New and old peroneal palsy.
- Lumbar disc herniation L5/S1.
- Lumbar sciatica.
- Sciatica.
- Lower back pain.
- Regional pain in the lower extremities in the L5-S3 segment.

L5 Spinal Nerve Injection [10–12]

The L5 spinal nerve injection involves precisely targeting the L5 spinal nerve to treat radicular pain and other neurological symptoms caused by irritation or inflammation of this nerve. The injection is performed by introducing the needle into the perineural space surrounding the L5 nerve, ensuring accurate delivery of the medication to alleviate symptoms and improve function (See Fig. 37.10).

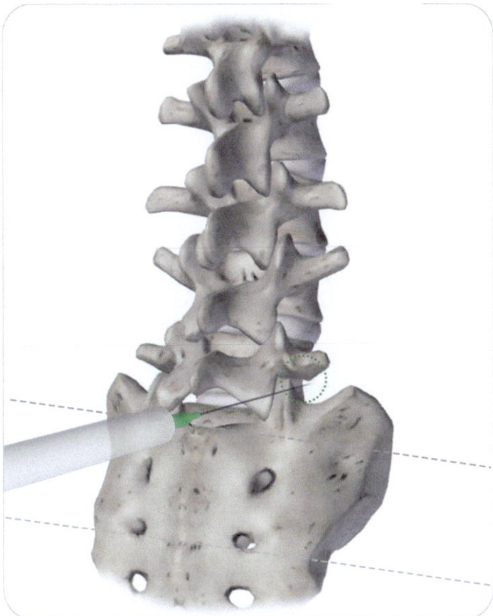

Fig. 37.10 Injection at the L5 spinal nerve: This illustration demonstrates the correct positioning of the needle for an injection at the L5 spinal nerve. The injection is precisely targeted into the perineural space to enable effective treatment of radicular pain and other neurological symptoms caused by irritation or inflammation of the L5 nerve. (Source: Own elaboration)

Injection site: Posterior spinous process of L5, 3 cm lateral to the sacroiliac (SI) joint (approximately 2.5 fingers lateral and 1 finger cranial).
Direction of injection entry: 10° caudal, 10° medial approach.
Injector: 60 × 0.60 mm or 80 × 0.60 mm needle.
Injection depth: 6–8 cm.

Sacral S1 Root Injection [10–12]

- *Injection site*: Approximately 1.5 fingers lateral and slightly cranial from the lower part of the S1 spinous process (2 fingers cranial and 1 finger medial to the posterior superior iliac spine) (See Fig. 37.11).
- *Direction of injection*: 30–45° caudal.
- *Injection depth*: 6 cm.
- *Materials to be used*: 80 × 0.60 mm needle.
- *Amount of local anesthetic* (LA) to be used: 4–5 ml of 0.5–1% Procain/Lidocaine.

Injection of the S2 Spinal Root [10]

The S2 spinous process is palpated. At this level, a 6 cm long needle is inserted 1 cm cranially and about 2 cm laterally at an angle of approximately 20° to the skin. At a depth of about 2–3 cm, the dorsal opening of the S2 foramen is reached. After advancing the needle by 0.5 cm and performing two aspiration attempts, 2–3 ml of procain solution is infiltrated. A sharp pain or pulling sensation in the S2 segment indicates that the injection is at the correct site.

Injection site: 2 cm lateral to the S2 spinous process.
Injection direction: Aim at the S2 foramen at an angle of about 20° to the skin.

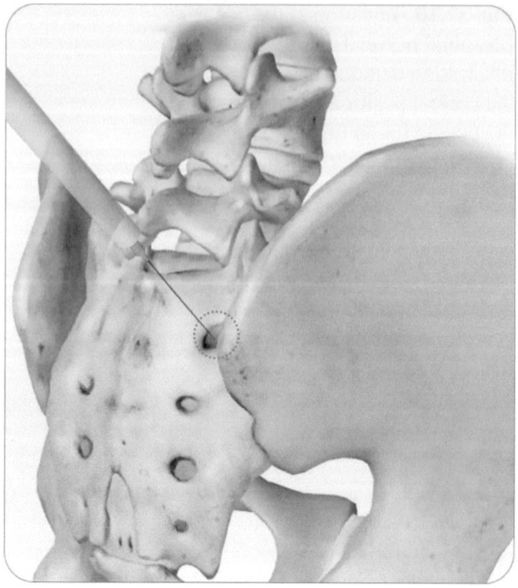

Fig. 37.11 Injection at the S1 spinal nerve: This illustration shows the correct positioning of the needle for an injection at the S1 spinal nerve. The injection is precisely targeted into the sacral area to effectively treat radicular pain and other neurological issues caused by irritation or inflammation of the S1 nerve. (Source: Own elaboration)

Injection depth: 2–3 cm.
Materials to be used: 40 × 0.40 mm needle.

Amount of local anesthetic (LA) to be Used: 2–3 ml of 0.5–1% Procain/lidocaine.
Sacral epidural injection [10, 13]:

The epidural space (also called the peridural space) is the space within the vertebral canal between the periosteum of the vertebrae and the dura mater ("sliding layer" for the dural sac). It consists of connective tissue, adipose tissue, supplying and draining vessels, and non-myelinated vegetative fibers of the sympathetic nervous system (providing sympathetic innervation to the periosteum, dura mater, and vessels of the vertebral canal).

Direction: Strictly median.
Injection point: Between the sacral cornua through the sacrococcygeal ligament into the sacral hiatus.

Summary
Sacral epidural injection:

- Blockade of the dorsal ramus of the sympathetic nervous system.
- Sympatholysis of the peridural vessels.
- Improved blood flow to the spinal cord and cauda equina, along with interruption of pain-conducting afferents from the dura mater and vertebral periosteum.
- Improvement of motor function and sensitivity.

References

1. Lippert H. Textbook of anatomy. 4th ed. Munich: Urban & Schwarzenberg; 1996. p. 107–80.
2. Bischoff HP, Moll H. Textbook of manual medicine. 6th ed. Balingen: Spitta; 2011. p. 97–123.
3. Dvorák J, Grob D. Thoracolumbar spine, diagnosis and therapy. Stuttgart: Thieme; 2010.
4. Nazlikul H. Lumbar vertebra syndrome: neural therapy approach to chronic Back and low Back pain. J Sci Complement Med Regul Neural Ther. 2013;19:10–7.
5. Özkan N, Nazlikul H. Functional and degenerative low Back complaints: neural therapy and manual medicine approach. Sci Complement Med Regulat Neural Ther J. 2017;11(3):1–8.
6. Böhni UW, Lauper M, Locher H. Manual medicine 1: practical application of diagnostic and therapeutic techniques. Lumbosacral transition and pelvic ring. Stuttgart: Thieme; 2012. p. 505–43.
7. Senlikci HB, Nazlikul FGU. Demonstrating the effectiveness of acupuncture and stabilization exercises in chronic non-specific low Back pain. Sci Complement Med Regulat Neural Ther J. 2020;14(3):59–63.
8. Aydın E, Nazlikul Ural FG. The effect of TENS on pain and quality of life in patients with low Back pain: pilot study. Sci Complement Med Regulat Neural Ther J. 2021;15(1):5–8.
9. Nazlikul H, Von Heymann W, Acarkan T, Fischer LO. Assessment of sacroiliac dysfunction with the combination of manual therapy and neural therapy. Sci Complement Med Regulat Neural Ther J. 2014;8(1):8–13.
10. Nazlikul H. Textbook of neural therapy. Istanbul: Nobel Kitabevi; 2010. p. 251–68.
11. Barop H. Textbook and atlas of neural therapy. 1st ed. Stuttgart: Haug Verlag; 1996. p. 236–45.
12. Fischer L. Textbook of neural therapy according to Huneke. 3rd ed. Stuttgart: Hippokrates; 2001. p. 110–5.
13. Barop H. Textbook and atlas of neural therapy. 2nd ed. Stuttgart: Haug Verlag; 2015.
14. Nazlikul F, Öztürk G, Dizdar D, Karabay I, Nazlikul H. Evaluation of the effectiveness of chiropractic manual treatment in patients with chronic low Back pain. Ankara Med J. 2021;21(2):250.
15. Nazlikul H, Babacan A. The role of neural therapy and injections. In: Babacan A, editor. Pain and injections. Ankara: Türkiye Klinikleri; 2019. p. 110–7.
16. Nazlikul H, Nazlikul FGU, Okur ŞÇ, Türk A, Tamam C, Firdin F, Tamam Y. Chiropractic approaches in locomotor system diseases. Sci Complement Med Regulat Neural Ther J. 2020;14(2):47–52.
17. Nazlikul H, Türk A, Nazlikul FGU, Tamam Y, Firdin F, Çağlar S. Diagnosis of sacroiliac dysfunction in athletes according to the principles of manual medicine and chiropractic. Germenica J Phys Educ Sports Sci. 2021;2(1):15–29.
18. Nazlikul H, Nazlikul FGU. The role of neural therapy and manual therapy applications in regulation medicine. Turkiye Klinikleri Sports Med Special Topics. 2023;9(1):8–14.
19. Nazlikul FGU, Dizdar D. Effectiveness of dry needling in myofascial pain syndrome: pilot study. Sci Complement Med Regulat Neural Ther J. 2020;14(3):64–8.
20. Nazlikul FGU, Şenlikci HB. Neural therapy in locomotor system diseases. Turkiye Klinikleri Tradit Complement Med Special Topics. 2022;3(1):61–6.
21. Karakan M, Nazlikul H. Disorders associated with non-specific chronic lower Back pain. Sci Complement Med Regulat Neural Ther J. 2015;9(2):26–8.
22. Acarkan T, Elmacıoğlu MA, Nazlikul H. Facet joint syndrome and clinical reflections. Sci Complement Med Regulat Neural Ther J. 2019;13(1):8–13.

Chapter 38
Sacroiliac Joint or Iliosacral Joint

Hüseyin Nazlikul and Fatma Gülçin Ural Nazlikul

1 Introduction and Biomechanics of the Pelvic Ring

Few joints are as controversial, enigmatic, and simultaneously mystifying as the sacroiliac joint (SIJ), often serving as an explanatory model for otherwise difficult-to-classify pain conditions and functional limitations.

2 Anatomy of the SIJ

The pelvic ring is composed of three bones that are uniquely connected: the sacrum (os sacrum) and the two hip bones (ossa coxae, each of which is a fusion of the ischium, pubis, and ilium). Of mechanical interest are the dorsal connections between the sacrum and each ilium—the two sacroiliac joints—as well as the ventral connection between the two ilia, the symphysis. The sacroiliac joints have purely passive mobility, ranging from 2° to 4°, which decreases with age (Klein, 2004). Although there are some muscles that span these joints (posteriorly:

H. Nazlikul (✉)
International Federation of Medical Associations of Neural Therapy – IFMANT, Schattenhalb, Switzerland

Nazlikul Naturel Foundation for the Development of Healthy Habitats, Istanbul, Turkey

Faculty of Medicine, Department of Biophysics, Istanbul University of Health and Technology, Istanbul, Turkey
e-mail: hnazlikul@web.de

F. G. U. Nazlikul
Faculty of Medicine, Physical Medicine and Rehabilitation, Istanbul Health and Technology University, Istanbul, Turkey
e-mail: fatma.nazlikul@istun.edu.tr

L. B. Pinilla Bonilla et al. (eds.), *Neuraltherapeutic Medicine*,
https://doi.org/10.1007/978-3-032-03257-7_38

quadratus lumborum, iliocostalis, gluteus maximus; anteriorly: piriformis, iliacus), their primary function is to move other joints. However, their tension always results in changes in tension within the SIJ. An active, voluntary movement of the pelvic ring without the leverage effect of other bones is not possible for humans [1].

There are many models regarding the axes of mobility of the sacroiliac joints (SIJ), but practically all of them have proven to be unrealistic. Today, it is believed that the movement in the two sacroiliac joints is best described by an oblique, helicoidal axis in three-dimensional space (see Figs. 38.1 and 38.2). Each joint has its own axis, meaning that they do not share a common axis; each joint is an individual entity (Klein 2004). The movement primarily occurs around two oblique,

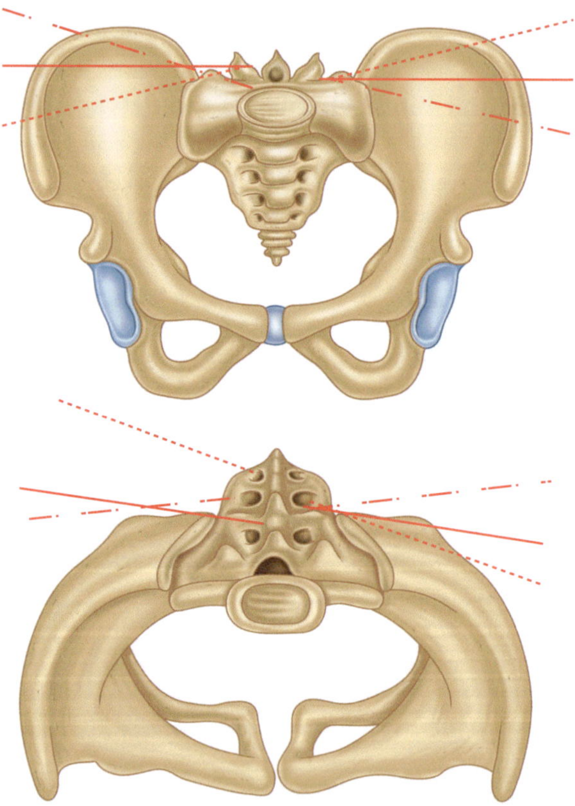

Fig. 38.1 The illustration shows a schematic representation of the helicoidal axes of movement of the sacroiliac joint (SIJ) viewed from both above and below. The red dashed lines highlight the oblique axes, illustrating the complex three-dimensional movements of the SIJ. It is shown that there is no common axis for both joints; instead, each sacroiliac joint has its own individual axis. A 3D representation of the effective helicoidal axes of sacroiliac joint movements during normal standing in extension as well as during single-leg standing on the right and left. (From studies by Jacob/Kissling 1995 and Klein 2004). Be aware that there is no common axis for the left and right sides. These points ensure that the redrawing is scientifically accurate and clearly conveys with the educational proposal from Bohni [2]

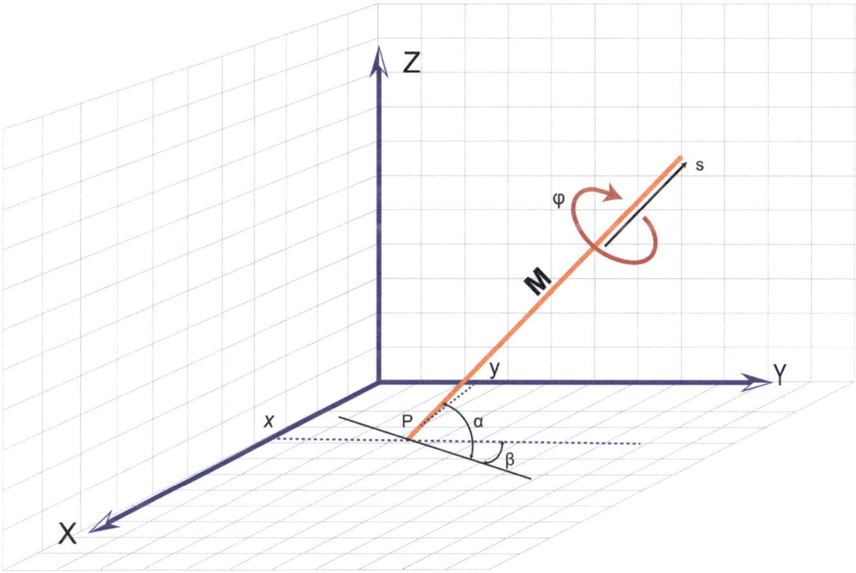

Fig. 38.2 The illustration shows a schematic representation of the helicoidal axis of mobility (M) in a three-dimensional coordinate system. The axis runs obliquely through space, defined by the angles α and β in relation to the X and Y axes. The angle φ represents the rotational movement around the axis. This depiction illustrates the complex motion sequences of the sacroiliac joint (SIJ) and is based on the biomechanical models from Böhni [2]

ventro-dorsal, horizontal, transverse axes, located dorsally to the joint, approximately in the region of the sacroiliac ligaments [1–3].

The sacroiliac joint is a strong, weight-bearing synovial joint located between the ear-shaped joint surfaces of the sacrum and ilium. These joint surfaces have indentations and protrusions that overlap each other. The sacrum is firmly connected to the ilium via the anterior and posterior sacroiliac ligaments and the interosseous ligament. The mobility of the sacroiliac joint is limited due to its role in transferring weight from the trunk to the hips (see Fig. 38.3) [1, 3, 4].

The movement of the sacroiliac joint is restricted by the overlapping joint surfaces of the bones, the thick interosseous ligament, and the posterior sacroiliac ligament, which adhere tightly to the bones. The movement of the sacroiliac joint is limited to minimal gliding and rotation. The sacrotuberous and sacrospinous ligaments allow for limited forward movement of the lower end of the sacrum [3, 4].

The sacroiliac joint is not an intervertebral joint. Phylogenetically, it is composed of the synovial tissue of the sacral vertebrae and the lower extremity plate. The proven maximum mobility of the sacroiliac joint ranges from 2 to 4°. This mobility is highly sensitive to restrictions, with the most common cause being the pseudoradicular sacroiliac joint syndrome. There is also no common axis for movement; each joint is an absolute individualist in its biomechanics [3–5].

The joint surfaces are surrounded by a large capsule and covered with hyaline cartilage, which is thinner and more fibrous on the iliac surface compared to the

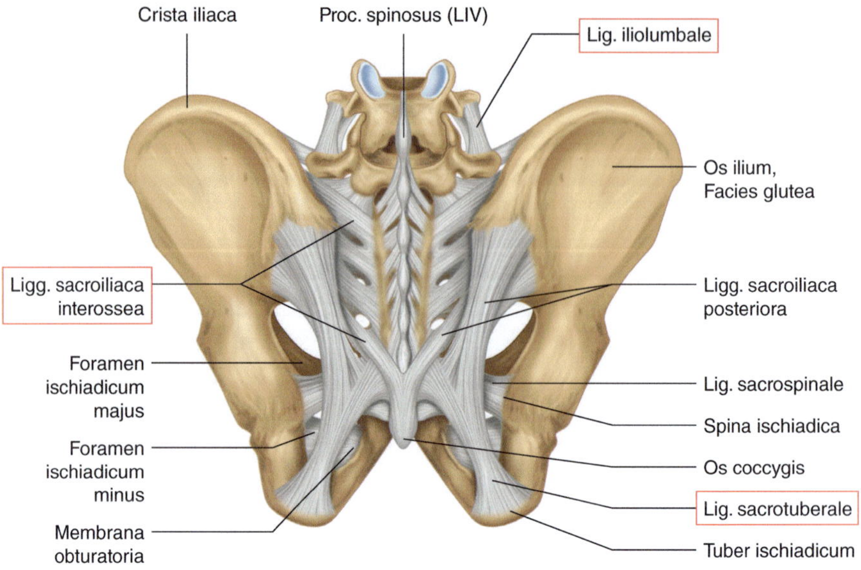

Fig. 38.3 This illustration shows the posterior view of the pelvis with a particular emphasis on the ligaments in the sacroiliac joint (SIJ) area. The key structures highlighted include the iliolumbar ligament, the interosseous sacroiliac ligaments, the sacrotuberous ligament, and the sacrospinous ligament. These ligaments play a crucial role in stabilizing the pelvis and restricting the mobility of the sacroiliac joint

sacral surface. Surrounding the joint are strong ligamentous structures that limit joint movements, including:

- Anterior sacroiliac ligament.
- Posterior sacroiliac ligament (Ligamentum sacroiliacum posterius).
- Interosseous sacroiliac ligament.
- Accessory ligaments (iliolumbar, sacrospinous, sacrotuberous).

3 Movements

Movements of the sacroiliac joint occur simultaneously with those of the hip and lumbosacral joints (L5-S1). Unlike other joints, there is no muscle that directly moves the sacroiliac joint. The joint exhibits a mobility range of 2–4°. Gliding, rotational, tilting, rocking, and translational movements have been observed within the joint. Mobility increases during childbirth and for up to 3 months afterward. It has been shown that mobility decreases in men between the ages of 40 and 50 and in women after the age of 50. The joint becomes sensitive to movement restrictions. The integrity of the joint is maintained through the mechanisms of “form closure” and “force closure.” “Form closure“refers to the stability provided by the bone structure, while “force closure“pertains to the stability provided by the myofascial structure. Due to mechanical injuries to the joint and weakness in the muscles surrounding it, “force closure“decreases, leading to increased ligament stress, resulting in pain and laxity [3–6].

Pain in the sacroiliac joint area is a common condition treated by neural therapy practitioners. Sacroiliac joint inflammation may result from acute or repeated trauma, spondyloarthropathies, degenerative arthritis, pregnancy, and rarely, infection of the joint. The injection of procaine using a neural therapy approach is an effective conservative option for treating this condition. By identifying reference points, this procedure can be performed with a level of safety and effectiveness comparable to image-guided techniques. In fact, patients undergoing periarticular injections may achieve similar or even better results, as there are significant extra-articular sources of pain in the sacroiliac region [6, 7].

In the literature, 18 different pain patterns have been described for the sacroiliac joint. Most of these are found in the gluteal region, with pain below the gluteal region (94%) and in the lower limbs (50%) being more common, although pain in the groin area and above L5 is not uncommon. For these reasons, the history-taking for pathology in the lumbar and hip regions is often limited (see Fig. 38.4).

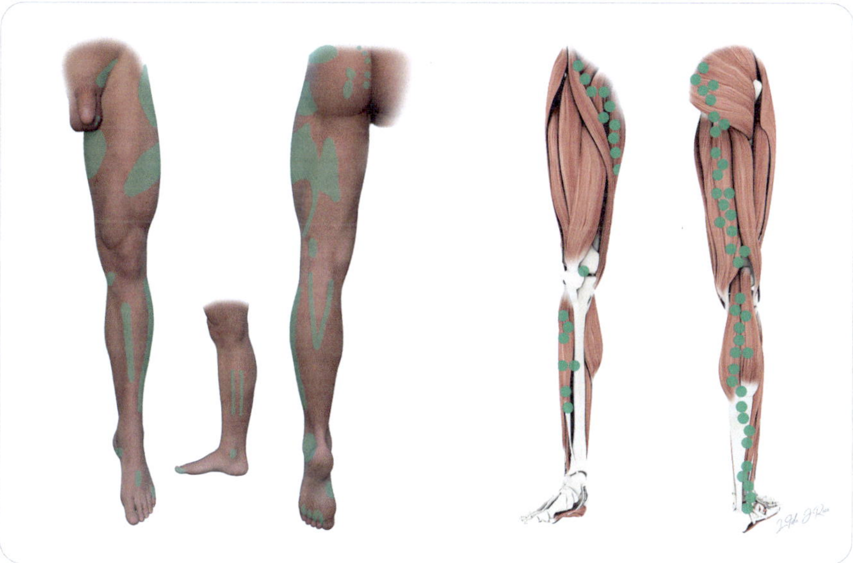

Fig. 38.4 The two illustrations show different pain distribution patterns associated with sacroiliac joint dysfunctions. On the left, a schematic representation with markings indicates typical pain points and affected areas in sacroiliac joint syndromes. On the right, common pain pathways are graphically displayed on an anatomical model of the leg. These images help to better understand pain projections and the effects of SIJ issues. A redrawing of these images could enhance clarity and precision in scientific publications or educational materials

Eighteen Different Pain Patterns Most commonly found in the gluteal region extending to the gluteal fold (94%) and in the lower extremities (50%). However, pain above L5 and in the groin area is also not uncommon. Distinguishing between pathologies of the lumbar spine and the hip joint is often imprecise and, in specific cases, nearly impossible.

4 Overview of SIJ Movements

- **Movement characteristics of the sacroiliac joint (SIJ)**: Movements in the sacroiliac joint primarily occur in the sagittal plane, revolving around a variable transverse axis that is positioned obliquely in space. This movement also involves a translational component, with a range of motion typically around 2–4°. However, in cases like ligamentous laxity syndrome, the range of motion can increase significantly, as demonstrated by a patient with a 9° rotation [8, 9].
- **Three-dimensional coupled movements:** Due to the unique topography and orientation of the SIJ surfaces, movement is three-dimensionally coupled, varying from side to side based on load and individual anatomical differences. Independent movement in one SIJ is not possible; movement in one joint necessitates movement in the other due to the closed kinematic chain [10].
- **Axes of movement**: While some theories propose additional axes (e.g., two oblique axes for sacral movements) [11], these are considered biomechanically implausible [12].
- **Nutation and counter-nutation:** During forward bending, the sacrum undergoes nutation (flexion), and the ilia move relatively posteriorly (ilium posterior). Conversely, as the body returns to an upright position, the sacrum performs counter-nutation or re-nutation, with the ilia moving relatively anteriorly (ilium anterior) (see Fig. 38.5).
- **Relative ilium movement:** In the transition from posterior to anterior movement of the ilium, the superior posterior iliac spine (SIPS) shifts from a posterior (dorsal), medial, and caudal position to an anterior (ventral), lateral, and cranial position. However, due to the proximity of the palpation point on the SIPS to the center of rotation, the range of motion in this area is minimal.
- **Translational movements**: Measured translational movements in the SIJ are minimal (<1 mm). Consequently, joint play tests such as the lift or shake test provide only qualitative results, typically based on pain response rather than quantitative measurement.
- **Dysfunctions and mobility:** Existing SIJ dysfunctions have not been found to cause a measurable reduction in mobility. In these cases, qualitative assessments, such as evaluating the "end feel," identifying signs of irritation, and conducting pain provocation tests, are essential for diagnosis.

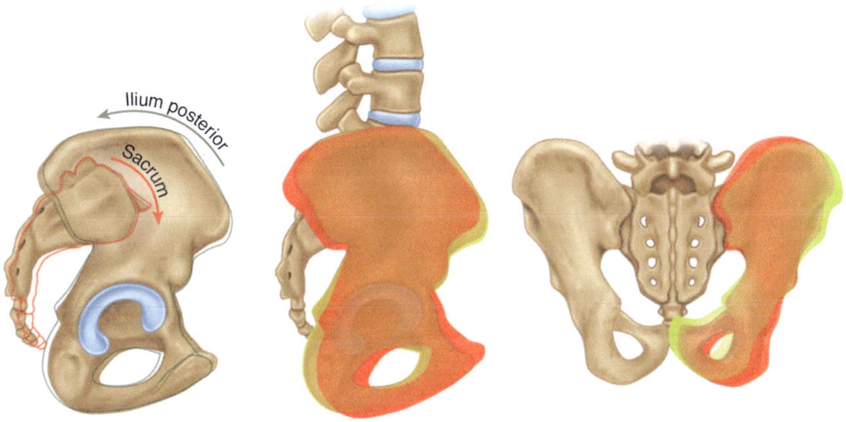

Fig. 38.5 Nutation movement: Nutation consists of the anterior flexion (forward) of the sacrum and the posterior movement of the ilium in the opposite direction. The ilium moves from the front (yellow) to the back (red). Due to the orientation of the joint surfaces, during nutation, the PSIS (posterior superior iliac spine) slides from an anterior-cranial-lateral position to a posterior-caudal-medial position. Counternutation occurs in the opposite direction (extension of the sacrum). The images illustrate the anatomy of the pelvis and the contact surfaces of the sacroiliac joint (SIJ). The highlighted areas (orange, yellow, red) emphasize the overlapping regions and surfaces involved in the biomechanical stability of the SIJ. This modified depiction helps to better understand the complex structures and spatial relationship of the pelvic bones

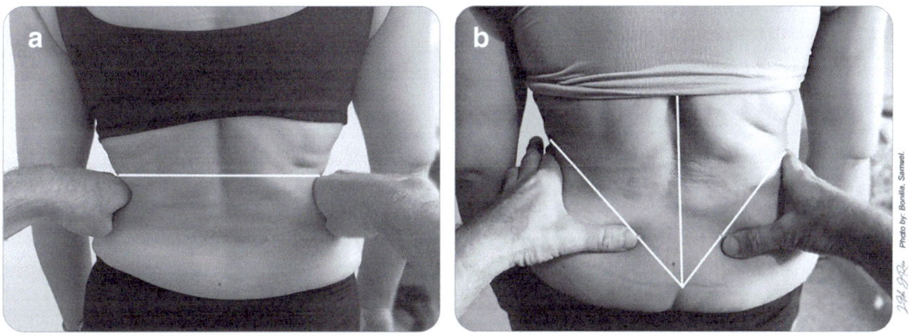

Fig. 38.6 The image shows the assessment of pelvic alignment in a standing patient. Image **a**, demonstrates the examination of the horizontal alignment of the posterior superior iliac spines (PSIS). Image **b**, illustrates the evaluation of pelvic torsion, where the height and position of the PSIS on both sides are compared. This assessment is a crucial part of the diagnostic evaluation of pelvic asymmetries

5 Assessment of Pelvic Alignment

The first step in the examination is the assessment of pelvic alignment. This involves evaluating the position of the anterior and posterior superior iliac spines as well as the iliac crests while the patient is standing (see Fig. 38.6). The patient should stand with feet hip-width apart, evenly distributing weight on both legs, with equal hip rotation, and with knees and hips as straight as possible.

In cases of unilateral hip and/or knee flexion contracture, the assessment should also be performed with both joints equally flexed to differentiate the effect of this condition on the observed pelvic misalignment. It is essential to distinguish between pelvic tilt and pelvic torsion. In a pelvic tilt, both the posterior iliac crests and the anterior superior iliac spines on the same side are lower. In a pelvic torsion, one side of the pelvis is lower dorsally, while the other side is lower ventrally [6, 7].

5.1 Specialized Joint Play Examinations

Specialized joint play examinations of the sacroiliac joint include the assessment of the forward-bending phenomenon and the Spine Test. In these examinations, it is important to recognize that the large palpable range of motion is only achieved by extending the range of movement to the body surface. The sacroiliac joint is an amphiarthrosis with very tight ligamentous support and correspondingly limited movement.

In vivo measurements of angular movements using tantalum markers between the ilium and sacrum have shown movements of 2–3°. For the nutation movement around the sagittal axis at the level of S2, values between 0.8° and 3.2° were recorded. This also applies to translational movements, which are greatest at the level of S1. These movements, contrary to the subjective perception of most examiners, measure only about 0.5 mm [3, 6, 7].

5.2 Assessment of the Forward-Bending Phenomenon

During the assessment of the forward-bending phenomenon, the patient stands with feet hip-width apart in front of the examiner. It is important to ensure that the weight is evenly distributed on both legs, hip rotation is equal on both sides, and the knees are as straight as possible. The examiner places both thumbs on the patient's posterior superior iliac spines and instructs the patient to slowly bend forward while keeping the knees as straight as possible. If there is unilateral hypo- or immobility in one SIJ (see Fig. 38.7), the sacrum on that side cannot glide cranially relative to the ilium. Therefore, the ilium on the affected side is pulled cranially earlier than on the opposite side ("runs forward"), which is indicated by the rising of the posterior superior iliac spine on the affected side [6].

However, this test has several potential sources of error. It is naturally unreliable in cases of bilateral dysfunctions in the SIJ and can also produce false results in patients with scoliosis. Additional sources of misinterpretation include unilateral or bilateral shortening of the hamstring muscles and blockages at the level of L4 and

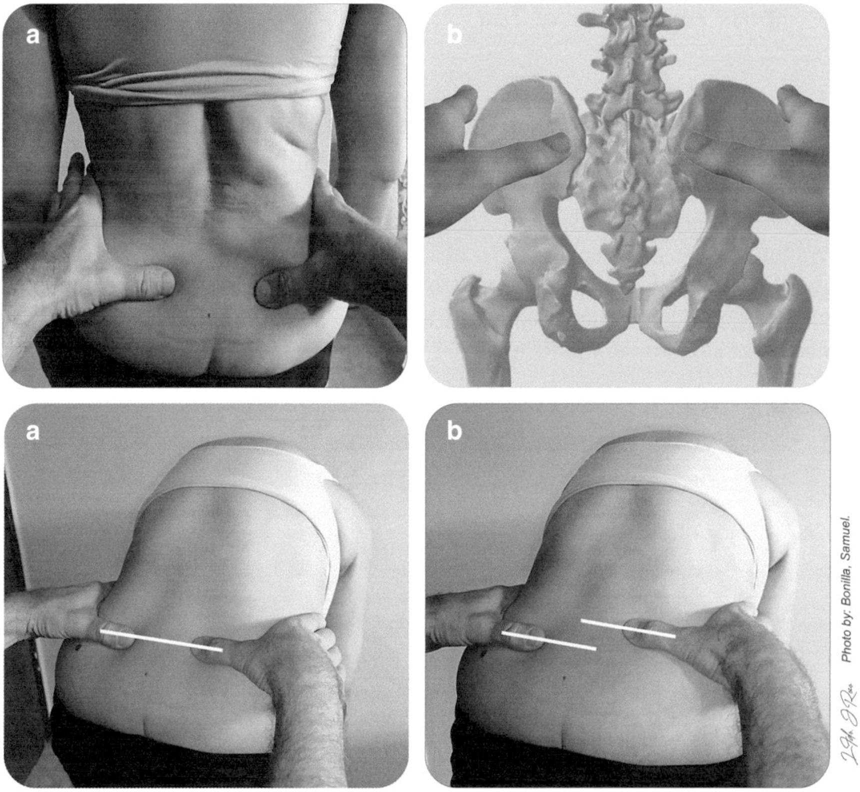

Fig. 38.7 Examination of the sacroiliac joint (SIJ) and forward-bending phenomenon according to H. Nazlikul. This image demonstrates the technique for assessing the forward-bending phenomenon, where the position of the posterior superior iliac spines (PSIS) is observed during the patient's forward bend. The images illustrate both the starting position and the changes that occur during the movement

L5 (where the ilium is carried along by the iliolumbar ligament on the affected side) [1, 3–7].

Summary

- The patient stands with feet hip-width apart, evenly distributing weight on both legs.
- The examiner places both thumbs on the PSISs (posterior superior iliac spines).
- The patient slowly bends forward.
- The PSIS on the impaired (possibly dysfunctional) side moves upward ("runs forward").
- Pitfalls: Lower lumbar spine blockages, scoliosis, shortened hamstring muscles, unilateral shortening of the quadratus lumborum muscle.

5.3 Spine Test (or Gillet Test)

The Spine Test is a side-specific functional assessment of the sacroiliac joints, allowing for a side-by-side comparison of movement in both SIJs.

For this test, the patient assumes the same starting position described in the forward-bending phenomenon test, standing in front of the examiner. The examiner places one thumb on the lower edge of the PSIS on the side being assessed and the other thumb at the same height on the sacral crest (between the spinous processes of S1 and S2). The patient is then asked to flex the hip and knee on the side being examined while keeping the other leg straight (see Fig. 38.8). The patient may use one hand for support during the test [1–4, 6].

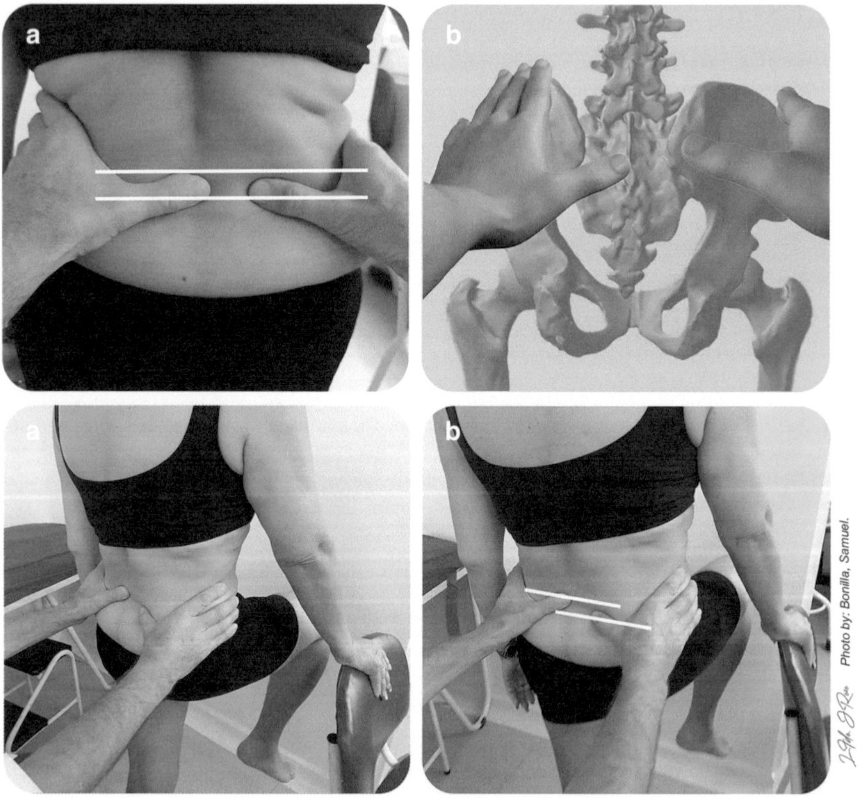

Fig. 38.8 Spine test (= return phenomenon = Gillet test) according to Nazlikul. This image demonstrates the technique of the Spine Test, which assesses the mobility of the sacroiliac joints (SIJ) through a side-by-side comparison (Top images (**a**) and (**b**)). The test detects SIJ dysfunctions by observing the movement of the posterior superior iliac spines (PSIS) as the leg is lifted (Bottom images (**a**) and (**b**)). (Photograph taken by: Samuel Bonilla)

Summary
- The patient stands with feet hip-width apart and legs straight in front of the examiner.
- The examiner places one thumb on the lower edge of the PSIS (posterior superior iliac spine) and the other thumb at the same height on the sacral crest.
- The patient lifts the leg on the side being examined.
- Pitfalls: Pelvic tilt and rotation in patients who lack sufficient postural stability.

Interpretation of Results
In this test, a free SIJ will immediately show a slight downward movement of the PSIS as soon as the movement begins. The absence of this small movement is already a clear indication of a dysfunction in the SIJ. As the hip joint continues to flex and reaches its range of motion, the PSIS on the examined side will more or less move downward, unless there is ankylosis or a significant blockage present. The onset of the ilium's movement is a measure of the hip joint's mobility, while the movement path indicates the function of the SIJ. The test is considered "positive" if the difference in movement is at least two centimeters. It is clear that this test allows not only an assessment of the function of the individual SIJ but also a comparison between both sides [1, 3].

6 Ligament Examination Is Very Important for Identifying SIJ Dysfunctions

Ligament tests are used to assess the SIJ and ligamentous conditions in the SIJ area. Such ligamentous conditions can arise due to either hypermobility or blockages. For example, as a result of a blockage in the SIJ or the costotransverse joint at T12, there can be a blockage-related hypertonicity of the quadratus lumborum muscle, which in turn leads to chronic stress on the iliolumbar ligament, resulting in ligamentosis [3, 6, 13].

6.1 Iliolumbar Ligament

The "ligament fan" test is used to assess the most important ligaments in the SIJ area. For this test, the patient lies on their back on the treatment table with their arms positioned alongside their body. The ligament is tested with the leg flexed at 90° in the hip and knee, with the opposite ilium stabilized. To assess for stretching pain in this ligament, the maximally flexed leg is adducted (see Fig. 38.9). A false result due to unintended pelvic movement is prevented by stabilizing the contralateral ilium. Applying pressure along the length of the thigh should be avoided, as this would fix the ipsilateral ilium on the surface and prevent the ligament from being stretched. Any pain occurring from such an error would primarily indicate involvement of the

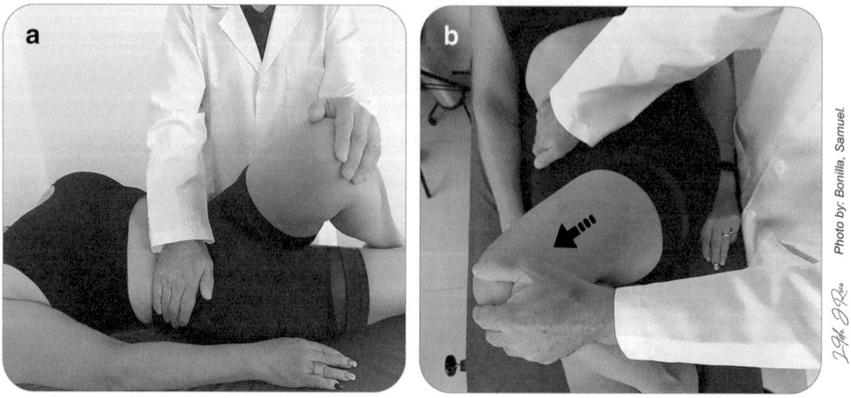

Fig. 38.9 Examination of the iliolumbar ligament according to H. Nazlikul. The image shows two different views of the test to assess the iliolumbar ligament. In image (**a**), the stretching of the ligament is performed by adducting the flexed leg while simultaneously stabilizing the pelvis. Image (**b**) illustrates the correct hand positioning and the direction of pressure to ensure an accurate assessment of the ligament

hip joint capsule, trochanteric tendinosis, or the piriformis muscle. Even with correct execution, the exact location of the pain must be identified, as the posterior ligamentous structures of the SIJ may also respond [7, 13].

6.2 Sacrospinous Ligament

To assess stretching pain in the sacrospinous ligament, the knee of the flexed leg is brought toward the contralateral elbow. The thigh of the contralateral leg is stabilized on the surface with an internal rotational counterforce (see Fig. 38.10) [7, 13].

6.3 Sacrotuberous Ligament

To assess the sacrotuberous ligament, the technique is similar to the previous one, but the leg on the side being tested is flexed at the hip and knee and then brought toward the contralateral shoulder (see Fig. 38.11). To accurately differentiate between the sacrotuberous and the previously mentioned ligaments, and to distinguish this from stretching pain in the hamstring muscles, topographical pain palpation is often necessary, as both tests (though to varying degrees) can elicit a response [7, 13].

Summary

- The patient lies on their back on the examination table.
- The therapist stands next to the table at the level of the SIJ.

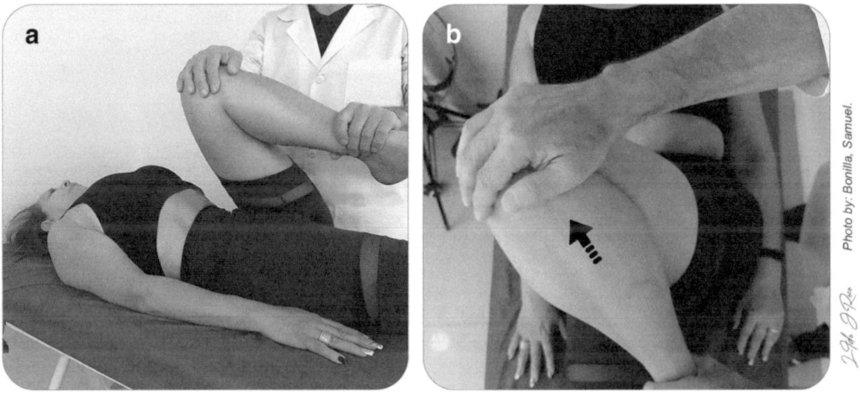

Fig. 38.10 Examination of the sacrospinous ligament according to H. Nazlikul. This image demonstrates the technique for assessing stretching pain in the sacrospinous ligament. In image (**a**), the patient's flexed leg is brought towards the contralateral elbow. Image (**b**) illustrates the exact hand positioning and direction of pressure needed to ensure an accurate assessment of the ligament

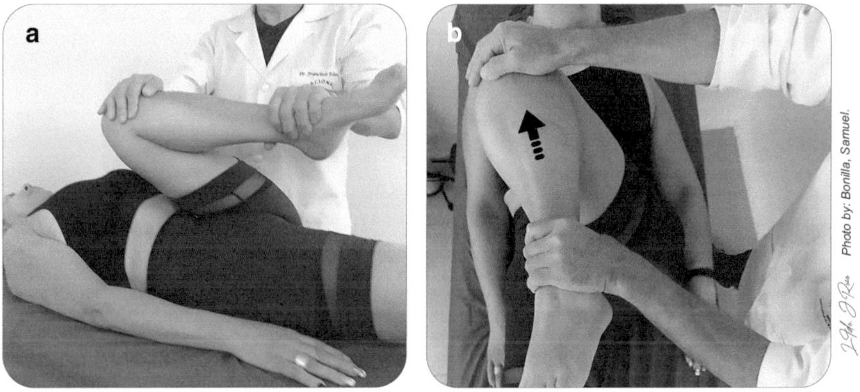

Fig. 38.11 Examination of the sacrotuberous ligament according to H. Nazlikul. This image demonstrates the technique for assessing stretching pain in the sacrotuberous ligament. In image (**a**), the leg on the side being tested is flexed at the hip and knee and brought toward the contralateral shoulder. Image (**b**) illustrates the exact hand positioning and direction of pressure required to ensure an accurate assessment of the ligament

- The patient's leg on the side being examined is flexed at the hip and knee, then adducted while stabilizing the pelvis.
- Pitfalls: Incorrect identification of the pain location.

Indications
- Low back pain.
- Joint blockages.
- Ankylosing spondylitis.
- Hip pain.

- Functional disorders of muscles associated with the axial skeleton.
- Chronic temporomandibular joint dysfunction.

7 Injections of Ligaments in the SIJ Area

- During ligament injections, the medication is not injected directly into the joint, but rather into the associated ligamentous structures. The examination of the ligaments has been described above. The goal is to eliminate irritated nociceptors in the fascia and ligaments. This technique was first described in neural therapy by Hüseyin Nazlikul in 2008 (see Fig. 38.12). The targeted diagnostic approach described above allows for differentiation of which ligament is causing pain [13].
- Targeted injection for isolated complaints in a specific ligament or unclear SIJ complaints provides rapid relief from symptoms [13].

Table 38.1 This table is the first draft describing injection sites and techniques for the ligamentous structures in the sacroiliac joint (SIJ) area, according to the author H. Nazlikul. The techniques focus on accurately targeting specific ligaments within the SIJ region.

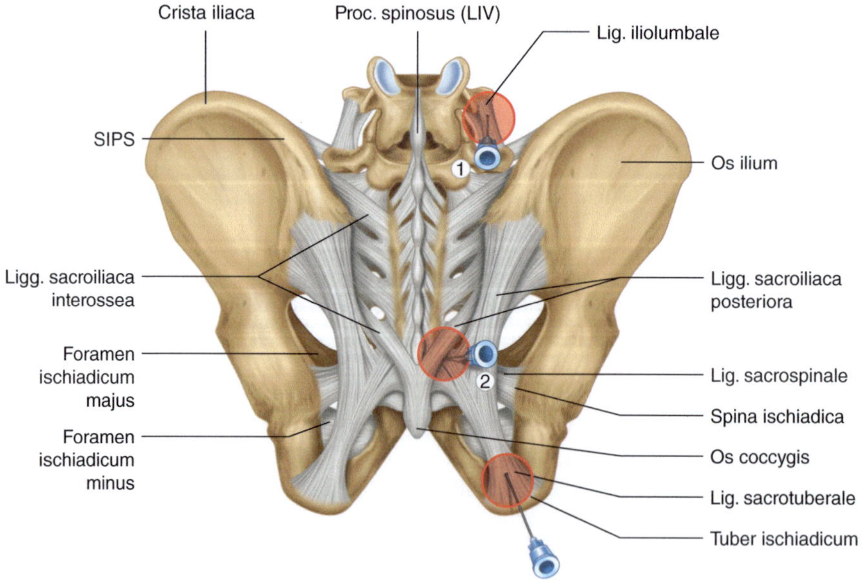

Fig. 38.12 Various injection sites for the infiltration of the ligaments of the sacroiliac joint (SIJ). This illustration highlights the ligamentous structures of the pelvis, with specific injection points marked according to the method of Hüseyin Nazlikul

Table 38.1 Injection sites and techniques for ligamentous structures in the SIJ region according to H. Nazlikul

Iliolumbar ligament	Sacrospinous ligament	Sacrotuberous ligament
Injection site		
Infiltration at the point of maximum pain	Mid-part of the iliac crest at the level of the medial sacroiliac joint (lateral) and the midline over the sacrum (medial)	In the ischial tuberosity, in the middle of the gluteus maximus muscle
Other injections are possible as needed	Fix the index and middle fingers on the site	The target structure is the insertion of the ligament into the ischial tuberosity
At the midpoint between the posterior superior iliac spine and the spinous process L4	Stretch the skin between your two fingers	Press the ischial tuberosity firmly with the finger
Left ligament: middle finger over iliac crest, index finger in the middle between spinous process L4/L5	Mark the insertion point	
With the finger firmly fixed		
Inject precisely between the two fingers		
Right ligament: upside-down fingers		
Injection technique		
2–4 cm perpendicular depth	Insertion perpendicular to the skin	

8 Injection at the SIJ

SIJ joint injection is possible by infiltrating the joint (see Figs. 38.13, 38.14, and 38.15). Avoid deep infiltration into the joint to prevent irritation of the periosteum, as periosteal injury or irritation is very painful.

8.1 Upper SIJ Joint Section

- *Injection site*: Position based on the posterior superior iliac spine (PSIS). Skin entry point is 2–3 cm cranial to the PSIS and 2–3 cm medial to the inner edge of the iliac crest.
- *Injection direction*: Proceed at a 45° angle laterally and 45° ventrally with firm pressure until a slight resistance is felt. At this point, you have reached the capsule.
- *Injection depth*: 2–3 cm.
- *Materials used*: 80 × 0.60 mm needle.
- *Amount of local anesthetic (LA) used*: 2–3 ml of 1% Procaine/Lidocaine [14–16].

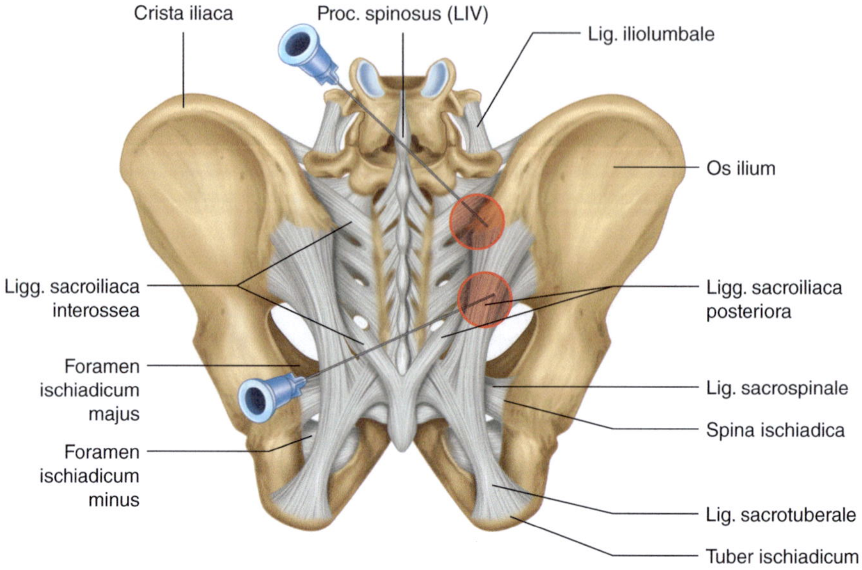

Fig. 38.13 This illustration shows the anatomical localization of the ligaments and the sacroiliac joint (SIJ) with marked injection points for both the upper and lower joint sections. The injection sites are specifically targeted for the treatment of the SIJ and surrounding ligamentous structures to carry out precise therapeutic interventions. The illustration highlights the positions of the iliolumbar ligament, the interosseous sacroiliac ligament, the posterior sacroiliac ligament, and the sacrotuberous ligament, along with their infiltration points. This image illustrates the injections according to Nazlikul

8.2 Upper SIJ Joint Section Injection According to Nazlikul

This injection technique was first described by the author (Nazlikul). It involves a combination injection that is more effective than a traditional joint injection. In more than 60% of SIJ issues, the iliolumbar ligament is also involved. Both the iliolumbar ligament and the upper part of the SIJ are infiltrated.

- *Injection site*: Midway between the PSIS and the L4 spinous process. Perform the injection targeting the iliolumbar ligament. For infiltrating the right ligament: Place the middle finger on the iliac crest and the index finger midway between the L4/L5 spinous processes. After advancing approximately 3–4 cm, the iliolumbar ligament is reached.

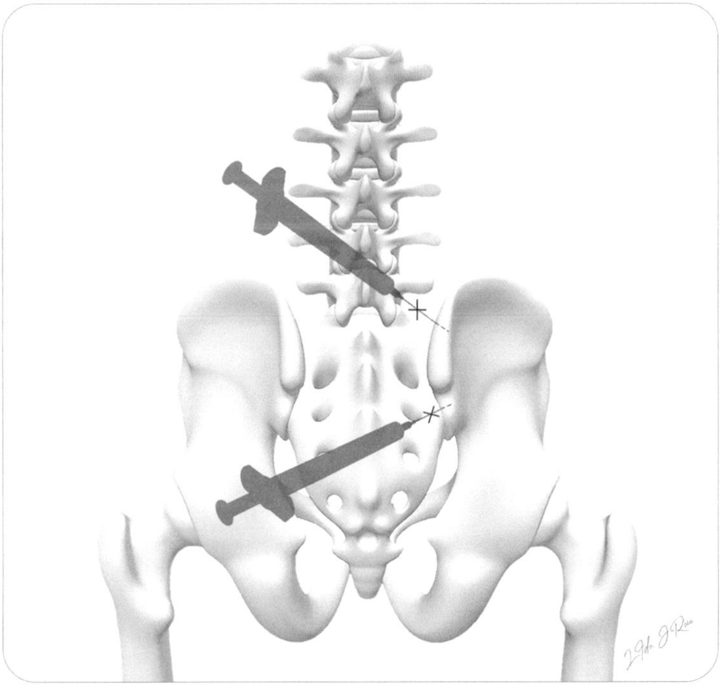

Fig. 38.14 The illustration shows injection techniques at the sacroiliac joint (SIJ) from above and below, as described by Lorenz Fischer. These injections target specific areas of the SIJ to achieve focused therapeutic effects

- *Injection direction*: After infiltrating the iliolumbar ligament, withdraw the needle 2–3 cm, change the direction to 45° laterally and 45° ventrally, and proceed with firm pressure until slight resistance is felt. At this point, you have reached the capsule.
- *Injection depth*: 4–6 cm.
- *Materials used*: 80 × 0.60 mm needle.
- *Amount of local anesthetic (LA) used*: 2–3 ml of 1% Procaine/Lidocaine.

8.3 Lower SIJ Joint Section

- Injection site: Palpate the joint space at the level of S1.
- *Injection direction*: From the joint space, proceed at a 30° angle laterally and 10° cranially, continuing with firm pressure until you reach bone or ligament contact.
- *Injection depth*: Infiltrate 1–3 cm caudally and 0.5 cm medially. Total depth is 2–3 cm.
- *Materials used*: 60 × 0.60 mm needle.
- *Amount of local anesthetic (LA) used*: 2–3 ml of 1% Procaine/Lidocaine [14–16].

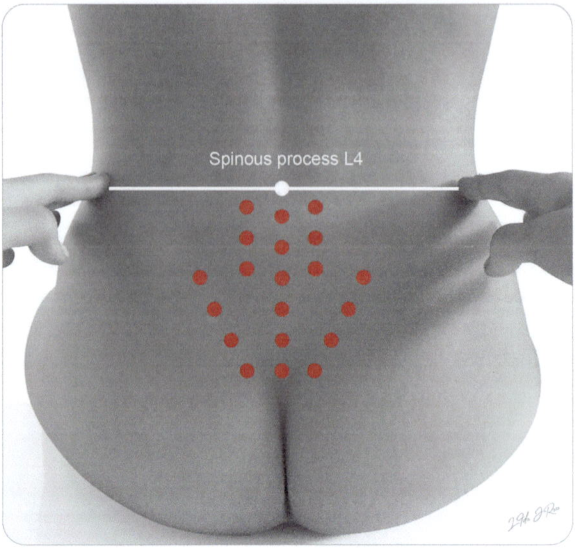

Fig. 38.15 This illustration shows injection techniques in the lower back, specifically targeting the region around the fourth lumbar vertebra (L4). The marked points indicate potential injection sites along the spine and sacral area

References

1. Heymann W, Moll H, Rauch G. Study on sacroiliac joint diagnostics: reliability of functional and pain provocation tests. Manual Med. 2018;56(3):239–48. https://doi.org/10.1007/s00337-018-0405-6.
2. Böhni UW, Lauper M, Locher H. Manual medicine 2: practical application of diagnostic and therapeutic techniques. Stuttgart: Thieme; 2012.
3. Nazlikul H, Heymann W, Acarkan T, Fischer L. Neural therapy and manual therapy combination at sacroiliac dysfunction. J Complement Med Regul Neural Ther. 2014;8(1):8–13.
4. Böhni UW, Lauper M, Locher H. Manual medicine 1: practical application of diagnostic and therapeutic techniques. Lumbosacral transition and pelvic ring. Stuttgart: Thieme; 2012. p. 544–602.
5. Dvorák J, Grob D. Cervical spine: diagnosis and therapy. Stuttgart: Thieme; 2010.
6. Bischoff HP, Moll H. Textbook of manual medicine. 6th ed. Balingen: Spitta; 2011. p. 54–70.
7. Nazlikul H. Lumbar vertebrae syndrome: a neural therapy perspective on chronic low back and back pain. J Sci Complement Med Regul Neural Ther. 2013;19:10–7.
8. Goode A, Hegedus EJ, Sizer P, Brismee JM, Linberg A, Cook CE. Three-dimensional movements of the sacroiliac joint: a systematic review of the literature and assessment of clinical utility. J Man Manip Ther. 2008;16(1):25–38.
9. Jacob HAC, Kissling RO. The mobility of the sacroiliac joints in healthy volunteers between 20 and 50 years of age. Clin Biomech. 1995;10(7):352–61.
10. Heymann WC. Considerations of a diagnostic test for sacroiliac (innominate) lesions. J Am Osteopath Assoc. 1968;67(9):1013–7.
11. Mitchell B, Verrills P, Vivian D. Sacroiliac joint pain: diagnosis and treatment. Australas Musculoskelet Med. 2012;17(1):15–24.
12. Klein J. Repair or replacement–a joint perspective. Science. 2009;323(5910):47–8.

13. Nazlikul H. Sacroiliac joint: infiltration of the ligaments in the region of the SIJ. In: Weinschenk S, editor. Handbook of neural therapy: therapy with local anesthetics. 2nd ed. Stuttgart: Thieme; 2020. p. 522–30.
14. Nazlikul H. Textbook of neural therapy. Istanbul: Nobel Kitabevi; 2010. p. 251–68.
15. Barop H. Textbook and atlas of neural therapy. 1st ed. Haug Verlag; 1996. p. 236–40.
16. Fischer L. Textbook of neural therapy according to Huneke. 3rd ed. Stuttgart: Hippokrates; 2001. p. 110–5.

Chapter 39
Gynecology

Stefan Weinschenk

1 Gynecological Pain: The Hidden Suffering

"Women don't complain"—worldwide genital pain is an underdiagnosed and undertreated complex of chronic diseases. NT is a simple, effective approach to many of these complaints. We can address all kinds of chronic pain in and around the small pelvis. Clinical research in the last decade has revealed several disorders well treatable by NT [10].

1.1 Acute Versus Chronic Pain

Acute pelvic pain is an emergency in most cases, which needs immediate help. Well-known examples are appendicitis, pedunculated ovarian cyst (ovarian torque syndrome), salpingitis, extrauterine pregnancy, intra-abdominal bleeding, or acute extragenital peritonitis.

In contrast, in clinics and practices, we often deal with chronic pain and chronic functional disorders, which require continuous, effective treatment over a longer time. Potential causes of chronic lower abdominal pain are listed in Table 39.1.

S. Weinschenk (✉)
Women's Hospital, Department of General Gynecology, Gynecological Pain Clinic, Heidelberg, Germany
e-mail: stefan.weinschenk@biogyn.de

L. B. Pinilla Bonilla et al. (eds.), *Neuraltherapeutic Medicine*,
https://doi.org/10.1007/978-3-032-03257-7_39

Table 39.1 Potential organs and disorders causing lower abdominal pain

Organ	Acute disease	Chronic disease	NT possible
Vulva	Vulvitis	Vulvodynia, vulva scars	++
Vagina	Vaginitis: Infectious or due to hormonal deficit	Vaginal pain, genital atrophy, scars	++
Uterus	Endometritis	Chronic pelvic pain syndrome (CPPS)	++
Adnexa	Pelvic inflammatory disease, salpingitis	CPPS	++
Bladder	Cystitis	Bladder pain syndrome (BPS), dysuria, interstitial cystitis, irritable bladder	+
Bowels	Ulcerous colitis, diverticulitis	Irritable bowel syndrome (IBS)	+
Douglas	Endometriosis	Endometriosis	(+)
Pelvic bones	Sacroiliitis	Blockades, such as SIJ blockade; pain after intervertebral disk surgery, or coccygeal trauma (skiing)	++
Peritoneum	Acute peritonitis, e.g., caused by appendicitis	Peritoneal dissemination of endometriosis	–

CPPS chronic pelvic pain syndrome, *EM* endometriosis, *IBS* irritable bowel syndrome, *SIG* sacro-iliacal joint, *S. p.* status post, history of. Acute diseases (column 2) are no subject of a treatment with NT

1.2 Chronic Lower Abdominal Pain

Lower abdominal pain (pelvic pain) can be acute or chronic. It may have many causes. The most common diseases associated with pelvic pain are listed in Table 39.1.

In the following section, we focus on patients with *chronic* discomfort and pain.

1.3 Pathophysiology of Genital Pain

Gynecological pain is based on a variety of pathophysiological conditions. In many cases, there are three main conditions underlying chronic gynecological pain: neuralgia, fascia tension, and silent inflammation (see Fig. 39.1).

We assume that many gynecological chronic pain disorders are associated with one or more of these conditions. Some disorders are more associated with neuralgia, some with fascial tension, and some with chronic silent inflammation. This new approach to gynecological pain allows a systematic therapeutic concept providing good success. This systematic approach applies NT on five levels. Each of these levels addresses one or more of the three conditions (see Table 39.2) [10].

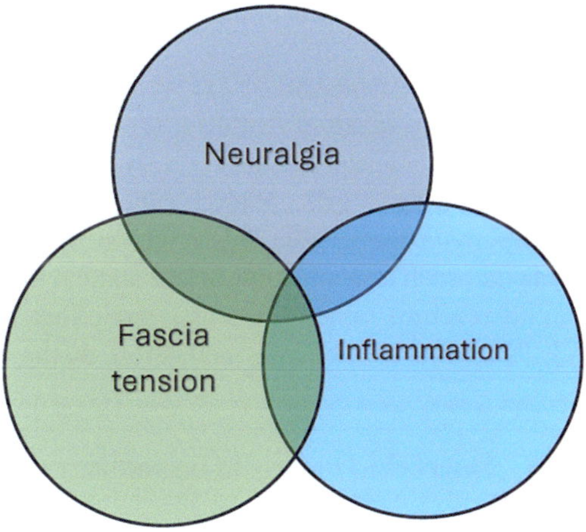

Fig. 39.1 The Triade of neuralgia, inflammation, and fascia tension in gynecological pain. (© S. Weinschenk 2024, with courtesy of the author)

Table 39.2 The five levels (approaches) of NT and their main focus in gynecology

Approach (level)	Neuralgia	Fascia tension	Inflammation
Local	+	++	+
Segmental	–	+	(+)
Regional	++	+	(+)
Remote	(+)	++	+
Systemic	(–)	(+)	++

1.4 General Considerations on Neural Therapy in Gynecology

Based on these five basic effects of local anesthesia (LA), NT exerts its clinical effects in three different mechanisms: desensitization, fascial release, and anti-inflammatory effects.

LAs are characterized by a variety of different molecular effects far beyond the blockade of the sodium channel. The latter is the best known of them and has been investigated for decades. Since 2000, an increasing number of molecular targets of LAs have been described (Lit.). The new *membrane theory of LA* explains this diversity of molecular effects [1].

1.4.1 Which Injection When?

The following disorders are the most prominent examples of a successful implementation of NT, the therapy with local anesthetics, into a multimodal therapy regime of chronic gynecological pain.

1.4.2 Adverse Effects of NT in Gynecology

Therapeutic local anesthesia (TLA) in gynecology is characterized by a remarkable low rate of severe adverse effects. The most common adverse effects are (a) a short, reversible hypotension with dizziness, (b) a special therapy effect occurring during the following 1–2 days called "reversible deterioration" (German: "*Erstverschlimmerung*"). This effect is well known in all methods of regulatory medicine, such as acupuncture, and manual therapy. It is supposed to be a sign of a healing reaction, rather than an adverse effect. It is frequently seen in gynecological NT. Patients should be informed before therapy on this and general adverse effects.

1.4.3 Stoerfield Therapy in Gynecology

The so-called **stoerfield** (German: Störfeld), or interference field, is a phenomenon well known to therapists in osteopathy and neural therapy. For a definition of the stoerfields, see Chaps. 13 and 24 in this book. There is little research on this phenomenon. The earliest hints of its existence came from an open field study, who found about 7% of remote effects [2]. In a study investigating neck reflex points, for the first time, a remote effect of NT (here: on neck disorders by LA injections to the pharyngeal region) could be demonstrated with a high reproducibility [3]. The lack of clinical studies hinders the distribution of knowledge on stoerfields in the medical community.

In gynecology, we distinguish between

1. Stoerfields affecting the genital region.
2. Genital stoerfields affecting other remote areas of the body.

An important source of the former are scars within the genital region itself, which are called segmental stoerfields. One of these is the umbilical scar (Fig. 39.2).

Such potential disruptive factors may induce and maintain genital disorders and chronic pain, and/or they may torpedo the therapeutic effect of an otherwise successful treatments.

Other scars within the genital region may also affect genital pain: Episiotomy scar on vulvodynia, abdominal cesarean section scar on CPPS, or coccygeal scars on chronic cystalgia.

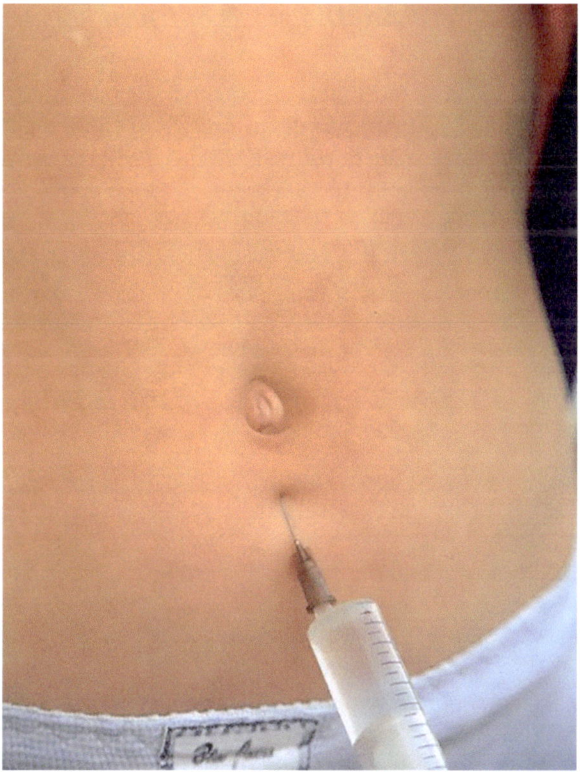

Fig. 39.2 LA treatment of the umbilical region as a potential stoerfield (interference field). (© S. Weinschenk 2010)

2 Chronic Pelvic Pain Syndrome (CPP, or CPPS)

2.1 Definition and Prevalence

Chronic pelvic pain syndrome (CPPS) is defined as "chronic lower abdominal pain without obvious origin for more than six months." It is an exclusion diagnosis in the absence of one or more of the diseases listed in Table 39.1. These disorders will be treated specifically, whereas chronic pain without an obvious origin is a domain of regulatory therapy such as neural therapy.

Dysmenorrhea is another frequent source of genital discomfort. In many cases, NT treatment is like that of CPPS.

2.2 *Differential Diagnosis of Chronic Pelvic Pain*

It is mandatory to exclude all potential organic or disorders by all possible means (see Table 39.1). A newly described sign of CPPS with a very high diagnostic value is the sign of parametropathy (PMP) [4]. PMP is a cervical motion tenderness found in bimanual examination. Its presence supports the diagnosis of CPP with a specificity of 92.5%. The PMP sign also serves as a therapy control for the effect of NT treatment of CPP, as it disappears after paracervical injections within 3–5 minutes (▶ Part 2.4).

2.3 *NT Treatment of Chronic Pelvic Pain*

CPP is a subject to effective NT treatment.

2.3.1 Local and Segmental Therapy

- Wheals in segment, "gynecological W".
- Wheals over the sacrum.
- Trigger point injections, e.g., oblique abdominal muscles.
- Scars in the segments L5–S4.
- Intravenous.
- Intrauterine instillation.

2.3.2 Regional and Ganglion Therapy

One of the most effective injections in the treatment of CPP are injections to the uterovaginal plexus.

- Uterovaginal plexus, abdominal.
- Uterovaginal plexus, vaginal.
- Parasympathetic centers S2–4.
- Lumbar sympathetic trunk.
- Sacral epidural injection.
- Ganglion impar.

2.3.3 Stoerfield Therapy

- Intestines: chronic malabsorption (malnutrition, dysbiosis).
- Tonsils, paranasal sinuses.

- Scars in segment: laparoscopy scars, appendectomy, status post conization, piercing.
- Teeth (in young individuals, occlusion disorders after jaw correction and tooth extractions, in older patients mostly tooth inflammations, periodontitis).

2.4 *Special Technique: Abdominal Approach to the Uterovaginal Plexus*

The abdominal injection technique to the uterovaginal plexus can be performed by every physician without special equipment. No gynecological chair is necessary. The patient lays in the spine position (see Fig. 39.3).

Neuroanatomical studies showed that the injection inflates the whole *ligamentum latum* of the uterus as well as a single branch of the pudendal nerve.

Some of the many effects of this injection are:

- Anti-inflammation.
- Pain reduction of the para-uterine ligaments.
- Improving circulation in the entire pelvis, especially bladder and genitals.
- Muscular relaxation in the pelvis (e.g., tension of the levator ani).
- Easing of the ligaments, including the sacro-uterine ligament.
- Relieving strain on the sacroiliac joint by relaxation of the sacro-uterine ligaments.

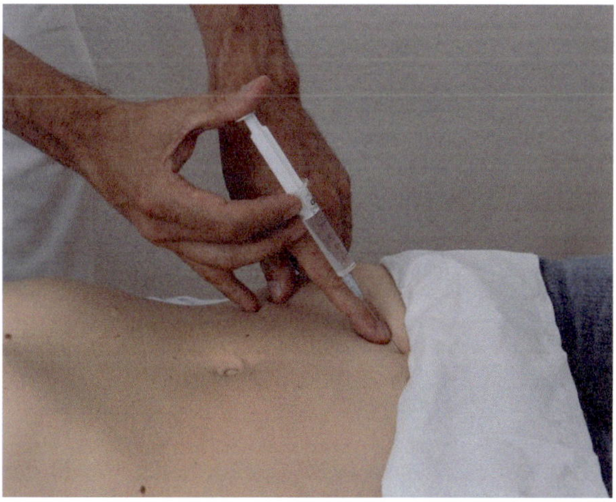

Fig. 39.3 Regional ganglia therapy. Suprapubic infiltration of the uterovaginal plexus. (© S. Weinschenk 2018, with courtesy of the author)

Material
Needle 0.6 × 80 (blue), 23G 3–5 ml LA per site, 1% procaine Cusco single-handed speculum Monitor with ultrasound during the injection not possible
Position of the patient
Very important: Empty bladder prior to the treatment Supine position with a knee roll. Gynecological chair not necessary
Point of injection
Palpate the pelvic rim 2–3 cm lateral of the midline Enter the needle 30° toward the midline and 45° vertically The needle follows the back side of the symphysis without touching the bone
Injection technique
Protrusion of the needle under continuous pressure, no aspiration (important for avoiding bleeding) The target region is reached as soon as the patient reports a short, flash-like pain in the vulva and lower part of the vagina (disappears again immediately) Injection of each 2–5 ml LA, e.g., procaine 1% Injection on both sides Screening of the pelvis with a curved ultrasound probe after injection, to detect possible bleeding of the retro-symphyseal region

3 Endometriosis

3.1 Definition and Prevalence

Endometriosis (EM) is caused by "dystopic endometrium," i.e., islands of endometrium (mucous membrane of the uterus) at atypical sites, such as the abdominal space. The ectopic tissue is also subject to the same cyclical fluctuations as eutopic endometrium, with growth and bleeding, and at the wrong sites, causes displacement (pain) and bleeding (scars, adhesions).

Common disease in females in childbearing age, prevalence in Middle Europe 10–20% stage I and II, approx. 1–5% stage III and IV.

3.2 Pathophysiology and Prevalence

EM is a frequent cause of chronic lower abdominal pain, cyclic and noncyclic, dysmenorrhea, dyspareunia, and dysuria. It is very important to detect this disease. The first step is "thinking of it."

Endometriosis is primarily viewed as an organic disease and is usually not associated with functional therapy methods like neural therapy. But endometriosis has a history that begins with a (subclinical) functional disorder, like many other diseases.

It presents as a severe organ disease only in the late stages with scarring and adhesions in the abdominal space (stage III according to EEC) or beyond (stage IV). Therefore, including NT in a multimodal concept is important in the early stages of the disease. Moreover, some patients with endometriosis continue to suffer from pain even after sufficient surgery and hormonal treatment.

The two known hypotheses regarding etiology are the metaplasia hypothesis, with spreading of endometrium through retrograde menstruation via the Fallopian tubes into the peritoneal space. A local immune deficiency of the peritoneum may foster the growth of endometrium on the peritoneal surface. Another hypothesis expands the spreading theory on an increased activity of the archimetra, the innermost layer of the uterus. Due to hyperperistalsis, "projection" of immature, actively growing cells from the deeper endometrial layers into the peritoneal space occurs [5, 6]. Hyperperistalsis of the archimetra may be caused by an increased sympathetic tone [7]. LAs are capable of reducing uterine contractility in vitro [8]. Sympathicolysis therefore may be one of the keys to the efficacy of neural therapy in endometriosis pain.

3.3 Indication for NT Treatment of Endometriosis

Endometriosis is treated according to the guidelines of the gynecology and endometriosis societies. In most cases, dysmenorrhea will lead to trace, but only invasive means, especially a laparoscopy, can fix the diagnosis.

Regular treatment consists of surgery (laparoscopy) and subsequent hormonal treatment. However, there is a remarkable number of patients which are not pain-free after standard treatment (see Table 39.3). These patients suffer from chronic pelvic pain even if they are operated on without residua and receive sufficient (anti-) hormonal treatment. Most probably, in this stage of endometriosis, the complaints are caused by a functional disorder rather than by the underlying organic disease. An elevated sympathetic tone must be assumed. NT offers a good perspective to these women. Indications of NT in endometriosis multimodal treatment are listed in Table 39.3.

3.4 NT Treatment of Endometriosis

3.4.1 Local and Segmental Therapy

- "Gynecological W"
- Muscular trigger points (mTrP) of the abdominal wall.
- Intrauterine instillation (10 ml Lidocaine 1%).
- This technique is an effective treatment for infertility in endometriosis [9].

Table 39.3 Indications for neural therapy in endometriosis, and possible indications for an add-on use of NT

Clinical situation	Indication	Add-on
Primary dysmenorrhea, therapy-resistant with HC	+	++
EM persistent pain with		
Previous sufficient surgery (R0)	++	++
Previous hormonal therapy (HT)	++	++
Current guideline-conform HT	++	++
Pat. rejects hormonal tx	+	+
Pat. rejects first explorative laparoscopy	0	(+) (limited trial)
Pat. suffers from adverse effects on HT	+	+
Pat. with contraindication against HT (e.g., oncological)	++	++
Pat. with family planning (no HT)	++	++

EM endometriosis, *HC* hormonal contraception, *HT* hormonal therapy, *Pat.* patient, *R0* complete surgery with removal of all endometriosis sites, *tx* therapy

3.4.2 Regional Therapy

- Injection into the uterovaginal plexus, vaginal approach, see part ▶ 3.5.
- Ganglion impar.
- Epidural sacral injection.

3.4.3 Stoerfield Therapy

Endometriosis is a systemic disease. There is some evidence pointing to a reduced immune defense. Therefore, stoerfields probably play a role. Stoerfield therapy of endometriosis may consider:

- Scars in segment: surgical scars in the genital region.
- Remote stoerfields. Every gynecological neural therapist should be able to examine the neck reflex points of the cervical spine (see ▶ Chap. 21) to find out remote stoerfields in the head and neck region.
- The thyroid gland is an important superior regulatory organ in genital pain and discomfort. It may function as a stoerfield to the genital region.

3.4.4 Special Technique: Paracervical Injection to the Uterovaginal Plexus

In endometriosis and CPPS, the infiltration of the plexus uterovaginalis Frankenhäuser plays a key role in successful NT. The vaginal technique allows a direct approach to this important plexus. This technique can be performed only on a gynecological chair.

The injection of LAs increases the regional perfusion of the organs of the pelvis, especially in chronic pelvic disorders.

A new approach with the bending of the needle in two directions of about 30° alleviates the injection (Fig. 39.4). It allows easy access to the lateral rim of the cervix. In the upper part of the lateral side of the cervix, the connective tissue is looser than in the lower cervical parts, which allows an easy flow of the LA into the *ligamentum latum*. For details of the techniques, see Table 39.4.

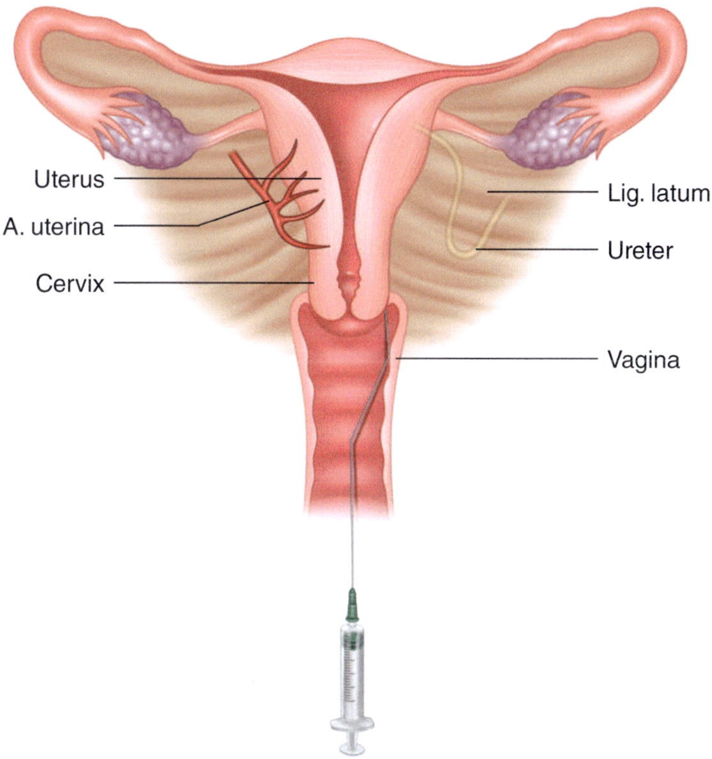

Fig. 39.4 Regional ganglia therapy with LA: paracervical infiltration of the uterine fascia and nerve ganglia

Table 39.4 Paracervical injection technique

Materials	
	Needle 0.8 × 60 (blue), 23G 4–5 ml procaine 1% per side
Position of the patient	
	Injection only possible in lithotomy position in gynecological chair Empty bladder Vaginal disinfection Speculum necessary, preferably a one-handed *Cusco*-type speculum
Injection site	
	Identify the lateral side of the cervix Insert the needle at 4 h and 8 h, respectively
Injection technique	
	Insert the needle with low resistance, about 0.1–0.2 cm deep Aspiration Infiltrate 2–3 ml each Important: Do not inject *into* the cervical muscle, but in the lateral soft vaginal tissue Cave: Bleeding of about 1–3 ml per side is possible. Use a swab to compress for a few minutes, if necessary

4 Vulvodynia

4.1 Definition and Prevalence

Vulvodynia is defined as "chronic vulvar pain or discomfort of >6 months without an identifiable cause," i.e., not associated with infectious, inflammatory, neoplastic, or hormonal disorders. For further details on the subgroups and covariates, see [11, 12].

4.2 Pathophysiology

There is increasing evidence that the main cause of vulvodynia is a hypersensitization of one or several genital nerves. The high success rate of TLA/NT supports this view in an impressive way [11]. In most cases, a neuralgia of the pudendal nerve is the cause of vulvodynia.

The five NANTES criteria [13] explicitly use the *success of a diagnostic injection with NT* for their definition of vulvodynia: (a) pain within the area of the pudendal nerve; (b) worsened by sitting; (c) no sensory impairment; (d) pain does not wake the patient at night; and (e) pain relieved by a diagnostic block of the pudendal nerve with local anesthetics (!).

Repeated blockades with LA obviously induce a de-sensitization of the affected nerves. This process is seen in Fig. 39.5. We therefore subsume vulvodynia to the pathophysiological group where neuralgia is a major part of the triad described in Fig. 39.1.

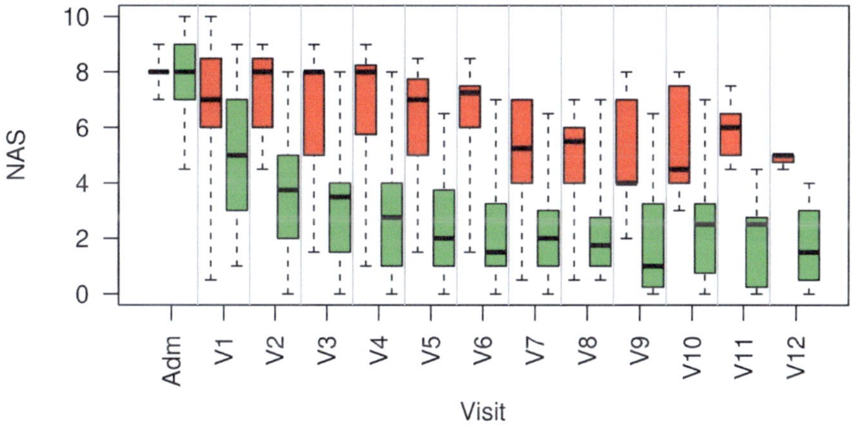

Fig. 39.5 Step-by-step de-sensitization of genital nerves in vulvodynia. The complaints of patients in the responder group (80% of the patients) continuously improve, beginning from the second TLA treatment session (green bars). Nonresponders (red bars) also experience a significant improvement, but less and later than responders. (From [11], © by the authors)

4.3 NT Treatment of Vulvodynia

Before the era of TLA treatment, vulvodynia was considered to be untreatable. Now we can offer patients an effective, evidence-based therapy with repeated LA blockades.

4.3.1 Local and Segmental Therapy

- Wheals over the sacrum.
- Scars in the segments L5–S4.
- Intravenous.

4.3.2 Regional and Ganglion Therapy

- Uterovaginal plexus, abdominal.
- Uterovaginal plexus, vaginal.
- Parasympathetic centers S2–4.
- Sacral epidural injection.
- Ganglion impar.

The key to success is the blockade of the pudendal nerve, see ▶ part 4.4, special technique. The repeated neural blockades with LA alleviate the desensitization of the affected nerve. In some cases (20–25%), other genital nerves are also affected, such as the genitofemoralis nerve. They also need to be treated with therapeutic blockades.

4.3.3 Stoerfield Therapy

- Intestines: chronic malabsorption (malnutrition, dysbiosis).
- Tonsils, paranasal sinuses.
- Scars in segment: laparoscopy scars, appendectomy, status post conization, piercing.
- Teeth (in young individuals, occlusion disorders after jaw correction and tooth extractions, in older patients, mostly tooth inflammations, periodontitis).

Stoerfield Therapy

VD is associated with genital scars, such as peripartal episiotomy, vaginal lazerization, or cervical conization surgery. The co-treatment of these scars is crucial for the successful therapy of VD.

4.4 Special Technique: Injection to the Pudendal Nerve

The pudendal nerve infiltration with LAs was a difficult procedure before 2017. It was performed either via the gluteal muscles under CT control or via the vagina with an IOWA trumpet. Both methods were unsatisfactory, as well as in efficacy, as in the rate of adverse effects. In 2017, we introduced the perineal injection technique, which allows easy access to all inferior branches of the pudendal nerve and provides anesthesia in 90% of the injections [14] (see Fig. 39.6).

Effects of the pudendal nerve injection:

- Increased circulation in the outer genitalia and pelvic floor.
- Instant alleviation of pain.
- "Holiday from pain": downregulation of the peripheral pain memory after several injections.
- Tension is released in the pelvic floor connective tissue and muscles.

The injection technique is described in detail in Table 39.5.

5 Scar Pain and Discomfort

5.1 Prevalence

Scars in the genital region are a frequent reason for discomfort and pain. They often are correlated with a trauma experience, or even PTPS (PTBS). This close connection to psycho-social disorders needs to be kept in mind when treating genital scars.

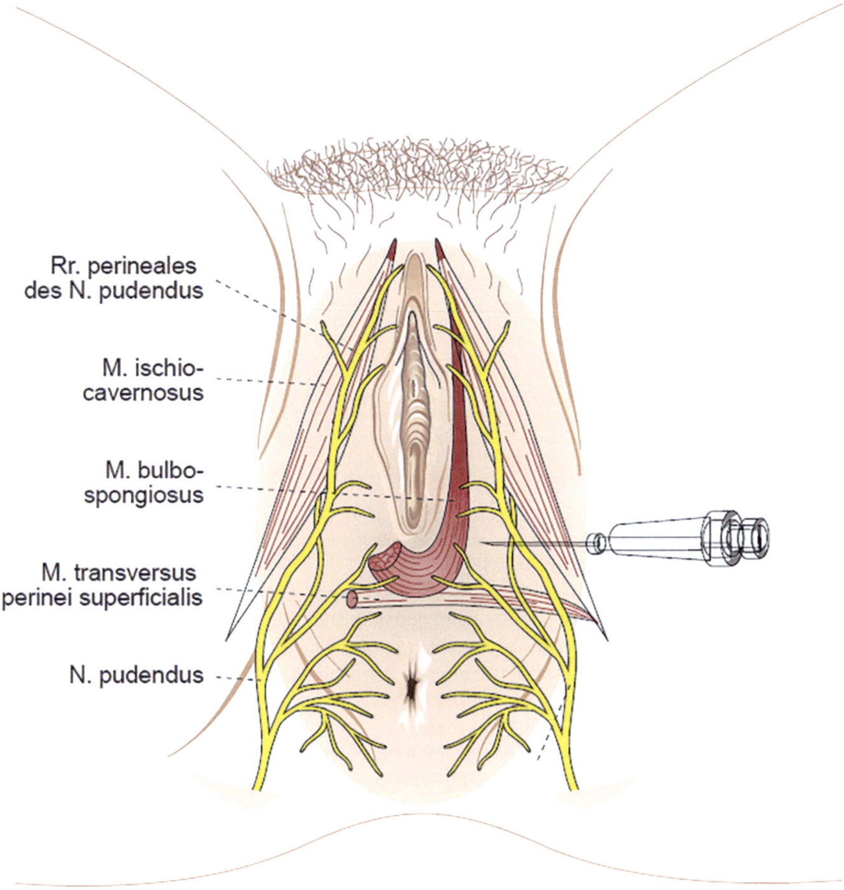

Fig. 39.6 Regional neural therapy with infiltration of the pudendal nerve. (© S. Weinschenk 2020, with courtesy of the author)

Table 39.5 Perineal injection to the pudendal nerve

Perineal method (see Fig. 39.6)
Materials
Needle 0.4 × 40 (grey), 27G In patients with BMI > 30, a 0.6 × 60 (blue), G23 needle may be used 5 ml procaine 1% or lidocaine 1% per side
Positioning patient
On a gynecological chair. No colposcope nor speculum is needed **Important: The gynecological chair should allow a deflection of the thighs of at least 90°** Perineal disinfection lateral of the vulva, cave: Do not apply alcohol directly on the introitus of the vagina, this is painful!
Injection site
Lateral to the labia majora (easily identifiable by its darker color), in the lower third, in line with the posterior commissure
Injection technique
Injection must be as painless as possible! This will be achieved by: Vertical injection, sagittal needle direction (towards the head) Slightly press the syringe stamp to inject a small amount when proceeding with the needle ("*injection under pressure*" technique) Important: Carefully insert the needle, use the "stop & go" method: The patient determines the speed of injection. If she expresses pain, do not further insert the needle, but inject a few drops; as soon as there is anesthesia, continue to insert the needle Inject 5 ml per side, half of it should be deposited around the main pudendal branch Injection is successful if the patient describes superficial hypesthesia or anesthesia of the perineum on swab test (in about 90% of cases) In the case of insufficient anesthesia, repeat the injection once, or use lidocaine 1% or Mepivacaine 1% (better infiltration into the surrounding tissue due to higher lipophilicity) Inject both sides

5.2 Pathophysiology of Genital Scars

Genital scars are located in one of the most innervated and emotionally most important regions of the body. Genital scars may derive from iatrogenic or traumatic events (see Table 39.6).

5.3 Treatment of Genital Scar Complaints

Local therapy of the scars themselves is the key to improvement of scar pain and discomfort. Treatment with LAs may also result in a better cosmetic result, for instance, in keloid-type scars, even if this is not the main goal of this approach.

The instillation of 1% or 2% Procaine into and under keloids and hypertrophic scars is a noteworthy therapy option with few side effects and a high success rate. The infiltrated scar becomes markedly flatter, softer, more elastic and approximates

Table 39.6 Potential sources of genital scars

Surgery or other trauma	Examples
Breast surgery	Reduction or enlargement breast surgery; mastectomy, breast Ca
Laparoscopy	In endometriosis surgery, cave: Large interior scars possible
Open abdominal surgery	Cesarean section, hysterectomy, other lower abdominal surgery
Vaginal surgery	Hysterectomy (LASH), descensus surgery,
Pelvic floor surgery	Colporrhaphy; sacral suspension surgery; MESH implants
Cervix	Punch biopsy, conization
Vulva	Episiotomy, punch biopsy
Violation	Stupor, genital mutilation
Bladder and urethra	Biopsy, urethra surgery, cystoscopy
Bowels	Hemicolectomy
Peritoneal surgery	In endometriosis or ovarian cancer
Vertebra	Trauma, e.g., fall on the coccygeal region (STURZ)
Lower vertebra surgery	Intervertebral discs
Car accident trauma	Pelvic fracture

the color of the surrounding skin. This occurs at different times in therapy, often after 4–5 therapy sessions. If the scars are more than 10 years old, ten or more treatments may be necessary.

5.3.1 Local Neural Therapy

- Injections into keloids may be painful. Thus, it is recommended that the scar area first be injected for the purpose of local regional anesthesia.
- The direction of insertion ranges from slightly tangential to 45°. The keloid begins to fade under injection. Procaine also diffuses from the keloid into the surrounding skin area.
- The actual bulge is hard and barely distensible. The high pressure necessary is best applied with a dental syringe. With the screwed-on cannula, the potential for the needle to bounce off is avoided. After the first few treatments, the tissue will become softer and the injection easier.

5.3.2 Segmental Therapy

In most genital scars, wheals cannot be applied. 1 ml 1% Procaine i.v. on the affected side may also serve as a segmental therapy.

Regional Therapy

Only applicable in special situations, when local or segmental therapy cannot be applied. Important injection techniques are the uterovaginal plexus (see ▶ part 2.4) and the stellate ganglion blockade (SGB) (see ▶ Chap. 35).

Stoerfield Therapy

Scar complaints and pain can be maintained by all closely located *stoerfields*, including other scars, especially those in the same segment.

5.4 Special Technique: Genital Scar Injections

Genital scars especially require a thorough and careful injection technique. Sometimes unexpected reactions on infiltration can occur, such as a sudden *emotional release*. Therefore, for scar injections, an informed consent should be obtained before.

For the special genital scar injection technique, see Table 39.7.

Two points should be considered:

- Infiltration from the inert surrounding tissue toward the scar (e.g., see Fig. 39.7).
- Integrate infiltration of the deeper parts of the scar, often located in the fascia, and easily identifiable by an exactly located tender point.

Scar treatment requires a gentle and thorough approach in order not to retraumatize the patient. Also, *flash-back* reactions occasionally occur during injection, and must be kept in mind.

Table 39.7 Genital scar injection techniques

Materials
Needle 0.4 × 20, 0.4 × 40 (grey), 27G In highly innervated regions, such as the vulva, also needles 0.3 × 13 (yellow), 30G may be used 5–10 ml procaine 1% or lidocaine 1% per scar
Position of the patient
Relaxed position, usually spine position Thorough disinfection of the scar area Cave: Do not apply alcohol directly on the introitus of the vagina
Injection site
Lateral to the scar in the healthy tissue, toward the subcutaneous tissue, undermining the scar
Injection technique
Injection must be performed as painlessly as possible! This will be achieved by: Slow injection technique, smallest needle diameter possible Slightly press the syringe stamp to inject a small amount when proceeding the needle ("*injection under pressure*" technique) Important: Carefully insert the needle, use the "stop & go" method: The patient determines the speed of injection. If she expresses pain, do not further insert the needle, but inject a few drops; as soon as there is anesthesia, continue to insert the needle Inject 5–10 ml per scar, half of it should be deposited around the scar in the healthy tissue Injection is successful if the scar and its surrounding tissue is numb In the case of insufficient effects, use lidocaine 1% or Mepivacaine 1% in the next sessions

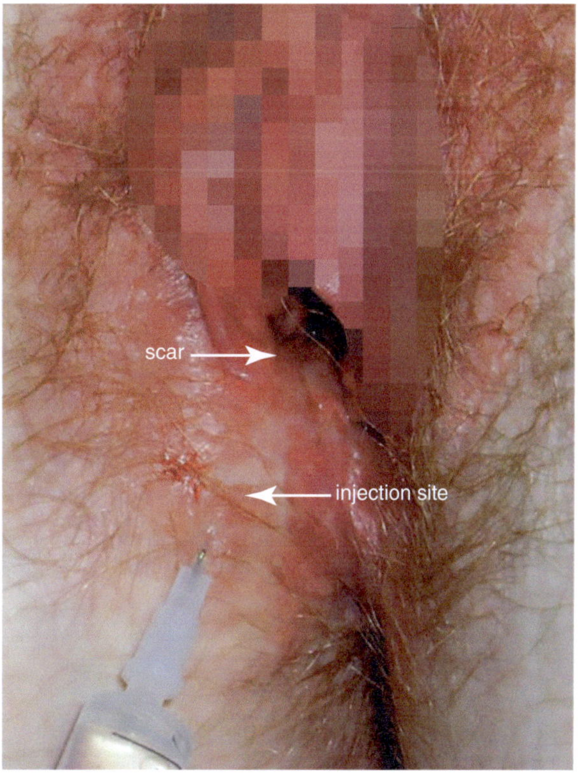

Fig. 39.7 Injection into an episiotomy scar of the right vulva. (© S. Weinschenk 2017)

References

1. Grage SL, Culetto A, Ulrich AS, Weinschenk S. Membrane-mediated activity of local anesthetics. Mol Pharmacol. 2021;100(5):502–12.
2. Ratschow M. Efficiency of therapeutic anesthesia. Acta Neuroveg (Wien). 1951;3(1–2):198–210.
3. Weinschenk S, Hollmann M, Göllner R, Picardi S, Strowitzki T, Diehl L, et al. Injections of local anesthetics into the pharyngeal region reduce trapezius muscle tenderness. Forsch Komplementmed. 2016;23(2):111.
4. Weinschenk S, Strowitzki T, Topbas Selcucki F, Gerhardt A, Feisst M. Paracervical tenderness (parametropathy) has a high diagnostic value in chronic pelvic pain. Submitted for publication; 2025.
5. Leyendecker G, Kunz G, Herbertz M, Beil D, Huppert P, Mall G, et al. Uterine peristaltic activity and the development of endometriosis. Ann N Y Acad Sci. 2004;1034:338–55.
6. Kissler S, Hamscho N, Zangos S, Wiegratz I, Schlichter S, Menzel C, et al. Uterotubal transport disorder in adenomyosis and endometriosis – a cause for infertility. BJOG. 2006;113(8):902–8.
7. Weinschenk S. Endometriosis, dysmenorrhea, and the autonomic nervous system. Erfahrungsheilkunde. 2004;53:523–32.
8. Weinschenk F, Dittrich R, Müller A, Beckmann MW, Weinschenk S. Change of uterine contractility in the perfused swine uterus model after application of the local anesthetics procaine, lidocaine, and ropivacaine. Am J Obstet Gynecol. 2018;13
9. Wickstrom K, Bruse C, Sjosten A, Spira J, Edelstam G. Perturbation with lignocaine as a new treatment of dysmenorrhea due to endometriosis: a randomized controlled trial. Hum Reprod. 2012;27(3):695–701.
10. Weinschenk S, editor. Handbook of neural therapy: diagnostics and therapy with local anesthetics (Textbook of therapy with local anesthetics). 1st ed. München: Elsevier, Urban & Fischer; 2010.
11. Weinschenk S, Benrath J, Kessler E, Strowitzki T, Feisst M. Therapy with local anesthetics to treat vulvodynia. A pilot study. Sex Med. 2022;10(2):100482.
12. Gerhardt A, Feisst M, Strowitzki T, Zivanovic O, Weinschenk S. Vulvodynia and chronic vulvar pain – influencing factors and long-term success after therapeutic local anesthesia (TLA). Pain Therapy. 2025;14:1025.
13. Labat JJ, Riant T, Robert R, Amarenco G, Lefaucheur JP, Rigaud J. Diagnostic criteria for pudendal neuralgia by pudendal nerve entrapment (Nantes criteria). Neurourol Urodyn. 2008;27(4):306–10.
14. Weinschenk S, Hollmann MW, Strowitzki T. New perineal injection technique for pudendal nerve infiltration in diagnostic and therapeutic procedures. Arch Gynecol Obstet. 2016;293(4):805–13.

Chapter 40
The Systemic Use of Procaine

Ralf Oettmeier and Laura Bibiana Pinilla Bonilla

1 The Systemic Use of Procaine in History

Since the synthesis of procaine in 1905 by Alfred Einhorn, this molecule has undergone a process of progressive discovery [1], from considering it a local anesthetic to discovering different properties that go beyond the effects of mere anesthetic blockade.

At the beginning, it was believed that procaine could be toxic or have adverse effects if it entered the general circulation. In 1909, Bier, for the first time, applied procaine intravenously to produce local anesthesia on the limbs; however, the entry of procaine into general circulation was avoided [2]. Since 1920, procaine history has begun to change: Leriche described the use of intra-arterial procaine for the treatment of migraine by irrigation of the temporal artery.

Five years later, the Huneke brothers introduced intravenous procaine to explore different ways to administer the procaine, searching for therapeutic effects but no anesthetics [3].

After the decade of the 1920s, the intravenous administration of procaine began to be a common exploration for several researchers (see Fig. 40.1). In the 1930s, Leriche and Fontaine described a successful treatment of endarteritis obliterans [2] and Lewy used it for the treatment of tinnitus [4].

R. Oettmeier (✉)
Alpstein Clinic, Gais, AR, Switzerland
e-mail: dr.oettmeier@alpstein-clinic.ch

L. B. Pinilla Bonilla
Faculty of Medicine, Master in Alternative Medicine, Neural Therapy Area,
Universidad Nacional de Colombia, Bogotá, Colombia

Integrated Health Services Subnetwork of the South, Research and Innovation Center,
Bogotá, Colombia
e-mail: lbpnillab@unal.edu.co

L. B. Pinilla Bonilla et al. (eds.), *Neuraltherapeutic Medicine*,
https://doi.org/10.1007/978-3-032-03257-7_40

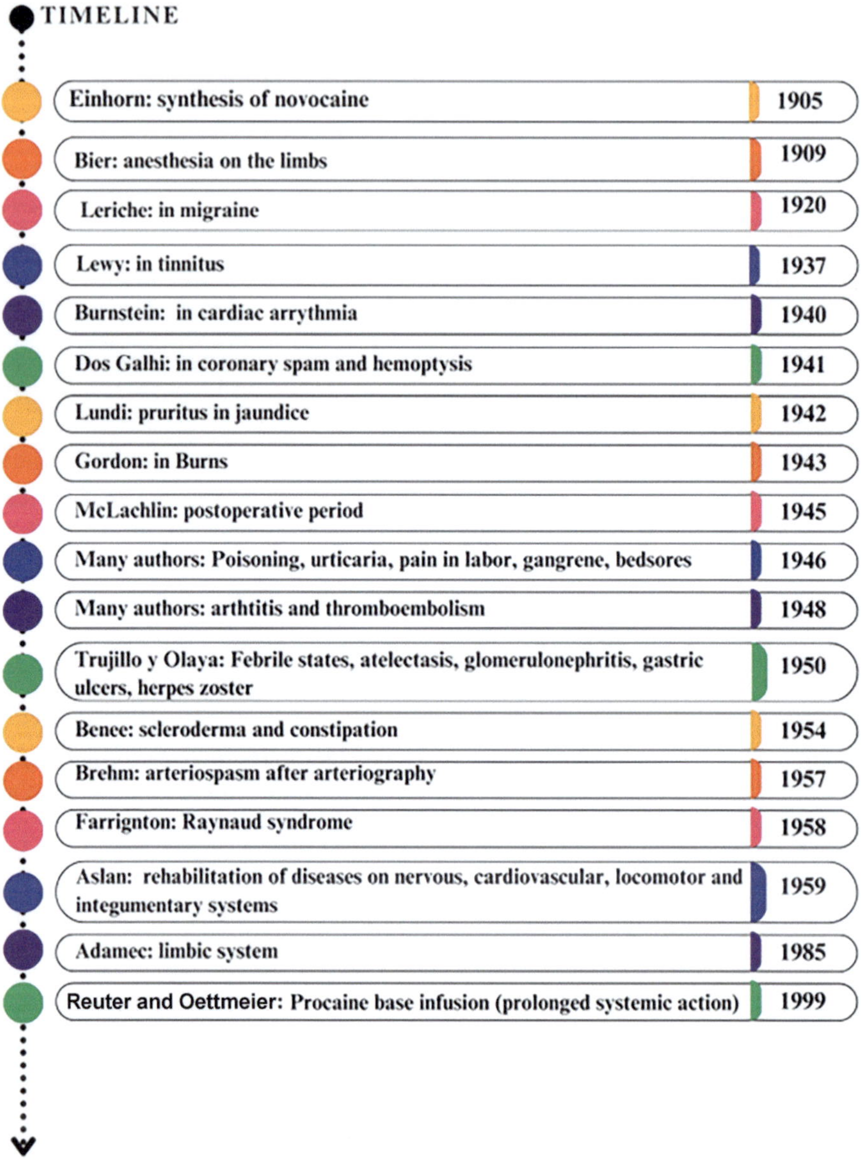
TIMELINE
Einhorn: synthesis of novocaine
1905
Bier: anesthesia on the limbs
1909
Leriche: in migraine
1920
Lewy: in tinnitus
1937
Burnstein: in cardiac arrythmia
1940
Dos Galhi: in coronary spam and hemoptysis
1941
Lundi: pruritus in jaundice
1942
Gordon: in Burns
1943
McLachlin: postoperative period
1945
Many authors: Poisoning, urticaria, pain in labor, gangrene, bedsores
1946
Many authors: arthtitis and thromboembolism
1948
Trujillo y Olaya: Febrile states, atelectasis, glomerulonephritis, gastric ulcers, herpes zoster
1950
Benee: scleroderma and constipation
1954
Brehm: arteriospasm after arteriography
1957
Farrignton: Raynaud syndrome
1958
Aslan: rehabilitation of diseases on nervous, cardiovascular, locomotor and integumentary systems
1959
Adamec: limbic system
1985
Reuter and Oettmeier: Procaine base infusion (prolonged systemic action)
1999

Fig. 40.1 Timeline about the milestone related to the therapeutic effects of procaine reported for the first time

The 1940s came with a lot of findings in the intravenous use of procaine: its use was described as a treatment for different diseases like cardiac arrhythmia [2], coronary spasm, coma, hypertension, enuresis, asthma, and hemoptysis. Lundy, from the Mayo Clinic, reported the use of intravenous procaine for relieving the pruritus in jaundice [2, 4] and, for similar conditions, its use was reported for the treatment of poisoning and urticaria [5, 6]. Continuing with its institutional use, procaine was reported for the treatment of a wide range of painful conditions in the City Hospital of New York, such as radicular pain, gangrene, bed sores, angina, fractures, and gallstones [7], and even as an analgesic for labor [2]. In Colombia and Argentina, the use of endovenous procaine was also described for the treatment of atelectasis, glomerulonephritis, sprains, herpes zoster, dislocations, gastric ulcers, toxic, and febrile states [5].

Since the fifties, the history of procaine use has begun to have a greater reach. Ana Aslan, a Romanian scientific woman who was a disciple of the neurologist George Marinescu, started to observe the impact of procaine administered intravenously in several cases that Leriche had reported between 1946 and 1949. After that, she tested the intra-arterial and intravenous action in arthritis, arthrosis, acrocyanosis, trophic disorders, the integumentary system, and the psychic state. In 1951, she started a study that lasted 8 years in which she investigated the possible effects of the process of aging at the C. I. Parhon Institute of Geriatrics on 7600 patients. In 1956, a pharmaceutical formula with a pH of 3.3 called Gerovital/GH3 that allowed more procaine to be metabolized more slowly was launched [1, 8]. The promotion of Gerovital was created under the financing of communist politician Nicolae Ceausescu (due to his declared interest in immortality), facilitating the administration of Gerovital in 144 clinics across Romania. Many celebrities came to their clinics to be treated [9], such as John F. Kennedy, Marlene Dietrich, Kirk Douglas, Salvador Dalí [10] Pablo Neruda, Charlie Chaplin, Indira Gandhi, Charles de Gaulle, Nikita Khrushchev, and Aristotle Onasis [11]. However, this phenomenon was met with disapproval within a segment of the scientific community: "With such celebrity and no reasonable scientific basis for such a panacea-like effect, the mainstream medical scientific community became increasingly incredulous" [9].

In the sixties, the National Institute on Aging commissioned a thorough evaluation of the studies and claims surrounding Gerovital H3. That commission concluded that "there was no scientifically credible evidence supporting the claims that procaine is beneficial in treating age-related diseases or syndromes" [9]. Additionally, another study from an evidence-based medicine perspective concluded that "there is no convincing evidence that procaine has any value in the treatment of elderly diseases" [12]. Even though it was a source of national pride for Romania [10] and Ana Aslan gathered a lot of experimental evidence regarding the beneficial effects on various areas [1, 8], other things probably played a bigger role in the West's thinking about this issue. Firstly, the rejection of communist ideas [9]; and secondly, the support for the pharmaceutical industry, which has been kept strong by swaying the scientific community's research and rules to keep its market niche [13] by discrediting any other options that might be competitors.

The effect on regulations may be clearly appreciated in the fact of the ban on Gerovital for "anti-aging" and associated claims issued by the Food and Drug Administration (FDA) in 1982 in the United States. Curiously, starting in the eighties, multiple studies emerged in various areas in the following years that ended up verifying the findings previously observed by Ana Aslan. Additionally, Oettmeier and Reuter developed a fresh idea for the use of procaine in combination with sodium bicarbonate at the turn of the century known as "infusion neural therapy," which supported and outperformed Aslan's findings [14]. These facts probably made it easier for the use of procaine to be allowed in 2011 by the FDA, but they issued an alert about false advertising in the market and in some literature [9]. These studies and others will be reviewed in the next section.

2 Reported Effects of Systemic Administration of Procaine

This review is based on scientific papers from 1946 to 2019 from authors in Africa, Canada, Colombia, England, Germany, Hungary, Poland, Romania, and the United States discussing the therapeutic effects of procaine intravenously or intra-arterially. However, other therapeutic effects and action mechanisms related to procaine through other ways of administering it can be found in Chap. 26.

In general, therapeutic effects in a wide spectrum of diseases have been reported. Table 40.1 shows the therapeutic effects reported on pain [2, 4, 5, 14, 15, 18–20], rheumatic diseases [2, 5, 8, 14, 15, 17, 21], musculoskeletal trauma [5, 18], integumentary system diseases [8, 15], mental and psychic effects [22, 27–32], allergic and toxic reactions [2, 4–6], and other symptoms and diseases [5, 14, 15, 18].

Other effects were also reported for the improvement and treatment of some visceral diseases and the nervous system, as Table 40.2 shows. There were reported therapeutic effects in cardiovascular diseases [2, 4, 5, 8, 14, 24–26], pulmonary diseases [2, 4, 5, 8], gastrointestinal diseases [5, 8, 14, 16], genitourinary diseases [4, 5, 14], diseases in the head [2, 4, 14, 16], and in the nervous system [8].

Among the published studies, there is an important reference to pain management in different disorders. Related to this, Bartolini et al. [33] investigate the antinociceptive effects of systemically administered procaine in mouse experimental models. They discovered that procaine produced significant antinociception, which was inhibited by atropine and hemicholinium-3. They also believe that the favorable effects of procaine on orientation, attention, memory, psychic depression, libido, appetite, euphoria, and various forms of pain, which Aslan first recorded, could be attributed to improved cholinergic system function.

Likewise, another of the common effects observed by Aslan and other authors has been on the mood. Several studies about the action mechanism of procaine on the brain have been made [27–32, 34]. Most of these investigations in the field of neuropsychiatry have studied the action of procaine on various structures of the limbic system, finding changes in its activation in a dose-related fashion. The data found indicates that procaine increases limbic excitability in part by interfering with local recurrent inhibition, not only reducing recurrent inhibition but also diminishing the response to excitatory input [35]. Also, it has been found that procaine inhibits conditioned fear in rats, affecting their avoidance behavior when faced with electric shock [32]. However, another recent study, supporting Aslan's research, reported an improvement in mood, sleep, and energy loss after repeated applications of endovenous procaine, even 6 months later [22].

Table 40.1 Therapeutic effects of the systemic administration of procaine in general diseases and systems

Therapeutic effects reported	Authors
Pain caused by	
Burns	Mushin and Rendell-Baker [2]
Postoperative pain	Mushin and Rendell-Baker [2]; Winter [4]; Oettmeier et al. [14]
Radicular pain / facet pain syndrome	Allen et all [18]; Oettmeier et al. [14]
Gallstones	Olaya [5]; Allen et all [18]
Urolithiasis	Olaya [5]
Migraine	Dosch [3]; Olaya [5]; Oettmeier et al. [14]
Labor	Olaya [5]
Herpes zoster/postherpetic neuralgia	Olaya [5]; Shanbrom [19]
Acute pancreatitis	Layer et al. [20]
Complex regional pain syndrome	Gordon [15]; Oettmeier et al. [14]
Other neuralgia	Oettmeier et al. [14]
Rheumatic diseases	
Arthritis	Mushin and Rendell-Baker [2]; Olaya [5]; Aslan [8]; Oettmeier et al. [14]
Osteoarthritis	Aslan [8]; Gordon [15]; Oettmeier et al. [14]
Balanitis xerotica	Farrington [17]
Morphea/scleroderma	Farrington [17]; Oettmeier et al. [14], Benee [21]
Raynaud syndrome	Farrington [17]
Lupus eritematosus	Oettmeier et al. [14]
Multiple sclerosis	Oettmeier et al. [14]
Musculoskeletal trauma	
Fractures	Allen et all [18]
Sprains	Olaya [5]
Dislocations	Olaya [5]
Integumentary system diseases	
Keloid scars	Gordon [15]
Psoriasis	Aslan [8]
Vitiligo	Aslan [8]
Lichen planus	Aslan [8]
Alopecia	Aslan [8]
Mental and psychic effects	
On psycho-vegetative symptoms	Hahn-Godeffroy et al. [22]
On limbic system	Kellner et al. [27]; Ketter et al. [28]; Servan-Schreiber and Perlstein [29]; Adinoff et al. [30] [31]; Matulewicz et al. [32]

(continued)

Table 40.1 (continued)

Therapeutic effects reported	Authors
Allergic and toxic reactions	
Pruritus of jaundice	Mushin and Rendell-Baker [2]; Winter [4]
Penicillin-sensitive reactions	Mushin and Rendell-Baker [2]; Moor [6]
Poisoning	Winter [4]
Urticaria and anaphylactic reactions	Moor [6]; Olaya [5]
Other symptoms and diseases	
Hiccups	Gordon [15]
Gangrene	Allen et all [18]
Bedsore	Allen et all [18]
Acute infectious diseases	Olaya [5]; Oettmeier et al. [14]
Osteoporosis	Oettmeier et al. [14]
Complementary cancer therapy	Oettmeier et al. [14]

Source own elaboration

Table 40.2 Therapeutic effects of the systemic administration of procaine in visceral diseases and nervous system

Therapeutic effects reported	Authors
Cardiovascular diseases	
Angina pectoris and coronary spasm	Mushin and Rendell-Baker [2]; Winter [4]; Olaya [5]; Aslan [8]; Allen et all [18]
Ventricular fibrillation	Mushin and Rendell-Baker [2]; Moor [6]
Endarteritis obliterans	Mushin and Rendell-Baker [2]
Thrombophlebitis	Mushin and Rendell-Baker [2]
Hypertension	Winter [4]
Peripheral vascular disease	Edwards et al. [23]; Oettmeier et al. [14]
Arteriospasm caused by arteriography	Howland et al. [24]; Brehm et al. [25]; Ng and Miller [26]
Pulmonary diseases	
Pulmonary embolism	Mushin and Rendell-Baker [2]
Edema	Winter [4]
Asthma	Mushin and Rendell-Baker [2]; Olaya [5]; Aslan [8]
Atelectasis	Olaya [5]
Gastrointestinal diseases	
Constipation	Benee [16]; Oettmeier et al. [14]
Gastric ulcers	Olaya [5]; Aslan [8]
Chron's disease	Oettmeier et al. [14]
Ulcerative colitis	Oettmeier et al. [14]
Genitourinary diseases	
Anuria	Winter [4]
Glomerulonephritis	Olaya [5]

(continued)

Table 40.2 (continued)

Therapeutic effects reported	Authors
Dysmenorrhea	Oettmeier et al. [14]
Diseases on the head	
Tinnitus	Mushin and Rendell-Baker [2]
Rhinitis	Winter [4]
Aphthous stomatitis	Benee [16]
Sudden deafness	Oettmeier et al. [14]
Nervous system diseases	
Parkinson's disease	Aslan [8]
Pseudobulbar palsy	Aslan [8]
Sequelae of cerebrovascular disease	Aslan [8]

Source own elaboration

Other studies have reported procaine's activity on many biochemical systems such as dopamine, norepinephrine, serotonin, and glutamate. For these reasons, procaine is considered useful for studying the limbic system and emotions [36].

3 Intramuscular Administration of Procaine

Brodie and coworkers demonstrated in 1948 that the intramuscular injection of 10 ml of a two percent solution of procaine (= 200 mg) was absorbed completely over a period of ten minutes. The studies also showed that the human being metabolizes procaine at a rate of approximately 20 mg per minute or more [37].

Using a two percent procaine solution, the team of Aslan established in Bucharest (Romania) the well-aging therapy due to intramuscular administration [38, 39]. They called it "rejuvenation therapy," using a dosage of 100 to 200 mg of procaine three times weekly.

In her original report [38], *Aslan* claimed phenomenal improvement in the psychic functioning of 109 elderly subjects who had undergone procaine therapy. She underlined that the intramuscular injections should be continued long enough to achieve therapeutic effects (three months to one year). *Bucci* and *Saunders* [40] studied 25 chronically psychotic women between the ages of 40 and 80 who had been hospitalized and failed to respond to phenothiazine drugs. The patients were given procaine hydrochloride three times per week in doses of 100 mg, for six months. Then they were given 160 mg three times a week for the next three months. The results showed alleviation of depression as well as a decrease in psychotic symptoms associated with schizophrenia. There was improvement in both the physical and mental status of the patients. Kral et al. [41] found similar results, with 32 inpatient patients (average age 81.1 years) with senile arteriosclerotic psychosis and 20 outpatients (average age 72) being treated for functional organic psychiatric illnesses. A temporary improvement in depression was noted, as well as an increased level of activity during the injection period.

Smigel et al. [42] studied 60 nursing home patients (ages 35–98) who had arthritis, nervous disorders, and senile mental disturbances. The double-blind study has shown that of 29 patients receiving procaine, 25 showed improvement in 5 months. Of the controls (placebo injections), nine showed improvement. Similar results focused on depression during senility are reported from other working groups [43, 44].

Several studies have examined the efficacy of procaine intramuscular injections in senile dementia and cerebral arteriosclerosis. In a study made by *Pascal* and *Bezusso* [45], 19 of 29 elderly patients showed a slight improvement in senile psychosis; 11 of 29 felt better, and 3 of 30 hallucinated less frequently. Giore [46] observed that 7 out of 10 elderly women treated with procaine improved on a vocabulary test, and 8 out of 10 performed better on the Progressive Matrices Test. Balganon [47] mixed procaine with PABA and observed significant improvement in around one-third of a sample of patients. Almost half of the group improved moderately. *Oury* and *Delvaille* [48] treated over 100 inpatients and 16.200 outpatients and observed similar results, especially increased memory and attention span.

In 1951, Aslan began to use procaine intramuscularly for the severe degenerative diseases of old age, including arthritis disease, both degenerative and rheumatic. The usual dosage schedule consisted of 5 ml of a 2 percent solution three times weekly in a series of 12 injections with a ten-day interval between. By 1960, several hundred arthritic patients had been treated. Restoration of joint mobility, reduction of pain, decrease of contractures, increase in muscle strength, and improvement in periarticular function were reported [39, 49, 50, 38–].

Finally, a lot more diagnostic groups from the intramuscular Procain injection series, according to the Aslan dosing, are described. These include the improvement of hypertension, diseases of the skin and hair, or the balance of endocrinological problems and sexual function. In general, procaine presents a wide spectrum of possible therapeutic actions, with its role as a geroprotector being the most relevant [1].

4 Doses, Dosages, and Secondary Effects of Procaine Administered Intravascularly

Since procaine began to be used intravenously in the first half of the twentieth century, the doses were applied both in a "bolus" and an infusion scheme lasting approximately 30–60 min. In the case of the bolus, the dose could range from 30 mg to 200 mg, injected very slowly [2, 6, 15, 16]. In the case of procaine administration under the infusion scheme, the dose varied from 100 mg to 1000 mg [2, 4, 5, 15, 17, 20, 21]. Sometimes the schedule was calculated based on weight, using the 4 mg/kg formula [2]. In other cases, the infusion is included in a treatment plan or "courses" that have a lot of variations: a daily application for six days, every six weeks, or a weekly application until a maximum of 10–12 courses [17, 19, 21]. In the vast majority of studies published in this period of time, no adverse effects were reported from the application of procaine at moderate doses [2, 7, 21]. However, when the dose exceeded or equaled 1000 mg, there were observed reactions such as a sensation of warmth, dizziness, a slight headache, buzzing in the ears, and sweating [4]. Other effects reported have been light-headedness, limb heaviness, blurred vision, accentuated noises, and, in rare cases, slight anginal pain or tremors. These effects were generally transient and manageable, for example, diminishing the rate of infusion [16, 19].

During the second half of the twentieth century, the application of procaine continued, in part, with the same infusion scheme that had been used, applying from 100 mg to 2000 mg administered over 30 to 75 minutes [12, 20, 22]. However, when the activity in the limbic system was discovered, other schemes for infusion were described. In the last case, doses were selected depending on the activation level of brain structures, considering the cerebral flow response evaluated by SPECT, which could range from 0.46 to 2.3 mg/Kg [27, 28, 30, 35]. The doses under 0.5 mg/Kg induced minimal changes in brain activity, while 1.0 induced global brain activation (limbic and nonlimbic structures), and doses higher than 1.38 mg/Kg could induce a specific activation of the limbic system [30]. In the case of intra-arterial application, which was especially used to avoid spasms secondary to arteriography, the doses used ranged from 30 to 200 mg of procaine [24–26]. In this last case, the authors found it better to use lower doses of procaine, beginning from 30 until reaching 100 mg, administered slowly to avoid symptoms of cortical irritation, apnea, or hypopnea [24, 26].

New schemes for treatment with procaine and bicarbonate were developed at the end of the twentieth century [14]. We will go over these schemes in more detail below.

5 The Combination of Procaine and Bicarbonate for Infusion

In 1930, the use of procaine with alkaline salts was mentioned for the first time [51]. In 1997, the first research, known as "neural infusion therapy" was published to combine the well-known pure alkaline infusion [52, 53] and pluripotent procaine.

Very quickly, the technique became popular in German-speaking countries and was incorporated into textbooks on neural therapy and pain following impressive positive outcomes in chronic pain patients [54]. By employing an animal model, Glusa et al. were also able to verify the vasodilation effect of the procaine-base mixture [55]. In animal studies, the addition of sodium bicarbonate also showed an accelerated initial effect and an increase in intra-cellular procaine concentration [56–58]. In numerous severe cases of inflammation and pain, the persistent application of Procaine-Base via a medical pump showed remarkable results [59–61]. The anti-rheumatic and joint-protective effects of Procaine-Base were also clearly superior to those of Dexamethasone in the osteoarthritic model of rats [62]. Recently, a summary of the experience with procaine-base infusion—which has been over two decades—was published [14].

Because of the effect of serum esterase, the plasmatic degradation of procaine was the main purpose of adding the natural buffer-base sodium bicarbonate. The characteristics of general build-up and ionization are common in all local anesthetics. They function on the voltage-dependent sodium channels because of these attributes. The transporting structure that can permeate is represented by the unloaded procaine molecule. Procaine-H+ (ionized form), which is loaded, binds to the sodium channel receptor, preventing an impulse from spreading. The ionized and nonionized forms of procaine can be affected by altering the pH value of the solution and the terrain [63].

Important properties like solubility and membrane penetration can be affected by changing the pH value, as can be seen in Fig. 40.2. By adding an alkaline additive, the relationship between the form of action and the form of transport is altered. Only 0.1% of procaine was found in the lipid-soluble form [63] when the pH value was low (<6). It is also known that various concentrations of sodium bicarbonate can affect the intracellular pH [64].

Initially, it was hypothesized that in an alkaline environment, the transformation of procaine into para-aminobenzoic acid (PABA) and diethylaminoethanol (DEAE) would be significantly diminished. Contrary to this assumption, it is believed that the intravenous injection of procaine-base results in its dilution within the bloodstream of major vessels, causing a rapid decrease in pH until it reaches normal physiological levels. Furthermore, the pulmonary circulation will induce a respiratory response to counteract alkalosis. The deceleration of procaine degradation can be elucidated in the following manner: The previously described pH-dependent dissociation shift will lead to higher quantities of transport forms that can penetrate well. Typically, this applies to all local anesthetics, resulting in the presence of 3–40% of the released base, determined by the pKa value of the anesthetic agent. It's crucial to consider the distribution's speed in addition to its steady-state distribution. The rate at which the substance diffuses through the membrane is the decisive factor in the speed of distribution [65]. Hence, the spreading is directly influenced by the lipophilicity of the substance. By altering the pH, the characteristics related to the affinity for lipids are modified. Elevated free base also means increased permeability, which is instantly absorbed by the surrounding tissue and

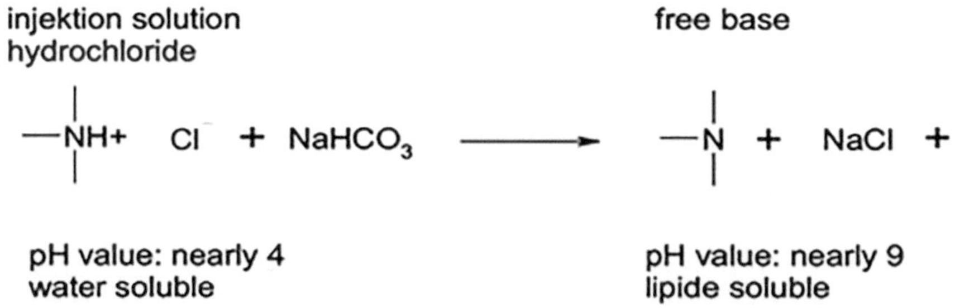

Fig. 40.2 Principle of change of the solubility and ability to penetrate depending on the pH value. (Taken from: Oettmeier et al. 2019 [14])

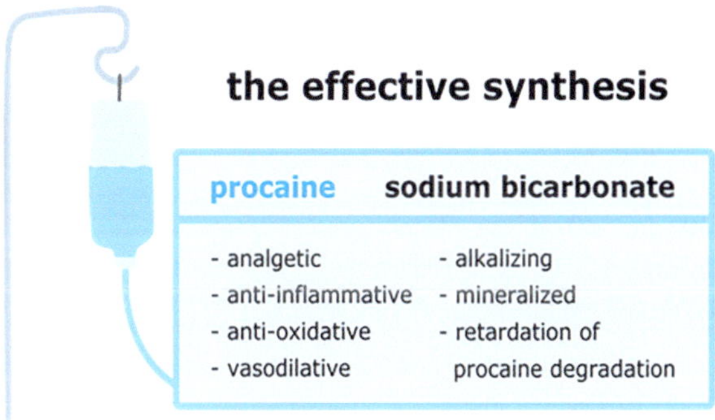

Fig. 40.3 The main effects of the action of procaine-bicarbonate combination. (Souce: own elaboration)

makes it more difficult for serum esterase to metabolize [64]. The following figure showcases the efficient combination of procaine and the naturally occurring buffer bicarbonate (see Fig. 40.3).

5.1 *Procedure for Infusions with Procaine-Base*

It is advised to perform a test application of one drop of 1% procaine into the conjunctiva if there is no prior knowledge regarding procaine tolerance before the infusion. Typically, the patient may experience numbness, acute redness from increased blood flow, and occasionally a brief burning sensation from HCl. If the intense sensation of burning continues for many minutes, it is advisable to refrain from receiving a parenteral infusion. It is crucial to emphasize that only procaine-HCl, which has been authorized for intravenous (IV) usage in the pharmaceutical industry and does not contain any preservatives, such as parabens, should be utilized [14].

It is recommended to initiate the treatment with a dose of 50–100 mg of procaine-HCl and 20 ml of sodium hydrogen carbonate (8.4%) that has been diluted in a carrier solution of 250 to 500 ml. Alternatively, the isotonic sodium chloride solution, which has been often used for an extended period, can be substituted with a comparable electrolyte solution to avoid hypernatremia. About 45 to 60 minutes pass during the infusion. The procaine-base infusion will be adjusted by gradually increasing the dosage of 50 mg procaine-HCl and 10 ml sodium bicarbonate (8.4%) until the appropriate therapeutic outcome is achieved. The maximum dosage of procaine-HCl for an individual with a normal weight is 300 mg, as indicated the dosing Tables 40.3 and 40.4.

For individuals who have risk factors for cardiovascular issues, it is advisable to employ a monitoring method such as electrocardiography (EKG) or oximetry when administering doses over 300 mg of procaine-HCl. An observation period of 30 min following treatment is advised. Additionally, it is recommended to refrain from operating a vehicle for approximately one hour following the therapy. Due to the instability of the procaine-base mixture, it is recommended to use it within a maximum of two hours, since procaine tends to degrade over time [14].

Table 40.3 Dosage in the case of using procaine 1%

Procaine dosage 1%	Sodium bicabonate dosage 8,4%	Sodium chloride 0,9%	Total volume
100 mg = 10 ml	20 ml	500 ml	530 ml
200 mg = 20 ml	40 ml	500 ml	560 ml
300 mg = 30 ml	*60 ml*	*500 ml*	*590 ml*
400 mg = 40 ml	80 ml	500 ml	620 ml
500 mg = 50 ml	100 ml	500 ml	650 ml

Taken and modified from Oettmeier et al. [14]

Table 40.4 Dosage in the case of using procaine 2%

Procaine dosage 2%	Sodium bicabonate dosage 8.4%	Sodium chloride 0.9%	Total volume
100 mg = 5 ml	20 ml	500 ml	525 ml
200 mg = 10 ml	40 ml	500 ml	550 ml
300 mg = 15 ml	*60 ml*	*500 ml*	*575 ml*
400 mg = 20 ml	80 ml	500 ml	600 ml
500 mg = 25 ml	100 ml	500 ml	625 ml

Taken and modified from Oettmeier et al. [14].

In the absence of acid-base diagnostic testing, it is recommended to limit the administration of procaine-base infusion to a maximum of three times per week, with at least one day of rest between each treatment. A range of 6 to 10 infusions, contingent on the medical situation, has received approval.

It is expected that blood markers of inflammation, like erythrocyte sedimentation rate and C-reactive protein (CRP), will get better after a course of procaine-base infusions. Patients often see a significant improvement in mood and overall condition after receiving four to six treatments. If a patient has a favorable response to the treatment, known as "responders" in approximately 80% of cases, it is recommended, particularly for chronic conditions, to continue with long-term therapy utilizing the effective dosage at longer intervals, such as once or twice a month [14].

5.2 *Experiences Reported with Procaine-Base Infusion*

The reported hypersensitivity to procaine, also known as "para-group allergy," with an elevated allergy rate mentioned in older textbooks has not been substantiated. A meta-analysis was conducted on 5698 patients to monitor important data during procaine-base infusions. This analysis included a thorough documentation of blood pressure, oximetry, and pulse rate before, during, and after the infusion. The results of the analysis did not reveal any statistically significant differences between the main groups [66]. A minimal inclination toward elevated mean blood pressure was observed when administering a high dose of procaine (exceeding 500 mg) and particularly sodium bicarbonate (at a concentration of 8.4%, exceeding 100 ml).

Moreover, it is noteworthy that there was no statistically significant discrepancy in the measured blood pressure between 15 and 30 minutes following the initiation of the infusion [14].

After administering approximately 800,000 procaine therapy infusions following the recommended scheme, according to Oettmeier, a single instance of long-term or severe side effects has not been found. There were no reported cases of a severe allergic emergency, confirming Becke's observations about the high level of therapeutic safety of procaine [67]. The more common symptoms reported have been:

- Heart palpitation (6%)
- Profuse sweating (5%)
- Short-term reduction in blood pressure and vasovagal syncope situations (6%)
- Sleep disorders (5%)
- Hyperactive feeling up to one day (5%)
- Temporary headaches and slight vertigo (4,5%)

It has been observed that patients who are taking nitro compounds, calcium antagonists, and beta-blockers appear to be more prone to experiencing these side effects [14].

5.3 *Indications and Contraindications of Procaine-Base Infusions*

After more than twenty years of experience using procaine-base infusions, Oettmeier et al. [14] have observed clinical improvements in several cases. The primary focus is on addressing acute and chronic pain, inflammatory and autoimmune diseases, vegetative imbalances, as well as providing complementary cancer treatments (see Table 40.5).

Table 40.6 summarizes the few contraindications that should be addressed in practice.

5.4 *Current Status: Procaine-Base Infusion Adapted to the Acid-Base Balance*

In a study conducted by Saha, it was found that 3 out of 13 patients exhibited clinical symptoms of metabolic alkalosis after receiving a total of seven procaine-base infusions. The dosages of procaine-HCl and sodium bicarbonate were gradually increased daily, reaching a maximum of 300 mg and 120 ml of 8.4% concentration, respectively. The base excess (BE) was measured through arterial blood gas analysis before and after the series of infusions. In all cases, the base excess was found to be greater than plus two, indicating the presence of a confirmed metabolic alkalosis [68].

Table 40.5 Main indications of procaine-base therapy

Acute situations	Radicular syndrome, pseudoradicular syndrome, acute infection, early stage of algodystrophy, sudden deafness, inflammation, migraine, activated osteoarthrosis, postoperative pain treatment
Chronic pain	Multiple arthralgias, chronic radicular–/pseudoradicular syndrome, algodystrophy, all kinds of neuralgia, facet pain syndrome
Chronic inflammations	Lupus erythematosus, rheumatoid arthritis, psoriatic arthritis, scleroderma, neurodermatitis, multiple sclerosis, Crohn's disease, ulcerative colitis, polymyalgia rheumatica, post-COVID-19 and postvaccination COVID-19 syndrome, Lyme disease
Cancer	To reduce side effects of tumor-destructive treatments (chemotherapy, radiation), as an important part of complementary oncology and immunotherapy, pain management of cancerous diseases
Others	Peripheral circulatory disorders, constipation, dysmenorrhea, clinical and paraclinical hints for tissue acidosis, osteoporosis, complementary cancer therapy, pre- and postoperative

Taken and modified from Oettmeier et al. [14].

Table 40.6 Contraindications for procaine-base infusions

Patient	Hypersensitivity towards procaine, Neurosis or Psychosis with unclear compliance, see also expert information at Procaine and Na-bicarbonate producers
Therapist and staff	Lack of knowledge in handling local anesthetics, inadequate educated staff, under-resourced rooms and lack of adequate emergency equipment

Taken and modified from Oettmeier et al. 2019 [14].

It is crucial to highlight that, based on the aforementioned procaine-base infusion procedure, the daily administration of such a large amount of sodium bicarbonate is not acceptable. This type of daily treatment is only suitable for patients who have a sufficient acid-base balance. Essentially, it is important to avoid overwhelming the body's inherent buffer system. Nevertheless, the number of patients experiencing metabolic alkalosis with a diminished capacity to compensate for acid-base imbalances is on the rise. Frequently, this occurs in situations involving excessive protein intake, advanced cancer, liver impairment, and dysbiosis of the large intestine leading to putrefaction. Moreover, the utilization of antacids, alkaline powders, loop diuretics, and excessive sodium consumption amplifies the alteration in the acid-base equilibrium, leading to alkalosis [69, 70].

Traditional blood gas analysis for the practical assessment of the acid-base balance could be advisable [71]. The test provides highly informative data regarding the base excess and precisely indicates the required amount of base. Metabolic alkalosis may also arise in cases of hyponatremia, hypokalemia, and elevated ammonia levels (in EDTA plasma).

On the other hand, metabolic acidosis is commonly observed in cases of inflammation, cardiac and renal dysfunctions, rheumatic diseases, and pain-related diseases [72]. These patients require a higher amount of buffer base and should be administered sodium bicarbonate in the range of 20–100 ml (8.4% solution) in addition to procaine.

Unlike instances of metabolic alkalosis, as depicted in Fig. 40.4, there is minimal or no requirement for additional base therapy. For this situation, administering infusions of procaine-HCl in conjunction with a carrier solution could be recommendable.

Depending on the BE result of the acid-base test, it should be advisable to make the adaptations to the bicarbonate amount for the infusion shown in Table 40.7.

To get an impression of the potency of procaine-base infusion, it is recommended to study the well-documented case reports in the overview article by Oettmeier et al. [14].

Analyte	Result		Reference range
pH	7.433		7.350 - 7.450
pCO2	31.0	mmHg	35.0 - 48.0
pO2	82.2	mmHg	83.0 - 108.0
Na+	138	mmol/L	138 - 146
K+	4.2	mmol/L	3.5 - 4.5
Cl-	109	mmol/L	98 - 107
Ca++	1.18	mmol/L	1.15 - 1.33
TCO2	20.3	mmol/L	22.0 - 29.0
Glu	90	mg/dL	74 - 100
Lac	0.71	mmol/L	0.36 - 0.75
BUN	7	mg/dL	8 - 26
Urea	2.6	mmol/L	2.9 - 9.3
Crea	0.80	mg/dL	0.51 - 1.19
Hct	40	%	38 - 51
cHgb	13.6	g/dL	12.0 - 17.0
cHCO3-	20.7	mmol/L	21.0 - 28.0
BE(ecf)	-3.6	mmol/L	-2.0 - 3.0

Fig. 40.4 Findings of metabolic acidosis (system EPOC, Siemens Healthcare AG). (Source: own elaboration)

Table 40.7 Adaptations of the bicarbonate amount depending on the acid-base test

Base excess (BE) mmol/l)	Bicarbonate (mmol/l)	Amount of 8.4% bicarbonate
>0	*>25*	*20 ml*
–1 – 0	*22–25*	*40 ml*
–2 – –1	*19–22*	*60 ml*
–3 – –2	*17–19*	*80 ml*
< –4	*< 17*	*100 ml*

Source own elaboration

6 Conclusion and Remarks

- There has been a progressive development of the therapeutic effects of procaine in several areas of medicine that began in the twenties, and it has continued until this millennium.
- Systemic use of procaine has included intravenous, intra-arterial, and intramuscular routes for administration.
- According to reports, procaine has therapeutic effects on a wide range of diseases, including the improvement of pain from various causes, rheumatic diseases, musculoskeletal trauma, integumentary system diseases, mental and psychic effects, allergic and toxic reactions, and other symptoms and diseases.
- Other effects were also reported for the improvement and treatment of some visceral diseases and the nervous system, such as therapeutic effects in cardiovascular diseases, pulmonary diseases, gastrointestinal diseases, genitourinary diseases, diseases in the head, and the nervous system.
- The so-called *Aslan injection* using 100 mg of procaine intramuscularly three times a week (for a minimum of three months) could be taken into consideration in cases in which the patient is not able to visit the neural therapist for a long time, and it can also be administered in conjunction with the classic treatment of Neuraltherapeutic medicine.
- Recently, a new proposal for the action of procaine for a longer time was developed using it in combination with sodium bicarbonate. Procaine-base infusion has a wide spectrum of indications for acute situations, chronic pain and inflammation, and complementary treatment in cancer.

References

1. Gradinaru D, Ungurianu A, Margina D, Moreno-Villanueva M, Bürkle A. Procaine-the controversial Geroprotector candidate: new insights regarding its molecular and cellular effects. Oxidative Med Cell Longev. 2021;31(2021):3617042. https://doi.org/10.1155/2021/3617042.
2. Mushin WW, Rendell-Baker L. Intravenous procaine; a review. Lancet. 1949;1(6554):619. https://doi.org/10.1016/s0140-6736(49)91716-x.
3. Dosch P, Dosch M. Chronological survey. In: Dosch P, Dosch M, editors. Manual of neural therapy according to Huneke. 2nd ed. Stuttgart: Georg Thieme Verlag; 2007. p. 4–8.
4. Winter L. Intravenous procaine infusions in the postoperative period. Ann Surg. 1950;132(1):143–6.
5. Olaya M. Uses and therapeutic possibilities of intravenous procaine. Rev la Fac Med. 1950;XIX(4):155–63.
6. Moor FB. A resume of intravenous procaine therapy. Med Arts Sci. 1948;2(4):401–10.
7. Allen FM, Crosmann LW, Lyons LV. Intravenous procaine analgesia. Dent Dig. 1946;52(11):611.
8. Aslan A. Procaine therapy in old age and other disorders (Novocaine factor H3). Geront Clin. 1960;2:148–76.
9. Perls T. The reappearance of procaine hydrochloride (Gerovital H3) for antiaging. J Am Geriatr Soc. 2013 Jun;61(6):1024–5. https://doi.org/10.1111/jgs.12278.

10. Grigoras A. 30 things that make us proud of Romania [internet]. Romania J. 2015; [cited 2024 Jun 12]. Available from: https://www.romaniajournal.ro/travel/30-things-that-make-us-proud-of-romania/.
11. Enciclopedia României – prima enciclopedie online despre România. Ana Aslan [Internet]. enciclopediaromaniei.ro. [cited 2024 Jun 12]. Available from: https://enciclopediaromaniei.ro/wiki/Ana_Aslan.
12. Ostfeld A, Smith CM, Stotsky BA. The systemic use of procaine in the treatment of the elderly: a review. J Am Geriatr Soc. 1977;25(1):1–8.
13. Dickinson J. Deadly medicines and organised crime: how big pharma has corrupted health-care. Can Fam Physician. 2014;60(4):367–8.
14. Oettmeier R, Reuter U, Pinilla-Bonilla L. The Procaine-Base-infusion: 20 years of experience of an alternative use with several therapeutic effects. J Altern Complement Integr Med. 2019;5:061.
15. Gordon RA. Intravenous procaine; clinical applications. Can Med Assoc J. 1948;59(6):534.
16. Benee J. Intravenous procaine (2%) in the treatment of constipation and aphthous stomatitis. Can Med Assoc J. 1954 Jan;70(1):54–6.
17. Farrington J. Intravenous procaine in the management of some cutaneous manifestations of collagen diseases. South Med J. 1958;51(11):1426–31. https://doi.org/10.1097/00007611-195811000-00013.
18. Allen FM, Crossman LW, Lyons LV. Intravenous procaine analgesia. Dent Dig. 1946;52(11):611.
19. Shanbrom E. Treatment of herpetic pain and Postherpetic neuralgia with intravenous procaine. JAMA. 1961;176(12):1041–3. https://doi.org/10.1001/jama.1961.63040250024020d.
20. Layer P, Bronisch HJ, Henniges UM, Koop I, Kahl M, Dignass A, Ell C, Freitag M, Keller J. Effects of systemic administration of a local anesthetic on pain in acute pancreatitis: a randomized clinical trial. Pancreas. 2011;40(5):673–9. https://doi.org/10.1097/MPA.0b013e318215ad38.
21. Benee J. Scleroderma treated with 2% procaine intravenously. Can Med Assoc J. 1954;70(1):71.
22. Hahn-Godeffroy JD, Mangold S, Bernert M, Bartelt A, Herdegen T. Long-lasting improvement of somatic and psychovegetative disorders under procaine infusions: a multicenter observational study. Compl Med Res. 2019;26(1):13–21. https://doi.org/10.1159/000491692.
23. Edwards JW, Jones NB, McConnell RB, Pemberton HS, Watson DC. Intra-arterial injections in the treatment of peripheral vascular disease. Br Med J. 1952;2(4788):808–11. https://doi.org/10.1136/bmj.2.4788.808.
24. Howland WJ, Curry JL, Wheeler PP. Intra-arterial administration of procaine hydrochloride after arteriography. Potential value in preventing arteriospasm and thrombosis. JAMA. 1967;201(11):813–6.
25. Brehm WF, King A, Coughlin J, Young J. Use of intracarotid arterial procaine during cranial arteriography. Surg Forum. 1957;8:540–5.
26. Ng AC, Miller RE. Intraarterial injection of procaine. Am J Roentgenol Radium Therapy, Nucl Med. 1971;111(4):791–3. https://doi.org/10.2214/ajr.111.4.791.
27. Kellner CH, Post RM, Putnam F, Cowdry R, Gardner D, Kling MA, Minichiello MD, Trettau JR, Coppola R. Intravenous procaine as a probe of limbic system activity in psychiatric patients and normal controls. Biol Psychiatry. 1987;22(9):1107–26. https://doi.org/10.1016/0006-3223(87)90053-9.
28. Ketter TA, Andreason PJ, George MS, Lee C, Gill DS, Parekh PI, Willis MW, Herscovitch P, Post RM. Anterior paralimbic mediation of procaine-induced emotional and psychosensory experiences. Arch Gen Psychiatry. 1996 Jan;53(1):59–69. https://doi.org/10.1001/archpsyc.1996.01830010061009.
29. Servan-Schreiber D, Perlstein WM. Pharmacologic activation of limbic structures and neuroimaging studies of emotions. J Clin Psychiatry. 1997;58(Suppl 16):13–5.
30. Adinoff B, Devous MD, Best SE, Alexander D, Kelly Payne J, Williams M. Dose-response measures of rCBF and subjective changes following procaine in healthy female volunteers. Psychiatry Res. 2002;114(3):123–35. https://doi.org/10.1016/s0925-4927(02)00008-2.

31. Adinoff B, Devous MD Sr, Best SE, Chandler P, Alexander D, Payne K, Harris TS, Williams MJ. Gender differences in limbic responsiveness, by SPECT, following a pharmacologic challenge in healthy subjects. NeuroImage. 2003;18(3):697–706. https://doi.org/10.1016/s1053-8119(03)00008-9.
32. Matulewicz P, Orzeł-Gryglewska J, Braszka Ł, Zawistowski P, Jurkowlaniec E. Hippocampal theta rhythm after local administration of procaine or amphetamine into the ventral tegmental area in fear conditioned rats. Neurosci Lett. 2015;4(589):132–7. https://doi.org/10.1016/j.neulet.2015.01.049.
33. Bartolini A, Galli A, Ghelardini C, Giotti A, Malcangio M, Malmberg-Aiello P, Zucchi PL. Antinociception induced by systemic administration of local anaesthetics depends on a central cholinergic mechanism. Br J Pharmacol. 1987;92(4):711–21. https://doi.org/10.1111/j.1476-5381.1987.tb11375.x.
34. Scheinberg P, Jayne HW, Blackburn LI, Rich M. Studies of cerebral circulatory functions following intravenous administration of procaine hydrochloride. AMA Arch NeurPsych. 1952;68(6):815–8. https://doi.org/10.1001/archneurpsyc.1952.02320240090009.
35. Adamec RE, Stark-Adamec C, Saint-Hilaire JM, Livingston KE. Basic science and clinical aspects of procaine HCl as a limbic system excitant. Prog Neuro-Psychopharmacol Biol Psychiatry. 1985;9(2):109–19. https://doi.org/10.1016/0278-5846(85)90073-9. PMID: 4001428
36. Benson B, Carson R, Kiesewetter D, et al. A potential cholinergic mechanism of procaine's limbic activation. Neuropsychopharmacol. 2004;29:1239–50. https://doi.org/10.1038/sj.npp.1300404.
37. Brodie BB, Lief PA, Poet L. The fate of procaine in men following its intravenous administration and methods for the estimation of procaine and diethylaminoethanol. J Pharmacol Exp Ther. 1948;94:359.
38. Aslan A. A new method for the prophylaxis and treatment of aging with Novocain—eutrophic and rejuvenating effects. Therapiewoche. 1956;7:14.
39. Aslan A. Recent experiences on rejuvenating action of Novocaine together with experimental, clinical and statistical findings. Therapiewoche. 1957;8:10–9.
40. Bucci L, Saunders JC. A psychopharmacological evaluation of 2-diethylamino-ethyl-paraminobenzoate (procaine). J Neuropsych. 1960;1:276.
41. Kral V, Cahn C, Deutsch M, et al. Procaine (Novocaine) treatment of patients with senile arteriosclerotic brain disease. Can Med Assoc J. 1962;87:1109.
42. Smigel JO, Piller J, Murphey C, et al. H-3 (procaine hydrochloride) therapy in aging institutionalized patients: an interim report. J Am Geriatr Soc. 1960;8:785.
43. Cohen S, Dittmann KS. Gerovital H3 in the treatment of the depressed aging patient. Psychosomatics. 1974;14:15.
44. Sakalis G, Oh D, Gershon S, et al. A trial of Gerovital in depression during senility. Curr Ther Res Clin Exp. 1974;16:59.
45. Pascal E, Bezusso CP. The therapeutic possibilities of novocaine in senile psychoses. Neuropsichiatria. 1960;3:502.
46. Giore R. Effects of prolonged novocainic treatment on intellectual efficiency in subjects of advanced age. Bull Soc Med Chir Pisa. 1959;27:1.
47. Balganon J. Trial of the combination procaine PABA in the prophylaxis and treatment of involution processes. Med Clin (Barc). 1962;8:44.
48. Oury P, Delavaille C. Treatments for senility Vie Méd. 1960;41:924.
49. Aslan A, Vrebiescu A. Procaine treatment in arthritis and arthrosis. Bull Sci Acad Roum P Repub. 1950;T11(7):891.
50. David C. Experiences with the treatment of the aging person. Zschr Ges Inn Med. 1960;15:820.
51. Rusu C, Borsa C, Gradinaru D, Ionescu C. Antioxidant and lipid-lowering effects of the original procaine-based products. Rom J Geront Geriatr. 1996;3:47–61.
52. Worlitschek K. Practice of acid-base household. Germany: Haug Publisher; 2012.

53. Reuter U, Oettmeier R. Regulation and pain treatment with infusion neural therapy. German Natura Med. 1997;12:20–5.
54. Reuter U, Oettmeier R. The high-dosed Procaine-Base-Infusion Ärztezeitschrift f. Naturheilverfahren. 1999;11:776–83.
55. Glusa E. Spasmolytic action of Procaine-Base on the aorta of rats. ID-Pharma, Research material; 1999.
56. Ibusuki S, Katsuki H, Takasaki M. The effects of extracellular pH with and without bicarbonate on intracellular procaine concentrations and anesthetic effects in crayfish giant cells. Anesthesiology. 1998;88:1549–57.
57. Yung E, Lahoti T, Jafari S, Weinberg JD, Schianodicola JJ, et al. Bicarbonate plus epinephrine shortens the onset and prolongs the duration of sciatic block using chloro-procaine followed by bupivacaine in Sprague-Dawley rats. Reg Anesth Pain Med. 2009;34:196–200.
58. Stevens RA, Chester WL, Grueter JA, Schubert A, Brandon D, et al. The effect of pH adjustment of 0.5% bupivacaine on the latency of epidural anesthesia. Reg Anesth. 1989;14:236–9.
59. Oettmeier R, Reuter U. The continuous Procaine-Base infusion/perfusion: new ways for systemic influencing regulation, inflammation, and pain. Erfahrungsheilkunde. 2000;2:75–84.
60. Iudenkov N. Intra-arterial infusion of penicillin and procaine in treatment of suppurative inflammations and open trauma. Voen Med Zh. 1959;86:77–9.
61. Fuzaylov G, Kelly TL, Bline C, Dunaev A, Dylewski M, et al. Post-operative pain control for burn reconstructive surgery in a resource-restricted country with subcutaneous infusion of local anesthetics through a soaker catheter to the surgical site: preliminary results. Burns. 2015;41:1811–5.
62. Bräuer et al. The anti-rheumatic and joint-protective effect of a defined Procaine-Base mixture. Presentation German Pain Congress. 2000.
63. Kasch H, Engert B, Reuter U, Oettmeier R. Internal research materials. JenCluster GmbH Jena; 2009.
64. Levraut J, Labib Y, Chave S, Payan P, Raucoules-Aime M, Grimaud D. Effect of sodium bicarbonate on intracellular pH under different buffering conditions. Kidney Int. 1996;49(5):1262–7.
65. Langguth P, Fricker G, Wunderli-Allenspach H. Biopharmacy. Weinheim, Germany: Wiley-VCH Verlag GmbH & Co. KGaA; 2004.
66. Oettmeier R, Reuter U. High-dosed Procaine-Base-infusions - is the risk calculable? Company product information-ID-Pharma: Metaanalysis of surveillance data from important parameters; 2000.
67. Becke M. Procaine and the discussion concerning the allergy. Ärztezeitschrift f Naturheilverfahren. 1996;37(12):908–12.
68. Saha FJ. Procaine-infusions in neural therapy—with or without alkalic additive? In: Presentation Medical Week Baden-Baden; 2016.
69. Oettmeier R, Reuter U. Examinations concerning the importance of metabolic alkalosis in cancer patients. Umwelt, Medizin, Gesellschaft. 2017;30:15–8.
70. Luke RG, Galla JH. Does chloride play an independent role in the pathogenesis of metabolic alkalosis? Semin Nephrol. 1989;9(2):203–5.
71. Cao J, Edwards R, Chairez J, Devaraj S. Validation of capillary blood analysis and capillary testing mode on the EPOC. Point of care system. Pract. Lab Med. 2017;9:24–7.
72. Shapiro JI. Pathogenesis of cardiac dysfunction during metabolic acidosis: therapeutic implications. Kidney Int Suppl. 1997;61:47–51.

Chapter 41
Mental and Emotional Therapeutic Approach

Laura Bibiana Pinilla Bonilla and Leonardo Morales-Hernández

1 Introduction

In Chap. 22, the theoretical and practical bases for the initial approach to the mental and emotional environment of patients have been described. Likewise, the epistemological bases and an explanatory model for the FADEt technique, which generates processes of restructuring networks of meaning in patients, have been presented.

The focus of this chapter will be on the specific description of the therapeutic approach with the FADEt technique. The authors of this chapter suggest this approach preferentially when the conditions to be treated in patients have a clearly emotional origin of a traumatic type. Generally, when this stage has been reached, the therapist has already exhausted all therapeutic resources from the approach of Neuraltherapeutic medicine. In other words, the therapist has been treating the irritative and dominant foci, which could also be influencing the emotional aspects of that human being. When the neuraltherapist observes that, despite having carried out a thorough approach reducing irritative loads in that organism, the mental and emotional symptoms persist, the therapeutic approach with the FADEt technique could be the line of management of choice in these cases.

L. B. Pinilla Bonilla (✉)
Faculty of Medicine, Master in Alternative Medicine, Neural Therapy Area,
Universidad Nacional de Colombia, Bogotá, Colombia

Integrated Health Services Subnetwork of the South, Research and Innovation Center,
Bogotá, Colombia
e-mail: lbpnillab@unal.edu.co

L. Morales-Hernández
Universidad Nacional de Colombia, Faculty of Medicine. Master in Alternative Medicine,
Neural Therapy Area, Bogotá, Colombia

Santa Clara Hospital. Psychiatry Department, Bogotá, Colombia

L. B. Pinilla Bonilla et al. (eds.), *Neuraltherapeutic Medicine*,
https://doi.org/10.1007/978-3-032-03257-7_41

In the event that these mental and emotional changes were caused by something that affected the person's visceral physiology, such as an acute respiratory or cardiac infection, gastrointestinal infection, genitourinary infection, or an infection of the paranasal sinuses, tonsils, or ear, and there isn't a clear emotional trigger or trigger in the person's life history [1], it is suggested that the segmental approach (Chap. 30) or the approach of ganglia, plexuses, nerve trunks, or sympathetic chains (Chap. 25) be used to treat the viscera.

Another aspect to take into account is that, even if the patient comes with a specific diagnosis, with the aim of achieving a true transformative process, it is important not to focus on this diagnostic label.[1]

When we talk about diagnosis, in this chapter we refer to the *patient's problem in its integral context*. In other words, how their life history is linked to their way of reacting, their neurological traits, their coping mechanisms, their attempted solutions, and other factors are structured in a specific way of presenting symptoms or getting sick, and not just in a label. This refers to the process that each person follows in their life history and the meaning that the symptoms have not only from the cognitive, emotional, visceral, and neurological but also in the meaning they have for their life.

In Chap. 13, some theories that are the base for mental and emotional processes, such as the Theory of Conditioned Reflexes [2] and the theory of functional systems [3], are reviewed, as well as more recent theories that emerged in the context of the complexity sciences (such as the theory of nonlinear dynamic systems and chaos theory) (see Chap. 7). Understanding that there are no states in living systems, but rather dynamic and nonlinear processes, is crucial. A neuroscientist from the United States named Walter Freeman applied these ideas to the nervous system and found that the brain has adaptable and flexible behavior that lets it create new patterns permanently [4]. This concept resembles Speransky's proposal (approximately 60 years earlier) of the reorganization that the organism undergoes with each new stimulus (or information) that it perceives and integrates, making it a new organism with a new pattern at each moment [5].

In this chapter, the first section aims to show the initial and middle stages of the interview, which will then allow us to move on to the application of the FADEt technique itself. It details how the traumatic memory is selected to initiate the desensitization process and the process of reevaluation of this traumatic memory after the intervention. Similarly, the chapter demonstrates the identification of central memories that could act as foci of pathological dominance in each organism. The chapter concludes with five clinical cases that demonstrate the application of this technique and their corresponding follow-ups.

[1] In reference to the sciences of complexity, the metaphor of "the map is not the territory; the name is not the thing named" has been revised.What the patient brings as a complaint is only one aspect of the entire complexity of their problem in the individuality of their characteristics. On the other hand, according to "second-order cybernetics," each observer in his or her process of care with the patient causes different contents to emerge, which reevaluates that initial diagnosis both in the diagnostic (nosographic) nomination and in the comprehensive understanding of the phenomenon.

2 Initial Patient Approach

I. **Initial Approach and Preparation: Initial Stage of the Interview**
It must have a private space for the patient's care that guarantees their sense of security and where they can flow openly.

Try to implement strategies that facilitate the establishment of trust and rapport with the patient, such as synchronizing the breathing of the therapist and the patient; identify whether it is visual, auditory, or kinesthetic, and, according to this, use this channel preferentially to communicate with the patient, as expanded in Chap. 22.

II. **Middle Stage of the Interview**
As already mentioned in Chap. 22, a strategic interview and a life story allow us to find, together with the patient, the therapeutic objective that corresponds to what is worth healing.
Next, one can perform targeted relaxation exercises or imagery that, although it is advisable to apply them to all patients, are considered essential in cases of extreme anxiety, emotional lability, or any other type of emotional crisis.

Relaxation Technique or Imagery
Place the patient in a comfortable place, such as a reclining chair or a stretcher in a lying position. Ask the patient to preferably keep their eyes closed to make it easier to conduct the exercise. It can be therapeutic for the patient to visualize a real or imaginary place that brings peace, security, and/or happiness. In the event that they do not identify any place, one can also suggest that they visualize themself doing some activity or sharing with nature or pets whose experience especially provides a feeling of security or tranquility. This exercise can take about 5 or 10 min to last.

III. **Application of the FADEt Technique (Fast Desensitization of Emotional Trauma)**

Once the therapeutic objective has been identified clearly, the following steps are carried out in this phase:

1. *Create an environment of relaxation/release*

While the patient is comfortable in a chair or stretcher, several strategies are used to induce the patient toward a state of relaxation. This approach can consist of making the patient aware of the present moment, the sounds of the environment, the ambient temperature, their breathing, their heartbeat, among other strategies. The therapist may also lead a relaxation with visualization of colored rays, specific sounds, or flavors.

Example: *"Take a deep breath… Please look at the right side, now the left, now up, now the front; now it's easy for you to close your eyes… Breathe and notice that your heartbeats are slower and exhales, and you will only perceive how the air enters a little colder and comes out a little warmer, slowly… Listen to the sounds in the air, and now you just hear my voice. Imagine a lemon… Green of a very pleasant color… And feel how the lemon drops fall on your tongue and now under your tongue. Breathe deeply, and now that saliva passes… Breathe again, and a white light enters your head and descends through your body… Healing light passes through your head, through your arms, forearms, and hands… move your fingers slowly as the light passes through them in your hands… and now all over your chest and abdomen, pelvis, thighs, and your feet, and now slowly move your toes and fingers and feel the tensions move away from your body."*

At this stage, the suggestion process guides the patient into a state of relaxation that amplifies their resources. For this, it is essential to have an attitude that respectfully makes the patient accept being taken to this state of trance or attention focused on their resources and the present time [6].

Adequate induction allows the patient to emerge with content related to what *is worthy of healing* more easily, since "when inhibition of the higher centers has been suppressed, suggestibility and other reflex tendencies increase. This allows for acertain ease in carrying out specific actions that would otherwise be impossible to perform" [7].

It is important to always individualize the relaxation process since, for example, not all patients could feel relaxation with a technique of observing their breathing. If the patient consults for a trauma related to a situation in which he felt "drowned" or was short of breath, an exercise of observing their breathing will probably not lead them to a state of relaxation. So the selection of the relaxation strategy must take into account the individuality of each being, their life history, and their culture.

2. *Selection of traumatic memory as a gateway according to the interview and approach*

Based on the life history and the strategic interview, the traumatic memory or memory networks that are "worthy of healing" are identified. This memory may correspond to a focus of emotional dominance, or it may correspond to a secondary memory that is associated by similarity with the dominant focus. In the event that the person does not yet remember the central, primary, or dominant traumatic memory that triggered their current situation, it is necessary to start with the most recent or most intense memory that they can remember as a gateway. The process for identifying the dominant focus or root focus will be explained later.

3. *Initial approach to traumatic memory*

   (a) The person is asked to recall the traumatic memory (an image of a scene). The person is free to verbalize it or simply remember it mentally.
   (b) From the entire scene, the person is asked to select the most difficult, most painful, or most disturbing part.

(c) Sometimes, some patients evoke this memory and generate negative thoughts about themselves. It is important to identify if this is the case and verbalize this negative thought.
(d) Evoking memory, the patient is asked to identify the emotion or emotions that trigger this remembrance: anger, fear, sadness, etc.
(e) Once the emotion is identified, the patient is asked to become aware of the sensation or body anchorage that generates that emotion. For example, there are fearful emotions that patients may feel in the chest or in the solar plexus, emotions of sadness that patients point to as a broken heart and feel in their chest.[2] These sensations can have different descriptions, such as "an emptiness," "a pressure," "a sting," "a tingling," "a tic or fasciculation," among others. The metaphor of the words of these sensations in itself can be a therapeutic element at another time because they are related to the "personal map"[3] or life history.
(f) For follow-up purposes, it may be helpful to ask the patient to rate the intensity of the emotion generated by memory recall on a visual analogue scale of 0–10.
(g) Proceed with the inhibition or desensitization of that memory.

4. *Process of inhibition/desensitization of traumatic memory*

According to what was reviewed in Chap. 22, there is a wide range of tools that can be used to inhibit or desensitize the traumatic memories (pathological reflexes) of patients, inspired by Pavlov's description of conditioned inhibition agents[4] [2, 8].

It should not be forgotten that the application of any of these stimuli must be carried out while the patient is recalling the traumatic experience in accordance with the rules enunciated by Pavlov to generate a conditioned inhibition [2].

The association[5] between the different stimuli and the internal emotional and neurological state that each person presents is the way to understand how the changes are consolidated. This happens as a new learning in which the dysfunctional

[2] The bodily locations of sensations are absolutely individual and linked to their life history. By way of illustration, the case of a patient who experienced a feeling of shame with an emotion of sadness in his thighs and knees is cited. When his life history is reviewed, it is found that when he served in the military, on one occasion he was humiliated by his superiors, who forced him to perform "squats", which made him feel deep shame. From this moment on, the feeling of shame was associated with the muscle groups that performed the squats.

[3] As an example, if a patient has associated their bodily sensations with a "tingling" or a "butterfly flapping," these descriptions can later be used as therapeutic metaphorical tools through the suggestion by the therapist: "It is easy for you to notice how these butterflies leave your body, and it feels lighter."

[4] Another way to understand it is that a memory circuit learned with a certain threatening pattern can change to another neutral or even positive pattern.

[5] The epistemological perspective from which these contents are structured is associationism, which maintains that memory is a function of three primary processes: [1] contiguity (phenomena that occur close in time or space are linked in the "mind"), [2] process of similarity, and [3] the process of contrast [9], which allows them to be resembled or distinguished.

or pathological way in which they were consolidated is changed by a new form of cognitive, emotional, neurological, or neurohumoral.

As Cobian explains, quoting Pavlov, conditioned reflexes are temporary connections associated with internal or external factors that are maintained by reinforcement or repetition; this becomes a system.

This organization functions as a system when it is structured as a whole, where the contents of experiences (physical, bodily, emotional, cognitive, or sensory) converge with the derived knowledge and their respective connections. This is the basis of human learning with its conditioned reflexes and subsequent interactions together with the elaboration of new connections acquired gradually according to the nuances of changing circumstances and/or contexts [6].

An exciting external stimulus such as that provided by neural therapy together with internal stimuli—which emerge when performing the psychotherapy process with bilateral brain stimulation—generates a focus of new activity as an association. This would be the basis of the focus of inhibition or reciprocal excitation of induction with this integral and dynamic process.

From this physiological approach, inhibition is also an active process of cessation of activity induced by other associations with complementary dynamics [6].

To induce cognitive, sensory, and ideational or other contents, it is important to take into account that any phenomenon or symptom presented by the patient—which is used by them to maintain the problem—can also be used indirectly to use it in their own "healing" process (Pereira, 2023) [10]. That is, the sensory or cognitive symptoms that the patient presents are those that must be taken directly into account to induce the emergence of contents and carry out the therapeutic process. These are known as Zeig's laws and are part of the teachings drawn from Milton Erickson.

The therapist can explore different tools in the patient, but preferably only one tool should be applied in each desensitization cycle, although during the entire session more than one tool can be used. This in order not to generate overstimulation that can generate the opposite effect of desensitization. Pavlov insisted that these agents must be characterized by a "low intensity" to act as inhibitors. If two stimuli are presented at the same time, one or both stimuli may lose their inhibitory potential.

These agents can enter through the different visual, auditory, olfactory, or tactile channels. The channels most explored by other therapeutic tools, such as Neurolinguistic Programming [11] or the Eye Movement Desensitization and Reprocessing technique [12], have been visual, auditory, and tactile. As an example of the different inhibitory stimuli, the following can be cited:

(a) Visual channel: eye movements[6] and moving colored lights [12]. In a desensitization cycle, about 30 cycles of movements are performed.

[6] Shapiro describes that the patient is asked to follow with his or her eyes the movement of the therapist's fingers in a horizontal, vertical, diagonal, circular direction or by drawing the number 8 or infinity sign in the air [12].

(b) Auditory channel: low-intensity sounds can be used, such as a snap of the fingers applied to both ears alternately or headphones that can perform binaural acoustic stimulation.
(c) Tactile channel: One of the best known is the gentle tapping[7] of places on the body, such as the knees, in an alternating manner [12]. However, depending on the life history, some patients have marked inhibitory responses (they relax deeply), for example, by doing a light massage on the scalp or back. In a desensitization cycle, approximately 30 taps can be performed or, in the case of massages, these could be performed for a time of 60 seconds. It is important to mention that some patients do not tolerate being touched on their body by another person; in this case, tapping can be done by self-stimulation guided by the therapist.
(d) Tactile-biochemical channel (dual action): At this point, special reference is made to the combination of a tactile stimulus with a stimulus that is generated thanks to the gentle injection of procaine through very short and thin needles (30G in diameter and half an inch in length). Chapter 22 introduces the reader to the effects of procaine on the limbic system, and Chap. 26 provides basic information on its pharmacokinetics and pharmacodynamics. The application of procaine is performed at the sites indicated by the patients where they feel the location in the body of the sensation associated with the emotion and traumatic memory.[8] A desensitization cycle is completed after the application of procaine to the patient-designated site.
(e) Compound channel (creation of internal images): This channel corresponds to a suggestion made to the patient to change one or more aspects of the traumatic memory scene in an imaginary way.[9] For example, a patient is reliving a scene where they are trapped in a dark room; the suggestion may be that they imagine there is a window they missed or a hidden place with a key to escape.[10]

    Likewise, a technique derived from hypnosis proposes that the person associate their emotion or pain with a certain shape/figure that has a certain size and color. Then, in an imaginary exercise guided by the therapist, the patient is

[7] There are other therapeutic procedures that perform stimulation in body areas corresponding to acupuncture points, but their description is beyond the scope of this chapter.

[8] It can be a very specific site on the patient's body, as well as an area. In this way, a single wheal is applied to the indicated spot, or wheals are distributed in the patient's referred area, respectively. Sometimes, patients may have locations at the level of the mucous membranes, such as the nasal mucosa, the oral mucosa, or the anal, vaginal, or vulvar mucosa. In the case of the oral or nasal mucosa, moderate irrigation with procaine in these places may be useful. In the case of the anal, vulvar, or vaginal mucosa, it is important first that only properly trained medical personnel apply procaine and that the patient trusts the application and does not view it as threatening.

[9] This technique is used in hypnosis and allows the narrative of the experiences to be changed from the resources of the person themselves; it is based on the fact that what is really important for the brain is the narrative that sustains it.

[10] The important thing is to make sure that the person has the necessary resources to transform the experience through the emotions, sensations, and experiences that they are living in the consultation; it is required that the person enter a level of trance.

asked to transform the shape, color, and size of the initial figure into ones that the patient previously associated with peace, joy, or security.

At this point, the range of possibilities expands considerably since, on the imaginary plane, everything is possible. There are some schools of alternative psychology, such as the school of humanistic psychology according to Silo, that propose changes as big as imagining that the traumatic event never happened or that it had a positive outcome under the name of "conversion of tense biographical images" [13]. A cycle of desensitization is fulfilled after having made a change in the patient's scene that imaginatively generated a different result and perception.

Once a cycle of desensitization with any of the tools is completed, a memory reevaluation is carried out.

Depending on the characteristics of each person with their story, there may be moments of "catharsis"[11] of different degrees of intensity (intense crying, body contractions, screams, foul words, among others) in which the therapist must be present, avoiding direct body intervention and facilitating the emergence of the contents that each one needs to express.

5. *Reevaluation of traumatic memory*

After each desensitization cycle, the patient is asked to recall the memory and the exact scene that was formerly worked on. Once it is being remembered, the patient is asked to identify if something has changed. If it changes in the way they remember or in the way they "feel" when they remember it (see Chap. 20). After a cycle of desensitization, the person may mention that they can no longer remember the scene as clearly, losing detail or depth. They may remember it in the third-person perspective,[12] or they may not be able to remember it at all. A cycle of desensitization may cause the patient to see the image the same way, but the intensity of the emotion decreases until the patient no longer feels any emotion associated with that memory.

It may be useful to ask the patient to rate again from 0 to 10 (on the visual analog scale) the intensity of the emotion they feel associated with the memory of the traumatic experience, to compare with the previous rating and assess the progress of desensitization.

The following are the possible outcomes after each cycle of sensitization, and suggested behaviors to be followed by the therapist:

[11] Catharsis, or abreaction, is an ancient medical term that refers to the flow and externalization of the affective contents that the person presents. Originally, this term, which also meant "purgation," referred to the digestive system, but it was appropriated by hypnotic techniques.

[12] The third-person perspective refers to a change that occurs spontaneously during the desensitization process in some patients, where they perceive as if the event is happening to a third person. For instance, they perceive themselves as a child, detached from the event, observing it without any emotional connection. They no longer feel like themselves, the victims of the traumatic scene.

(a) Total change (disturbance rated as 0, total change in perspective,[13] no longer perceives sensations or body anchors): final check-up, recommendations and closure are carried out.
(b) Partial change (decrease in felt body intensity): body anchorage sites are re-evaluated, and a new desensitization cycle is performed.
(c) No change: reassess whether the body anchor site is correct. Reassess whether there is a dominant focus on this disturbing memory that does not allow memory transformation to take place. It is advisable to change the desensitization tool.
(d) In the case of b or c, desensitization should continue until the disturbance reaches almost 0 or < 2 and/or until a total change of perspective is achieved.
(e) If within the process a positive belief arises spontaneously from the patient himself, such as "I am valuable," "I am brave," "I have the right to make mistakes," "I can always learn," "I deserve to be loved," it is advisable to proceed to reinforce this belief through repetition out loud, making aware of the positive emotion that it generates and the bodily location that it has (positive anchoring).

6. *Central or root memory identification*

During the desensitization process, it may happen that, while the process of recalling the traumatic memory is being carried out, the patient automatically remembers a previous or stronger and similar event, or that there is no evidence of progress in the desensitization of the memory for which it was decided to initiate the therapeutic process.

These two situations indicate a need to address the central memory or root of the problem, which in physiological terms would correspond to a dominant focus or center [14] (see Chap. 13). In the event that this dominant memory is not remembered spontaneously, the therapist can direct the patient by asking them to identify in the past of their life if there is any experience where they have felt or thought in a similar way. Another way to approach it can be to ask the patient: have you felt this before? This question is especially directed toward the way the patient thinks about himself, the emotions that it generates, and the related bodily sensations.

An example to illustrate this can be with a patient who, after ending an affective relationship with a partner, feels a deep abandonment and a deep emotion of sadness anchored in their chest. When asked, in the state of relaxation, if they had felt something similar before, the patient spontaneously remember when they were 3 years old and their mother, for the first time, took them away from the family nucleus and left them in a kindergarten at the hands of strangers. That day, that being thought that their mother and their family had abandoned them, and that memory remained

[13] A total change in perspective is identified when, prior to desensitization, the patient related what had happened to them with negative cognitions and emotions, and after the desensitization cycle, the patient may experience the following: no longer feels negative emotions, considers that what happened to them no longer corresponds to something for which they are responsible, they identify within themselves their own positive values that they were not able to observe before, they are no longer able to perceive the previous situation as threatening, among other changes.

there, making it easier for similar events to be interpreted from the perspective of that same abandonment. It is important to understand that, for the psyche, similar events are linked to the same memory network; what unites them is the feeling-thought and the bodily anchorage. In the same sense that Freud mentioned, "it is not the experiences themselves that have a traumatic effect, but only their reanimation as a memory" [15].

In general, when the dominant or root memory of the memory network has been identified, the work of desensitizing this memory can cause the other memories belonging to the same network to be desensitized in the same way. This can be verified in a very simple way: once the complete desensitization of the central or root memory is verified, the patient is asked to remember a more recent or less intense memory that belongs to the same memory network, and is asked to rate the disturbance generated by remembering it from 0 to 10.

Another way to identify memories that belong to the same network is to ask the patient to write a short autobiography, days before the session, trying to identify the age at which the events occurred. It is important to identify if a negative belief is generated about themselves with that memory, identify the emotion it generates, and the sites of body anchorage. At the end, they could rate each memory globally on a scale of 0 to 10 according to the intensity of the emotion generated by remembering it. This autobiography will be analyzed together with the therapist to identify similar memories, and thus, build the map of memory networks of that patient.

During the analysis of this autobiography, several conflicting memory networks may emerge that are worthy of healing. The decision of which memory network to work on first is a decision that must be made by the therapist-patient set. It will depend on which one is more significant and important for the patient at that moment, or which memory destabilizes the patient more at that moment, leading them to risky situations or behaviors[14] such as substance abuse, habits that deteriorate their health or other behaviors that may threaten their own life.

It is advisable, if the patient agrees, to work on all memory networks that are dysfunctional or poorly adapted within the patient's psyche in a therapeutic scheme of several sessions. In general, during the therapeutic process, the same patient expresses the need to work on other memory networks different from those that were being intervened. It is entirely feasible that once a memory network is desensitized, the patient experiences, in the intersession periods, spontaneous memories of other memory networks that can be revealed both during sleep and consciously during the day. It is important that the therapist be attentive to these manifestations

[14] From hypnosis or different ways of understanding the human being, it is known that there are three tendencies to handle risky situations: one of them is to try to control everything, the other is to evade; these two usually do not have a result in terms of solving problems but only relieve temporarily. In this way, behaviors are developed that, as attempted solutions, end up complicating the problem further.

The other trend is that of facing and seeking to solve with the patient's resources, which is the one that is processed in therapy and that can be encouraged so that patients also perform autonomously in their personal spaces.

and be willing to go at the pace set by the patient himself. Memory that arises spontaneously during the therapeutic process is meaningful to the patient and, therefore, worthy of healing.

7. *How to manage sessions*

The length of each individual session depends on each therapist. It is recommended that sessions last no less than 45 min to allow sufficient time for initial dialogue, physical examination, several desensitization cycles, evaluation of progress, closure, and recommendations.

Since it is a rapid desensitization technique, especially when a procaine injection is used, it may be possible to completely desensitize from one to three traumatic memories in the same session. However, given the individuality of each patient, if a memory is highly anchored with a very deep life-threatening meaning, it is possible that desensitization time may take more than one session.

IV. **Closing of the Interview and Intervention**

(a) *Emotional stabilization of the patient with a safe place and/or other hypnotic or NLP techniques* [6, 11].

At the end of each session, it is important that the patient finishes with a sense of accomplishment and tranquility. For this, they are asked to rate the final state of disturbance. If stabilization is necessary, we can use different tools.

There are possibilities of stabilizing with suggestions that can allude to the shape, size, or sensation of the discomfort that the patient presents; the following is one example that could be used:

> *Please indicate the part of the body in which you feel the discomfort at this time… Give it a color… And now take that color and pull it out with your hands completely out, totally out, deep outside [phrase repeated three times slowly, suggestively, monotonously] … Now shake your hands so that you have them completely cleansed of that and select a color that is healing for you… Now, place your hand again on top of the place where you felt it was, and now it's going to fill it with that completely blue color, totally blue, deep blue.*

In the same way, different activities can be carried out with metaphors. One could be the "emotion container" (which can also be done physically with a paper envelope), with elements of nature that help or clean, such as a light bulb that comes from the top or with water or sounds, among other resources that depend on the imagination, strategy, or training of each therapist.

(b) *Explanation of the individualized management plan. Assess the need for interdisciplinary management or referral*

It is important that the following points are defined so that there is a good connection with the patient and a true therapeutic contract:

(i) Avoid interpreting according to a single scheme. It is to understand that each patient has a different map and a way of interpreting and giving meaning to their symptoms and experiences in a particular way; finally, this conception allows us to approach them.

(ii) Avoiding judgment, understanding that the behaviors or symptoms that the person presents are the best attempt at a solution that they have been able to do with the resources that they had developed up to that moment.

(iii) Provide the patient with an empathetic response that includes:

1. An understanding of the problem (what was understood of the problem, feedback, paraphrasing)
2. To make explicit what can be solved and what cannot be solved, with the commitment to accompany in any possible circumstance.
3. Establish a plan according to their resources and in their language.
4. Talk openly about what can be expected from this approach.
5. Identify the patient's internal support resources and reinforce them, as well as external resources or family and/or social-community support networks.

(c) Strategic emotional management work at home

I. Self-hypnosis: There are different strategies that can be used with the patient depending on the type of problem; self-hypnotic audios can be directed and used at home.
II. Emotional release through writing (journaling), painting, etc.
III. Observe dreams and repetitive thoughts: write them down.
IV. Audio.
V. Selected readings according to the patient's worthiness of healing.
VI. Medication formulation if relevant.

3 Clinical Cases

Next, five summarized clinical cases that were managed using the FADEt technique will be presented. This corresponds to patients of various ages, genders, and diagnoses according to the DSM-5. Despite the diagnosis, the patients were approached with the aim of achieving a transformation of their memory and meaning networks. Over the course of treatment, patients were uninstalling many of their symptoms that were part of the diagnostic criteria, while their traumatic memories were desensitized.

All patients agreed to the publication of the case under anonymization of their personal information and signed informed consent.

3.1 Clinical Case: Post-Traumatic Stress Disorder

Reason for Consultation A 19-year-old female patient who attended the Neuraltherapeutic Medicine clinic in March 2019. The patient experienced daily abdominal, pelvic, and perineal pain, with a VAS of 10/10. Additionally, she has had headaches, nausea, vomiting, tachycardia, depression, insomnia, and auditory and tactile hallucinations at night for five months of evolution.

Background Two years earlier, she had presented with an episode of severe pelvic pain (VAS 10/10) after appendectomy. Ultrasound, gynecological evaluation, CT scan of the abdomen and pelvis were performed with the only finding being "polycystic ovaries," and surgical management for the cysts was proposed. The general surgery service is referred at the Hospital to the Neuraltherapeutic Medicine Service, where initial management was carried out with significant improvement after 3 months of treatment.

Among other antecedents: pyelonephritis in 2010, wisdom tooth extraction in 2018.

On Physical Examination Extreme shyness. She does not talk about her past. She does not hold her gaze. She does not make eye contact with the doctor. Just crying. Face of pain, manifesting pelvic and perineal pain.

Initial Therapeutic Approach Initially, the approach was carried out from Neuraltherapeutic medicine with injections in the tonsils, abdominal scar, scalp, multiple interventions in the lower hypogastric plexus, sacral roots, pudendal nerve, intravaginal points, cauda equina, with partial improvement (improvement for only 15 days). A follow-up TV ultrasound was performed in July 2019, which no longer reported polycystic ovary.

After several failed attempts with Neuraltherapeutic medicine, the patient is urged to clarify whether there are any psychologically traumatic events that would be important to review and treat. At the insistence, the patient communicates in a very brief way, indicating that "Something happened to me with a man." "I just want to die." From this event, she manifests fear of men.

A clear blockage of communication is observed, with no eye contact, only crying. A joint management by psychiatry and psychology is proposed, in the face of which the patient manifests a categorical refusal to this type of treatment. Management with the FADEt technique is proposed, to which the patient initially manifests resistance for fear of remembering the traumatic event.

A couple of sessions later, the patient finally confessed in writing that she had been a victim of sexual abuse in September of the previous year. She would rather not talk to anyone, and she was afraid to go to the consultation for fear of having to talk. Since the event, she had been experiencing nightmares where she relived the traumatic moment, which generated insomnia and permanent flashbacks. She would rather not have any close relationship with any man, much less sexual relations.

Treatment with the FADEt Technique In October 2019, for the first time, she accepted to be treated with the FADEt technique. Memory networks reveal childhood and adolescent traumas, including psychological and sometimes physical violence, that require healing. These traumas include permanent acts of exclusion that make her feel rejected and abandoned by her family. For this reason, the patient developed untreated and unidentified early depression. The focus of the sessions was on the traumatic event of sexual abuse.

Evolution During the development of the treatment, the patient was able to accept the approach of someone of the male gender by starting a relationship in November 2019, initially without sexual relations.

The last session was held in January 2020 for a total of 6 sessions. By this time her facial expression had changed completely. She manifested being free of pelvic pain, and she dialogued fluently. She could make eye contact. For the first time, she made jokes, she indicated having a restful sleep without hallucinations. She had a dialogue about her future professional plans and indicated an improvement in her family relationships by talking more easily about her childhood and the traumatic event without discomfort.

In April 2020, she was able to start her sexual life with peace of mind, and to date, the patient remains asymptomatic with respect to post-traumatic stress syndrome.

3.2 Clinical Case: Bipolar Affective Disorder, Bulimia Nervosa, Dissociative Identity Disorder

Reason for Consultation and Background A 35-year-old female patient attended the consultation for the first time on February 2, 2022, due to aggravation of bipolar affective disorder. Although the diagnosis of this disorder was made when she was 19, since she had COVID a year ago, the symptoms have worsened, without mention of a manic crisis. She went to a psychiatry consultation, where the doctor prescribed lithium. The patient decided not to start the proposed pharmacological treatment. She went to the Neural therapy consultation because she does not want to be hospitalized or have to agree to take medication. She has been undergoing treatment for psychology for several years. Additionally, since the age of 11, she has been presenting eating disorders due to anorexia and bulimia.

The patient had attempted to schedule the appointment multiple times, but she had canceled it herself. After attending, she abruptly stood up, spoke loudly to the secretary, and left without waiting for her appointment with no apparent reason.

Physical Examination The attitude during the first appointment was defiant. She crossed his arms and stated that she did not want to be in consultation, that she wanted to leave.

Initial Approach In February, a neuraltherapeutic approach focused on post-COVID syndrome was carried out, considering it a symptomatic aggravating factor. Interventions were carried out on tonsils, trigeminal branches, and lung segment.

The following are the reported symptoms and the memories that arose spontaneously in the patient. From March 14, intervention with the FADEt technique begins in each of the sessions:

Date	Findings
14-March-2022	Depression and insomnia manifest themselves: "I have to chase others to be loved"
23-March-2022	Bulimic behavior reset. Memories of the 5-year-old emerge: "I'm the worst for my mom," "it's my fault that all the problems with my parents were," "that's why my dad left home," "my father tells me he became an alcoholic because of me," the parents didn't attend their kindergarten grade "My brother beat me a lot," "if I am the way I am, no one will love me"
9-April-2022	Conflict due to current partner: Did not attend her master's degree
30-April-2022	The so-called "disconnections" return. These disconnections had occurred 5 months ago and 1 year ago (during Christmas). These are episodes where there is a trigger, for example, a man who intends to make her fall in love or a family argument. During the event she is aggressive verbally, she can destroy things and hit others, and she has ended up in the police for it. She refers to not remembering those events or having control of them, as a kind of "mental blackout." "another self" is identified that lives in it. She knows her name and identifies her as "P." "I'm very scared" The patient identifies "P" as a teenager, P dresses in black, is impolite. is bored by people, almost everyone dislikes her. She imagines her locked in a room beating everything: "They left us alone a lot," "she wants to protect me."
25-May-2022	Memories that P tells her are reviewed: Father beating the mother, the girl crying
10-June-2022	Another memory arises: Her brother beating her and tells her "you are crazy, you are hysterical." P was born to tell you "you are strong."
25-June-2022	Vomiting has not been induced again. The disconnections have not returned. "P is already integrated into me," but I still see myself as fat. The memories of school bullying arise: "They called me Libretón," "they call me a pig and pinch me," "they got out of the door." "everyone leaves me if I'm fat."
6-August-2022	She has been without dissociations for almost a month, but the insomnia continues. Feels estranged from parents
22-September-2022	New COVID infection. Again she feels sadness, but without vomiting, without P. This time there is no FADEt but two sessions of NTM to stabilize
11-November-2022	The FADEt sessions are restarted: "I'm eating a lot." memories of adulthood begin to express themselves: "I'm sad about my partner's infidelity." she remembers several relationships suffering from infidelity. At 19, my boyfriend cheated on me with my best friend

(continued)

Date	Findings
Nov 20, 2022	Memory of 30 years, separation from husband. She had a mistress. She had a memory with another couple who didn't know he was married. She became pregnant; she must terminate the pregnancy. During the session, she relives exactly the moment of abortion with misoprostol; after the session, the patient begins with vaginal bleeding that lasts a few days
December-2022	She has been able to sleep, physical symptoms in resolution; she describes herself as "self-empowered." "these have been quiet celebrations. I have drunk alcohol, and I have shared happily with my friends. This month, which I was so terrified of, I have been able to go through it calmly and with love."

Evolution From 2023 onward, the patient has consulted for minor issues such as work stress, love disappointments, and infections. One of the most complex episodes was the death of her pet that was her companion for a long time. She supported herself during the mourning, which lasted about two months. During 2023 she did not present episodes of dissociation or bulimic behavior, and emotionally she has been much more stable. Strategies for emotional self-management have been recommended that she have begun to apply autonomously. During the year 2024, she became pregnant again, before which she decided to terminate it, requiring emotional support during the mourning. However, these new events never triggered episodes of bulimia, BAD, or dissociations. They were short-lived and naturally reactive depressive episodes. Currently, she is more focused on emotional self-management.

3.3 Clinical Case: Anxious Depressive Disorder, Dissociative Identity Disorder

Reason for Consultation A 45-year-old male patient. He initially attended the Neuraltherapeutic Medicine consultation for post-COVID syndrome in February 2022, consisting of headache, nasal congestion, dysgeusia, photophobia, otalgia, and weakness.

Among his Antecedents There was only a bilateral inguinal herniorrhaphy, a rib fracture, and a hip dislocation due to a traffic accident.

Initial Approach It is initially approached as a typical post-COVID case, and several NTM sessions are performed until the resolution of physical symptoms. However, at 2 months, when the physical symptoms had already resolved, he began presenting depression and irritability, a feeling of chest tightness with dyspnea. He attended a psychiatry consultation who prescribed antidepressants and bupropion. He remembered many events from his childhood that depressed him.

Beginning of the Application of the FADEt Technique He accepted the proposal to use the FADEt technique to approach these memories in light of the findings. During the scan, the following memory networks were found:

- Emotional memories of abandonment from the age of 6 by the mother: with "wanting a hug, but she was not there." Anger and sadness
- 6 years old: "They left me at grandma's house." "I don't want my mother." Anger and sadness
- 9 years old: I had to prepare lunch, and it burned. My father hit me. Anger and sadness
- Adulthood: economic losses, migration to other countries: "I have been stupidly innocent."

Each of these traumas was addressed with the technique described, and the depressive state subsides. In the month of June, a new event appears that totally disconcerts the patient. On June 8, 2022, he had a very severe episode of anger during the physical training he had for a marathon, and after that: "In a car traffic, someone closed me in, and I went to blows with him. I almost killed him; I had no control of myself. If I had had a gun, I would have killed him. I'm terrified."

He identifies "another self" within the same patient that he calls "the madman." The patient's madman is between 8 and 9 years old. Networks of memories that "madman" has are reviewed:

- The father always carry a gun, highly violent, sometimes fired the gun, repeated child violence and is too rigid and inflexible with the patient
- "I failed my dad," "I'm incapable," to which he experiences frustration and anger.

Sessions continue to be held through the FADEt technique until the last session that takes place on August 29. In total, eight sessions were held. After this, an asymptomatic patient was observed in the controls, and the progressive suspension of bupropion and antidepressants was carried out. To date, the patient is asymptomatic.

3.4 Clinical Case: Primary Tokophobia and Anxiety Disorder

Reason for Consultation and Background Female patient, 45 years of age, with a history of eating disorders during her youth and obesity. She attends the Neuraltherapeutic medicine consultation with the diagnosis of anxiety disorder and primary tokophobia, which is manifested by panic about getting pregnant. This fact has led her to make the decision never to start her sexual life and to avoid sexual relations and approaches to men at all costs. She presents concomitantly anxious and panicked thoughts at the idea of forming a family.

She exhibits challenges in interpersonal relationships, including socialization issues with both the opposite sex (including verbal aggression) and the female gender, an obsession with work (without setting boundaries), and feelings of being undervalued in the workplace.

In recent years she had attended other types of therapies trying to find a solution to her phobia, such as cognitive behavioral therapy, psychiatry, biological decoding, and neurolinguistic programming.

Other Symptoms Trigeminal neuralgia that has been managed with the neurologist with imipramine and sometimes with sumatriptan.

Other Antecedents UTI, Urolithiasis, Mandibular osteotomy, multiple extractions.

Physical Exam at the First Visit She uses clothing with a tendency to be unicolor; she makes sure to look as serious as possible to create distance from others.

- A logorrheic patient with extreme and paroxysmal mood swings (from laughter to crying).
- Extreme anxiety (permanent changes in position: sitting, standing, walking, looking out the window).
- Sudden communication blocks: "I don't want to talk about what's happening to me, but I do." She looked out the window and said: "When I see that mountain, I would like to go and live there, like a hermit, where I don't have to interact with anyone or have to talk about this."

Initial Approach Given the active symptomatology of trigeminal neuralgia, neural therapy management is prioritized by performing intervention on tonsils, performing an orthopantomography study, and treating of dental and trigeminal foci.

Start of Treatment with the FADEt technique (September 2019) Several important elements were identified within her life history, such as domestic violence during her childhood, the traumatic separation of her parents at the age of 13, the death of her mother at the age of 20, from which a compulsive eating disorder began. The FADEt technique initially focused on addressing the following memory networks:

- Conflict due to domestic violence and separation from parents that makes her feel afraid to live a family life.
- She has experienced traumas with the opposite sex that have made her distrustful and afraid to enter into a relationship.

During the sessions, spontaneously and uncontrollably, the following traumatic memories arise, which become desensitized:

- Traumas at the time of birth.
- Family tree traumas (female line): the patient remembers as if she were her grandmother and mother, the traumas they had with the male gender.

Evolution After 10 sessions of the FADEt technique, the following changes were observed:

- Slower speech, fluid dialogue.
- She used makeup and jewelry, and used bright colors in her clothing: "I vindicated myself with my uterus and my femininity."
- Change at work: "Now I think of myself first; I learned to set limits."
- Interpersonal relationships: "Now I advise women," "I can now talk to men without attacking them."
- Restart of an old romantic relationship.
- First sexual intercourse in May 2020.
- "I want more than anything to be a mother and form a family."

3.5 *Clinical Case: Anxiety and Suicidal Behavior Disorder*

A 15-year-old female patient, a high school student, attended the Neuraltherapeutic medicine consultation on 06/05/2023 for migraine, rhinitis, dysmenorrhea, anxiety, and depressive disorder.

Among the pathological antecedents are infectious mononucleosis that generated hepatomegaly, left pyelocalyceal dilation without urinary tract infections, COVID during 2021 that presented with nasal pain and rhinitis.

Within her psychological history, the mother reported that since she was 3–4 years old, she had some social anxiety behaviors because she experienced bullying at school. These patterns of anxiety worsened at 8–9 years of age after the mother decided to move in with the father, manifested with bruxism, constant movements of the legs, and dyspnea. Currently, she lives only with her mother; her parents have been separated for 3 years.

From 2021 on, during the pandemic, anxious behaviors increased considerably. The patient continued to experience nervousness, a persistent sense of fear and anxiety, as well as chest pressure and dyspnea. During June 2021, she also required hospitalization for a suicide attempt due to the ingestion of many tablets of a drug. Since hospitalization, the patient began to attend psychotherapy. During 2022, she presents cutting behaviors in her arms. Since March 2023, she has been prescribed escitalopram for the management of anxiety disorder and valproic acid for migraine.

During the first two sessions, a neuraltherapeutic approach is performed for the treatment of physical irritations by performing injections on the tonsils, ear segment, branches of the trigeminal site vaccinations, area of the head of the uterus.

From the third session onward, the treatment with the FADEt technique starts by identifying the following memories:

Date	Finds
27/05/2023	9 years old: "We are in a taxi. My dad was fighting with my mom. I feel like we are going to crash. I feel terrified." 12 years: "My dad is kicking my grandmother's diapers; my grandmother is crying."
10/06/2023	6 years old: "I was doing homework; my dad yelled at me. I'm very scared." 8 years old: "I'm at my grandparents' house, and my dad comes to pick me up," "I would rather not stay with my dad." my dad arrived; I'm crying. He asked me: Why are you crying?" 9 years old: "I have a problem at school; my dad found out through a call and a note in the school agenda. When he hung up, he yelled at me and threw the agenda. I'm terrified." 13 years old: "I took some pills, and my dad banged on the door violently when he realized it; he took me to the hospital, and I was hospitalized." 14 years old: "My dad forced me to take off my sweatshirt and noticed the wounds on my arms (cutting). He grabbed my arm very tightly; I was scared."
24/06/2023	All memories were reviewed, and a slight disturbance was found with the memories of the 8, 13, and 14-year-olds. Again, there is a cycle of desensitization. The memories of the 6- and 9-year-olds no longer generate disturbance Physical symptoms: The VAS 9/10 headache still continues; it occurs daily. She no longer has rhinitis, she no longer has neck pain, and anxiety has been decreasing. From this month on, she will voluntarily suspend psychotherapy.
08/07/2023	The headache decreased considerably; in fact, she voluntarily decided to suspend valproic acid. She has not presented cutting behaviors again; the anxiety has been much better (subjective scale 4/10); however, she still perceives some sensation of pressure in the chest. The final FADEt session has taken place
27/01/2025	A virtual medical consultation (control) appointment has been scheduled with the patient's mother. They say that she has been asymptomatic and leads a much calmer life since September 2023 (more than 16 months ago). In fact, for this date, they decided to progressively suspend Escitalopram. By December of 2023, escitalopram had been completely suspended. Nor is she attending psychological treatments. She is making plans for her future studies at university. For about 8–10 months, the relationship with the father has improved

References

1. Head H. Certain mental changes that accompany visceral disease: the Goulstonian lectures for 1901. Brain. 1901;4(3):345–429.
2. Pavlov IP. Conditioned reflexes: lessons on the function of great hemispheres. 3rd ed. Madrid: Ediciones Morata; 2021. p. 433. [Spanish]
3. Sudakov KV. Theory of functional systems: a keystone of integrative biology. In: Nadin M, editor. Anticipation: learning from the past. The Russian/soviet contributions to the science of anticipation, Cognitive systems monographs, vol. 25. New York: Springer; 2015. p. 153–73. Available from: https://doi.org/10.1007/978-3-319-19446-2_9.
4. Kozma R. Reflections on a giant of brain science: how lucky we are having Walter J. Freeman as our beacon in cognitive neurodynamics research. Cogn Neurodyn. 2016;10(6):457–69. Available from: https://doi.org/10.1007/s11571-016-9403-3.
5. Speransky AD. A basis for the theory of medicine. New York: International Publishers; 1943.

6. Cobian A. Hypnosis and its therapeutic applications. Barcelona: Costa Llibreter; 2004.
7. Martinez-Perigod B, Asís M. Hypnosis, theories, methods and techniques. Havana: Scientific and Technical; 1995.
8. Konradi G. Activity of the nervous system. In: Bykov KM, editor. Textbook of physiology. Moscow: Foreign Languages Publishing House; 1960. p. 516–70.
9. Lawson R, Anderson D, Cepeda-Benito A. History of psychology. Mexico: Trillas; 2022.
10. Pereira A. Ericksonian hypnosis module. Bogotá: Colombian Association of Clinical Hypnosis (ACHC); 2023.
11. O'Connor J, Seymour J. Introduction to NLP. Barcelona: Ediciones Urano; 2007.
12. Shapiro F. EMDR eye movement desensitization and reprocessing. Mexico City: Editorial Pax; 2004.
13. Ammann LA. Lesson 8. In: Self-liberation. Barcelona: Ediciones León Alado; 2015.
14. Zueva EY, Zuev KB. The concept of dominance by AA Ukhtomsky and anticipation. In: Nadin M, editor. Anticipation: learning from the past. The Russian/soviet contributions to the science of anticipation, Cognitive systems monographs, vol. 25. New York: Springer; 2015. p. 13–35. Available from: https://doi.org/10.1007/978-3-319-19446-2_2.
15. Freud S. New clarifications on the Neuropsychoses of defense. In: Complete works, vol. III. Buenos Aires: Amorrortu Editores; 1976.

Part IX
Fields of Action of Neuraltherapeutic Medicine

Chapter 42
Clinical Applications of Neuraltherapeutic Medicine/Neural Therapy

Andrés Felipe Bermúdez and Jazmín Ariza-Tarazona

1 Warning

Before starting this chapter, the authors would like to recommend reading the previous chapters, which address the philosophical and historical aspects of neuraltherapeutic medicine and the contributions to a theory of health. We do not seek the validity of this complex medical system from the methodological framework of double-blind randomized clinical trials and systematic reviews, but we do seek a broad critical reflection on the various forms of research and knowledge production. The intention is to create a coherent process in the development of methodologies that respond to the complexity of life.

We hope that in this process, Cartesian thought and its discourse of method, which underlies the foundations of biomedicine, will lose its mantle of naturalness for the reader and that, behind the mist of the apparent, the essence of what is, one of the ways of relating to reality that is the product of specific historical-concrete conditions and that, therefore, it is not the ideal or the only possible one.

It is likely that you will be somewhat uncomfortable seeing the application of this type of study designs and methodologies to the field of neuraltherapeutic medicine. But don't worry, that will be a symptom that you have delved into the complexities of this medical system and will never see medicine with the same eyes again.

A. F. Bermúdez
Department of Internal Medicine, Clínica Reina Sofía, Bogotá, Colombia

J. Ariza-Tarazona (✉)
Master in Alternative Medicine, Neural Therapy Area, Faculty of Medicine, Universidad Nacional de Colombia, Bogotá, Colombia
e-mail: jsarizatarazona@gmail.com

L. B. Pinilla Bonilla et al. (eds.), *Neuraltherapeutic Medicine*,
https://doi.org/10.1007/978-3-032-03257-7_42

2 Introduction

Neuraltherapeutic medicine in the evolution of its existence, has been reporting therapeutic benefits in patients, regardless of the conditions for which they have consulted, which allows us to consider its versatility, allowing it to provide benefits in all types of patients, regardless of the medical system under which they are being managed or the medical specialty within conventional therapy. This chapter presents the studies published in the field of neuraltherapeutic medicine/neural therapy (NTM/NT) that are found in the databases of PubMed, Cochrane, Lilacs and Scielo, without the intention of making an exhaustive analysis of the methodological strengths and weaknesses. At the end, some philosophical reflections are generated and on the research methods most in line with the principles of NTM.

The way in which the various studies are grouped seeks to respect, on the one hand, the neuraltherapeutic conception, which uses diagnostic strategies typical of its philosophy of thought considering the self-eco-organizational processes of human beings that are expressed as what we know as disease and, on the other, the design of the study and the way of presenting the results by the authors. For which it was decided to group them more with a syndromatic intention, since this concept still has a space for singularity.

3 Osteo-Myofascial-Articular Conditions

A retrospective cohort study compared conventional physical therapy with neural therapy for fibromyalgia management, using a local painful point and segmental approach. The primary outcomes changed in VAS, SF-36, and FIQ scores after treatment. VAS, FIQ, and nearly all SF-36 parameters were found to improve significantly in the neural therapy group compared to the physical therapy group ($P < 0.001$) [1].

In a randomized controlled clinical trial of patients with low back pain due to piriformis syndrome, the effect of neural therapy on pain and function was evaluated. All patients received stretching exercises for the piriformis muscle. The neural therapy group received six sessions that included segmental therapy T11-S2, trigger points in the piriformis muscle, and application in the sacral canal. The visual analogue scale (VAS) and the Oswestry Disability Index (ODI) were assessed before and after treatment in both groups. There was improvement in both groups; however, it was higher in the neural therapy group [2].

In another prospective study of 50 patients with chronic low back pain of at least 3 months' duration, the effects of neural therapy (local, segmental and interfering field approach) and physical therapy were evaluated. For pain, the visual analog scale (VAS) was used, for disability the Roland Morris Disability Questionnaire (RMDQ), for quality of life the Nottingham-Health-Profile (NHP), for depression and anxiety the Hospital Anxiety-Depression Scale (HADS). These scales were used before and after treatment. Significant improvement was found in VAS, RMDQ, NHP-Pain, NHP-Physical activity, and HADS in both groups. In addition, there was a significant improvement in NHP-Energy and NHP-Social only in the neural therapy group [3].

In another randomized clinical trial where the effectiveness of neural therapy was determined in patients with chronic low back pain resistant to medical and physical therapies, the variation in VAS and RMDQ (Roland Morris Disability Questionnaire) scores was evaluated, finding that they were significantly lower at 3 and 6 months ($P < 0.05$) in the neural therapy group compared to the control group [4].

In a randomized clinical trial of patients with acute myofascial pain syndrome, one group was treated with kinesiological taping, another with neural therapy in trigger points, and a third group with neural therapy in trigger points, chest segment, and periosteum of the sternum. At the end of the treatment, there was improvement in pain and disability in all groups, with no difference between them [5].

In an interventional study, 70 patients with acute mechanical lumbosacral pain were treated with up to 10 sessions of segmental and interfering field neural therapy. At the end of the study, 57.2% of patients were pain-free and 61.4% were free of functional impotence. In both cases, the differences between before and after treatment were significant ($P < 0.01$) [6].

In a case report, a 31-year-old woman with bruxism and left low back pain VAS 7/10, secondary to sacroiliac joint dysfunction, was treated with neural therapy in the temporomandibular joint, trigger point in the masseter and C4 segment; post-intervention, pain decreased to VAS 1/10 and improvement persisted at 3 months of follow-up [7].

An athlete patient with plantar fasciitis who reported pain of 1.5 years of evolution, with an intensity of VAS 10/10 when walking, was treated with neural therapy in a plantar fasciotomy scar; After the first session, the pain decreased by 90% and at the end of the third intervention the pain had disappeared without recurrence after 2.5 years of follow-up [8].

A case report of myofascial pain syndrome, manifested as non odontogenic mandibular molar pain referred from the masseter muscle, was relieved by a combination of trigger point injection and stellate ganglion block. He had undergone pulpectomy under local anesthesia without improvement. Physical examination did not reveal any dental abnormalities. An approach was performed at the tender point of the masseter muscle with partial control of pain for 7 h. As it is considered to be derived from the sympathetic nerve, a block of the stellate ganglion is performed, which abolishes pain in the patient [9].

In an intervention study, 64 patients with musculoskeletal pain underwent neural therapy of 2 and 5 sessions, with different approaches according to their life histories. The SF-36 quality of life questionnaire was applied to each patient before and after treatment; Overall, a significant improvement in the score was found on the physical activities, physical performance, and general health subscales [10].

In another study with similar methodology, 47 patients with humeral epicondylitis were treated with several sessions of segmental and painful point therapy. The

VAS and BARTHEL scales were applied before and after treatment. Regarding pain, high values of improvement were obtained between the fifth and tenth session of treatment, while functional improvement was slower but noticeable. These findings are similar to those found in meta-analyses that included other techniques such as ultrasound and physical media [11].

An open-label, multicenter, prospective intervention study that included 34 patients diagnosed with nonspecific low back pain evaluated the efficacy of neural therapy, with a local and segmental approach, in improving pain and disability. The evaluation instruments used were the VAS for low back pain and sciatica, specific quality of life questionnaires: Oswestry and RolandMorris for pain and disability due to low back pain, respectively. A reduction in VAS for low back pain of 5.23 points and for sciatica of 3.88 points was obtained, the Oswestry showed a 36.1% reduction in pain and the RolandMorris 11 points less in disability due to low back pain than at the beginning of treatment [12].

4 Tenosinovial Conditions

In a randomized clinical trial, 36 patients with De Quervain's tenosynovitis were randomized to neural therapy (local approach, segmental C5-T8, trigger points, and stellate ganglion) and control group. All were indicated a splint for thumb and rest of the hand. VAS and the Duruöz Hand index (DHI) were used to measure pain and function at baseline, 1 month, and 12 months after the end of treatment. Both groups showed improvement compared to baseline ($P < 0.001$). The VAS score was significantly lower at one month and twelve months compared to baseline in the neural therapy group ($P < 0.001$, $P = 0.002$, respectively). The DHI score was lower in the neural therapy group at one month ($P = 0.009$), and at twelve months there were no significant differences between the two groups ($P = 0.252$) [13].

5 Urogynecologic Conditions

In one case series, five women with localized vulvar pain were treated with local neural therapy on painful spots. Two presented complete relief and three had significant improvement with an initial VAS greater than 70, which decreased to less than 30. Improvement was maintained over time with a minimum follow-up of 6 months [14].

Ten women with irritable bladder were treated with neural therapy using paraurethral applications. After the third injection, three were symptom-free and six reported marked improvement and slight improvement. The mean bladder volume at the first sensation of urinating increased significantly ($P = 0.02$) and there were no changes in other urodynamic parameters [15].

Stellate ganglion block (SGB) is an alternative for the management of severe menopausal symptoms, such as hot flashes. Data suggest that hormone replacement therapy has side effects, but it is suggested that blocking the stellate ganglion may be useful for the treatment of hot flashes. The per-protocol analysis included 19 women. One woman was excluded due to the absence of Horner's syndrome after SGB. Four weeks after SGB, the mean blushing score had decreased by 34% ± 7.4% (95% confidence interval (CI) 18–49%; $P < 0.005$). Nine women had a decrease in blushing score between 40% and 90%, with a mean response of 65 ± 4.9% (95% CI 53–76%). The other ten women did not respond to treatment, with a decrease in blushing score between 0% and 11%. Quality of life and sleep, both assessed using a questionnaire, improved significantly. The results of this study support the observation that stellate ganglion block may be a useful therapy for a subset of women with severe postmenopausal flushing [16].

Another similar study shows that breast cancer survivors undergoing endocrine therapy (ET) suffer side effects such as hot flashes and sleep disturbances accompanied by poor quality of life. SGB has been shown to be safe and effective, and has been proven to work better than pregabalin, with no side effects. Twenty-nine breast cancer survivors with severe hot flashes and sleep disturbances under ET received procaine SGB. The diaries recorded hot flashes and sleep quality scores through week 24. All patients participated and none refused the SGB. Each patient received a SGB every 4 weeks with no side effects observed. Weekly scores were reduced from baseline by 33.6% ($P < 0.01$) (hot flashes) and 22.3% ($P < 0.01$) (sleep disturbances) after 4 sessions, and by 58.8% ($P < 0.01$) (hot flashes) and 50.8% ($P < 0.01$) (sleep disturbances) after 20 weeks. Significant reductions in hot flashes and sleep disturbances were found after 1 and 6 months [17].

There are numerous reports of the use of SGB for climacteric psychosis, which is considered a sympathicotonic response to stress. In a case series, three women underwent SGB three times a week with 5 mL of 1% lidocaine, and symptom improvement was observed after the fifth block. Patients reported psychological relaxation after receiving SGB therapy. Changes in serum concentrations of ACTH, LH, FSH, and catecholamines (epinephrine, norepinephrine) before and after SGB were quantified in 8 patients suffering from climacteric psychosis. There was a significant decrease in norepinephrine concentration after blockade. There were no significant changes in ACTH, LH, FSH, and epinephrine. It was concluded that SGB therapy may be effective for climacteric psychosis due to sympathetic blockage, but the influence of the endocrinological response to SGB could not be clarified [18].

A descriptive, prospective, and longitudinal study was carried out for 10 months to test the efficacy of neural therapy in pelvic disease. The sample consisted of 72 adolescent patients and older women who were admitted to the gynecology service with the diagnosis of pelvic disease or who voluntarily attended the neural therapy consultation. Variables such as age, quality of the technique, complications, and disease evolution were used. The main objective was to demonstrate the efficacy of neural therapy in the treatment of pelvic inflammatory diseases. The predominant age was 16–20 years. The technique was good. Burning pain was the most frequent complication and the evolution was favorable, as 72.2% were asymptomatic [19].

6 Nervous System and Neuromuscular Conditions

A pilot study ($n = 40$) followed by a randomized, double-blind, placebo-controlled clinical trial ($n = 21$) included 61 patients with various variants of multiple sclerosis. The operated group underwent neural therapy on trigger points in the ankles and around the skull, while the placebo group was given saline solution. The primary outcome was improvement in the Kurtzke scales and the DSS or EDSS. At the end of the first week, there was a statistically significant improvement ($P < 0.01$) in the intervention group. In the second week, the two groups received neural therapy with lidocaine and later on acupunture needle. In total, 65% of patients in the pilot study ($n = 40$) and 76% in the double-blind study ($n = 21$) showed improvement. In the long term, from 2 to 3.5 years, more than 50% of patients continued to show improvement [20].

In another multiple sclerosis study, 28 patients with neurogenic detrusor hyperactivity underwent weekly neural therapy for 5 weeks. In each session, T10-L1 urogenital segment, gynecological plexus, vaginal and sacral epidural were applied. They received clinical and urodynamic evaluation 1 month before and 3, 9, and 12 months after neural therapy. The multiple sclerosis quality of life inventory (MSQL-54) and bladder control scale (BLCS) were also applied. Significant improvement was observed after 3 months in volume at the first involuntary contraction of the bladder, maximum detrusor pressure during filling, and maximum bladder cystometric capacity. There was also improvement in MSQL-54 scores at 3 months after treatment, but regression was observed from month 9 onward and after 12 months it was observed to be slightly above baseline [21].

In a letter to the editor, they report a case of notalgia paresthetica successfully treated with segmental neural therapy of T2-T10, which resulted in a reduction in pain in VAS from 7 to 1 [22].

A case report of progressive facial hemiatrophy was treated with SGB in a Japanese girl, affecting the soft tissue of the left buccal region, with onset at the age of 6 years after minor local trauma. He consulted at 9 years of age and left SGB was started. Local injection of lidocaine was performed in multiple episodes over a period of 1 year and 4 months. During therapy and subsequent 4-year follow-up, the atrophy state remained unchanged and did not progress. Stellate ganglion block as a therapy against progressive facial hemiatrophy was considered to merit further evaluation due to its results [23].

In a retrospective study with a total of 361 cases of acute, chronic peripheral, acute central, and chronic central facial paralysis, the authors sought to compare two types of management that included SGB in one group and conventional therapy in the other group. The Sunnybrook Facial Grading System (SFGS) score obtained before and after treatment in the groups with and without SGB was used to assess the outcome. In addition, the blood glucose level in acute peripheral facial paralysis was measured. SFGS in the group with SGB was superior to that of the group without block after treatment in peripheral facial nerve palsy, while blood glucose in the group without ganglion block increased and was higher than in the block group during treatment in acute peripheral nerve palsy. Therefore, the finding suggests that the group with stellate ganglion block has a better therapeutic effect than conventional treatment in acute and chronic peripheral facial nerve palsy in patients with type 2 diabetes mellitus [24].

A case report describes the use of SGB in the treatment of epileptic pain in a patient with severe paroxysmal pain in the right upper limb with a diagnosis of drug-resistant partial epilepsy. The patient received SGB with lidocaine for two cycles for 2 weeks and oral carbamazepine once daily. The dose of carbamazepine was gradually reduced until it was discontinued, and epileptic pain seizures became less and less frequent, until they finally disappeared [25].

In another case report, a 32-year-old woman with peripheral facial paralysis without response to corticosteroids had presented multiple inflammatory processes throughout her life that compromised areas innervated by the trigeminal. A chronic periapical inflammatory process was documented by means of an X-ray. He showed clinical improvement once the extraction of the compromised tooth was performed, which shows from the conception of neural therapy that this source of irritation was closely related to his condition [26].

7 Vascular Conditions

In a prospective, nonrandomized, interventional clinical cohort study under real-life conditions over 6 months, palliative neural therapy was performed to reduce ischemic pain secondary to lower limb occlusive arterial disease, where a revascularization intervention was not feasible and their pain was VAS $\geq$7. The decrease in the intensity of pain in the extremities in the post-treatment period was significant ($P = 0.001$), as was the quality of life ($P = 0.004$). A significant improvement ($P \leq 0.005$) was also evidenced in changes in skin temperature and ankle/brachial index [27].

8 Subacute and Chronic Pain

In a study that included 280 patients with severe chronic pain of more than 3 months without response to conventional treatment, most of them with low back pain, neural therapy was performed using a local and segmental approach in 56%, an interfering field approach in 2% and a mixed approach in 42%. At 1 year of follow-up, 41 patients were pain-free, 126 had considerable improvement, 52 had a slight improvement, and in 60 patients the pain did not change [28].

In a case series, 51 patients with chronic pain of several years of evolution of various etiologies (spondyloarthrosis, periarthritis, coxarthrosis, arthritis, migraine, intermittent claudication and abdominal pain) received interfering field treatment (scars). In 39 cases there was instant relief (phenomenon in seconds); in 15 of them there was no recurrence of pain; In 24 cases, pain decreased in each session with long intervals between recurrences until the final disappearance of the pain. There were 12 unsuccessful cases; 10 of them improved with segmental therapy [29].

In an intervention study, 82 patients with subacute and chronic pain predominantly of osteomyoarticular origin, without response to conventional analgesics, were treated with neural therapy, showing a progressive decrease in pain with a mean pre-intervention VAS of 7.94 and 3.48 at 6 months. Drug use decreased by 74.4% at 2 weeks and 80% at 6 months [30].

Case report of a patient who developed severe persistent rectal pain following a gunshot wound without improvement during more than 10 years of analgesic treatment. Rectoscopy performed procaine infiltration of the scar; post-surgery, pain disappeared [31].

In a prospective pilot study of 10 patients with chronic pain who were treated with neural therapy during three visits, quality of life was assessed using the SF-12 health questionnaire and serum NGF and BDNF levels were measured. The median serum levels of both neurotrophins showed a tendency to decrease and an improvement in quality of life was observed [32].

A randomized, double-blind, placebo-controlled study to compare the analgesic efficacy of preoperative SGB in relieving postoperative pain after orthopedic upper limb surgery. Patients were given a 3 mL injection during ultrasound-guided SGB; 15 patients received 2% lidocaine and 15 patients received 0.9% saline. After block, all patients received standardized general anesthesia. Patients were observed at 0, 2, 4, 6, 8, 12, and 24 h after surgery. The mean hourly consumption of tramadol was significantly reduced in the SGB group compared to the saline group, with statistical significance. The present study has demonstrated a postoperative analgesic and tramadol-sparing effect of preoperative SGB in patients undergoing orthopedic upper limb surgery under general anesthesia [33].

A case report of severe trigeminal neuralgia treated with procaine SGB describes the successful treatment of a patient with refractory neuralgia. This study also discusses the role of the sympathetic nervous system and the possible mechanisms of action [34].

An experimental phase II, controlled, single-center clinical trial study aimed to evaluate the efficacy of neural therapy in the treatment of pain as a manifestation of grade II cyclic breast dysplasia compared to conventional therapy. A total of 240 patients were studied, who were divided into 4 groups according to the type of treatment: neural therapy (group I), vitamin E (group II), progesterone (group III), and non-steroidal anti-inflammatory drugs (group IV). Pain improvement was observed in more than 60% of group I and was similar with the use of progesterone. There were significant differences with nonsteroidal anti-inflammatory drugs and vitamin E [35].

9 Psychiatric Conditions

One patient developed acute stress disorder, panic disorder, following the resection of an abdominal mass secondary to lymphoma. On physical examination, hypersensitivity points were found in the sternal cost region (corresponding to the Head zone of the heart), scar in the right iliac fossa, and occipital and vertical region of the skull (Head areas of the liver and intestine). Procaine injections were performed on two occasions at these sites, which showed improvement in her symptoms [36].

10 Craniofacial Organ Conditions

A case report showing that due to toxic doses of quinine, there was a deterioration in vision due to amaurosis, which improved with the intervention of SGB with lidocaine, based on the premise that SGB has been shown to cause dilation of retinal vessels, even in cases of embolism of the central retinal artery [37].

Symptoms such as tinnitus were managed with SGB. The efficacy of lymph node block was assessed using the five-step patient self-assessment method and the audiometric method. The efficacy rates of lymph node block for tinnitus were 62.5% by self-assessment and 68.8% by audiometric assessment. Hearing acuity was partially recovered and was associated with partial relief of tinnitus. An 18-month follow-up study revealed that SGB's efficacy for tinnitus persisted [38].

In cases of atrophic rhinitis, the rate of symptom relief with SGB has been found to be much higher than with conservative treatment. Therefore, it is believed that if SGBs are used as the first line of treatment rather than wasting weeks and months on conservative treatment, we may be able to obtain cases in their earliest stages when vasodilation can help reverse histopathology [39].

A prospective, experimental, and descriptive study was conducted to determine the results of neural therapy in 71 patients with chronic pharyngitis examined in the clinic for a period of 2 years, where 52 patients and women (41 women) predominated. The most frequent symptoms were burning, throat clearing, and pharyngeal stinging, with a marked improvement after treatment. It was shown that 53 patients (74.6%) treated with neural therapy responded satisfactorily to this treatment [40].

A prospective, descriptive, cross-sectional study was carried out of 50 patients diagnosed with acute alveolar abscesses in anterior teeth with a history of having started pulporradicular treatment (PRT) in devitalized teeth, in addition to the fact that during the course of the treatment it failed. The results were evaluated according to the number of sessions applied, observing that 45 patients (90%) presented a good response with only 1 or 2 sessions of segmental neural therapy in the week. Compared to the conventional method of leaving the duct open again for 5 to 7 days for pus drainage, together with analgesic and antibiotic treatment, washing and drying of the duct, which entails a long stay [41].

11 Visceral Functions

Forty patients with thoracolumbar fracture scheduled for subsequent spinal surgery were randomly assigned to 2 groups: ultrasound-guided SGB and control group. Ultrasound-guided SGB (n = 20) or a sham procedure ($n = 20$) was performed after induction with an injection of 6 mL of 1% lidocaine or 0.9% saline, respectively. Return of postoperative gastrointestinal function, including auscultation of bowel sounds, incidence and degree of abdominal distention, time of flatulence, and paralytic ileus, was assessed. Patients in the SGB group had better gastrointestinal function compared to those in the control group, as indicated by more regular bowel sounds at 24 and 36 h postoperatively (80% vs. 40%, $P = 0.024$, and 95% vs. 60%, $P = 0.023$), less bloating (10% vs. 45%, $P = 0.034$), and a slightly shorter flatulence time (mean [SD], 12.0 [4.4] vs. 14.7 [4.6] hours, $P = 0.068$). Analysis based on regular bowel sounds found a significant difference between the 2 groups ($P = 0.004$). In addition, more patients had higher satisfaction after SGB (85% vs. 45%, $P = 0.020$). There was no postoperative ileus or mortality. In this preliminary study, ultrasound-guided SGB accelerated the return of gastrointestinal transit, relieved bowel symptoms, and improved patient satisfaction after thoracolumbar spine surgery [42].

Thirty-six patients with paroxysmal atrial fibrillation (AF) were randomly assigned in a 2:1 ratio to temporary transcutaneous SGB with lidocaine or placebo prior to pulmonary vein isolation. Lidocaine was randomly infused in a 1:1 ratio into the right or left node. Before and after randomization, the effective refractory period (ERP) of both atria, the difference between right and left atrial ERP, intra- and interatrial conduction time, AF inducibility, and duration of AF were evaluated. Unilateral SGB temporarily prolonged atrial ERP, reduced the inducibility of atrial fibrillation, and decreased its duration. An equivalent effect of right and left GBS was observed in both atria [43].

A study of a group of 120 patients, with chronic ulcerative colitis for 2 years, with a control group with the use of oral sulfasalazine and an experimental group of stellate ganglion block performed with 10 ml of lidocaine. Clinical symptoms and disease activity in these two groups were compared before and after endoscopic treatment. In addition, blood measurement of IL-8 (interleukin 8) was performed. After treatment, clinical symptoms and disease activity were shown to be relieved by endoscopy in both the control and experimental groups. However, patients in the control group did not have obvious relief from abdominal pain. In addition, the degree of pain relief in the experimental group was statistically better than in the control group ($P < 0.05$). Ten days after treatment, the IL-8 level was found to be significantly lower in the experimental group than in the control group, and the difference was statistically significant ($P < 0.05$). In addition, adverse events were significantly higher in the control group than in the experimental group, and the difference was statistically significant ($\chi 2 = 33.215$, $P = 0.000$) [44].

12 Autoimmune Conditions

In a case report, a 43-year-old patient with rheumatoid arthritis, who presented with multiple physical and emotional symptoms and had discontinued management with conventional treatment, was treated with neuraltherapeutic medicine over 3 years. A total of 21 interventions were performed with a focus on possible interfering fields, painful points, and segmental therapy, presenting complete remission of their symptoms [45].

13 Infectious Conditions

An 82-year-old male patient with COVID-19, with severity criteria, who was diagnosed by the emergency department with multilobar pneumonia and pulmonary thromboembolism, in addition to conventional management, underwent neuraltherapeutic medicine with a segmental approach. The patient showed an improvement in less time than expected, which allowed an early exit from the hospital (9 days) due to lower oxygen requirement [46].

14 Other Conditions

SGB has been used to improve blood flow. A study was carried out to measure the change in tissue oxygenation in the mandibular region after the block and the therapeutic effect of the same for postoperative mandibular nerve hypoesthesia. To determine the variation in tissue oxygenation in the mandibular region, tissue oxygen index (TOI; percentage of oxygenated hemoglobin in total hemoglobin) in the skin near the mental foramen bilaterally, at the primary site of unilateral block, was measured using 6 mL of 1% lidocaine for the treatment of postoperative bilateral mandibular nerve injury. Thirteen patients were included in this study. On both the blocked and contralateral sides, TOI was significantly increased compared to that prior to lymph node block (ΔTOI at 15 minutes after SGB, 5.87% ± 2.89%, $P < 0.001$, 95% CI 4.122–7.617% on the blocked side, 1.88% ± 2.73%, $P = 0.005$, 95% CI 1.877–2.725% on the contralateral side). It is concluded that unilateral blockade with 6 ml of 1% lidocaine produces an increase in tissue oxygenation in the mandibular region [47].

A series of cases carried out by SGB for arrhythmia control. Lidocaine, bupivacaine, or a combination of both were injected in the vicinity of the left stellate node. In total, 18 blocks were performed in 11 patients. Seven patients received only one block; three underwent two procedures and one required three blocks and two continuous infusions to control ventricular (VA) arrhythmias. The mean ventricular arrhythmia load, 1 h after each block, was zero compared to five in the previous hour ($P < 0.001$); 83% of patients were VA-free; efficacy at 24 h increased with repeated blocks. Anatomy-based stellate ganglion block is a safe and rapidly effective treatment for refractory thunderstorms [48].

A prospective clinical trial was carried out for 1 year, where the sample consisted of all patients with renal lithiasis who attended medical consultation. The sample of 60 patients was divided into two groups of 30 each (control and experimental group). The selection of patients in each group was carried out randomly, after controlling the variables that were studied to ensure homogeneity between both groups. The renal silhouette scheme (papules in the renal area) was applied to the experimental group. The results showed that patients were able to expel lithiasis from the fifth treatment session, regardless of location and up to a diameter of 12 mm [49].

An intervention study was conducted in 88 patients between the ages of 20 and 50 years with the diagnosis of alopecia areata. The sample was divided into two groups with an equal number of patients. One group was operated on with neural therapy and the other with conventional treatment (phenol and alcohol touches, sedatives and vitamins). At the third week of treatment, satisfactory results were shown in the neural therapy treatment with significant differences ($P = 0.05$), which became more evident at the sixth week [50].

15 Discussion and Conclusions

The reviewed articles show a benefit of the use of strategies based on NTM/NT compared to other conventional management, which allows us to conclude the benefit of their use in a variety of disease states.

The databases reviewed found 49 studies described in this chapter. There are many other publications in university databases around the world, but it is impossible to access all of them. It would be important for all this research to be available in databases with open access in order to be able to dimension the totality of the research produced in the field of NTM/NT.

Within the studies, the local, segmental, and mixed approach predominates, while the interfering field approach is a minority (see Table 42.1).

The analysis of Table 42.1 shows that the segmental approach adds a greater amount, because node blockages are counted here; only one study described as an interfering field is reported, but in mixed studies, it can be read that local, segmental, and/or interfering field interventions are carried out.

Table 42.1 Distribution of approaches in neural therapy/neuraltherapeutic medicine

Total studies	50 studies
Segmental approach	21 studies
Mixed approach	19 studies
Interfering field approach	1 study
Local approach studies	9 studies

Although the articles reviewed describe the use of local anesthetics with good therapeutic results, most of them do not describe a methodology based on neuraltherapeutic thinking.

It is considered that research processes in neuraltherapeutic medicine should be based on a methodology anchored in its philosophical principles, from the theory of complexity, with an integrative approach aimed at capturing the symptomatic totality and the meaning of the conditions that a human being may experience at a given point in his or her existence, in such a way that the complexity of life and its self-eco-organizational processes are valued so that decisions can be made in order to make decisions Therapeutic measures are not standardized, but depend on the meticulous analysis of each patient's life history and the complete physical examination, understanding that the whole is more than the sum of the parts.

16 Final Thoughts

As stated in the introduction, the intention of this chapter is not to make a conventional critical analysis of the studies cited. On the contrary, it is considered necessary to generate questions from philosophical criticism (understanding criticism as the analysis of the conditions of possibility) that discuss the hidden dwellings that condition the production of this type of studies and their implication for the essence of neuraltherapeutic medicine.

It should not be forgotten that no clinical measurement instrument is neutral and that every research method conditions the results obtained. The scientific method of biomedicine is Cartesian; it is not concerned with the historical-concrete conditioning of the knowing subject; it artificially fragments reality into apparently independent units and is ultimately an expression of the forms of production of the material life of reality in modernity. Therefore, it is not something natural, although it is apparently presented to us as such; it has a historicity and it is not the only way to relate to reality.

That is why one of the questions that should be asked when researching neuraltherapeutic medicine is whether there is any clinical research method that captures the complexity of life and its self-eco-organizational processes. Paradoxically, case reports (lower level of evidence for biomedicine) allow, from the theory of complexity, an integrative approach aimed at capturing the totality and meaning of the conditions that a human being may experience at a given point in his or her future. In this review there are some examples of case reports that, based on the elaboration of a detailed life history of the patient, account for what has been said above.

On the other hand, the following reflections remain: what are the implications of assuming the research methods of biomedicine in the field of neuraltherapeutic medicine, if for the former it is vital to make an artificial cut of reality to measure one or a few variables and to be able to control possible biases, while neuraltherapeutic medicine does not intend to sacrifice the whole and understands that the whole is more than the sum of the parts? Is it possible that a methodology that serves other research interests, where the homogenization of the sample and the control of the variables is vital, when transferred to the field of neuraltherapeutic medicine, in a certain way, does not necessarily impoverish it, constrain it, and blur it? Finally, doesn't neuraltherapeutic medicine end up becoming just another tool to be had, ignoring its worldview and principles?

References

1. Balevi Batur E, Atan T. Neural therapy for fibromyalgia: myth or improving quality of life? Int J Clin Pract. 2021;75(4) https://doi.org/10.1111/ijcp.13719.
2. Nazlikul H, Ural FG, Oztürk GT, Oztürk ADT. Evaluation of neural therapy effect in patients with piriformis syndrome. J Back Musculoskelet Rehabil. 2018;31(6):1105–10. https://doi.org/10.3233/BMR-170980.
3. Atalay NS, Sahin F, Atalay A, Akkaya N. Comparison of efficacy of neural therapy and physical therapy in chronic low back pain. Afr J Tradit Complement Altern Med. 2013;10(3):431–5. https://doi.org/10.4314/ajtcam.v10i3.8.
4. Yilmaz E. The determination of the efficacy of neural therapy in conservative treatment-resistant patients with chronic low back pain. Spine. 2021;46(14):E752–9.
5. Ay S, Tur BS, Karakaş M, Gökmen D, Altinbilek T, Evcik D. Comparison of Kinesio taping, trigger point injection, and neural therapy in the treatment of acute myofascial pain syndrome: a randomized controlled study. Agri. 2023;35(3):134–41. https://doi.org/10.14744/agri.2022.39259.
6. Trevín Fernández G, Palma Febres A, Santoya Varela V, Expósito Reyes O, Sánchez Manduley Manzanillo Granma C. Effectiveness of neural therapy in acute mechanical lumbosacral pain. Multimed. 2012;16(Suppl 1):723–32.
7. Boluk Senlikci H, Ozen S. Sacroiliac joint dysfunction treated using neural therapy to the temporomandibular joint: a case report. Complement Med Res. 2021;28(4):379–81. https://doi.org/10.1159/000513131.
8. Fleckenstein J, König M, Banzer W. Correction to: neural therapy of an athlete's chronic plantar fasciitis: a case report and review of the literature. J Med Case Rep. 2018;12(1):1–5. https://doi.org/10.1186/s13256-018-1852-3.
9. Handa T, Fukuda K, Ichinohe T. Effect of combination of trigger point injection and stellate ganglion block on non-odontogenic mandibular molar pain referred from masseter muscle: a case report. Bull Tokyo Dent Coll. 2013;54(3):171–5. https://doi.org/10.2209/tdcpublication.54.171.
10. Enrique J, Garzón R. Changes in the quality of life of patients with musculoskeletal pain treated with neural therapy in outpatient care. Rev Fac Med. 2012:1–74.
11. Peraza Morelles R, Hernández Barrios D, Gil García V, Garrido PR. Efficacy of neural therapy in the treatment of patients with humeral epicondylitis. Rev Arch Med Camagüey. 2011;15(2):271–83.
12. Medrano García R, Varela Hernández A, de la Torre Rosés M, Mendoza Cisneros R, Acosta Davison Y. Results of applying neural therapy in nonspecific low back pain. Arch Med Camagüey. 2011;15(1):1–11. Available from: http://scielo.sld.cu/pdf/amc/v15n1/amc070111.pdf
13. Bölük Şenlikci H, Odabaşı ÖS, Ural Nazlıkul FG, Nazlıkul H. Effects of local anaesthetics (neural therapy) on pain and hand functions in patients with De Quervain tenosynovitis: a prospective randomised controlled study. Int J Clin Pract. 2021;75(10):1–8. https://doi.org/10.1111/ijcp.14581.

14. Rey Novoa M, Muñoz-Sellart M, Catalán Soriano M, Vinyes D. Treatment of localized vulvar pain with neural therapy: a case series and literature review. Complement Med Res. 2021;28(6):571–7. https://doi.org/10.1159/000514945.
15. Spernol R, Riss P. Urodynamic evaluation of the effect of neural therapy in motor and sensory urgency. Geburtshilfe Frauenheilkd. 1982;42(7):527–9. https://doi.org/10.1055/S-2008-1036911.
16. Van Gastel P, Kallewaard JW, Van Der Zanden M, De Boer H. Stellate-ganglion block as a treatment for severe postmenopausal flushing. Climacteric. 2012;16(1):41–7. https://doi.org/10.3109/13697137.2012.709889.
17. Soecknick S. Stellate ganglion block with procaine in breast cancer survivors with hot flashes and sleep disturbances undergoing endocrine therapy. Medicine (United States). 2024;103(2):E36848. https://doi.org/10.1097/MD.0000000000036848.
18. Ikeda K, Isshiki A, Yoshimatsu N, Oumi A, Ito S, IT. Three case reports of the use of stellate ganglion blocks for climacteric psychosis. Masui. 1993;42(11):1696–8. Available from: https://pubmed.ncbi.nlm.nih.gov/8254884/
19. Corona LR, Reytor Gutiérrez R, Castellanos AC. Neural therapy for the treatment of IPC. Multimed. 2009;13(2) Available from: https://revmultimed.sld.cu/index.php/mtm/article/view/1681
20. Gibson RG, Gibson SLM. Neural therapy in the treatment of multiple sclerosis. J Altern Complement Med. 1999;5(6):543–52. https://doi.org/10.1089/acm.1999.5.543.
21. Tamam Y, Özdemir HH, Gedik A, Tamam C, Nazlıkul H. Efficacy of peripheral lidocaine application (neural therapy) in the treatment of neurogenic detrusor overactivity in multiple sclerosis patients. Neurourol Urodyn. 2017;36(7):1832–8. https://doi.org/10.1002/nau.23191.
22. Mülkoğlu C, Nacir B, Genç H. An alternative in the treatment of notalgia paresthetica: neural therapy. Int J Dermatol. 2018;57(9):e70–1. https://doi.org/10.1111/ijd.14086.
23. Mizuguchi M, Komiya K. Stellate ganglion block therapy against progressive facial hemiatrophy. No To Hattatsu. 1989;21(6):574–8. Available from: https://pubmed.ncbi.nlm.nih.gov/2803814/
24. Luo G, He J, Wu T, Huang Y, Miao Z, Zhao Z, Wang X, Wang Y. The therapeutic effect of stellate ganglion block on facial nerve palsy in patients with type 2 diabetes mellitus. Eur Neurol. 2015;74:112–7. https://doi.org/10.1159/000435834.
25. Wang S, Zhu Y. A case report of stellate ganglion block in the treatment of epileptic pain. Medicine (United States). 2017;96(6):2016–8. https://doi.org/10.1097/MD.0000000000006044.
26. Kawano-Hokama M, Shiratori-Tusita LN, Pinilla-Bonilla LB, Cruz-Rodríguez Y. The potential role of trigeminal nerve irritation in the pathophysiology of Bell's palsy. A case report from a neural therapy perspective. Case Rep. 2022;8(2):1–8. Available from: https://revistas.unal.edu.co/index.php/care/article/view/93840
27. Istvan M, Zsolt DB, Gabriella H, Zoltan K, Gabor K, Henrik S. Effects of neural therapy on quality of life in patients with inoperable lower extremity artery disease. Ideggyogy Szle. 2018;71(11–12):393–402. https://doi.org/10.18071/ISZ.71.0393.
28. Egli S, Pfister M, Ludin SM, Puente de la Vega K, Busato A, Fischer L. Long-term results of therapeutic local anesthesia (neural therapy) in 280 referred refractory chronic pain patients. BMC Complement Altern Med. 2015;15(1) https://doi.org/10.1186/s12906-015-0735-z.
29. Gerzner LF. Management of intractable pain by neural therapy. Med J Aust. 1970;1(21):1051–4. https://doi.org/10.5694/j.1326-5377.1970.tb84399.x.
30. Lóriz Peralta O, Raya Rejón A, Pérez Morales D, Girona Amores A, Vinyes Casajoana D, De La Vega P, Costa K. Intervention study on subacute and chronic pain in primary care: an approach to the effectiveness of neural therapy. Aten Primaria. 2011;43(11):604. https://doi.org/10.1016/J.APRIM.2010.10.004.
31. Saha FJ, Komhard V, Langhorst J. Successful endoscopic neural therapy of a patient with chronic pain syndrome after rectum gunshot injury. Forsch Komplementmed. 2006;21(5):310–3. https://doi.org/10.1159/000367719.

32. Garzón C, Caminos JE, Alzate JP, Eslava-Schmalbach JH, Garcés MF, Beltrán-Dussan EH. Effect of neural therapy on NGF and BDNF serum levels in patients with chronic pain. A pilot study. Rev Fac Med. 2021;69(4):1–7. https://doi.org/10.15446/REVFACMED.V69N3.80142.
33. Kumar N, Thapa D, Gombar S, Ahuja V, Gupta R. Analgesic efficacy of pre-operative stellate ganglion block on postoperative pain relief: a randomised controlled trial. Anaesthesia. 2014;69(9):954–60. https://doi.org/10.1111/anae.12774.
34. Lopes CA, Fischer L. A case of severe trigeminal neuralgia: recovery by means of stellate ganglion block with procaine. Discussion of possible mechanisms of action. J Int Med Res. 2023;51(4) https://doi.org/10.1177/03000605231164479.
35. Expósito Reyes OR, Vargas LaO F, Alba Verdecia E, Roselló Salcedo O, Tornés Salgado C. Neural therapy as treatment for pain in grade II cyclical mammary dysplasia. Rev Cubana Cir. 2007;46(3)
36. Ruiz-Mejía AF, Beltrán-Dussán EH, Morales-Hernandez LA, Pinilla-Bonilla LB. Neural therapy approach in a hospitalized patient with acute stress disorder. Case report. Case Rep. 2020;6(1):25–32. https://doi.org/10.15446/CR.V6N1.79132.
37. Bricknell PP, Middleton HG, Hollingsworth A, Evans EML. Stellate ganglion block in treatment of total blindness due to quinine. Br Med J. 1967;4(5576):400–1. https://doi.org/10.1136/BMJ.4.5576.400.
38. Matoba T, Sakurai T, Noguchi I, Noguchi H. Stellate ganglion block for the relief of tinnitus in vibration disease. Kurume Med J. 1984;31(4):295–300. https://doi.org/10.2739/KURUMEMEDJ.31.295.
39. Sharma AN, Sardana DS. Stellate ganglion block in atrophic rhinitis. J Laryngol Otol. 1966;80(2):184–6. https://doi.org/10.1017/S0022215100065129.
40. Álvarez Urbay MA, Conejero Alvarez HF, Boudet Ávila M, Ferrer Murgas G, Santana ÁJ. Results of neural therapy in chronic pharyngitis. Rev Arch Med Camagüey. 2007;11(2) Available from: http://scielo.sld.cu/scielo.php?script=sci_arttext&pid=S1025-02552007000200010&lng=es&nrm=iso&tlng=es
41. Paneque Gamboalez MR, González García AM, Rodríguez Martínez BM. Use of neural therapy in root canal sepsis 2008-2009: polyclinic type III. MULTIMED. 2009; Available from: http://www.multimedgrm.sld.cu/articulos/2009/v13-3-4/4.html
42. Peng K, Zhang J, Chen W, Liu H, Ji F. Ultrasound-guided stellate ganglion block improves gastrointestinal function after thoracolumbar spinal surgery. Clin Ther. 2017;39(11):2322–30. https://doi.org/10.1016/j.clinthera.2017.09.008.
43. Leftheriotis D, Flevari P, Kossyvakis C, Katsaras D, Batistaki C, Arvaniti C, Giannopoulos G, Deftereos S, Kostopanagiotou G, Lekakis J. Acute effects of unilateral temporary stellate ganglion block on human atrial electrophysiological properties and atrial fibrillation inducibility. Heart Rhythm. 2016;13(11):2111–7. https://doi.org/10.1016/j.hrthm.2016.06.025.
44. Zhao HY, Yang GT, Sun NN, Kong Y, Liu YF. Efficacy and safety of stellate ganglion block in chronic ulcerative colitis. World J Gastroenterol. 2017;23(3):533–9. https://doi.org/10.3748/WJG.V23.I3.533.
45. Ballén-Vanegas AE, Pinilla-Bonilla LB, Amaris-Peña OE. Symptomatic remission in a patient with rheumatoid arthritis treated with neural therapy. Case report. Case Rep. 2023;9(1) https://doi.org/10.15446/CR.V9N1.92936.
46. Bustamante C, Pinilla L, Amaris O. An approach to acute SARS-CoV-2 management with complementary neural therapeutic medicine: a case report. Clin Med Insights Case Rep. 2023;16:2–7. https://doi.org/10.1177/11795476231159584.
47. Yasuda M, Kuroda H, Suzuki K, Takahashi S, Morimoto Y, Sanuki T. Impact of stellate ganglion block on tissue blood flow/oxygenation and postoperative mandibular nerve hypoesthesia: a cohort study. J Oral Maxillofac Surg. 2022;80(2):266.e1–8. https://doi.org/10.1016/j.joms.2021.08.161.
48. Savastano S, Dusi V, Baldi E, Rordorf R, Sanzo A, Camporotondo R, Fracchia R, Compagnoni S, Frigerio L, Visconti LO, De Ferrari GM. Anatomical-based percutaneous left stellate

ganglion block in patients with drug-refractory electrical storm and structural heart disease: a single-Centre case series. EP Europace. 2021;23(4):581–6. https://doi.org/10.1093/EUROPACE/EUAA319.
49. de la Torres Rosés MM, Mendoza RL. Neural therapy: an alternative in the treatment of kidney stones. Rev Arch Med Camagüey. 2008;12(2) Available from: http://scielo.sld.cu/scielo.php?script=sci_arttext&pid=S1025-02552008000200003&lng=es&nrm=iso&tlng=es
50. Díaz Alcorta T, Batallán Jérez MP, Acosta Martínez B. Neural therapy in the treatment of alopecia areata: January 2000-June 2002. Correo Cient Med Holguín. 2004:1–7. Available from: http://www.cocmed.sld.cu/no84/n84ori6.htm

Chapter 43
Neurofocal Dentistry

Lucy Naomi Shiratori Tusita and Sandra Lucia Patiño Niño

1 The Relationship Between the Oral Cavity and the Whole Body

1.1 Introduction

Medicine and dentistry have been working apart, but scientific development and clinical observations have increasingly shown the importance of the mouth in systemic health. Based on concepts of classical physics and linear mathematics of Descartes and Newton, which often guided the evolution of Medicine among other areas, the body has been understood as separate parts.

Nowadays the current neurophysiological and neuroanatomical knowledge recognizes that there are no segmental boundaries and that the human body works as an integrated system, where it has to be considered as a whole. The neuroanatomical circuit, the occurrence of sensitization processes between segments, neuroplastic alterations, immune processes, and neurogenic inflammation, reinforce that the segments go beyond the anatomical limit previously [1].

In Neural Therapy, the concept of interference field, first described by the Huneke brothers as written in Chap. 2, it is also defined as "neuromodulatory trigger" by Engel et al. [1]. They are a chronic irritative condition in any part of the body and usually there are no direct symptoms in the region itself. The pathological impulses which come from this region represent chronic stimuli for the nociceptive and

L. N. Shiratori Tusita (✉)
Private Practice, São Paulo, Brazil
e-mail: lushiratori@gmail.com

S. L. Patiño Niño
Faculty of Dentistry, Universidad Nacional de Colombia, Bogotá, Colombia
e-mail: slpatinon@unal.edu.co

L. B. Pinilla Bonilla et al. (eds.), *Neuraltherapeutic Medicine*,
https://doi.org/10.1007/978-3-032-03257-7_43

sympathetic fibers and stress the basic system. As a result, the interconnected control circuits become unstable, and the systems no longer function according to the principle of homeostasis and economy. If other stress factors are added (other neuromodulatory triggers, intestinal dysbiosis, heavy metals, exogenous electromagnetic load, etc.), the body's regulatory mechanisms can fail [2].

Approximately 70% of neuromodulatory triggers (interference fields) are found in the oral and dental region [2]. The great influence of this region on systemic health can be explained primarily by the neuroanatomical connections of the trigeminal nerve, embryological aspects of oral cavity, and the role of the sympathetic nervous system.

The trigeminal nerve is the largest and most complex of the cranial nerves. As well as being the largest conductor of afferent stimuli in the face and it provides motor innervation for the masticatory muscles.

Pathological processes in the orofacial, temporomandibular, infratemporal, and pterygopalatine regions can influence all organs and organ systems [1]. Therefore, diagnosis and treatment are so important but are unfortunately often overlooked in medicine.

1.2 Embryological Aspects of Oral Cavity

During the embryonic development process in the gastrulation phase, the three embryonic leaflets are formed where the cells reorganize to form the layers that will give rise to the different tissues and organs of the body. They are called endoderm, mesoderm, and ectoderm.

The endoderm, the innermost layer of the embryo, gives rise to internal organs such as the digestive system, lungs, bladder, and endocrine glands (such as the pancreas and liver).

The mesoderm, which lies between the ectoderm and the endoderm, gives rise to muscles, bones, the circulatory system (heart and blood vessels), the kidneys, and other internal organs.

The ectoderm is formed from the outermost layer of the embryo. Its cells undergo differentiation and form the ectodermal epithelium and the neural plate, which has two main divisions: neural tube and neural crest. The ectodermal epithelium gives rise to the epidermis, hair, nails, skin and mammary glands, anterior pituitary gland, inner ear, retin and tooth enamel.

The neural tube gives rise to the central nervous system and the neural crest to the peripheral nervous system, which consists of the sensory and cranial nerves and ganglia, adrenal medulla, dentin-pulp complex (odontoblasts and dentin), periodontal ligament, cementum, and alveolar bone.

Therefore, the dental organ originates from the ectoderm, with the tooth enamel coming from the ectodermal epithelium and the dentin-pulp complex from the neural crest.

Odontoblasts are responsible for the formation of dentin. Their cell body is intrapulpal, and their extension is inside the dentin canaliculi. The cell bodies are organized in a single layer along the interface with the dentin.

The dentin-pulp complex is made up of two tissues (dentin and pulp) that are totally interconnected and function as a structural unit where the extensions of odontoblasts are included in the dentin and as a functional unit where the pulp maintains the vitality of the dentin and the dentin protects the pulp. What affects the pulp affects the dentin and vice versa (physiological, pathological, or iatrogenic factors), as well as having the same embryological origin.

The peripheral nervous system and the dentin-pulp complex have the same embryological origin. In addition to the odontoblast being a sensory cell, the presence of the extracellular matrix with fibers from the sympathetic nervous system and sensory fibers from the trigeminal nerve connect the teeth and adjacent structures (oral cavity) to the entire organism [3].

Special characteristics of the odontoblast extension (cytoplasmic extension): poor in organelles, abundant microtubules (similar in quantity to neurons), presence of S-100 protein (glial cells), and its embryological origin is the neural crest, the same as the peripheral nervous system [4].

1.3 Anatomical and Neurophysiological Aspects of Trigeminal Nerve and Trigeminal Nucleus

The trigeminal nerve, V cranial nerve, is a mixed nerve. Predominantly sensory, with a small motor portion. It has three main divisions:

The ophthalmic branch (V1) is responsible for sensitivity in the upper region of the face, such as the forehead, eyes, and scalp.

The maxillary branch (V2) is responsible for the sensitivity of the middle region of the face, including the lower part of the eyes, the cheeks, and the upper teeth.

The mandibular branch (V3) is responsible for sensitivity in the lower region of the face, including the mandible and lower teeth.

The motor fibers originate in the motor nucleus of the trigeminal nerve, located in the brainstem, and are responsible for the innervation of the muscles of mastication (masseter, temporal, and pterygoid muscles).

The trigeminal ganglion is one of the largest sensory ganglia of the cranial nerves and is located in the temporal fossa. It contains the cell bodies of the sensory neurons, which axons make synapses with the trigeminal sensory nuclei in the brainstem (main sensory nucleus, spinal trigeminal nucleus, and mesencephalic nucleus).

The teeth, maxilla, and mandible are connected to the nervous system by the trigeminal nerve (and also by sympathetic fibers). Afferent stimuli from the trigeminal nerve stimulate the trigeminal nucleus.

Regarding the trigeminal nucleus, there are further relevant neuroanatomical aspects.

The trigeminal nucleus is in the brainstem and upper cervical spinal cord. It is divided into three main parts: the main, the spinal, and the mesencephalic. In the spinal nucleus of the trigeminal nerve (SNTN) there is a convergence of afferent fibers from various cranial nerves (VII, IX, and X) as well as from the upper cervical nerves [5–10]. The functional structure of the SNTN in the superior cervical spinal cord corresponds, in principle, to that of the posterior column (see Fig. 43.1) [7].

In the spinal nucleus of the trigeminal nerve and nucleus tractus solitarius, some afferent fibers from the glossopharyngeal nerve (IX pair) and the vagus nerve (X pair) terminate among them. The SNTN and nucleus tractus solitarius extend to the cervical spinal cord and there are connections between them [2, 11].

Nociceptive afferent fibers from the spinal nerves that are directed to the posterior column of the upper cervical segments are intermingled with those of the SNTN (see Fig. 43.1).

Considering the neuroanatomical connections discussed above, there are some pathophysiological aspects related to the spinal nucleus of the trigeminal nerve. These connections explain our clinical observations of the dependency of oral pathologies and visceral disorders. As well as that, pathologies of the teeth/mandibular region can influence the muscular and articular structures of the cervical spine (pain, tension, blockage). And even disturbances in the cervical spinal area may be attributed to tonsillitis and/or pharyngitis.

The pathological impulses represent chronic stimuli for the nociceptive and sympathetic fibers. These impulses can come from the teeth (trigeminal inervation region). The stimulus is subliminal; usually, there are no direct symptoms in the region itself but can stress the basic system. The common efferent signals in the

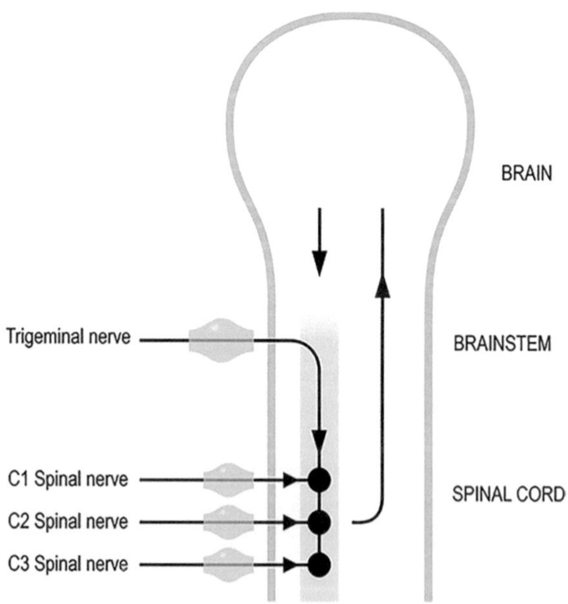

Fig. 43.1 An example of connection between trigeminal nerve and cervical nerves in the spinal nucleus of the trigeminal nerve (SNTN). (Taken from: © Shiratori and Fischer [9])

SNTN (see Fig. 43.2) and nucleus solitarius could explain the concept of neuromodulatory trigger (interference field) [1, 2].

1.4 The Role of the Sympathetic Nervous System

Teeth are connected to the nervous system via the trigeminal nerve and also contain fibers of the sympathetic nervous system.

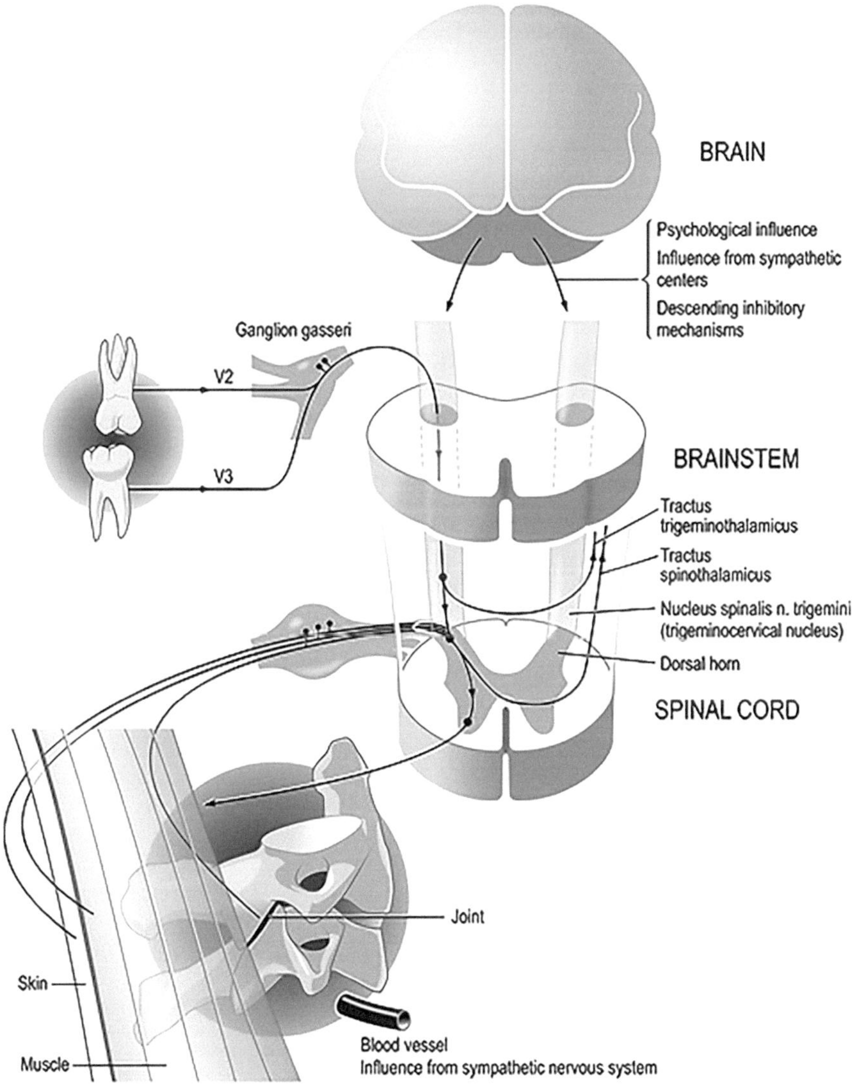

Fig. 43.2 An example of a neuroanatomical connection among trigeminal nerve, cervical nerves in the SNTN and brain/brainstem. (Taken from: © Shiratori and Fischer [9])

In the periphery, the sympathetic nerve fibers consist of an intertwined network of fine fibers with their extremities immersed and integrated in the basic system known as the terminal reticulum [12]. As the basic system and the sympathetic nervous system are ubiquitous, a stimulus in the teeth/jaw region can reach anywhere, which in turn can influence all organ systems of the body [1, 5, 7, 9, 13–16].

In the central nervous system, the SNS modulates pain perception through its influence on the descending modulation system [15]. In case of chronic stress and negative emotions, which activate the SNS, can lead to a dysfunction of this system, resulting in increased sensitivity to pain (see Fig. 43.2).

Therefore, the sympathetic nervous system can influence pain and also inflammation and microcirculation, including the processes of the trigeminal-cervical complex, which can be amplified by feedback mechanisms through the brainstem and brain (see Chap. 16).

2 Dental Pathologies and Systemic Health

2.1 Introduction

The relationship between oral health and general health has been recognized since ancient times. Historically, the first relevant record mentioning the importance of oral health for general well-being dates to ancient Egyptian medicine, around 1550 BC, with references to treatments for oral diseases and suggesting that the teeth were considered important for the general health of the body.

In ancient Greece, Hippocrates, considered the father of medicine, wrote about the relationship between oral diseases and other health conditions.

Medicine and Dentistry are amid a major transition where there is growing evidence from concepts of neurophysiology that the complex human body has a holistic way of being; therefore, diagnostic and therapeutic management in health care requires an interdisciplinary approach.

Experiments in Neural Therapy [17] show that inflammation and mechanical problems in the oral-dental region can lead to referred pain or systemic changes [2, 5, 13, 17, 18]. As explained above, these disturbances are called neuromodulatory triggers [1], also known as interference fields [17], which are a chronic irritative condition in any part of the body. The stimulus is subliminal; usually, there are no direct symptoms in the region itself.

2.2 Potential Neuromodulatory Triggers (Interference Fields) in the Oral Region and Their Influence on Systemic Health

There are several alterations in the oral region, most of them with no pain, which can trigger pathological information to the basic system, immune system and nervous system, consequently having an impact on the systemic health. Some examples are endodontically treated teeth, mechanical forces related to third molars with space problems, impacted and/or lack of space problem teeth, teeth filled in with different metals generating an electrical potential, periodontal diseases, pulp chronic inflammation, pulp necrosis, apical osteitis, cysts and/or scars that could be neuromodulatory triggers/interference fields.

Periodontitis is one of them, which is a chronic non-communicable disease (NCD) with a high prevalence, being severe periodontitis, affecting 11.2% of the world's population, the sixth most common human disease [19].

Periodontitis affects the supporting tissues of the teeth, such as the gums, the periodontal ligament, and the alveolar bone, and can lead to tooth loss and other health problems. It causes a local inflammatory response, releasing substances such as cytokines and prostaglandins, which also act systemically, affecting metabolic processes, for instance, increasing insulin resistance [20, 21].

Some studies have shown the existence of a bidirectional link between periodontal health and systemic pathologies like cardiovascular diseases and diabetes. Diabetes increases susceptibility to infections, increasing the likelihood of developing periodontitis. Likewise, cardiovascular diseases are aggravated by periodontitis [20, 22].

Evidence suggests that periodontal inflammation triggers systemic inflammation, which, together with damage mediated by antibodies that cross-react between periodontal pathogens and intimal wall components and direct damage by bacteria that enter the circulation, promotes the development of atherosclerosis [23].

Another common pathological alteration is the periapical lesion, which generates inflammation. Sometimes, initially, the body responds with acute inflammation, characterized by vasodilation, increased vascular permeability, and migration of inflammatory cells. If the causative agent is not eliminated, the acute process evolves into a chronic process, which is characterized by the predominant presence of macrophages, lymphocytes, and plasma cells. Bone destruction occurs due to the action of inflammatory mediators and cells such as osteoclasts, activated by inflammatory cytokines (e.g., IL-1, IL-6, TNF-α, and prostaglandins) [24, 25]. Most chronic periapical lesions are asymptomatic, but the chronic inflammatory process is perceived by the nervous and immune systems, which try to repair the tissue damage.

In dental practice, third molars (3 M) often remain included/semi-included or poorly positioned due to problems of lack of space. This condition can lead to the increase of dental plaque, which promotes the occurrence of localized inflammations such as gingivitis, pericoronitis, and caries. These teeth may be locally asymptomatic, but that doesn't mean that they are always free of disease. There may be chronic inflammatory processes and silent pathologies in them that affect systemic health [26–28].

The scars following surgeries, for instance, from tooth extractions, should also be considered as possible neuromodulatory trigger/interference fields because the tissue contains collagen fibers which behave similar to electrical dipoles. If mechanically stimulated, they may generate action potentials that are transmitted centrally via the trigeminal nerve. Another possibility for action potentials to appear is the ectopic type emerging from neuromas in the scar tissue [9, 14, 15, 29–31].

Changes in oral health can also increase the risk of autoimmune diseases [32], heart disease [33], myocardial infarction [34], premature birth and low birth weight babies [35, 36], and diabetes [20, 21].

The pathologies in the oral region are perceived by the nervous system [2, 5, 13, 18]. Its sensory input from the region (via trigeminal nerve and sympathetic fibers) stimulates the trigeminal nucleus, where there are several anatomical connections with cervical nerves, vagus nerve, facial nerve, etc. (see Sect. 1.2). The common efferent signals can explain the strong influence of the trigeminal nerve region on systemic health [9, 11, 37].

Besides the neuroanatomical connections, the basic system as a ubiquitous synapse and terminal reticulum with sympathetic fibers in the extracellular matrix explains that pathological information in the oral region can influence any part of the body.

3 Effects of Mastication and Malocclusion on the Systemic Health

3.1 Introduction

The close relationship between the mouth and the entire body is evident, considering the connections between the trigeminal nerve and the vagus, glossopharyngeal, facial, and cervical nerves, as well as with sympathetic fibers of the autonomic nervous system that are distributed in the extracellular matrix, forming what is known as a ubiquitous synapse.

The importance of this area for systemic health is clear, which afferent stimuli originating from the trigeminal nerve and sympathetic fibers can influence any part of the body through these connections.

3.2 Mastication and Malocclusion in Relation to Systemic Health

Efficient chewing stimuli can also be related to good systemic health. There are numerous studies that show the relationship between good occlusion, good mastication and the prevention of dementia [38, 39].

Chewing to facilitate the effective processing of food by enzymes is called mastication. The semi-autonomic activity involves the brainstem and various regions of the brain that control and create the complex masticatory patterns under the coordination of the CNS [40].

The masticatory process stimulates various regions of the brain, increasing cerebral oxygenation in the hippocampus and prefrontal cortex (PFC), which can act on the learning and memory process of chewing, stimulating cognitive functions [38, 41, 42].

There are multiple neural circuits that connect the teeth to the central nervous system, and particularly during an adequate mastication, the afferent stimuli also act on the hippocampus and can contribute to maintaining cognitive functions [38, 39, 41, 42].

Chewing stimulates neurogenesis and synaptic plasticity in the hippocampus. This is due to the activation of neural circuits that increase blood flow and brain oxygenation [43].

In addition to the hippocampus, the hypothalamic-pituitary-adrenal (HPA) axis has been linked to chewing, which reveals connections between oral function, brain and stress regulation [44].

Chewing has been shown to reduce stress-induced damage to the hippocampus. Regular chewing activities can decrease glucocorticoid production, protecting hippocampal neurons from the excitotoxicity caused by stress [45]. In addition, it attenuates the HPA axis response to stress by reducing the release of cortisol. Stress regulation is considered to be related to afferent signals from oral mechanoreceptors to brain regions [44].

The interactions between these systems create a feedback loop, where chewing not only improves the function of the hippocampus, acting on memory and learning, but also moderates the stress response [43].

The relationship between chewing, the hippocampus, and the HPA axis highlights the importance of oral health, the preservation of an efficient chewing function and its systemic effects on brain health and stress regulation. However, future research is still needed to explore therapeutic applications, especially for elderly populations and individuals with chronic stress or neurodegenerative conditions [43, 44].

Hence, masticatory disorders and occlusal malfunctions, which lead to mastication dysfunctions, have gained interest in the prevention of cognitive alterations [38, 41, 42, 46].

4 Clinical Aspects

4.1 History of Life

Make sure you have a life history that includes medical, dental (previous treatments, dental materials, dental creams, rinses), dietary, and environmental information which can play a role in the pathophysiology of the disease. Ask also the patient about medical, psychiatric, emotional, social, cultural, and other diagnoses. Correlate all these data with the reason for the dental consultation.

4.1.1 History of Teeth

Teeth are of particular importance in people's lives, and it is vital to understand how they develop. The eruption processes of primary and permanent teeth are directed by nerve signals, with sympathetic innervation being crucial for normal tooth eruption [47]. Tooth eruption involves the dental follicle, derived from neural crest cells, which regulate osteoclastogenesis and osteogenesis generated by gene expression both chronologically and spatially [48]. Parathyroid hormone-related peptide (PTHrP) and its receptor (PTH1R) have also been found to be molecules involved in signaling pathways in the different phases of eruption [49].

There are three stages in the history of teeth: the primary dentition (0–6 years), the mixed dentition where the primary teeth exfoliate and the permanent teeth erupt (6–12 years), and the permanent dentition (12 years and older). The eruption and exfoliation processes are intense in the mixed dentition and coincide with peaks of maxillomandibular growth, cognitive, and socio-affective development. It is vital to identify anomalies in the eruption and exfoliation processes in chronology, sequence, and tooth position, as these could be the effects of irritations to the nervous system. Further research is needed.

4.2 *Physical Examination*

4.2.1 Introduction

Identify the clinical scenario in which you are going to act. To do so, confirm dental, periodontal, endodontic, temporomandibular joint, occlusal diagnoses and sleep disorders or presence of oral habits. Basic semiological tools of observation, intraoral and extraoral palpation are part of the clinical exam. The areas of pain at the craniofacial level based on the cartographies offered by Adler, Mackenzie and Head (see Chap. 15) might be detected, and if necessary, the algometer could be used. Emotional states like anxiety and fear should be observed during the consultation. Use complementary examinations such as X-rays, CT scans, digital models, salivary tests, photographs, videos or any other exam that you consider appropriate and diagnostic methods of Galvanism (see Chap. 44). The objective of this process is to identify the neuromodulatory triggers, the symptoms and signs of dystrophy, the reactions that the organism has generated and their biological significance, the synchronicity in time and space of irritations.

4.2.2 Extraoral Inspection and Palpation (Neck and Head Region)

Extraoral Inspection

The extraoral inspection initially evaluates the patient's posture, including the alignment of the head in relation to the trunk, to check for postural deviations. The presence of muscle contractures (hypertonia, stiffness, trigger points), facial asymmetries, skin alterations (color, texture, lesions, scars, nevi, telangiectasias, pigmentary alterations, or other dermatoses) on the face and neck are observed. The identification of edema, erythema, and other tissue alterations is also relevant. It also identifies possible movement restrictions or pain.

The evaluation of cervical mobility is fundamental for the differential diagnosis of several conditions, such as neck pain, stiff neck, cervical disc hernias, temporomandibular disorders (TMD) and neurovascular compressive syndromes. Cervical range of motion (ROM) is evaluated by the movement of the head in the different planes:

- Flexion: Anterior inclination of the head, bringing the chin closer to the sternum (physiological ROM: 45–60°).
- Extension: Posterior inclination of the head, directing the gaze towards the upper plane (physiological ROM: 60–75°).
- Rotation: Lateral rotation of the head, directing the eyes towards the lateral plane (physiological ROM: 70–90° on each side).
- Lateral inclination (lateral flexion): Lateral inclination of the head, bringing the ear closer to the ipsilateral shoulder (physiological ROM: 40–45° on each side).

Extraoral Palpation

Extraoral palpation is complementary to inspection, and it should be systematically performed on both sides for evaluation of pain on palpation (POP), areas of hypertonia, muscle spasms, trigger points and changes in skin texture. Fundamental areas include:

- Muscles: Temporalis muscle, masseter muscle (superficial and deep portions), sternocleidomastoid muscle, trapezius muscle, scalene muscles, and other cervical muscles.
- Ligaments: Stylomandibular ligament, retrodiscal ligament.
- Temporomandibular joint (TMJ): Lateral pole, retrodiscal region, and capsular ligaments. Evaluate the presence of crepitation, clicking, blockage, or pain on palpation.
- Lymphonodes: Palpate the preauricular, retroauricular, occipital, submandibular, submental, superficial and deep cervical lymphnodes, evaluate size, consistency, and sensitivity.

4.2.3 Intra-Oral Inspection, Palpation, and Percussion

Intraoral Clinical Examination: Importance and Methodology

The intraoral clinical examination is an indispensable tool in dental practice, given the interrelationship between the oral cavity and systemic health. It allows for a visual and tactile assessment of intraoral structures, making it possible to identify alterations or pathologies that may have an impact on the patient's general health.

Interdisciplinary collaboration between dentists and doctors is essential, especially to familiarize the doctor with the particularities of the intraoral region.

Inspection

During the inspection, the color, texture and presence of lesions or alterations in structures such as the lips, buccal mucosa, tongue, palate, and floor of the mouth are thoroughly evaluated. In relation to the teeth, characteristics such as color, shape, size, position, as well as the presence of cavities, restorations, fractures, wear, or stains are analyzed. The gums, on the other hand, should be examined for color, contour, and texture, as well as signs of bleeding, swelling, or retraction. In the oropharynx, the tonsils, posterior pharyngeal wall, and uvula should be examined in detail.

Important note: In patients wearing dentures, these should be removed beforehand for a proper evaluation.

Palpation

Palpation complements inspection, providing additional information on the integrity of intraoral structures. It should be carried out gently, using the index finger, and is aimed at identifying alterations such as edema, sensitization, pain, etc.

Percussion

The dental percussion test is a basic clinical examination in dentistry that evaluates the sensitivity of the periodontal ligament (the tissue that connects the tooth to the bone). It consists of lightly touching the tooth with an instrument in different directions (vertical and horizontal), observing the patient's reaction and comparing it with adjacent healthy teeth.

It indicates inflammation in the area around the root of the tooth, caused by deep caries, trauma, root canal treatments, or other infections. Also can suggests the presence of periodontal disease, tooth fractures, or even maxillary sinusitis.

The test gives complementary information to clinical examination and helps in diagnosis and treatment planning.

4.3 *Diagnostic Images*

4.3.1 Orthopantomography

Orthopantomography is an X-ray examination that provides a comprehensive view of the oral structures, thus allowing a general assessment of the patient's oral condition, in order to support diagnosis and planning.

This X-ray exam provides an overview of teeth, bones, TMJ, and other areas:

- In the teeth: Extensive caries, included/impacted teeth, dental anomalies, and root resorption.
- In the bones: Periodontal bone loss, fractures, chronic periapical lesions, cysts, osteitis, tumor.
- In the TMJ: Degenerative changes (shape and structure of the condyles and fossae) and signs of disc displacement.
- Other areas: Sinusitis (changes in the maxillary sinuses) and calcifications in soft tissues (salivary calculi, etc.).

Important
The medical doctor may also recommend an orthopantomography whenever, on inspecting and palpating the oral area, he/she suspects the presence of neuromodulatory triggers/interfering fields in the region. Symptoms such as pain, sensitivity, and clinical signals such as swelling and others described above in 4.2.3 should be observed.

Interpretation and treatment planning should be performed in collaboration with the dentist, in a multidisciplinary approach due to the importance of the oral region for systemic health.

4.3.2 Periapical and Computed Tomography

There are other complementary exams that are possible, such as periapical X-rays, indicated to examine one or more teeth and the surrounding bone in detail. In addition, computed tomography is used to provide detailed three-dimensional images of the teeth, jawbone, and adjacent structures, assisting with implant planning, surgery, orthodontic treatment, and pathology and trauma diagnosis, providing a more complete view than conventional radiographs. It is important to note that the need for these X-rays exams must be assessed by the dental doctor, in order to determine the most appropriate type of exam for each case, as well as its interpretation and treatment planning.

4.4 Diagnosis in Neurofocal Dentistry

The diagnostic approach for neurofocal dentistry has the same basis as the general approach of Neuraltherapeutic medicine, since both share the same theoretical and experimental foundations.

This diagnosis is based on a scheme of irritation stages or neurodystrophic phases, as can be seen in Chap. 24. These stages or phases are inspired by the diagnostic scheme from Huneke School, the classification of the dystrophies according to Speransky, and the rules that Head described for the extension of the pain (see Table 43.1).

Table 43.1 The stages of an irritation or neurodystrophy in the organism. An example in dentistry is shown following these classifications

Stage	Description	Example in dentistry
Local irritation or dystrophy	It happens when, after specific irritation, the organism keeps it under control, avoiding its extension to other structures.	A tooth extraction that recovers normally without the existence of any symptom occurring in other parts of the mouth, parts of the trigeminal nerve, or parts of the cervical segment neither.
Segmental irritation or dystrophy	It occurs when an irritation is extended by contiguity or symmetrization to other parts of the same segment.	Following a tooth extraction, the patient has started exhibiting symptoms such as caries on another tooth, gingivitis, or toothaches. In the segment, the patient could present with keratitis, conjunctivitis, otitis, rhinitis, and sinusitis. On the cervical segment, the patient could exhibit neck pain and superior limb pain (in the shoulder, arm, elbow, wrist, hand, and fingers).
Meta-segmental irritation or dystrophy	It takes place when the initial irritation caused the excitation to spread to other parts of the same segment as well as parts of the organism that are less resistant or that are part of a conditioned reflex.	A tooth extraction after which the patient started to exhibit pain or any other disease in a part of the body previously affected in his/her history of life.
Corticalization or generalization of an irritation or dystrophy	An organism's altered inhibitory mechanisms allow the irritation to spread even throughout the entire cortex. Clinically, we could recognize it when an organism exhibits an alteration of more than three segments.	After having a tooth extraction, a long process of progressive neurodystrophy began. This affects not only the trigeminal and cervical segments but also more than three segments, such as the cardiopulmonary area, the gastrointestinal area, and the lower limbs or lumbosacral segment.

Source: own elaboration

Dental Test As it was described first by Huneke, there is a diagnostic test that could be made if there is a suspicion that one tooth could be the cause of a distant or local pathology in the body. The injection with local anesthetic is made submucosally, directed towards the root of the tooth. This test could result in a Huneke phenomenon or phenomenon in seconds, which means that the pain or pathological condition could disappear for at least 8 h. From the classical point of view, if this phenomenon occurred, this tooth was considered an interference field [50]. However, clinical experience has shown that even when the Huneke test is negative for a suspicious tooth, there is a high incidence (around 50%) of false-negative results in the oral region. It should not be discarded that the suspicious tooth is a neuromodulatory trigger. In addition, when a Huneke test is negative (in the first 8 h), it is possible that after the injection on the suspected tooth, the patient begins to feel better even 48 h later. Within the neuratherapeutic diagnostic approach, it is essential to consider each patient's individual response.

4.5 General Therapeutic Guidelines for Dental Treatment

4.5.1 Introduction

From bioethics, humanism, and patients' rights, you can generate an approach to the patient. Build safe spaces during the consultation where the patient can feel confident and calm. Try to reach consensual decisions with the patient based on prudence, respect for others, honesty, beneficence, and non-maleficence, supported by validated technical and scientific criteria. When faced with difficult decisions, consider the Ottawa Decision-Making Guide for Patients [51] or others. Ensure that a fully informed consent process is carried out.

The aim of these interventions is to interrupt the reflexes that the patient has created by the presence of multiple irritations in the stomatognathic system.

If it is difficult or totally impossible to remove irritants because they are established and irreversible treatments in the oral region, opt at first for lowering the loads of collateral irritants based on the Barrel of Fischer theory [52] and then proceed with the irritants that are considered to generate greater irritation to the system. In all cases, maintaining communication with the consultant and their doctor is crucial for follow-up and monitoring potential local or systemic reactions.

4.5.2 Recommendations for the Procaine Administration

Administer procaine as the sole injectable solution at a concentration of 0.5%, applying it in the form of papules in areas adjacent to the sites of irritation. When necessary, employ intraoral truncal techniques for the pterygopalatine ganglion, inferior alveolar, mental, infraorbital, greater palatine, or nasopalatine nerves. Opt for short 27–30 gauge or extracorporeal needles.

For extraoral techniques, target structures such as the infraorbital nerve, nasociliary nerve, temporoauricular nerve, Gasserian ganglion, scalp, occipital nerve, and others. Select short or long 27–30 gauge needles, ensuring that you have certified training and legal authorization in your country.

Remember that procaine can be used to come into contact with mucous membranes, dentine, or dental cement, so it can be irrigated at the time of cavity preparations, endodontic, periodontal, or surgical treatments (see Chap. 26).

4.5.3 Dental Treatment

Based on the anamnesis, clinical examination, and complementary exams, identify the irritant that generates symptoms or dystrophic tissues for the stomatognathic system. Remember that it can be of chemical origin (materials), electrochemical (metals in the mouth), biological (inflammatory or infectious processes), mechanical (occlusal disharmony or occlusal trauma), or traumatic (surgical procedures or dental or maxillofacial trauma).

On the understanding that excitatory or inhibitory reflexes are generated by irritants in the stomatognathic system, which may be unknown to the clinician, it is suggested that the therapeutic processes be slow and adjusted to the systemic conditions of the patient.

In contemporary dentistry, minimally invasive procedures and the implementation of non-invasive strategies and soft technology for the management of caries and periodontal disease are the most prevalent diseases.

In case the irritant is chemical and is associated with the use of a material, you may consider replacing it with biocompatible and tissue-regenerating materials that have the most extensive evidence [53]. Minimize or avoid contact with chemical substances that may cause intoxication.

When the irritant is electrochemical, you can replace the metal filling with a non-metallic one [54, 55]. Follow the protocol for the removal of amalgam [56] and metallic materials faithfully to avoid poisoning the patient and contaminating your practice. Should this not be possible, consider contact and friction isolation between metallic materials.

In cases where the irritant is biological, educate the patient on controlling dento-gingival plaque and modifying the environment to reduce plaque colonization and growth through operative, periodontal, endodontic, or orthodontic treatment.

When the irritant is mechanical, aim to achieve occlusal stability using techniques such as myorelaxation plates, selective grinding, dental alignment, or orthodontics, depending on the patient's needs. Ensure that the maintenance of occlusal stability is correlated with the patient's posture while at rest, standing, sitting, and walking [57].

Should the irritant be traumatic, adjust and relieve pressure from the prosthesis. Keep in mind that areas affected by surgical trauma may remain active sources of irritation and should be treated with procaine. If tissue trauma is linked to harmful oral habits, consider an interdisciplinary approach involving a physiotherapist, psychologist, and physician for intraoral management.

In case of sleep apnea and bruxism, medical and dental management is imperative. One of the therapeutic tools used is the mandibular protrusion plates, and sleep hygiene.

In all cases, consider *occlusal stability* as a priority because it reduces the effects of occlusal trauma during chewing, swallowing, and rest. There are reports of relationships between occlusal disharmony with joint and head pain [58, 59]. Also, deficiency of mastication has been related with dementia (see Sect. 3).

Complement the treatment with dietary suggestions according to the chewing abilities of the patient and the physiological needs of the patient with an emphasis on the prevention of caries and chronic non-communicable diseases. Use other complex medical systems or alternative or complementary therapeutic tools that have therapeutic validation and fit the patient's morbid condition.

Possibility of Interdisciplinary Work and Follow-Up It is imperative to work in interdisciplinary teams that allow consensual and coordinated actions. It is necessary to create clearly established work routes and communication flows with the patient and their support network in the event of acute reactions after neural therapy interventions.

5 Review of Clinical Cases

Case reports provide a valuable contribution to a better understanding of the multiple complex interactions between oral and systemic health. They offer useful clinical data on diagnosis, management, and treatment efficacy. These examples emphasize the need for a multidisciplinary approach to improve patient outcomes.

Case 1

From the perspective of Neural Therapy and Neurofocal Dentistry, Kawano-Hokama et al. [37] reported a clinical case in which they support the hypothesis that irritations in the trigeminal nerve innervation area may be related to the pathophysiology of Bell's facial paralysis. They reinforce the role of the nervous system as a physiological basis functioning as a unit. Where a previous dystrophy or alteration, in the case described, of the trigeminal nerve may, through its different branches, accumulate over time, end up affecting the nerve tone or trophism of the facial nerve by anastomosis (see Fig. 43.3).

During the treatment, no concurrent interventions were done, only Neural Therapy and Dentistry treatment.

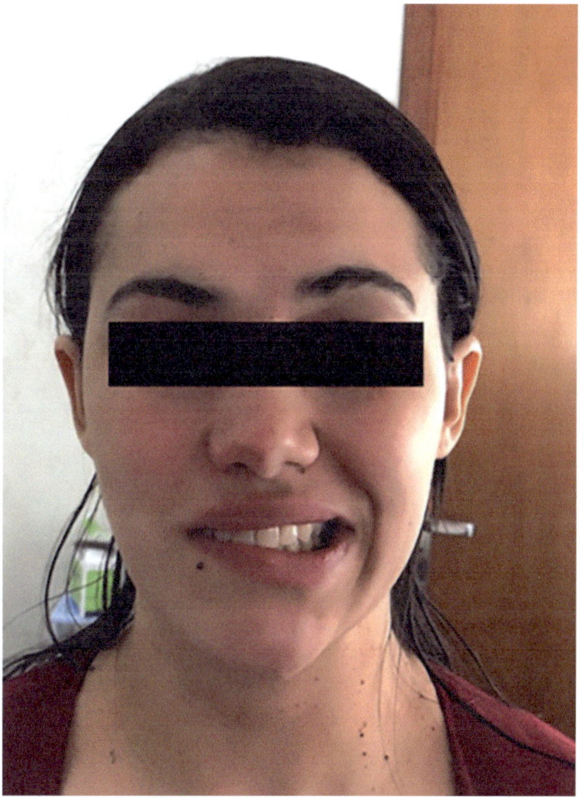

Fig. 43.3 Right incomplete facial asymmetry—Grade III (House Brackman scale). (Taken from: Hokama et al. [37])

Medical and dental approaches for the improvement of Bell's palsy treating trigeminal irritations were made (see Figs. 43.4 and 43.5).

Case 2

Shiratori and Fischer [9] reported a case of refractory chronic neck pain, the cause of which was found in the tooth/jaw region, more specifically, in wisdom teeth with space problems and partially impacted (see Fig. 43.6). The tooth/jaw region itself

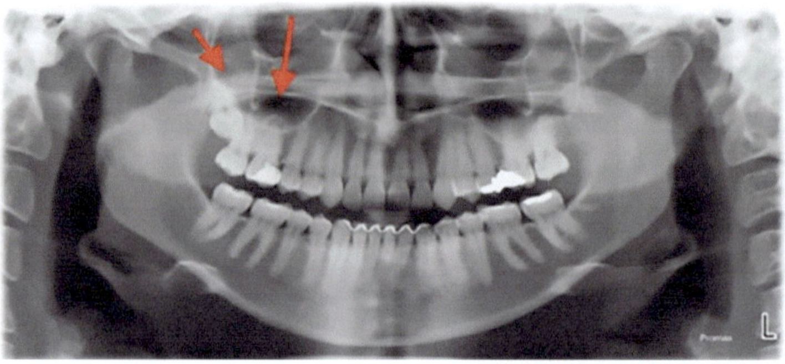

Fig. 43.4 Orthopantomography—tooth 16 with periapical lesion and tooth 18 included. (Taken from: Hokama et al. [37])

Fig. 43.5 Within 48 hours of performing endodontic treatment on tooth 16, Bell's palsy improved from grade III to grade I on the House–Brackmann score, and facial mimicry symmetry was recovered. (Taken from: Hokama et al. [37])

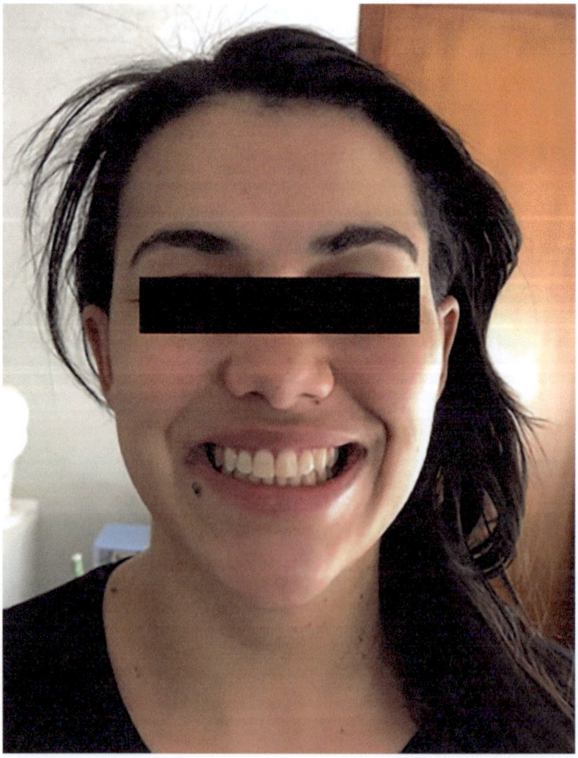

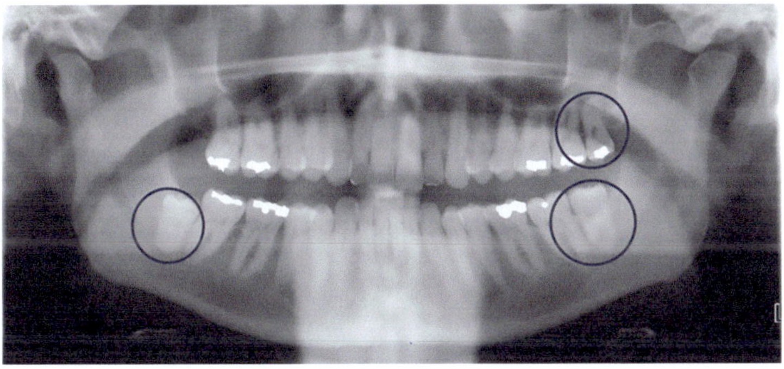

Fig. 43.6 The close vicinity between semi-included tooth 4.8 and the mandibular ramus of the trigeminal nerve can generate sensory input to the nervous system by mechanical pressure, and its partial eruption can generate chronic gingival inflammation. The left mandibular ascending ramus is very close to the erupted teeth 2.8 and 3.8. The lack of space around the two teeth could originate gingival chronic inflammation because of difficult daily oral care. (Taken from: Shiratori, Fischer [9])

Fig. 43.7 Tooth 36 RX (2017 Oct)

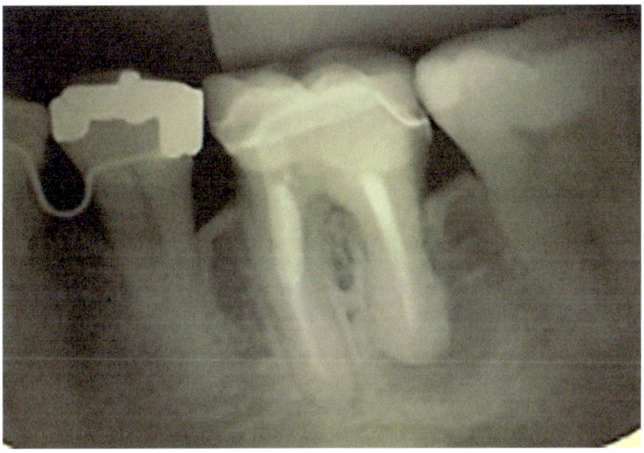

was not painful, but the neck pain developed through the n. trigemini spinal nucleus, which extends to the cervical spinal cord. Surgical removal of the wisdom teeth and subsequent neural therapy treatment of the extraction scars provided permanent pain relief.

In the case of chronic neck pain that is resistant to therapy (among others), it is worth looking for interfering fields (neuromodulatory triggers) in the dental/jaw area, which could allow for causal therapy. Do not limit yourself only to degenerative findings obtained by imaging in the area of pain but look for possible chronic irritations in the trigeminal zone.

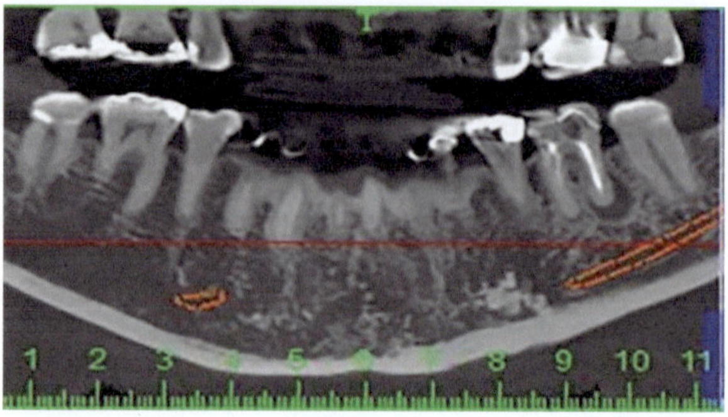

Fig. 43.8 Computed tomography—Tooth 36 (2017 Oct)

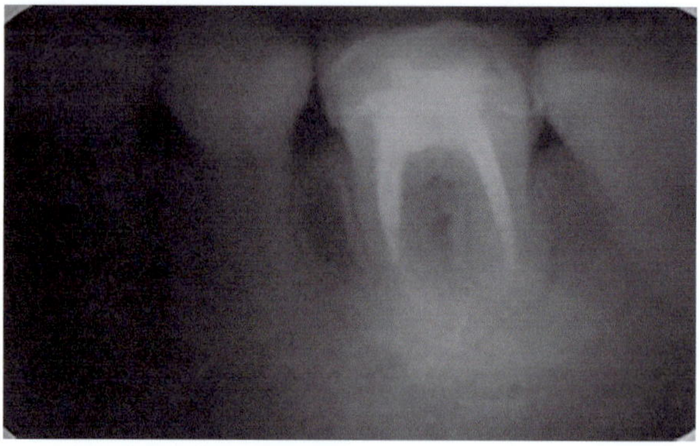

Fig. 43.9 Tooth 36 (2018 Jul)

Case 3

An example of vagal and trigeminal correlations with the next clinical case,[1] shows the close relationship between visceral disorders and irritation in the trigeminal area (interference fields/neuromodulatory triggers). The patient had irritable bowel syndrome, with symptoms of insomnia, diarrhea, weight loss, and hair loss. In the clinical and radiographic dental evaluation, a periapical lesion was observed (asymptomatic on tooth 36) (see Figs. 43.7 and 43.8) and the presence of centric bruxism, with several muscle trigger points in the masseter and temporal muscle region. The canal of tooth 36 was re-treated and 1% procaine was applied to the trigger points on the face, as well as a gluten-restricted diet. The patient showed a significant improvement in all symptoms and radiographic control was carried out on the lesion, which disappeared 8 months after root canal treatment (see Fig. 43.9).

[1] which was presented as an abstract in the International Forum of Neural therapy in Vienna of 2019, and count with a previous approval from the patient and signed informed consent.

Remarks on Orthodontic Treatments

In dental practice, orthodontic treatments are very common, not only to achieve better occlusion, but also for aesthetic reasons. Vinyes et al. investigated the relationship between orthodontic treatment and chronic neck pain or gonalgia, which often does not respond to conventional treatments and impairs patients' quality of life. The study involved six orthodontic patients with long-term chronic pain (VAS 6 to 10) refractory to conventional treatments [60].

After the exclusion of concomitant pathologies, all patients were diagnosed with chronic musculoskeletal pain.

The patients received injections of 0.5% procaine in specific areas of the oral mucosa (areas of tension and/or sensitivity) and extraoral myofascial regions. All reported significant improvement in chronic pain, with no residual pain during the six-month follow-up.

The pathophysiological mechanism involved is related to the induction of tension in the muscle fasciae, which have many sympathetic fibers, generating disturbances in microcirculation and muscle tension. The muscle fasciae are loose connective tissue and connect all the muscles in the body to each other.

According to the principle of mechanotransduction, where biomechanical stimuli generate biochemical responses in the tissues, tension stimuli can generate pain anywhere in the body. The use of procaine was considered due to its safety profile, rapid metabolization and favorable effects on microcirculation and acting as a short-reset on nerve fibers, thus being able to improve chronic pain.

Other additional considerations are the complex interrelationship between oral structures and cervical muscles, highlighting how activation of the trigeminal nerve can influence neck pain, reinforcing the relationship of the cervical trigeminal complex. As well as identifying myofascial trigger points and treating them with procaine injections. This investigation shows that injections of local anesthetics, such as procaine, can be an effective intervention for post-orthodontic musculoskeletal pain.

Some clinical reports reinforce that functional anatomy and modern neurophysiology are leading us more and more towards a holistic view where medical and dental doctors have to work together for a better and long-term result [1, 14].

References

1. Engel R, Barop H, Giebel J, Ludin SM, Fischer L. The influence of modern neurophysiology on the previous definitions of "segment" and "interference field" in neural therapy. Complement Med Res. 2022;29(3):257–67. https://doi.org/10.1159/000522391.
2. Fischer L. Neural therapy: neurophysiology, injection technique, therapy suggestions. 5th ed. Stuttgart: Thieme; 2019.
3. Nerves LE. Tooth, mouth, jaw. Berlin: Verlag für Zahnmedizin; 1994.
4. Magloire H, Couble ML, Romeas A, Bleicher F. Odontoblast primary cilia: facts and hypotheses. Cell Biol Int. 2004;28(1):93–9.

5. Barop H. Textbook and atlas of neural therapy: diagnosis and therapy with local anesthetics. Stuttgart: Thieme; 2018.
6. Caous CA, de Sousa BH, Lindsey CJ. Neuronal connections of the paratrigeminal nucleus: a topographic analysis of neurons projecting to bulbar, pontine and thalamic nuclei related to cardiovascular, respiratory and sensory functions. Auton Neurosci. 2001;94(1–2):14–24. https://doi.org/10.1016/s1566-0702(01)00338-1.
7. Neuhuber WL. Functional neuroanatomy of the craniovertebral junction. In: Hülse M, Neuhuber WL, Wolff HD, editors. The upper cervical spine: pathophysiology and clinic. Heidelberg: Springer; 2005. p. 55–71.
8. Schmidt M, Hennke T, Knöchel M, Kürten A, Hierholzer J, Daniel P, et al. Can chronic irritations of the trigeminal nerve cause musculoskeletal disorders? Forsch Komplementmed. 2010;17(3):149–53. https://doi.org/10.1159/000315338.
9. Shiratori T, Fischer L. Chronic therapy-resistant neck pain in a fifty-year-old man: the role of partially impacted third molars – case report and new pathophysiological insights. Complement Med Res. 2023;30(3):270–4. https://doi.org/10.1159/000529293.
10. Weinschenk S, Hollmann MW, Göllner R, Picardi S, Strowitzki T, Diehl L, Hotz L, Meuser T. Heidelberg University neural therapy education and research group (the HUNTER Group). Injections of local anesthetics into the pharyngeal region reduce trapezius muscle tenderness. Forsch Komplementmed. 2016;23(2):111–6. https://doi.org/10.1159/000444665.
11. Henssen DJHA, Derks B, van Doorn M, Verhoogt NC, Staats P, Vissers K, Cappellen V, van Walsum AM. Visualizing the trigeminovagal complex in the human medulla by combining ex-vivo ultra-high resolution structural MRI and polarized light imaging microscopy. Sci Rep. 2019;9(1):11305. https://doi.org/10.1038/s41598-019-47855-5.
12. van der Zypen E. Electron microscopy findings on the final spread of the autonomic nervous system and their interpretation. Acta Anat. 1967;67:431–515.
13. Adler E. Focus and foci in the trigeminal area. 4th ed. Heidelberg: Verlag für Medizin Dr. E. Fischer; 1990.
14. Fischer L, Barop H, Ludin SM, Schaible HG. Regulation of acute reflex hyperinflammation in viral and other diseases by means of stellate ganglion block: a conceptual view with a focus on Covid-19. Auton Neurosci. 2022;237:102903. https://doi.org/10.1016/j.autneu.2021.102903.
15. Jänig W, Baron R. Pathophysiology of pain. In: Fischer L, Peuker E, editors. Textbook of integrative pain therapy. Stuttgart: Haug; 2011. p. 35–71.
16. Ommerborn M, Raab W. Odontalgia. In: Hugger A, Göbel H, Schilgen M, editors. Facial and headache pain from an interdisciplinary perspective. Heidelberg: Springer; 2006. p. 51–63.
17. Huneke F. Neural therapy, phenomenon in seconds, and surgery. Therapiewoche. 1955;5:286–94.
18. Weinschenk S, editor. Handbook of neural therapy. 2nd ed. Stuttgart: Thieme; 2020.
19. Nazir M, Al-Ansari A, Al-Khalifa K, Alhareky M, Gaffar B, Almas K. Global prevalence of periodontal disease and lack of its surveillance. Scient World J. 2020;2020:2146160. https://doi.org/10.1155/2020/2146160.
20. Herrera D, Sanz M, Shapira L, Brotons C, Chapple I, Frese T, Graziani F, Hobbs FDR, Huck O, Hummers E, Jepsen S, Kravtchenko O, Madianos P, Molina A, Ungan M, Vilaseca J, Windak A, Vinker S. Association between periodontal diseases and cardiovascular diseases, diabetes and respiratory diseases: consensus report of the joint workshop by the European Federation of Periodontology (EFP) and the European arm of the World Organization of Family Doctors (WONCA Europe). J Clin Periodontol. 2023;50(6):819–41. https://doi.org/10.1111/jcpe.13807. Epub 2023 Mar 22
21. Sanz M, Marco Del Castillo A, Jepsen S, Gonzalez-Juanatey JR, D'Aiuto F, Bouchard P, Chapple I, Dietrich T, Gotsman I, Graziani F, Herrera D, Loos B, Madianos P, Michel JB, Perel P, Pieske B, Shapira L, Shechter M, Tonetti M, Vlachopoulos C, Wimmer G. Periodontitis and cardiovascular diseases: consensus report. J Clin Periodontol. 2020;47(3):268–88. https://doi.org/10.1111/jcpe.13189. Epub 2020 Feb 3

22. Liccardo D, Cannavo A, Spagnuolo G, Ferrara N, Cittadini A, Rengo C, Rengo G. Periodontal disease: a risk factor for diabetes and cardiovascular disease. Int J Mol Sci. 2019;20(6):1414. https://doi.org/10.3390/ijms20061414.
23. Carrizales-Sepúlveda EF, Ordaz-Farías A, Vera-Pineda R, Flores-Ramírez R. Periodontal disease, systemic inflammation and the risk of cardiovascular disease. Heart Lung Circ. 2018;27(11):1327–34. https://doi.org/10.1016/j.hlc.2018.05.102. Epub 2018 Jun 2
24. Ye L, Cao L, Song W, Yang C, Tang Q, Yuan Z. Interaction between apical periodontitis and systemic disease: review. Int J Mol Med. 2023;52(1):60. https://doi.org/10.3892/ijmm.2023.5263. Epub 2023 Jun 2
25. Stashenko P, Wang CY, Tani-Ishii N, Yu SM. Pathogenesis of induced rat periapical lesions. Oral Surg Oral Med Oral Pathol. 1994;78(4):494–502. https://doi.org/10.1016/0030-4220(94)90044-2.
26. Blakey GH, Jacks MT, Offenbacher S, Nance PE, Phillips C, Haug RH, et al. Progression of periodontal disease in the second/third molar region in subjects with asymptomatic third molars. J Oral Maxillofac Surg. 2006;64(2):189–93. https://doi.org/10.1016/j.joms.2005.10.014.
27. Campbell JH. Pathology associated with the third molar. Oral Maxillofac Surg Clin North Am. 2013;25(1):1–10. https://doi.org/10.1016/j.coms.2012.11.005.
28. Offenbacher S, Beck JD, Moss KL, Barros S, Mendoza L, White RP Jr. What are the local and systemic implications of third molar retention? J Oral Maxillofac Surg. 2012;70(9 Suppl 1):S58–65. https://doi.org/10.1016/j.joms.2012.04.036.
29. Athenstaedt H. Pyroelectric and piezoelectric properties of vertebrates. Ann N Y Acad Sci. 1974;238:68–94. https://doi.org/10.1111/j.1749-6632.1974.tb26780.x. PMID: 4531280
30. Fischer L, Ludin SM, Puente de la Vega K, Sturzenegger M. Neuralgia of the glossopharyngeal nerve in a patient with post-tonsillectomy scarring: recovery after local infiltration of procaine – case report and pathophysiologic discussion. Case Rep Neurol Med. 2015;2015:560546. https://doi.org/10.1155/2015/560546. Epub 2015 Apr 16. PMID: 25960898; PMCID: PMC4415660
31. Michels T, Ahmadi S, Michels D. Physiological-anatomical aspects in neural therapy. Treatment results of acute and chronic pain. Deutsche Zeitschrift für Akupunktur. 2011;54(2):6–9.
32. Julkunen A, Heikkinen AM, Söder B, Söder PÖ, Toppila-Salmi S, Meurman JH. Autoimmune diseases and oral health: 30-year follow-up of a Swedish cohort. Dent J (Basel). 2017;6(1):1. https://doi.org/10.3390/dj6010001.
33. Bahekar AA, Singh S, Saha S, Molnar J, Arora R. The prevalence and incidence of coronary heart disease is significantly increased in periodontitis: a meta-analysis. Am Heart J. 2007;154(5):830–7. https://doi.org/10.1016/j.ahj.2007.06.037.
34. Rydén L, Buhlin K, Ekstrand E, de Faire U, Gustafsson A, Holmer J, et al. Periodontitis increases the risk of a first myocardial infarction: a report from the PAROKRANK study. Circulation. 2016;133(6):576–83. https://doi.org/10.1161/CIRCULATIONAHA.115.020324.
35. Khader YS, Ta'ani Q. Periodontal diseases and the risk of preterm birth and low birth weight: a meta-analysis. J Periodontol. 2005;76(2):161–5. https://doi.org/10.1902/jop.2005.76.2.161.
36. Manrique-Corredor EJ, Orozco-Beltran D, Lopez-Pineda A, Quesada JA, Gil-Guillen VF, Carratala-Munuera C. Maternal periodontitis and preterm birth: systematic review and meta-analysis. Community Dent Oral Epidemiol. 2019;47(3):243–51.
37. Kawano-Hokama M, Shiratori-Tusita LN, Pinilla-Bonilla LB, Cruz-Rodríguez Y. The potential role of trigeminal nerve irritation in the pathophysiology of Bell's palsy: a case report from a Neural Therapy perspective. Case Rep [Internet]. 2022;8(2). [cited 4 February 2025]. Available from: https://revistas.unal.edu.co/index.php/care/article/view/93840
38. Krishnamoorthy G, Narayana AI, Balkrishanan D. Mastication as a tool to prevent cognitive dysfunctions. Jpn Dent Sci Rev. 2018;54(4):169–73. https://doi.org/10.1016/j.jdsr.2018.06.001.
39. Nakamura T, Zou K, Shibuya Y, Michikawa M. Oral dysfunctions and cognitive impairment/dementia. J Neurosci Res. 2021;99(2):518–28. https://doi.org/10.1002/jnr.24745.
40. Hasegawa Y, Sakagami J, Ono T, Hori K, Zhang M, Maeda Y. Circulatory response and autonomic nervous activity during gum chewing. Eur J Oral Sci. 2009;117(4):470–3. https://doi.org/10.1111/j.1600-0722.2009.00637.x.

41. Onozuka M, Fujita M, Watanabe K, Hirano Y, Niwa M, Nishiyama K. Mapping brain region activity during chewing: a functional magnetic resonance imaging study. J Dent Res. 2002;81:743–6.
42. Onozuka M, Fujita M, Watanabe K, Hirano Y, Niwa M, Nishiyama K. Age-related changes in brain regional activity during chewing: a functional magnetic resonance imaging study. J Dent Res. 2003;82:657–60.
43. Chen H, Iinuma M, Onozuka M, Kubo KY. Chewing maintains hippocampus-dependent cognitive function. Int J Med Sci. 2015;12(6):502–9. https://doi.org/10.7150/ijms.11911.
44. Azuma K, Zhou Q, Niwa M, Kubo KY. Association between mastication, the hippocampus, and the HPA axis: a comprehensive review. Int J Mol Sci. 2017;18(8):1687. https://doi.org/10.3390/ijms18081687.
45. Kubo KY, Iinuma M, Chen H. Mastication as a stress-coping behavior. Biomed Res Int. 2015;2015:876409. https://doi.org/10.1155/2015/876409. Epub 2015 May 18. PMID: 26090453; PMCID: PMC4450283
46. Okamoto N, Morikawa M, Okamoto K, Habu N, Iwamoto J, Tomioka K, Saeki K, Yanagi M, Amano N, Kurumatani N. Relationship of tooth loss to mild memory impairment and cognitive impairment: findings from the Fujiwara-kyo study. Behav Brain Funct. 2010;6:77. https://doi.org/10.1186/1744-9081-6-77. PMID: 21194415; PMCID: PMC3024962
47. Chidiac JJ, Kassab A, Rifai K, Saadé NE, Al Chaer ED. Modulation of incisor eruption in rats by sympathetic efferents. Arch Oral Biol. 2018;89:31–6.
48. Wise G. Cellular and molecular basis of tooth eruption. Orthod & Craniofac Res. [Internet] 2009;12(2):67–73. [cited 31 January 2025]; Available from: https://onlinelibrary.wiley.com/doi/abs/10.1111/j.1601-6343.2009.01439.x
49. Richman JM. Shedding new light on the mysteries of tooth eruption. Proc Natl Acad Sci USA [Internet]. 2019 [cited 31 January 2025];116(2):353–5. Available from: https://pnas.org/doi/full/10.1073/pnas.1819412116.
50. Dosch P, Dosch M. Manual of neural therapy according to Huneke. 2nd ed. Stuttgart: Georg Thieme Verlag; 2007.
51. Ottawa Personal Decision Guides—Patient Decision Aids—Ottawa Hospital Research Institute [Internet]. Ottawa: Ottawa Hospital Research Institute; [cited 20 January 2025]. Available at: https://decisionaid.ohri.ca/decguide.html
52. Fischer L. Bases of neural therapy. Self-organization in biology [Internet]. 2006 [cited 20 January 2025]. Available at: https://terapianeural.com/articulos/16-de-las-teorias/74-bases-de-la-terapia-neural-autoorganizacion-en-la-biologia
53. Nuñez-Lucio EI. Electrogalvanism in neurofocal dentistry [Internet]. [cited 20 January 2025]. Available at: https://odontologosecuador.com/espanol/artodontologos/odontologia_neurofocal.htm
54. Rost A. Dental foci. Sanitation and therapy [Internet]. [cited 20 January 2025]. Available at: https://terapianeural.com/publicaciones/29-articulos-y-publicaciones/odontologia-neurofocal/134-focos-odontologicos-saneamiento-y-terapia.
55. Kim SM. Oral galvanism related to dental implants. Maxillofac Plastic Reconstr Surg [Internet]. 2023 [cited Dec 27, 2024];45(1):36. https://doi.org/10.1186/s40902-023-00403-8.
56. International Academy of Oral Medicine & Toxicology. The safe technique for mercury amalgam removal (SMART). [Internet]. [cited 20 January 2025]. Available at: https://es.iaomt.org/recursos/extracci%C3%B3n-segura-de-empastes-de-amalgama/
57. Tardieu C, Dumitrescu M, Giraudeau A, Blanc JL, Cheynet F, Borel L. Dental occlusion and postural control in adults. Neurosci Lett. 2009;450(2):221–4. https://doi.org/10.1016/j.neulet.2008.12.005. Epub 2008 Dec 6. PMID: 19070652
58. Casañasa R, González-Esmorís I, Cabrera J, Pérez-Candela V, Saavedrae V, Larena-Avellaneda J. Temporomandibular joint involvement as a cause of acute and chronic headaches and other otoneurological symptoms. Medicina de Familia. 2021;47(3):151–60. https://doi.org/10.1016/j.semerg.2020.12.004.

59. Gómez García JP, Garcés Machado N. Relationship between neurofocal dentistry and cervical and shoulder pain. Acta Méd Centro. 2017;11(3):31–8. Available at: https://revactamedicacentro.sld.cu/index.php/amc/article/view/848
60. Vinyes D, Traverso PH, Murillo JH, Sánchez-Padilla M, Muñoz-Sellart M. Improvement in post-orthodontic chronic musculoskeletal pain after local anesthetic injections in the trigeminal area: a case series. J Int Med Res. 2023;51(11) https://doi.org/10.1177/03000605231214064.

Chapter 44
Effects of Some Metallic Dental Materials on Human Health: The View from Neurofocal Dentistry

Sandra Lucia Patiño Niño

1 The Impact of Metallic Dental Materials on Health

The development of conservative dentistry is aimed at preserving the coronal tissues and restoring them with materials suitable for their functional and aesthetic requirements. Metallic dental materials are widely used in dentistry. The most commonly used metals are titanium, zirconium, palladium, silver, cobalt-chromium, nickel, and copper. Nonetheless, the presence of these metals can impact human physiology because of their electrochemical characteristics in a liquid environment like saliva. The objective of this chapter is to review physical and chemical the interactions of main metallic dental materials and its effects on human health.

1.1 Galvanism

From the physical point of view, galvanism is defined as the electricity produced by a chemical reaction [1] or the electricity developed by the contact of two metals with the interposition of a liquid [2] while from the biological point of view it is the production of physiological phenomena by means of electric currents [1].

In galvanism, an electric current is produced by the difference of potentials between an anodic and a cathodic surface, i.e., one of the metals is negatively charged (anode) and generates oxidation and the other positively charged (cathode) which generates a reduction [3–5]. These processes are simultaneous and occur in aqueous media. After these oxidation and reduction reactions, equilibrium tends to be generated at the aqueous solution-metal interface [6].

S. L. Patiño Niño (✉)
Faculty of Dentistry, Universidad Nacional de Colombia, Bogotá, Colombia
e-mail: slpatinon@unal.edu.co

L. B. Pinilla Bonilla et al. (eds.), *Neuraltherapeutic Medicine*,
https://doi.org/10.1007/978-3-032-03257-7_44

The classification of metals in dentistry is electropositive (tends to give up or lose electrons) and electronegative (tends to gain or attract electrons). Gold, platinum, mercury, silver, and copper are electropositive, while tin, zinc, chromium, cobalt, nickel, magnesium, and aluminum are electronegative, the former exhibits greater cathodic properties, making it less susceptible to corrosion, while the latter is more anodic and prone to corroding corrosion [5–7].

1.2 How Does Galvanism Occur in the Oral Cavity?

The presence of various metallic materials in the mouth in an aqueous medium, such as saliva, can generate the phenomenon of galvanism. This effect is produced by the difference in electrical potential between the metals used in dental treatments [8] In the mouth, the metal alloys used in dental treatments come into contact in various ways and are bathed in saliva, which consists of a high percentage of water (99%) and has a pH ranging from 6.2 to 7.6, making it neutral or slightly acidic due to food components and the salivary buffer effect.

The different ways in which the Voltaic pile can be generated in the mouth were described by Bohorquez CE [1], where he found different ways of making contact between the different elements in the mouth to generate it (see Fig. 44.1).

Oral environment I (a): Two different metallic fillings in contiguous contact.

Oral environment II (b): Two antagonistic fillings in different metals or that are in direct contact at the moment of occlusion or that contact each other through the tongue or cheeks.

Oral environment III (c): Two restorations with dissimilar metals in jaws without direct contact (without being a direct antagonist). The circuit is closed by bone and muscle.

Another option occurs when different metals or alloys come into contact in the same tooth or when the same alloy can constitute a stack.

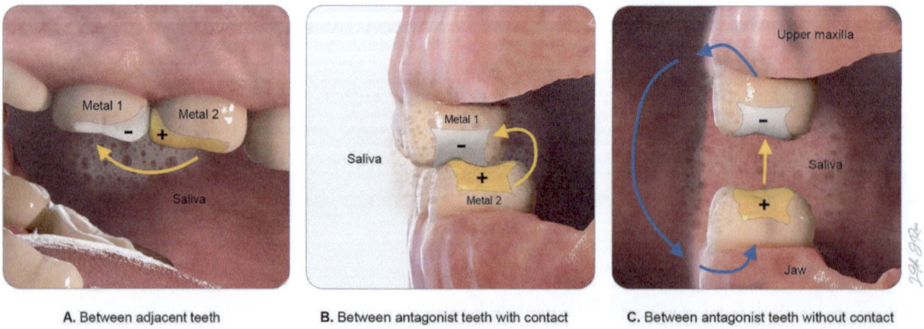

Fig. 44.1 Oral environment. (**a**) Between adjacent teeth. (**b**) Between antagonist teeth with contact. (**c**) Between antagonist teeth without contact

1.3 Oral Galvanism and Galvanic Corrosion

Oral galvanism (OG) or electro galvanism is a variable current flow in the oral cavity produced by different metals and anatomical structures that behave as conductors or insulators [3, 9]. This current is generated according to the polarity of the components and the differences in potential (from high to low potential) [3].

The material that has been most studied and that generates galvanic currents is dental amalgam, and more recently, it has been identified that the components of implant-supported rehabilitation can generate such currents due to the diversity of metals and alloys in each of them.

Kim et al. [3] identify both dental and non-dental factors contributing to galvanism. The primary oral causes include the biological incompatibility of materials, the stress roughness, and manufacturing issues homogenization. When there are problems with the biological compatibility of materials, bacterial adhesion may be altered, toxic effects may be increased, and allergic reactions may occur. Non-dental causes include the composition of saliva and its buffering capacity and temperature associated with food intake [3, 10].

Corrosion is a process of degradation of metallic materials; it is also defined as the "*destruction of a material by the electrochemical reaction of a metal with the surrounding medium and results in the release of ions into the environment*" [1]. Galvanic corrosion occurs as a result of the formation of the galvanic pile [2]. The less noble metal is destroyed when it comes into contact with the more noble metal in a medium that generates the electrochemical reaction with the subsequent passage of electric current [2, 8].

There are ways in which electrochemical corrosion can occur in the oral cavity [3, 9]. The most frequent kinds of corrosion are galvanic and pitting; and to a lesser extent, the corrosion caused by microorganisms. It can be inferred that the different types of corrosion, generated in the oral cavity, can interact and enhance each other [3].

Passivation of a metal is the "formation of a protective surface layer against corrosion from initial reaction products that inhibit further reactions" [4] it is a characteristic of some metals to slow down the rate of dissolution [2, 5]. There are two mechanisms to generate passivation: A thin, compact, adherent, low porosity oxide layer is generated, which isolates the metal from the medium; the second mechanism is by monoatomic layers of oxygen, which are absorbed on the metal surface [5]. When the oxide layer is lost again due to electrochemical environmental conditions, and the metal is left bare, a new passivation process is generated, called re-passivation [5].

1.4 Diagnosis of Galvanism in the Oral Cavity

The first diagnostic tool for the diagnosis of oral galvanism is a thorough anamnesis by a dentist, a family physician, an otolaryngologist, or an internist [3, 11]. The diagnosis of oral galvanism is a thorough anamnesis related to pain in the mucosa and tongue, atypical intraoral and/or extraoral nerve pain, exaggerated sensitivity to mild stimuli or discomfort from previous dental treatments [3]. Other symptoms that can be a reason for consultation are a burning sensation around the teeth, metallic taste, and pulp irritability [11].

A second diagnostic element is the intraoral clinical examination where the number and characteristics of the surfaces of the metal restorations, their location and contact forms can be identified according to the classification generated by Bohorquez [1]. The most important information to collect is the identification of the state of the soft tissues around the metal restorations where inflammation, lichenoid changes, and changes in the color of the mucous membranes can be found. The semiological process can be complemented with radiographs, and hematological and toxicological examinations in urine and feces [3]. Yin et al. report subjects under 6 years old with more than five Amalgam restorations had the highest blood inorganic mercury and urine mercury among all age groups [12].

Specialized hair tests for diagnosis of heavy metals and trace elements have been developed. It is understood that hair mineral analysis is used for a number of reasons, including the screening of metals such as uranium (U), lead (Pb), mercury (Hg), cadmium (Cd), arsenic (As), aluminum (Al), and nickel (Ni) [3], for toxicological purposes. Cabaña-Muñoz ME et al. [13] discovered that patients with long-term exposure to dental amalgam and titanium implants experience systemic oxidative stress, indicated by elevated levels of malondialdehyde (MDA). Their findings imply that higher cobalt (Co) levels may intensify oxidative stress in amalgam and implants studies [14].

Cells from the oral mucosa or adjacent implant tissues, such as epithelial cells and macrophages, could act as bioindicators for systemic conditions in both the short- and long-term contamination. Exfoliative cytology offers a straightforward, non-invasive, and cost-effective diagnostic approach for observing corrosion and patient clinical conditions follow-up [14, 15].

Changes in saliva can be recorded in patients with suspected galvanism [3]. Decreased levels of IgA1, IgA2, secretory IgA, and lysozyme and increased levels of IgA against heat-shock protein 60 (anti-hsp60 IgA) have been found [3, 16]. Other saliva elements such as Ca and Mg concentrations were lower and proteins, Na, Cl, and P were significantly higher [3]. Procházková [17]. reports that measuring the amount of metal content in the saliva of patients before and after restorative treatment is important because these particles in the saliva may be the etiology of local or systemic conditions of sensitive patients.

Methods and devices have been designed to measure galvanic currents between different alloys and oral tissues in order to detect galvanic currents that have a pathological effect; nevertheless, correlative significance is still unknown [3, 18, 19].

Kim et al. [3] present in their article a list of patents for methods and devices developed since 1999.

When the patient's main symptom is pain, it is necessary to confirm by separating the surfaces that are generating the galvanic currents with a non-conductive material, also the change of metallic material for a non-metallic one, to generate relief of the symptoms or discomfort in sensitive patients [3].

It is possible that other related psychological symptoms may be present, which could include reduced energy levels that may make it difficult to cope with day-to-day work or household duties, reduced quality of life, fatigue, anxiety, depression, an impaired ability to relax; sleep disturbances; and minor irritations [3, 20], which are diagnosed by psychiatrists or psychologists using a comprehensive battery of psychological tests [3].

1.5 Metallic Dental Materials That Report Galvanic Corrosion

Research indicates that certain metals and their alloys cause corrosion in the mouth environment. Greet G et al. indicated, "*Oral restorations made of gold have been widely used over time because this metal acts as a noble material and has high thermodynamic stability and high corrosion resistance*" [2]. Other restorative materials, such as palladium and silver alloys, showed low corrosion potential. The high costs of these materials have led specialists to manufacture alloys that have a higher tendency to corrode, some of them being nickel, copper, iron, and cobalt [2, 21].

To identify the metals and alloys used in dentistry, Table 44.1 shows the main metals used for coronal rehabilitation was constructed, except for titanium which is used for implants, as it will be dealt with in the following section.

Identifying the electrical potential of a metal restoration (EPR) is important for understanding the phenomenon of corrosion in the oral cavity and is significant in the origin of galvanism. This data can provide information on the galvanic corrosion tendency that could be generated at the time of rehabilitation treatment [2, 33]. A study by Castaño-Rivera P et al. [29] evaluated in the laboratory the galvanic interaction between amalgams and different metals such as titanium, gold-palladium alloys and nickel-chromium-molybdenum, and concluded that although there is similar galvanic interaction between the amalgam and the metals evaluated, the greatest galvanic interaction was generated between amalgams and titanium, so they recommend avoiding the use of this combination in vivo [29].

Carey et al. [8] show that under acidic conditions, the amalgam appears to suppress the release of titanium due to the redistribution of TiOx/SnOx on the titanium surface. This redistribution of SnOx appears to be a consequence of the amalgam releasing its components (Hg, Cu, Sn, Ag), with Sn demonstrating a thermodynamic preference for oxidation [8].

Table 44.1 Dental metals that have reported corrosion

Metal	Corrosion
Nickel	High corrosion has been reported and is considered to be a major clinical risk. The loss of the oxide layer compromise the alloy, which can lead to a variety of adverse reactions [22]
Copper	It was found that copper alloys are very sensitive to corrosion, and high corrosion currents can alter surfaces [21]
Silver	Although silver has a low corrosion potential, it has been shown that in comparison to metals such as gold it can be very corrosive [23]
Palladium	They generally have a low corrosion potential, however, being in an alloy with silver and copper can increase the level of corrosion [23]. When alloyed with gallium it can generate smaller surface pores and this decreases the possibility of corrosion [24]
Noble alloys with high gold content	They are considered highly corrosion resistant, although they are known to release copper, zinc, silver and gold to a small extent. Wright 1982, Pourbaix 1984, Moberg 1985 referenced by Bizar [4] and Mellado [24]
Silver—palladium noble alloys	They have been found to release silver and have been shown to be more resistant to corrosion the less silver they contain. Mezner1989, Lucas 1992 Referenced by Bizar [4]
Noble palladium—copper alloys	Those containing 15% copper by weight are found to release copper first. Goehlbich 1990 Referenced by Bizar [4]
Palladium—cobalt noble alloys	Those containing 19% cobalt by weight, the cobalt is released first, resulting in a more corrosion resistant surface. Goehlbich 1990 as referenced by Bizar [4]
Non-noble cobalt chromium and chromium nickel alloys	The corrosion resistance of these two alloys depends on the formation of the passivation and repassivation layer. It has been identified that chromium content between 16% and 27% gives the alloy significant resistance. If beryllium is added to these alloys, a phase of the alloy is generated which is particularly susceptible to corrosion [25]. On the other hand, if molybdenum is added at a percentage of 9%, corrosion resistance improves [24]. Chromium cobalt alloys have been found that there is a good passivation capacity, while the chromium nickel alloys have difficulty in repassivation if this protective layer is broken and therefore have a greater tendency to galvanic corrosion. Lucas L.C. Referenced by Bizar [4] has found that the passive layer of chrome-cobalt alloys can be altered by erosion and friction, exposing areas that react with oral fluids [26, 27]
Copper alloys	It is known to have a high corrosion capacity with a consequent release of ions into the oral environment [44]
Nickel, chromium, molybdenum, and titanium	This alloy is used as implant superstructure materials, a high corrosion rate has been found in vitro [24]

(continued)

Table 44.1 (continued)

Metal	Corrosion
Zirconium	A recent study found a moderate level of corrosion that increases with time when zirconium was introduced in sodium carbonate (Na2CO3), sodium chloride (NaCl), and citric acid (C6H8O7). It was identified that it corrodes more intensely when in contact with citric acid [28]
Amalgam	High corrosive capacity and generation of electrochemical currents when in contact with alloys such as titanium, silver-palladium, and nickel-cormo-molybdenum which generates the deterioration of the materials and nearby tissues [29]

Table modified and adapted from Greet [2]

1.6 Oral Effects of Ions and Metal Particles Release

Bizar J. in his doctoral thesis reports authors such as Bergman M. in 1986, Burrows D. in 1986 and MunKgaard E.C. in 1992 agree that there has been a growing concern about the possible local and systemic effects of the degradation of metals or alloys used in dentistry, showing that the effects can be mainly toxic or allergic [4]. Similarly in this thesis, Craig R.G. reported in 1990 that he carried out in vitro studies with fibroblasts in media impregnated with microparticles containing different metals, showing cytotoxic effects of the metals in order from lowest to highest: gold, palladium, titanium, silver, nickel, and copper [4].

Metal alloys used in oral restorations generally have good corrosion resistance. However, they are responsible for a high release of metal ions during years of use that may remain in living tissues. According to Chaturvedi [34], these ions alter some healing mechanisms when wounds are present, and Ti ions are also capable of preventing the growth of hydroxyapatite crystals in the surrounding bone [34].

Nickel-chromium alloys have a well-documented history of causing cellular damage and genetic mutations [35]. With Cr + 6 and Ni, many morphological, biochemical, and histological alterations have been observed in human gingival fibroblasts affecting its organelles in special rough endoplasmic reticulum and mitochondria [35].

The release of mercury particles resulting from oral galvanism in amalgam fillings "may generate a mercury- and antibiotic-resistant microflora" [36] Other findings lead to the inference that mercury particles may produce methylmercury in the mouth [2, 37].

In orthodontics, when is used metallic materials, galvanic corrosion could be produced with the consequent release of ions, leading to oral and systemic manifestations because they create a corrosive environment depending on treatment times. This situation is frequent in cases where arch wires and brackets are composed of different alloys or when different types of arch wires are used; among the most frequent combinations are: stainless steel with chrome-cobalt or nickel-titanium [2, 30, 31].

Nitinol is an alloy composed of Nickel-Titanium (NiTi) used in orthodontics, which has a nickel percentage of 50%, generating the possibility of release of this metal from corrosion phenomena in the oral environment. In healthy patients or those with a history of nickel allergy, it can cause oral allergic manifestations [2, 31, 32].

1.7 Oral Effects of Electro-Galvanism

The literature indicates that galvanic interactions among dental metal alloys may lead to both oral and systemic clinical issues manifestations. These symptoms are painful and uncomfortable for individuals [2, 38]. Symptoms such as metallic taste, sensation of burning in the mouth (burning mouth), punctiform pain of the tongue, dry mouth [11], galvanic pain [3, 9], xerostomia, hypogeusia or dysgeusia, burning pain [9] and signs such as glossitis, scaly lips, erythema, ulcerations on the mucous membrane of the mouth [1, 9], recurrent oral mucosal ulcerations, leukoplakia, gingival hypertrophy, dark pigmentation of tissues, pulp irritability and in other cases increased salivary secretion (sialorrhea) [9] diagnosed pathologies such as red lichen planus, squamous cell carcinoma, and trigeminal neuralgia [1–3, 11].

Oral burning syndrome has been defined as a chronic, idiopathic pain, characterized by a burning sensation in the oral cavity, which is not accompanied by mucosal lesions or other clinical signs [39]. This syndrome is currently classified within pathologies associated with psychogenic pain, with a higher prevalence in women of menopausal age and/or who present some psychiatric comorbidities [3, 39, 40].

Other relevant manifestations include erythema, whitening, and, in severe cases, ulceration of the mucous membranes adjacent to the teeth where the galvanic currents are produced. The latter may disappear and reappear, with a high possibility of turning into chronic ulcerations [1, 11].

Leukoplakia in the oral cavity has been clinically characterized as a white patch or plaque often located in contact areas and are associated with an increased risk of developing cancer, either in the area of the leukoplakia or elsewhere in the mouth, head, or neck [2, 41]. Studies have suggested that differences in electrical potential play an etiological role in the development of leukoplakia and oral lichen. The malignant transformation of leukoplakia varies depending on the type and size, with the sites at highest risk being the ventral tongue, the floor of the mouth, and the soft palate [2, 41–43]. A study by Bánóczy et al. [44] analyzed the relationship between metals and leukoplakia and concluded that eliminating the galvanic currents generated by metals in the mouth leads to the disappearance of not only leukoplakia but also lesions histologically and clinically related to oral lichen planus [2, 44].

Other frequent adverse effects are the migration of metal ions to adjacent tissues, which can cause toxic or allergic reactions such as dermatitis and stomatitis [9] Lehman et al. [45], cited by Rasul et al. [46], indicated that in repetitive contact with chromium and nickel, some individuals develop dermatitis as a hypersensitivity type IV [45]. They described a case involving an old woman with oral lichenoid lesions displaying Wickham's striae, a history of gold-containing dental implants, and allergic skin reactions to various medications. Following allergy testing, healthcare providers and dentists concluded that she had a gold hypersensitivity allergy [46, 47].

Sutow [48], reported by Greet [2], studied some patients affected by corrosion and found through anamnesis data that 39 patients suffered from some signs and symptoms, such as burning, salty or metallic taste, and dry mouth, among others. On physical examination of the oral cavity, various manifestations were observed, the most frequent being a fissured tongue and amalgam tattooing [2, 48].

Lucas and Von Fraunhofer cited by Mellado [24], consider that at the clinical level the phenomenon of galvanic corrosion translates into an electropositive environment as a consequence of the degradation of metals, which accumulate at the gingival level influencing the soft tissues and bone resorption.

1.8 Reported Systemic Effects of Oral Galvanism

A study conducted in Sweden by Herrstrom and Hogstedt in 1993 [20] took 218 patients diagnosed with galvanism and underwent clinical, dental, and medical examinations and surveys. The examinations included blood samples and examinations with medical specialists in orthopedics, gastroenterology, neurology, and psychiatry, among others, in order to relate the findings observed and found in the patients to the systemic diagnoses [2]. As a result, it was found that some patients presented mental disorders (anxiety, depression, sleep disorders), somatic diseases, and allergies (rhinitis and sinusitis) to some dental metallic materials [1, 20].

Other studies confirm that patients with galvanism present headache, insomnia, vertigo, nausea, pain in the arms, legs, back, neck, joint pain, and itching sensation [3, 9]. Additionally, there are distant symptoms in different parts of the body, such as eyes, muscle and joint pain, fatigue, and numbness of limbs [2, 49, 50]. Studies in Sweden report that galvanism is a predisposing factor for diseases such as multiple sclerosis, asthma, and fibromyalgia [2, 51]. Asthma was reported in adults who had high exposure to amalgam [52].

Case reports suggest that galvanic interaction between titanium dioxide and amalgam or gold metal restorations also leads to yellow nail syndrome, which is described as the triad of yellow nails, lymphoedema, and respiratory tract involvement [2, 53].

The release of metal ions from restorations causes problems of biocompatibility of the materials, especially when the material is in the oral cavity for prolonged periods of time. In the case of nickel, depending on the time of use, a greater or lesser quantity of nickel ions will be released, which can cause hypersensitivity effects, contact dermatitis, and even cytotoxicity when the maximum quantities that the body can admit are exceeded [2, 54].

Comparing the signs and symptoms of Alzheimer's disease to those of mercury poisoning, Silbreud et al. [55] studied whether Alzheimer's disease is related to mercury exposure. They informed inhibition in neurotransmitters like acetylcholine, dopamine, serotonin, glutamate, and norepinephrine in patients with

Alzheimer's disease and mercury toxicity [55]. Mercury exposure is linked to increased platelet activation, impaired odor identification, hypertension, depression, and a higher prevalence of chlamydia infections and herpes virus, as well as Alzheimer's disease [55]. "*This review of the literature strongly suggests that mercury may be a cause of Alzheimer's disease*" [55].

The most studied material is amalgam due to its high mercury content, which is a significant source of body contamination, despite being discontinued for use by the Minamata Convention [56], is essential to understanding its long-term effects on health. Understanding the signs and symptoms of galvanism is essential for a doctor or dentist to relate them to clinical, laboratory, toxicological, and electrical findings, thereby generating suitable treatments.

2 Impact of Dental Implants on Systemic Health

Dental implants are the most common way of replacing missing teeth [57]. An implant is a prosthetic solution for replacing a tooth or molar. Strategically placed implants are used to support prostheses involving segments or the entire maxillary or mandibular arch. In general, an implant is composed of three parts: implant (intraosseous), abutment (connection), and crown (see Fig. 44.2).

Metal implant surface modification and coating depositions improve the implant's performance biocompatibility and osseointegration [58]. Among the strategies for surface modification are microscale modifications [24] or methods aimed at

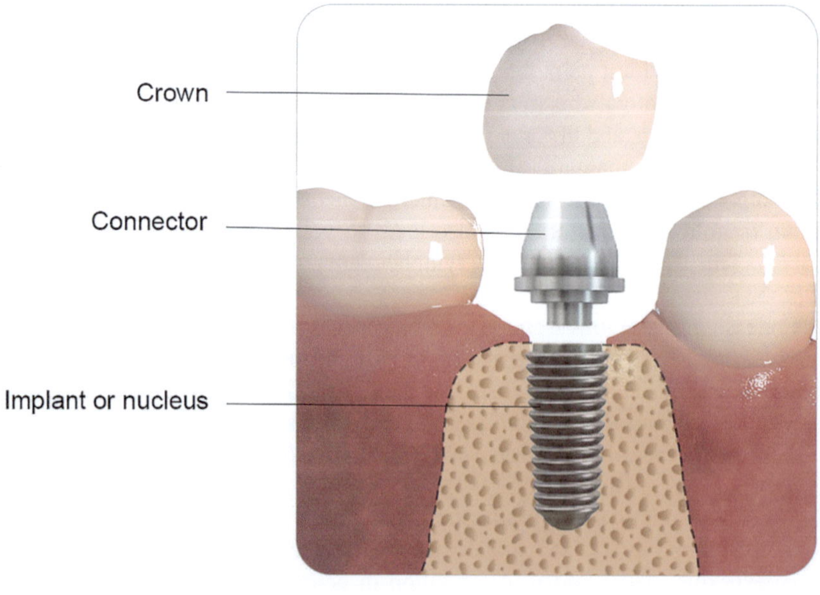

Fig. 44.2 Components of dental implant

changing the surface roughness of implants to improve their integration [57]. On the other hand, there are nanoscale modifications, mainly isotropic nanospheres and nanotubes [24, 59]. This nanoscale modification form protective and/or bioactive coatings on implants to improve their corrosion resistance, biocompatibility, biomechanical stability, and antibacterial properties and to promote bone tissue regeneration [57].

Gulati et al. [60] identified the main metallic ions/nanoparticles on/inside nanotubules: Calcium, Copper, Gallium, Gold, Lanthanum, Silver, Strontium, Tantalum, Zinc, Silicon, Calcium Phosphate-based materials (CAPS) [61], Hydroxyapatite, antibiotics, Peek, etc. [59, 62].

Figure 44.3 shows the conditions surrounding the implant. Notice how the implant features interact with micro- and nano-modifications, as well as different metal-doped implants such as Ca: calcium, Ga: gallium, Au: gold, Cu: copper, Ag: silver, Zn: zinc, La: lanthanum, Si: silicon, and P: phosphorus. Additionally, consider the metal degradation factors present in the oral cavity, including changes in salivary pH and bacterial accumulation.

A neurofocal dentist must be able to suggest this therapeutic option to a patient to rehabilitate function and esthetics in the oral cavity according to the characteristics of the implant and the needs of the patient. This section focuses on the biotribocorrosion of implants and its local and systemic effects,

2.1 *Biotribocorrosion*

Tribocorrosion is the process of deterioration of a metal due to corrosion in conjunction with metal wear [63]. Another definition refers to the combined study of the mechanical phenomena of impact wear or friction of the metal surface and electrochemical phenomena (corrosion) on the contact surfaces of metals. It is called biotribocorrosion when it includes a biological environment, as is the case with metallic elements used in the body [64].

As Gaur S et al. [14] defined, "*Bio-tribocorrosion is a phenomenon that combines the essentials of tribology (friction, wear, and lubrication) and corrosion with microbiological processes*" [14], which is more appropriate when examining implants in the maxilla and mandibular bones of the oral cavity, due to the environment being conducive to biofilm formation and growth [14, 63]. It is understood that for patients, biotribocorrosion phenomenon in the mouth, begins with the insertion of the dental implant [35]. In dentistry, corrosion and wear are two different forms of degradation with different consequences on materials; however, in a corrosive environment, a greater loss of material can be precipitated by being exposed to wear, while this same (wear) can increase the corrosion mechanism [63, 65].

Kunrath MF et al. suggested that mastication and deglutition involve the rupture and release of particles and ions from the implant surface caused by movements at the micro- and nanoscale [35, 66, 67]. Typically, saliva maintains a stable pH (between 6 and 7); however, factors such as hygiene, diet, and microbiota can lower

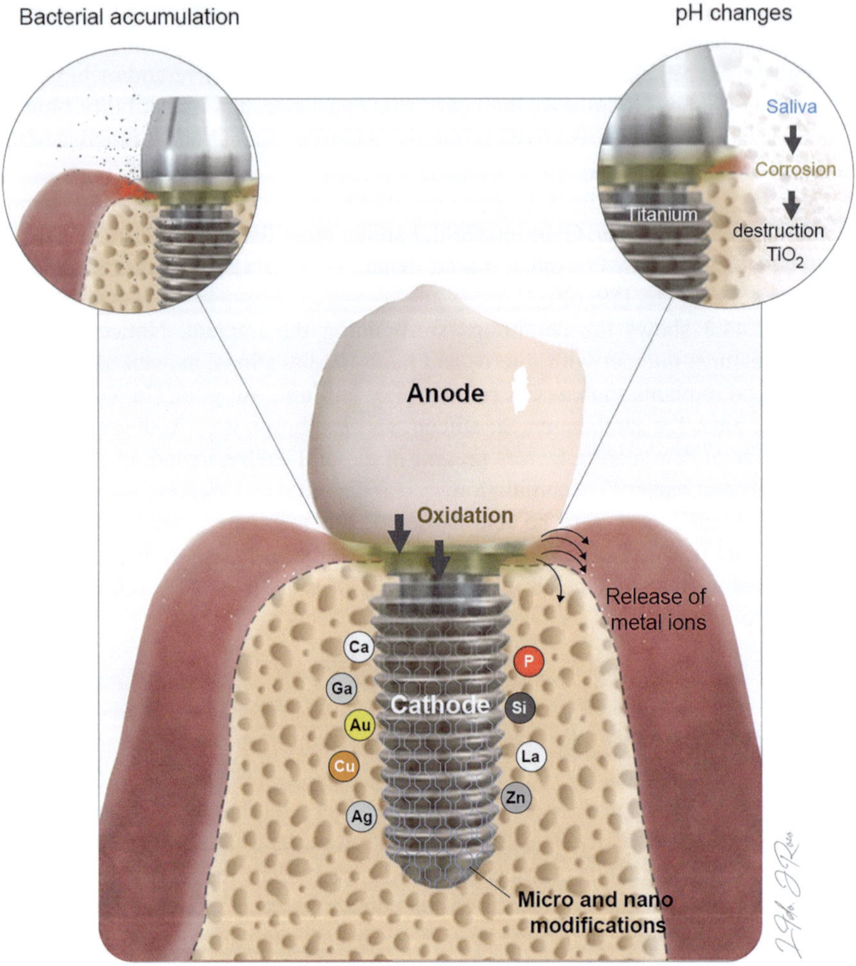

Fig. 44.3 Implant surrounding conditions

the pH, which stimulates degradation by decreasing resistance to corrosion [35, 68]. In the mouth, all considerations related to organisms associated with microbiological, metabolic, biochemical, and immunological processes generated in the microenvironment near dental implants affect their deterioration [14, 63, 68, 69].

2.2 *Toxic Implications of Metallic Ions and Nanoparticles Secondary to Biotribocorrosion*

Cytotoxicity is understood as the capacity of certain substances or cells to damage or destroy living cells [70]. In nervous tissue, neurotoxicants alter the structure or function depending on the toxic substance, dose, duration of exposure, and individual susceptibility. Consequently, permanent or reversible damage is caused, evidenced by general symptoms and neurological symptoms [71]. It is thought that genotoxic substances may potentially interact with the sequence and structure of DNA, which could result in damage to the genetic material of cells [72].

Metals existing as both free ions and nanoparticles (NPs), due to biotribocorrosion, interact with biological fluids. It is recognized that nanoparticles can bind to lipids, proteins, and nucleic acids, with their composition influenced by the tissue environment and the material's characteristics, including shape, structure, size, charge, and hydrophobicity [60]. According to Gulati K et al. [60], "*this binding process leads to the formation of a dynamic protein corona covering the NPs.*" Through mechanisms of phagocytosis or endocytosis, this corona facilitates the transport of metal ions into the cell, a process known as the Trojan Horse [60].

Goodman et al. [73] found that binding metals such as titanium, cobalt, chromium, aluminum, and vanadium to serum proteins can mediate immunological reactions. It has been identified that different metal-protein complexes are generated [71], and Ribeiro et al. [74] concluded that titanium nanoparticles interact with adjacent cells or can be transported by tissue fluids to distant bone cells. Such titanium oxide particles are covered by a bio-complex composed of calcium, phosphorus, hydroxyapatite, and proteins. This bio complex works as a Trojan horse that facilitates the internalization of these nanoparticles in bone cells, which can subsequently interact with organelles, leading to functional modifications and intracellular lesions [2, 74].

Once in the cytoplasm, metals can affect the mitochondrial membrane, disrupting energy production and generating reactive oxygen species (ROS). The exaggerated increase of ROS generates oxidative damage to proteins, lipids, and DNA. Additionally, they can alter cell signaling, lead to chronic inflammatory states, and finally, cell death [60].

2.3 *Human Toxicity of Titanium (and Alloy Titanium)*

According to Gaur et al. [14], Titanium (Ti) ions are highly insoluble and difficult to eliminate from the body. It has been observed that they are released gradually without causing a systemic disruption in the body, and their effects are often imperceptible [14]. Nevertheless, host bone osteoclasts and osteoblasts are affected by high concentrations of titanium particles, resulting in changes to homeostasis in superficial tissues, such as subepithelial connective tissue and oral epithelium tissue

[14, 75–77]. Kunrath et al. [35] noted that minimal degradation levels may have an effect on inflammatory signaling pathways, which could potentially impact the behavior of cells in the vicinity of the implants. This, in turn, could possibly lead to systemic toxicity.

During the degradation process at the implant-abutment connection, released metal ions and particles may trigger an inflammatory response in the peri-implant tissues. This could subsequently influence the sensitivity of the gingival epithelium cells [2, 78, 79]. On the other hand, it has been identified that metal debris is recognized as a foreign body by the immune system, which can stimulate the migration of polymorphonuclear leukocytes and macrophages that activate mediators associated with bone resorption and peri-implant disease [73].

2.3.1 Cytotoxic Effects of Titanium and Titanium Alloy in Oral Tissues

As Gaur S et al. described [14], "*The cytotoxic effects of Ti particles depend on their size and concentration in the surrounding tissues*" [14]. Ti ions released form implant enhanced the sensitivity of gingival epithelial cells to microorganisms and facilitated monocyte infiltration in tissues located in the interface between implant and gingival tissue resulting in higher inflammation and cytotoxicity [14, 80].

Bressan et al. [76], cited by Kunrath et al. [35], showed a reduction in cell viability for mesenchymal stem cells and fibroblasts when exposed to Ti nanoparticles. Furthermore, histological analysis indicated collagen fiber degradation and changes in blood vessels, which impede bone healing rates [35, 78]. In vitro experiments with periodontal ligament hTERT cells, exposed to high concentrations of titanium dioxide and zirconia nanoparticles could detect increased in intranuclear cell uptake ratio [81].

Biopsies of human oral mucosa from individuals who have contact with Ti revealed toxic involvement of osteoblasts, fibroblasts, lymphocytes, and monocytes, along with increased numbers of macrophages and T-lymphocytes [14, 82]. About 10 ppm of Ti ions inhibit osteoblastic growth and differentiation [14, 83].

In alloy Ti6Al4V, with clinical hindsight studies, report the dissolution of vanadium and aluminum after implant corrosion in vivo [84, 85]. Alumina and Vanadium in Ti6Al4V alloy caused cytotoxicity on human gingival fibroblast [14, 86]. Researchers concluded that vanadium affects organelles in cells (cytotoxic effect), and Aluminum shows neurotoxic effects and can generate peri-implant osteolysis and local inflammation [85, 87, 88].

As Kunrath et al. revealed, the toxicity of aluminum depends on high levels of Al3+, dosage, and solubility [35, 89]. At the cellular level, cytotoxicity arises from oxidative damage that impacts mitochondrial processes, cellular metabolic systems, and tissue survival [35, 90]. The systematic release of aluminum from corroded titanium implants may cause inhibition of peri-implant bone formation and mineralization by increasing osteoclastic activity while reducing osteoblastic activity [91, 92]. Following the same logic, research suggests that aluminum may play a role in triggering cell apoptosis and tissue necrosis [85, 93, 94].

Costa et al. [95] demonstrated the release of ions and Vanadium (V) particles from the Ti-6Al-V4 alloy. After exposure to high concentrations of V (like V2O5), they showed a reduction of cell viability and significant differences in cell morphology for MC3T3-E1 pre-osteoblasts and NIH3T3 fibroblasts [35, 95].

2.3.2 Proinflammatory Cytokines

Fretwurst et al. studied 12 patients and found elements such as titanium (Ti) and iron (Fe) in 9 of them in both hard and soft peri-implant tissues, which stimulate high levels of macrophages and lymphocytes [35, 96]. These Ti ions and their oxidized forms behave like foreign particles, triggering inflammation around the implant [14, 97, 98].

The main pro-inflammatory cytokines were produced by macrophages that include (e.g., interleukin [IL]-1β, IL-6, TNF-α, and RANKL), chemokines, growth factors, prostanoids, and degradative enzymes. [14, 97–99] "*which further promoted bone and soft tissue destruction, clinically visible as peri-implant mucositis or peri-implantitis*" [14, 100].

2.3.3 Bone Lose and Peri-Implantitis

Inflammatory processes act as accelerators of bone dissolution around the implants, and changes in the structure and diversity of the microbiome around the implant have been reported [14, 101]. *P. gingivalis* produces lipopolysaccharides (LPS) that promote inflammation around the implant [14].

The LPS increases Ti corrosion and tribocorrosion, further accelerating its adherence to the Ti surface at acidic pH [14, 102].On the other hand, the multinucleated giant cells and osteoclasts generated in the peri-implant region promote the osteolytic process [82].

When in contact with fibroblastic and mesenchymal stem cells, Ti particles, whether alone or under inflammatory conditions, evoked a time-dependent increase in ROS production that was associated with a decrease in osteogenic differentiation [35, 76]. Severino et al. [99] reported elevated levels of IL-17 in individuals affected by peri-implantitis, which contributes to bone loss. Daubert el al. concluded that the microbiota of peri-implantitis was possibly modified by high levels of titanium found in the submucosal plaque samples [35, 101].

2.3.4 Hypersensitivity and Allergy of Titanium

General signs of titanium allergy include pruritus, redness, skin eczema, and swelling. In studies of patients who have received dental implants and are found to be allergic, the primary symptom is eczema, often preferentially located on the face, and the reaction ceases after its removal [14]. Type IV hypersensitivity reactions to titanium at elevated levels may lead to gingival enlargement and mucosal hyperemia [103]. Moreover, continuous exposure to antigenic molecules is taken up by Langerhans cells, leading to a delayed hypersensitivity reaction [14, 34]. Titanium particles are linked to edema of the glottis and the spontaneous shedding of implants [14, 104].

2.3.5 Genotoxicity

Daubert et al. [105] studied a human case-control study on the impact of peri-implantitis caused by titanium dental implants and found a connection between peri-implantitis and epigenetic changes in the surrounding tissue. Moreover, they suggest that the concentration and dissolution levels of titanium could influence global tissue methylation levels produced [14, 105].

2.3.6 Neurotoxicity

Ti has a broad use in industry, daily life, and medicine [106]. Neurotoxicity nanoparticles (TiO_2-NPs) have been studied in various animal models, although evidence in humans is limited [106]. Symptoms of neurotoxicity observed in preclinical studies include alterations in cognitive and emotional behavior, as well as changes in brain biochemistry and oxidative stress [60, 106].

Shelly et al. [107] identified the potential toxicity of TiNP, particularly concerning the Central Nervous System. Their hypothesis suggested that prolonged exposure to TiNP might lead to disruptions in the blood-brain barrier, indicating that titanium prosthetic implants could serve as a potential source of this exposure. Additionally, they observed a linear relationship between the duration an implant remains in tissue and titanium levels, which points to a consistent release of titanium into the system body [107]. In the context of biomedical and dental implants, several factors affect the safety of titanium implants. These include the shape of the implant, its surface area, composition, the surgical insertion technique, and the inflammatory response that commonly occurs at the implantation site. Each of these factors can impact the quantity of particles released and the physiological state of the surrounding tissue organs [107].

While Ti is generally considered biocompatible, concerns have been raised about its potential effects on the central nervous system (CNS) when in nanoparticle form. The following is the list of content's main concerns:

- Cognitive and Behavioral Functions: Studies in animal models have demonstrated memory impairments following exposure to titanium nanoparticles, suggesting potential impacts on cognitive functions. Behavioral changes, such as alterations in locomotor activity and spatial recognition memory, have also been observed, indicating that TiO_2 nanoparticles may affect behavioral functions [107, 108].

- Oxidative Stress: Titanium dioxide nanoparticles have been shown to induce oxidative stress, which is a key mechanism of their neurotoxic effects. This is characterized by increased production of reactive oxygen species (ROS), leading to cellular damage and apoptosis in neuronal cells [109, 110].
- Neuroinflammation: Exposure to TiO2 nanoparticles has been associated with neuroinflammation, characterized by the activation of microglia and increased expression of pro-inflammatory cytokines such as IL-1β and IL-6. This inflammatory response can exacerbate neuronal damage and contribute to Central Nervous System (CNS) dysfunction [107, 111].
- Central Nervous System Effects: Impairments of nervous system have been associated with TiO2 NPs contacts [106, 107]. The ability of TiO2 nanoparticles to cross the blood-brain barrier (BBB) and accumulate in the brain has been documented, although the exact mechanisms remain under investigation [111]. This accumulation can lead to structural and functional impairments in the CNS, including synaptic dysfunction and neuronal apoptosis [106, 108].

Overall, the potential neurotoxic effects of titanium dioxide nanoparticles, particularly in high concentrations or prolonged exposure from a variety of sources (environment, food, medicaments, implants) and ways of contact (inhalation, digestion system, skin, mucous membrane, blood) [106]. Warrant further investigation to fully understand their impact on the CNS and related functions.

2.4 Zirconium Implants Reactions

Beger et al. [112] reported findings showing the presence of aluminum on the surface of zirconia-based (ZrO2) commercial implants, by means of energy-dispersive X-ray spectroscopy (EDX) [112] It is very significant in implanted patients to take into account the systemic effects of aluminum [85].Researchers and industry can optimize aluminum-doped zirconia to minimize aluminum release while maintaining the material's mechanical properties and biocompatibility implant [85].

Ti-Zr alloys demonstrate increased corrosion resistance in comparison with traditional titanium alloys, which can be associated with the formation of passivating ZrO2 film on the implant Surface [57].

2.5 Reactions to Implants in Cobalt-Chromium Alloys

In studies made in vitro, Kunrath MF et al. [35] cited the results of Hallab NJ et al. [113], who found that "*Degradation products from Cr and Ti alloys can display cytotoxic potential, leading to unwanted peri-implant and systemic effects*" [35]. Other studies point out that cobalt can lead to the highest release of harmful ions [114]. It may cause inflammatory reactions and hyperplasia [115–117].

In the case of CoCr alloy, its corrosion resistance was improved in the presence of fluorides, as already reported by Takemoto et al. [118]. They observed a corrosion resistance of CoCr alloy in a saline solution containing 0.1% sodium fluoride similar to the resistance shown by gold alloys [118, 119].

2.6 Nickel-Chromium Alloys Toxicity

Mellado Valero A et al. studied the electrochemical properties of five different dental alloys and discovered that these alloys show spontaneous passivation. However, the tendency for nickel-chromium-titanium alloys to passivate decreases when exposed to fluoride in the oral microenvironment [119].

Allergic reactions to dental implant alloys can vary depending on the specific metal involved. Among the alloys mentioned, nickel-chromium (Ni-Cr) alloys are particularly noteworthy due to the potential for nickel ion release, which can lead to hypersensitivity reactions, particularly in individuals with prior sensitization to nickel from non-dental sources [120].

2.7 Stainless Steel Implants Toxicity

This kind of implant can be used in short-term exposure in orthodontics mini implants. Szuhanek et al. [121] concluded that stainless steel implants developed a low cytotoxic effect that might have been non-detectable in clinical trials. However, the cytotoxic activity induced on Human Gingival Fibroblast cells was not very significant and blood contact impairment was also reduced, but vigilance is required in Ni-sensitive patients [121]. In addition, Saha S et al. commented that stainless steel alloys are susceptible to pitting corrosion because they contain a higher nickel content by weight. Therefore, caution should be exercised when using this material for implants as it may cause an allergic reaction [115, 122]. In some individuals, "*nickel and chromium from the alloy may cause hypersensitivity*" [115, 123].

In the oral cavity, various dental treatments employ different metallic materials. As shown in Fig. 44.4, which illustrates galvanism and biotribocorrosion, you can observe the options available for crowns, dental implants, and restorations.

2.8 Toxicity Generated by Implant Surface Modifications

The process of biotribocorrosion could be heightened depending on the treatment methods applied to the implant surface or the surrounding tissue environment applied [35]. Kunrath et al. [35] concluded that implant surface treatments have the possibility to create roughness in order to increase cell adhesion and enhance the

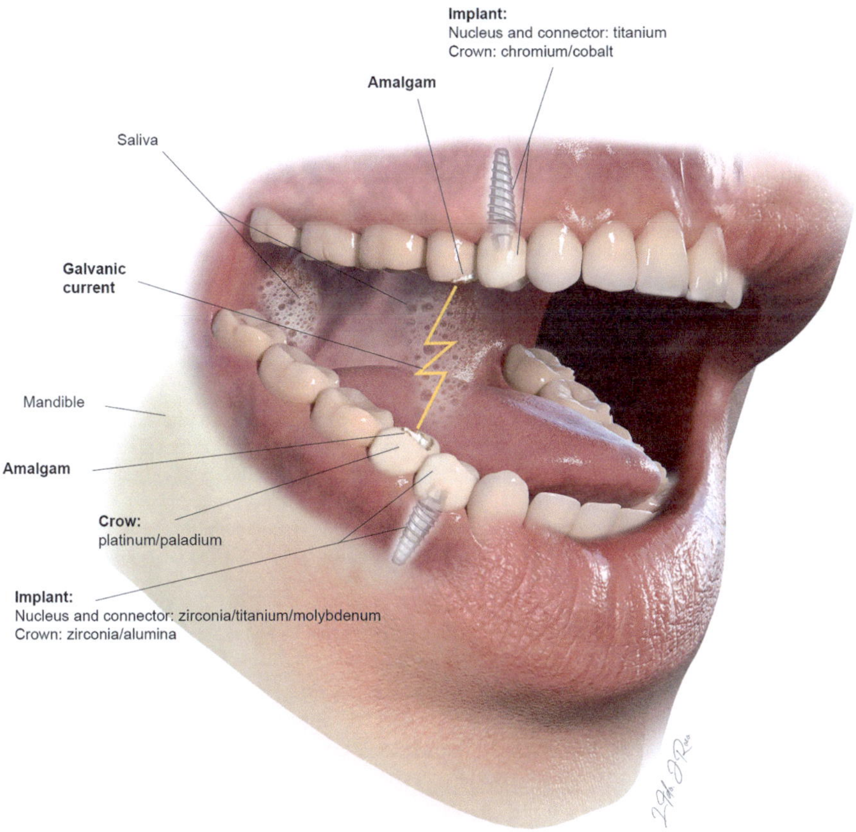

Fig. 44.4 Galvanism and biotribocorrosion representation

osseointegration process. However, these modifications in oral microenvironments where corrosion, friction, and wear occur and create breaks in the dental material that result in the release of particles and subsequent cytotoxicity and inflammation (see Table 44.2) [35].

2.9 Systemic Toxic Reactions of Different Metals

Metallosis is a rare condition characterized by the deposition and build-up of metal debris in the soft tissues of the body associated with metal-on-metal (MOM) prosthetic devices [134]. Souza et al. [98] informed that signs and symptoms like fever, swelling of the spleen and liver, suppression of biliary circulation, and acute renal failure can occur because enzymes such as proteases and metallothioneins may be involved in the metabolism of some metallic nanomaterials [98].

Table 44.2 Coating and its effects on human health

Coating	Effects
Ag nanoparticles	Cytotoxicity and toxic injury to the blood-brain-barrier, neurotoxicity [124]. AgNPs accentuate the release of IL-1β through inflammasome formation and caspase-1 activation [60, 125]
Ti particles	Ti particles induce ROS production in human stem cells. In vivo findings suggest that the release of Ti particles causes a possible gene deletion and consequently deregulation of the bone regeneration process [35, 76]
Al3O2 and SiO2 nanoparticles	Nanoparticles concentration high 200 g/mL caused cytotoxic and genotoxic to macrophages [35, 126]
Al3O2 and TiO2 nanoparticles	Nanoparticles caused viability decrease in UMR 106 cells after 96 h of culture. Suggested that events caused by cytotoxic effects can induce osseointegration failures [35, 127]
Carbon fibers-polyether ether ketone composite (CF-PEEK), carbon fibers reinforced-polyether ether ketone composite (CFR-PEEK)	In the in vitro cell evaluation, CFR-PEEK with interface strengthening by GO showed no cytotoxicity and exhibited significantly enhanced adhesion and proliferation of bone marrow mesenchymal stem cells (BMSCs) on the surface [128]. According to the results of cytotoxicity test and hemocompatibility assessment, it indicated that the two kinds of carbon fiber CF-PEEK composites showed mild toxicity and no hemolytic reaction. The histopathological section of systemic toxicity test showed that the CF-PEEK composites had no obvious acute toxicity to organisms [129]
Silica microparticles	Induced apoptosis of human periosteal cells and decrease in proliferation and viability [35, 130]
Silicon carbide nanoparticles	Silicon carbide nanowires are toxic to human MSCs (0.1 mg/mL). Possible toxic in the application situ [35, 131]
Silicon oxide	Marquardt et al. demonstrated dose-dependent cytotoxicity for silicone (SiO2) particles by evoking membrane disruption and death of the murine macrophages RAW 264.7. They also revealed that low concentrations of SiO2 nanoparticles are sufficient to activate autophagy [35, 132]
Mix of nanoparticles	AgNPs, au, and metal oxides, such as TiO2 or ZnO, act as DNA intercalators and generate ROS responsible for severe oxidative DNA damages [60, 133]

Information is taken from: Wang et al. [124], Gulati et al. [60], Kunrath [35], Qin [128], and Li [129]

Gaur et al. considered that Ti can diffuse to the lungs, liver, and kidneys [14]. Gulati et al. noted that TiO2 NPs have a high likelihood of nano-scale metallic species leaching into saliva and being absorbed by the digestive tract, primarily through intestinal enterocytes and Peyer's patches in the small intestine. The small size and positive charge of these particles enhance the rate of absorption and systemic distribution of nanomaterials [60]. NPs and degradation products can accumulate in the spleen, liver, kidney, heart, lungs, bone marrow, and central nervous system [60, 135].

In orthopedic literature, Shelly S. et al. stated that lymph nodes, the liver, and the spleen could experience fibrosis and structural changes as a result of cellular toxicity generated by TiNp [107, 136, 137].

Shah et al. [104] cited by Gaur et al. [14] reported that the International Agency for Research on Cancer (IARC) classifies TiO2 as a Group 2B carcinogen, indicating that it is a probable human carcinogen. They question the carcinogenic potential of dental implants, noting that titanium is associated with squamous cell carcinoma, plasmacytoma, and osteosarcoma mandible [14, 104].

Aluminum (Al) is a metal present in titanium and zirconium implants. Al will be linked to several significant dysfunctions such as neurodegeneration and endocrine disruptors, as well as major inflammatory disorders that can affect multiple organs. This includes ischemic strokes, which pose life-threatening risks to those affected [85, 138]. Furthermore, studies have identified a direct correlation between the onset of Alzheimer's disease and various encephalopathies characterized by high aluminum levels in brain tissue [139]. Late-onset epilepsy could be the result of aluminum present in the hippocampus and glial cells of certain persons [85, 140]. Increased levels of aluminum in the blood have been linked to Alzheimer's disease, Parkinson's disease, and diabetic encephalopathy [141, 142].

In Fig. 44.5, you can see a synthesis of the systemic effects of biotribocorrosion. Note that some effects are general, while others are localized or intraoral tissues. Over time, high concentrations of corrosion products can provoke reactions in various organs.

In conclusion, it is worth noting that titanium is the most studied material, followed by zirconium. A great deal of research has been conducted in vitro and in vivo (animal models), which has helped to identify the presence of biotribocorrosion and its local and systemic effects. There are a significant number of studies reporting toxicity involving titanium and zirconium alloys with aluminum, vanadium, and silver nanoparticle coatings.

The development of technologies to enhance materials, metal alloys, and techniques is driven by the aspiration to mitigate the impact of biotribocorrosion, thereby reducing the risk of peri-implantitis and subsequent implant loss. It is evident that, in clinical settings, a comprehensive understanding of the effects of various materials and metals that interact with the alveolar bone is becoming paramount for identifying patients who stand to benefit from implant-supported oral rehabilitation treatment.

It is important to understand that the biological and physicochemical phenomena that occur around a dental implant are complex processes with multiple variables and interactions involving a patient's physiology, pathophysiology, diet, and oral hygiene habits. Therefore, replicating in vitro research or animal models allows only a fractional understanding of what may occur when a variable such as material, metal alloy, or coating is changed. Extensive clinical research is essential to validate or challenge earlier findings research.

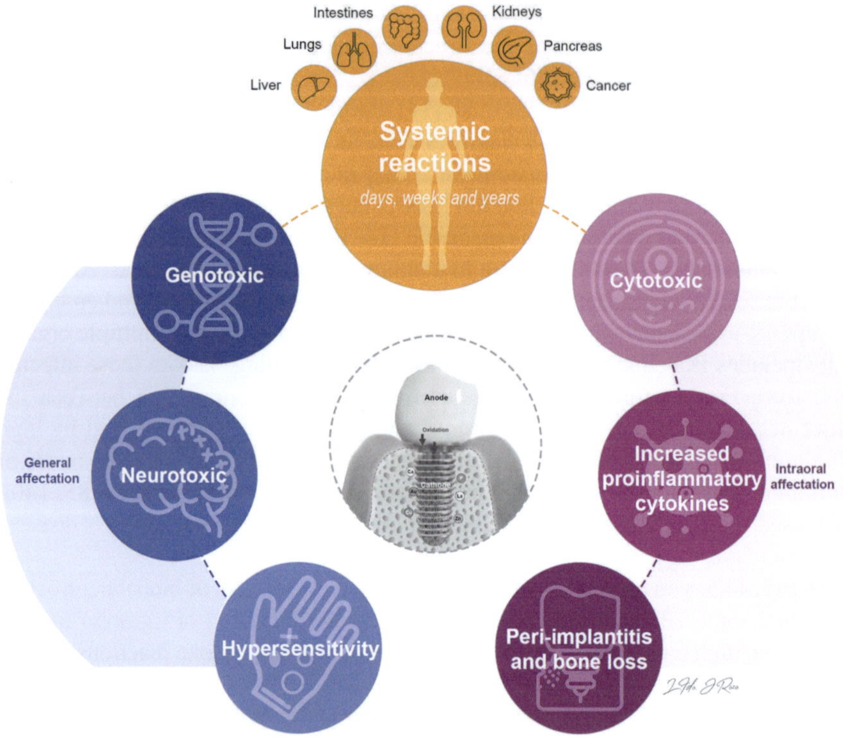

Fig. 44.5 Systemic effects of biotribocorrosion

3 Effects of Mobile Phone Electromagnetic Waves on Oral Soft Tissues

The relationship between electromagnetic radiation from cell phones and soft oral tissues has been investigated due to the close connection between mobile phones and buccal structures, along with their frequent daily use. Recent studies suggest that this radiation may affect oral health tissues in various ways.

3.1 Effects on Oral Mucosal Cells

3.1.1 Nuclear Abnormalities

Research indicates a minor rise in nuclear abnormalities, including micronuclei and binucleated cells, in the oral mucosa of individuals who frequently use cell phones [143, 144]. These effects were more noticeable in individuals who used their phones for over 60 min weekly and for over 8 years [144].

3.1.2 Cytotoxic Effects

Some studies suggest that radiofrequency electromagnetic fields (RF-EMFs) from mobile phones may cause cytotoxic effects [145]. Kundi et al. [145] realized under controlled conditions, a study involving human intervention trials examined chromosomal damage and acute toxic effects. The present study provides clear evidence of the induction of acute toxicity and disruption of the cell cycle (cytokinesis) resulting from exposure to a high radiation dose (1.6 W/kg). These effects may disrupt mitochondrial homeostasis and trigger inflammatory responses [145].

3.1.3 Genotoxicity and Mutagenicity

Some authors consider that the evidence for genotoxic effects is not clear [146]. However, Kundi et al.'s findings indicate that mechanisms beyond chromosomal damage may result in the neoplastic transformation of cells when exposed to certain high-frequency electromagnetic fields (HF-EMF) emitted by mobile phones [145].

3.2 Effects on Salivary Glands and Flow

Changes in salivary flow rates have been associated with cell phone radiation [144]. It is important to note what happens to people who have a very frequent use of mobile phones. Mishra et al. found that saliva flow is increased, and in turn, the expression profile of cytokines is altered [144]. In contrast, Siqueira et al. [147] report that a majority of the study subjects had significantly less stimulated salivary secretion ($P < 0.01$) compared to the control subjects [147].

Mishra S et al. concluded "*Cell phones do not cause tumor of the salivary gland, but since few studies had found adverse effects of cell phone on orofacial structures so uncertainties remain and a continued precautionary approach is recommended until the situation is clarified*" [144] Cell phone exposure to the parotid glands may change salivary IL-10 and IL-1β levels, indicating a pro-inflammatory microenvironment possibly linked to heat production [147].

3.3 Effects on Oral Health

3.3.1 Nickel Ion Release

Aisha A. found that comparing nickel levels in saliva over 4 weeks, both with and without earphone use, suggests that mobile phones may increase the release of nickel ions from orthodontic appliances. This increase could be related to electromagnetic radiation; however, earphones appear to reduce this effect [148].

3.3.2 Mercury Release

Mortazavi MS et al., cited by Mishra S., described, "*There was a significant release of mercury from dental amalgam restoration due to microwave radiation emitted from mobile phones.*" [144, 149].

3.3.3 Bone-to-Implant Osseointegration

In this regard, there are two distinct situations. Exposure to cell phone radiation may affect bone healing around dental implants, potentially delaying osseointegration [150]. In contrast, Jing et al. "*demonstrates that pulsed electromagnetic fields PEMF improve osteogenesis and osseointegration of porous titanium alloys by promoting skeletal anabolic activities…*" [151].

3.3.4 Thermal Effects of Metal Implant

A comparison between implants in Stainless steel 410 and Ti-6Al-4 V within human tissues under near-field electromagnetic induction revealed that the stainless-steel implants resulted in higher tissue temperatures. Larger spherical implants led to increased tissue temperatures compared to smaller ones, highlighting the need to factor in implant size when evaluating thermal effects [152].

3.3.5 Nerve Dysfunction

"*Cell phones increase the temperature of the surrounding tissues and cause facial nerve dysfunction*" [144].

3.3.6 Healing Process

Shojaee et al. in an experimental study concluded, "*The results of this study showed that intermittent exposure to high-frequency electromagnetic fields over a period of 20 hours has no significant effect on the healing process of alveolar socket after tooth extraction in rats*" [153].

While there is some evidence that mobile phone electromagnetic radiation may impact soft oral tissues, particularly regarding nuclear abnormalities, cytotoxicity, genotoxicity, and salivary changes, people with metallic restorations or appliances made of nickel and mercury should exercise caution due to the potential release of metallic ions. More research is necessary in this topic.

4 Perspective of Neurofocal Dentistry on the Phenomenon of Electrogalvanism

It is interesting to observe how from different paradigms the same problem can be studied: the effects of metals for dental use on human biology. On the one hand, there is the explanation generated by neurofocal dentistry associated with the concept of neural irritations that it generates, and, on the other hand, the explanations given by the scientific paradigm associated with the generation of toxins in situ or at a distance through research carried out mainly in vitro and in live models about corrosion. Although the observations have different explanatory arguments typical of their paradigm, what is clear to both is the need to improve the understanding of oral galvanism.

The information collected in the previous sections related to the effects of dental materials, the effect of implants and the effect of electromagnatism generated by cell phones makes sense to the extent that it can be understood from neurofocal dentistry and the different stages that have been evidenced in its historical development (see Chap. 5). Thus, we will begin with the characterization of the information found and its most important findings to end with an interpretation of these phenomena from the nerves.

Greet G[2]. found two stages in her work when making an analysis of the information collected on the subject of oral galvanism. The first from the 1970s to the 1990s, research concerns were generated in Europe and the United States, which began with live observations of the effects of oral galvanism in patients related to the use of metallic materials such as silver amalgam, high-gold alloys [11, 38, 50], silver palladium alloys, and nickel chromium [33, 50, 65, 154]. As a result, we found a study that glimpsed the toxic and allergic effects of metals such as nickel, chromium, and gold [155]. It was also possible to identify studies that reported the clinical effects identified in signs, symptoms and pathologies that could be related to the use of silver amalgam and the metallic materials that were being developed in those years such as silver-palladium, chromium-cobalt, and nickel-chromium [38, 43, 50]. Among the most frequent reactions found during these years were white lesions [44] and ulcerative lesions [1, 11].

A second phase began in the late 1990s and continues to the present, showing a notable rise in studies over the last two decades, likely due to the widespread use of titanium and zirconium as restorative materials in various dental appliances or devices. In this second phase, she found multiple in vitro and in vivo studies that simulate some of the characteristics that occur in the oral cavity, using basic science knowledge such as biochemistry, biology, and physics, incorporating methods and simulation systems, especially when it comes to identifying biochemical and electrochemical phenomena at the cellular and tissue levels, generated by the interactions of various metals like titanium, zirconium, chromium, cobalt, aluminum, nickel, among others, as well as galvanic and friction interactions that give rise to biotribocorrosion [2].

The effects of galvanism are framed in the redox phenomena of metals that generate electric currents due to the displacement of electrons from the metal acting as the anode to the metal acting as the cathode. A primary consequence of this electrochemical process is related to the production of electric currents of varying intensities, which are related to the subsequent corrosion rate and the passivation process of the metals [11, 41].

Additionally, a third phase has been identified in the last decade, recognizing the need to make micro and nano modifications to the structures of implants made from different metallic and non-metallic materials, to avoid corrosion, achieve antibacterial effects, and promote osseointegration. These coatings play an important role because they add biochemical effects to the implant rehabilitation processes. Simultaneously, research has been generated concerning the effects of electromagnetism produced by mobile phones on soft tissues, where cytotoxic effects and cellular alterations have been reported. These investigations are particularly relevant due to the increasingly frequent use of mobile phones near the face and neck daily.

With the historical development of neurofocal dentistry, it can be understood that the semiological tools that a neurofocal dentist possesses are in the field of thorough clinical observation of the oral cavity, general health, and systemic interrelations with the social and environmental milieu. Using these tools, authors such as Escalante [156], Osorio Y and Fajardo F [157], Núñez-Lucio E [158], and Osorio [159]., among others, have reported the relationship between the presence of electrogalvanism and corrosion with the prevalence of oral and systemic pathology. Among the most frequently observed conditions by dentists who practice this approach concerning galvanism are chronic inflammatory processes and allergic reactions [2]. Similarly, Rost A [160]. found that the corrosion of metallic materials in the oral cavity "*generates sensitization through the formation of metal-protein complexes due to the existing tension between metals of different electrical potential; generating interfering neural fields.*" This concept of the metal-protein complex was referred to by Ribeiro et al. [74], who considers it to behave like a "*Trojan horse*" that internalizes within the cell and leads to the impairment of bone cells' functions and intracellular dynamics [1, 3].

Cartagena Montalvo SL cited by Greet G [2]. reports that neurofocal dentists used voltmeters and potentiometers to identify the voltages of electric currents in the oral cavity, as well as the different electric potentials of restorations (EPR), finding differences in electrical potentials with the production of Hertzian waves up to 800mv that travel through the human neurovegetative system [161].

It is interesting to observe how the clinical findings reported by neurofocal dentists in Colombia and other regions in the 1980s and 1990s raised questions about galvanism and its effects, which were addressed from neurofocal dentistry by referring to the concepts of interfering fields due to the chronic inflammatory processes found in patients and the distant reactions observed in the reported clinical cases [43, 158].

With the advent of neuraltherapeutic medicine as a complex medical system (see Chap. 6) and the recognition of nervism as one of its paradigmatic cores, we are invited to interpret the phenomena described in relation to electrogalvanism, biotribocorrosion, and electromagnetism and their consequences in the oral cavity.

The dental rehabilitation process can be described as a history of visible and invisible irritations. The invisible irritations are those related to electrogalvanism and electromagnetism, which have implications at the cellular and tissue levels. The visible irritations are all interventions done on the teeth. Restorative dentistry proposes metallic or non-metallic fillings to control caries, maintain the tooth in the mouth, or replace it with an implant, thereby restoring aesthetics and masticatory function.

When fillings are placed in cavities generated by caries, dental materials or devices are used for endodontic or periodontal treatment, creating external stimuli or irritations to the oral tissues that vary in intensity, frequency, and duration depending on the diagnosed pathologies. According to Russian nervism (Séchenov), irritations can generate excitation or inhibition in the nervous system. Delov [162]. mentions that "All acts of the organism in response to stimulation of the receptors and involving the central nervous system are reflexes." Reflexes can be conditioned or unconditioned, using certain structures of the nervous system to capture information such as receptors, afferent fibers, nerve center, efferent fiber, and effector [162]. Thus, the stomatognathic system is one of the most innervated systems with a significant variety of specialized receptors in each of the tissues.

For nervism (see Chap. 13), it is recognized that the nervous system organizes and coordinates all the functions of the organism; it is not segmented but acts as a unit [163]. Thus, a masterful musical symphony is generated between excitations and inhibitions from the different organs and tissues of the body in order to fulfill basic functions.

According to Delov [162] excitation processes are basically mediated by afferent receptors of external stimuli, while inhibition processes are mediated by internal reactions to external stimuli, which are configured as a suppression of excitation or a decrease in excitability and conductivity; then inhibited nerve structures do not propagate excitation, one can understand that a stimulus from the outside world can remain unanswered. Inhibition is an important physiological regulatory process. Chewing and swallowing are examples of how excitatory and inhibitory processes are coordinated in the stomatognathic and respiratory systems to generate efficient function.

The irritations generated by dental treatments become specific stimuli that produce a series of biological reactions associated with basic responses such as acute or chronic inflammation, microbial infections and their consequences (abscesses, fistulas, cellulitis, etc.), conditions where soft tissue is lost (lacerations, ulcerations) or where tissue is increased (fibroids, papilloma), white lesions, erythematous lesions, loss of hard tissue (dental or bone demineralization), dental remineralization or increase in bone tissue (exostosis), alterations in the histological development of hard and soft tissues, degenerative processes, reactions to poisoning by metals or other elements, oral manifestations of autoimmune, hematological, viral and neoplastic diseases, among others, which can be considered as the consequence of irritations generated by various somatic, therapeutic, relational actors. They are the result of the symphony of excitations and inhibitions that were generated and coordinated by the nervous system in an attempt to adapt to fulfill the basic functions of chewing, swallowing, breathing, and speaking.

A second conceptual element to understand about nervism is trophism as a mechanism used by the nervous system to control metabolic processes and maintain the homeostasis of a complex organism [164] It follows that the nervous system has a trophic function, that is, tissue regulation, so dystrophy is a manifestation of tissues or cells when the nervous system is not able to adequately maintain integrity and their function. Speransky [164] quoting Charcot points out that not every injury to a nerve ended with dystrophic lesions in the tissues due to cessation of nerve function, but due to irritation to it; therefore he considered partial nerve injury more dangerous than total nerve section. Making a comparison with Speransky's experiments where he irritated the nerves with chemical substances and the result was chronic ulcers that he called trophic ulcers, in the anatomical areas of innervation of the affected nerve, we understand then that the effects of corrosion can generate dystrophic tissue areas at the local level, that is, areas that are not adequately regulated in their physiology and metabolism due to the irritation that is generated in the tissues surrounding the dental restoration or implant. Penarrocha M. and Bohorquez C.E. report the appearance of ulcers in the oral cavity associated with galvanism [1, 11].

On the other hand, Speransky found that when irritation reaches a particular intensity, it cannot be stopped even if the dystrophic tissue is excited and the agent causing the nervous irritation is removed [164]. He found that ulcers worsened even more when accompanied by infectious processes. This information allows us to understand that the system retains the irritation imprint for a period or permanently and can modulate future reactions to intense stimuli of another nature. Vishnesky A.S., referenced by Speransky [164] described that ulcerous lesions could recur when the subject came down with the flu, and once the viral infection subsided, the trophic ulcer disappeared. This information is relevant to be observed in the course of dental treatment.

A third conceptual element of nervism that can help us understand is the concept of Parabiosis, defined as a profound excitation that cannot extend [162]. A characteristic of parabiotic excitation is stability and continuity, meaning it deepens under the influence of new excitation impulses. Therefore, the impulses that come stronger and more frequently in the area of parabiosis prevent future nerve conduction. The parabiotic area is characterized by very low lability, becoming incapable of reproducing frequent and strong excitations [162] When electrochemical, electrical, electromagnetic, chemical, or mechanical stimuli are generated on rehabilitated or implanted oral tissues, we can consider that the intensity and frequency of these irritating agents lead to the phenomenon of parabiosis in the nervous tissue of the affected area, with the consequent inability to respond to new stimuli, whether strong or weak, due to the intense inhibition generated. The clinical consequence of this process is that the patient does not present painful symptoms and only perceives changes in the surrounding bone tissues when implant or tooth mobility occurs, occlusal discomfort, or severe damage to the tissues surrounding the restoration.

A fourth concept is the first hit and second hit, developed especially by Speransky [164], who considers that irritative stimuli or "hits" can be of different types: nervous traumas of a surgical nature, infectious processes, or contact with chemical substances. These irritative stimuli on a "nerve" affect the entire system as if putting it on alert and develop a series of barriers over the tissues along which the irritant has not yet passed. This initial defensive action of the nervous system preserves the organism's integrity and prevents the extension of the irritation to the segment.

Once it recovers from the first excitation, a latency period is generated that differs in each individual depending on the stimuli to which they are exposed. Speransky insists on remembering that "*the disappearance of pathological symptoms after the first trauma is not proof of the complete restoration of the nervous elements that have suffered*" [164]. It is likely that a new stimulus, very small or insignificant to the patient, could generate a new irritative event on the nervous system. The second irritative hit generates dystrophic symptoms in the system similar to the symptoms developed in the first hit, even if the site of irritation is topographically different. However, Speransky notes that the type of irritative stimulus can be similar [164].

Speransky recognizes that when a second hit is generated, it can be thought that the chemical or biological irritant has been transported from the primary focus by the blood or lymphatics, in which case the affection of those distant tissues is also direct. However, he refers to the concept of "*tropism*"to identify the special sensitivity or affinity of certain organs or entire systems for an irritant [164]. A galvanic affection can become the first or second hit to an organism, and the systemic affections generated in patients after dental treatment have been reported by neurofocal dentists [2, 160] and by academics [3].

On the other hand, the irritation process occurs in different degrees. It starts with local affections that do not extend beyond the limits due to the activation of the inhibitory mechanism; it can continue with lateral extension affecting contralateral nerve segments [164]; it extends to segmental irritations that can affect nerve pathways or embryonic development segments (see Chap. 15); a fourth degree involves metasegmental irritations when more than two segments are affected, and generalizations when the entire system is affected. It is important to consider this aspect specifically in late allergic reactions to metals. Rasul T F. reports the case of a patient with a gold allergy and manifestations of lichen planus associated with dental restorations [46].

Speransky states that "*the strength of an irritant agent lies in the degree of irritation, which is the sum of many processes developing one after another and which must be taken into account until the end, that is, until the real extinction of all phenomena*" [164]. This concept is definitive in the history of nervous system irritations because each new experience of the nervous system changes the tone of the local response and the overall outcome.

One last element to consider is the concept of dominance from nervism, developed by A.A. Ukhtomsky, defined as a guiding principle of brain functions that allows fulfilling a specific function [165]. A pathological dominance focus is created from a focal irritation of the nervous system, generating a conditioned reflex that has the ability to attract other excitations to itself and inhibit other nervous centers, which determines a behavioral orientation; it possesses excessive excitability due to a low excitation threshold, leading to a state of excessive inertia, producing stagnation.

Although the organism creates a focus of pathological dominance as a nervous phenomenon with an adaptive purpose, utilizing the plasticity of the structures and functions of the nervous system to its advantage, it is important to recognize that this is a complex process that is positively feedbacked to the extent that each new stimulus allows its permanence over time. Uncovering those foci that hold biological significance at a given moment in a patient's life is challenging for the clinician. On some occasions, all the restorative experiences a patient undergoes become a long series of irritations of diverse origins that contribute to the modulation of the tone of reactions and physiological outcomes. The treatment failure rate and the supporting tissues' implications can reflect this.

An additional observation regarding research is the limitations in conducting in vivo research or animal models that simulate the conditions of the oral cavity. Speransky managed to conduct in vivo experimentation with animal models with few restrictions due to the historical and epistemological context of the era, yet the questions regarding a more detailed explanation of how and what the pathophysiological pathways in local and systemic cells and tissues are, which generate the mentioned clinical effects, are yet to be answered.

Neurofocal dentists have the commitment to identify the materials to be used in restorative procedures. When it becomes necessary to use metals, it is crucial to know their physical, chemical, electrochemical, and mechanical characteristics to generate the best possible option according to the patient's history and oral characteristics, accompanied by a detailed mapping of the irritations to the nervous system and the local and systemic dystrophic reactions generated in each patient.

References

1. Bohorquez CE. Oral galvanism. Rev Colomb Dermatol. 1998;6(1):11–6.
2. Greet G. Oral and systemic effects of galvanism due to metallic dental materials: a look from integrative dentistry [thesis]. Bogotá: Universidad Nacional de Colombia; 2021.
3. Kim SM. Oral galvanism related to dental implants. Maxillofac Plast Reconstr Surg. 2023;45(1):36. https://doi.org/10.1186/s40902-023-00403-8.
4. Bizar RJ. Effect of thermal variations during the fusion of castings in fixed prostheses [Internet]. Universitat de Barcelona; 1999 [cited 2025 Jan 10]. Available from: https://dialnet.unirioja.es/servlet/tesis?codigo=74932.
5. ASTM International. Standard terminology relating to corrosion and corrosion testing [Internet]. 2007 [cited 2025 Jan 15]. Available from: https://www.scribd.com/document/362600832/ASTM-G15.
6. Amigó Borrás V. Laboratory notebook: foundation of materials science [Internet]. [date unknown] [cited 2025 Jan 10]. Available from: https://personales.upv.es/~avicente/material/Fcm/Pdf/Practicas/fcm12trb.pdf.

7. Mellado-Valero A, Muñoz AI, Pina VG, Sola-Ruiz MF. Electrochemical behaviour and galvanic effects of titanium implants coupled to metallic suprastructures in artificial saliva. Materials. 2018;11(1):171.
8. Carey PH, Hsu SM, Fares C, Kamenov G, Ren F, Esquivel-Upshaw J. The galvanic effect of titanium and amalgam in the oral environment. Materials (Basel). 2020;13(19):4425.
9. Bergman M, Ginstrup O, Nilner K. Potential and polarization measurements in vivo of oral galvanism. Scand J Dent Res. 1978;86(2):135–45.
10. Chaturvedi TP, Upadhayay SN. An overview of orthodontic material degradation in oral cavity. Indian J Dent Res. 2010;21(2):275–84. https://doi.org/10.4103/0970-9290.66648.
11. Peñarrocha M. Ulcerated lesions of the oral mucosa associated with intraoral galvanism. Av Odontoestomatol. 1992;3:181–5.
12. Yin L, Lin S, Summers AO, Roper V, Campen MJ, Yu X. Children with amalgam dental restorations have significantly elevated blood and urine mercury levels. Toxicol Sci. 2021;184(1):104–26.
13. Cabaña-Muñoz ME, Parmigiani-Izquierdo JM, Camacho Alonso F, Merino JJ. Increased systemic malondialdehyde levels and decreased Mo/co, co/Fe2+ ratios in patients with long-term dental titanium implants and amalgams. J Clin Med. 2019;8(1):86.
14. Gaur S, Agnihotri R, Albin S. Bio-tribocorrosion of titanium dental implants and its toxicological implications: a scoping review. ScientificWorldJournal. 2022;2022:4498613.
15. Domingo MG, Nalli GA, Tasat DR, Olmedo DG. Exfoliated oral mucosa cells as bioindicators of short- and long-term systemic titanium contamination. J Trace Elem Med Biol. 2023;76:127114.
16. Podzimek S, Tomka M, Sommerova P, Lyuya-Mi Y, Bartova J, Prochazkova J, et al. Immune markers in oral discomfort patients before and after elimination of oral galvanism. Neuro Endocrinol Lett. 2013;34:802–8.
17. Procházková J, Podzimek S, Tomka M, Kucerová H, Mihaljevic M, Hána K, et al. Metal alloys in the oral cavity as a cause of oral discomfort in sensitive patients. Neuro Endocrinol Lett. 2006;27(Suppl 1):53–8.
18. Lebedev KA, Maksimovskiĭ IM, Sagan NN, Mitronin AV. Principles of galvanic currents determination in the oral cavity and their clinical background. Stomatologiia (Mosk). 2007;86(3):11–6.
19. Kucerová H, Dostálová T, Procházková J, Bártová J, Himmlová L. Influence of galvanic phenomena on the occurrence of algic symptoms in the mouth. Gen Dent. 2002;50(1):62–5.
20. Herrström P, Högstedt B. Clinical study of oral galvanism: no evidence of toxic mercury exposure but anxiety disorder an important background factor. Scand J Dent Res. 1993;101(4):232–7.
21. Johansson BI, Lucas LC, Lemons JE. Corrosion of copper, nickel, and gold dental casting alloys: an in vitro and in vivo study. J Biomed Mater Res. 1989;23(Suppl A3):349–61.
22. Wataha JC, Drury JL, Chung WO. Nickel alloys in the oral environment. Expert Rev Med Devices. 2013;10(4):519–39.
23. Cortada M, Giner L, Costa S, Gil FJ, Rodríguez D, Planell JA. Galvanic corrosion behavior of titanium implants coupled to dental alloys. J Mater Sci Mater Med. 2000;11(5):287–93.
24. Mellado VA. Study of the electrochemical behavior and galvanic corrosion of biomedical alloys for dental implants and suprastructures [thesis]. 2016. [cited 16 January 2025] Available from: http://hdl.handle.net/10550/54553
25. Saji VS, Choe HC. Electrochemical behavior of co-Cr and Ni-Cr dental cast alloys. Trans Nonferrous Met Soc China. 2009;19:785–90.
26. Marti A. Cobalt-base alloys used in bone surgery. Injury, Int J Care Injured. 2000;31:18–21.
27. Crook P, Silence WL. Cobalt alloys. In: Uhlig's corrosion handbook. 2nd ed. Wiley; 2000. p. 717–28.
28. Soygun K, Ozer A, Ulucan MC, Bolayir G. An investigation of corrosive effects on zirconia with different crystal structures. Microsc Res Tech. 2020:1–8.

29. Castaño-Rivera P, Echavarría-Velásquez A, Gómez GJ, Arismendi J. Evaluation of the galvanic corrosion of high copper dental amalgams by means of electrochemical techniques. Revista Facultad de Ingeniería Universidad de Antioquia. 2008;45:77–86.
30. Muller A, Van Loon L, Davidson C. Electrical potentials of restorations in subjects without oral complaints. J Oral Rehabil. 1990;17(5):419–24.
31. Chaturvedi T. An overview of the corrosion aspect of dental implants. Indian J Dent Res. 2009;20(1):91–8.
32. Kunrath MF, Muradás TC, Penha N, Campos MM. Innovative surfaces and alloys for dental implants: what about biointerface-safety concerns? Dent Mater. 2021;37(10):1447–62.
33. Summers AO, Wireman J, Vimy MJ, Lorscheider FL, Marshall B, Levy SB, Bennett S, Billard L. Mercury released from dental "silver" fillings provokes an increase in mercury- and antibiotic-resistant bacteria in oral and intestinal floras of primates. Antimicrob Agents Chemother. 1993;37(4):825–34.
34. Sellars WA, Sellars R, Liang L, Hefley JD. Methyl mercury in dental amalgams in the human mouth. J Nutr Environ Med. 1996;6(1):33–6.
35. Udabe Pagola I. Changes in Salivary Composition in Orthodontic Treatment [Internet] [master's thesis]. Oviedo: Universidad de Oviedo; 2015 [cited 2025 Jan 17]. Available from: https://digibuo.uniovi.es/dspace/handle/10651/30921
36. Montañez N, Peña DY, Estupiñan H. Corrosion of nitinol wires in artificial saliva by electrochemical techniques. Rev ION. 2008;21(1):87–96.
37. Rishor-Olney CR, Gnugnoli DM. Nickel allergy. In: StatPearls [Internet]. StatPearls Publishing; 2023 [cited 2025 Feb 7]. Available from: https://www.ncbi.nlm.nih.gov/sites/books/NBK557638/
38. Nilner K, Glantz PO, Ryge G, Sundberg H. Oral galvanic action after treatment with extensive metallic restorations. Acta Odontol Scand. 1982;40(6):381–8.
39. López Carriches C, Martínez-González J, Gómez Font R, Leco Berrocal L, Donado RM. Clinical-epidemiological study on burning mouth syndrome. Av Odontoestomatol. 2003;19(4)
40. Bender SD. Burning mouth syndrome. Dent Clin N Am. 2018;62(4):585–96.
41. Lucas LC, Lemons JE. Biodegradation of restorative metallic systems. Adv Dent Res. 1992;6(1):32–7.
42. van der Waal I. Oral leukoplakia, the ongoing discussion on definition and terminology. Med Oral Patol Oral Cir Bucal. 2015;20(6):e685–92.
43. Villa A, Sonis S. Oral leukoplakia remains a challenging condition. Oral Dis. 2018;24(1–2):179–83.
44. Bánóczy J, Roed-Petersen B, Pindborg JJ, Inovay J. Clinical and histologic studies on electrogalvanically induced oral white lesions. Oral Surg Oral Med Oral Pathol. 1979;48(4):319–23.
45. Lehman JS, Tollefson MM, Gibson LE. Lichen planus. Int J Dermatol. 2009;48(7):682–94.
46. Rasul TF, Anderson J, Bergholz DR, et al. Gold dental implant-induced oral lichen planus. Cureus. 2022;14(2):e21852. https://doi.org/10.7759/cureus.21852.
47. Jerez E, Epifanio R. Oral manifestations of contact stomatitis: a literature review. Contacto Científico. 2018;2:9–16.
48. Sutow EJ, Maillet WA, Hall GC. Corrosion potential variation of aged dental amalgam restorations over time. Dent Mater. 2006;22(4):325–9.
49. Meyer RD, Meyer J, Taloumis LJ. Intraoral galvanic corrosion: literature review and case report. J Prosthet Dent. 1993;69(2):141–3.
50. Agerberg G. Signs and symptoms of mandibular dysfunction in patients with suspected oral galvanism. Acta Odontol Scand. 1987;45(1):41–8.
51. Molin C. Oral galvanism in Sweden. J Am Dent Assoc. 1990;121(2):281–4.
52. Geier DA, Geier MR. Reported asthma and dental amalgam exposure among adults in the United States: an assessment of the National Health and nutrition examination survey. SAGE Open Med. 2023;1(1):55–68.
53. Decker A, Daly D, Scher RK. Role of titanium in the development of yellow nail syndrome. Skin Appendage Disord. 2015;1(1):28–30.

54. Weinhold E, Viloria GJV. Release of metal ions in the oral environment due to alloy corrosion phenomena [Internet]. 2006 [cited 2025 Jan 17]. Available from: https://www.semanticscholar.org/paper/Liberaci%C3%B3n-de-iones-met%C3%A1licos-en-el-medio-bucal-por-Weinhold-Viloria/bdcf2cd5b03405e9c4567a0235d846b960688fed
55. Siblerud R, Mutter J, Moore E, Naumann J, Walach H. A hypothesis and evidence that mercury may be an etiological factor in Alzheimer's disease. Int J Environ Res Public Health. 2019;16(24):5152.
56. Minamata Convention. Minamata Convention Booklet [Internet]. Oct 2023 [cited 2025 Jan 21]. Available from: https://minamataconvention.org/sites/default/files/documents/information_document/Minamata-Convention-booklet-Oct2023-ES.pdf
57. Sotova C, Yanushevich O, Kriheli N, Grigoriev S, Evdokimov V, Kramar O, et al. Dental implants: modern materials and methods of their surface modification. Materials (Basel). 2023;16(23):7383.
58. Sharifianjazi F, Khaksar S, Esmaeilkhanian A, Bazli L, Eskandarinezhad S, Salahshour P, et al. Advancements in fabrication and application of chitosan composites in implants and dentistry: a review. Biomolecules. 2022;12(2):155.
59. Bokobza L. On the use of nanoparticles in dental implants. Materials. 2024;17:3191. https://doi.org/10.3390/ma17133191.
60. Gulati K, Scimeca JC, Ivanovski S, Verron E. Double-edged sword: therapeutic efficacy versus toxicity evaluations of doped titanium implants. Drug Discov Today. 2021;26(11):2734–42.
61. Mocanu AC, Miculescu F, Stan GE, Pasuk I, Tite T, Pascu A, Butte TM, Ciocan LT. Modulated laser cladding of implant-type coatings by bovine bone-derived hydroxyapatite powder injection on Ti6Al4V substrates – part I: fabrication and physico-chemical characterization. Materials. 2022;15:7971. https://doi.org/10.3390/ma15227971.
62. Ma Z, Zhao X, Zhao J, Zhao Z, Wang Q, Zhang C. Biologically modified polyether ether ketone as dental implant material. Front Bioeng Biotechnol. 2020;8:620537.
63. Dini C, Costa RC, Sukotjo C, Takoudis CG, Mathew MT, Barão VAR. Progression of bio-tribocorrosion in implant dentistry. Front Mech Eng. 2020;6:1.
64. Cruz HV, Souza JCM, Henriques M, Rocha LA, et al. Tribocorrosion and bio-tribocorrosion in the oral environment: the case of dental implants [Internet]. ResearchGate. 2011. Available from: https://www.researchgate.net/publication/259025605
65. Villanueva J, Trino L, Thomas J, et al. Corrosion, tribology, and tribocorrosion research in biomedical implants: progressive trend in the published literature. J Bio Tribo Corros. 2017;3(1):1. https://doi.org/10.1007/s40735-016-0060-1.
66. Suárez-López del Amo F, Garaicoa-Pazmiño C, Fretwurst T, Castilho RM, Squarize CH. Dental implants-associated release of titanium particles: a systematic review. Clin Oral Implants Res. 2018;29(11):1085–100.
67. Blum K, Wiest W, Fella C, Balles A, Dittmann J, Rack A, et al. Fatigue-induced changes in conical implant–abutment connections. Dent Mater. 2015;31(11):1415–26.
68. Liu X, Chen S, Tsoi JKH, Matinlinna JP. Binary titanium alloys as dental implant materials – a review. Regen Biomater. 2017;4(5):315–23.
69. Olmedo DG, Nalli G, Verdu S, Paparella ML, Cabrini RL. Exfoliative cytology and titanium dental implants: a pilot study. J Periodontol. 2013;84(1):78–83.
70. StudySmarter ES. Cytotoxicity: definition and apoptosis [Internet]. [date unknown] [cited 2025 Jan 2]. Available from: https://www.studysmarter.es/resumenes/medicina/oncologia/citotoxicidad/
71. Academia Lab. Neurotoxicity [Internet]. [date unknown] [cited 2025 Jan 2]. Available from: https://academia-lab.com/enciclopedia/neurotoxicidad/.
72. Academia Lab. Genotoxicity. [Internet]. [date unknown] [cited 2025 Jan 9]. Available from: https://academia-lab.com/enciclopedia/genotoxicidad/
73. Goodman SB. Wear particles, periprosthetic osteolysis and the immune system. Biomaterials. 2007;28(34):5044–8.

74. Ribeiro AR, Gemini-Piperni S, Travassos R, Lemgruber L, Silva RC, Rossi AL, et al. Trojan-like internalization of anatase titanium dioxide nanoparticles by human osteoblast cells. Sci Rep. 2016;29(6):23615.
75. Noronha Oliveira M, Schunemann WVH, Mathew MT, Henriques B, Magini RS, Teughels W, et al. Can degradation products released from dental implants affect peri-implant tissues? J Periodontal Res. 2018;53(1):1–11.
76. Bressan E, Ferroni L, Gardin C, Bellin G, Sbricoli L, Sivolella S, et al. Metal nanoparticles released from dental implant surfaces: potential contribution to chronic inflammation and peri-implant bone loss. Materials. 2019;12(12):2036.
77. Zhou Z, Shi Q, Wang J, et al. The unfavorable role of titanium particles released from dental implants. Nano Theranostics. 2021;5(3):321–32.
78. Noumbissi S, Scarano A, Gupta S. A literature review study on atomic ions dissolution of titanium and its alloys in implant dentistry. Materials. 2019;12(3):368.
79. Schunemannn WVH. Effect of metallic particles released from dental implants on peri-implant tissues [thesis]. Florianópolis: Universidade Federal de Santa Catarina; 2015.
80. Makihira S, Mine Y, Nikawa H, Shuto T, Iwata S, Hosokawa R, et al. Titanium ion induces necrosis and sensitivity to lipopolysaccharide in gingival epithelial-like cells. Toxicol In Vitro. 2010;24(7):1905–10.
81. Dhein J, Haller C, Reichl FX, Milz S, Hickel R, Kollmuss M, et al. Intranuclear cell uptake and toxicity of titanium dioxide and zirconia particles as well as bacterial adhesion on dental titanium- and zirconia-implants. Dent Mater. 2022;38(3):517–28.
82. Berryman Z, Bridger L, Hussaini HM, Rich AM, Atieh M, Tawse-Smith A. Titanium particles: an emerging risk factor for peri-implant bone loss. Saudi Dent J. 2020;32(6):283–92.
83. Zhu WQ, Ming PP, Qiu J, et al. Effect of titanium ions on the hippo/YAP signaling pathway in regulating biological behaviors of MC3T3-E1 osteoblasts. J Appl Toxicol. 2018;38(6):824–33.
84. Sridhar S, Wang F, Wilson TG, Palmer K, Valderrama P, Rodrigues DC. The role of bacterial biofilm and mechanical forces in modulating dental implant failures. J Mech Behav Biomed Mater. 2019;92:118–27.
85. Tchinda A, Lerebours A, Kouitat-Njiwa R, Bravetti P. Zirconia dental implants: a closer look at surface condition and intrinsic composition by SEM-EDX. Bioengineering. 2023;10:1102.
86. Chandar S, Kotian R, Madhyastha P, Kabekkodu SP, Rao P. In vitro evaluation of cytotoxicity and corrosion behavior of commercially pure titanium and Ti-6Al-4V alloy for dental implants. J Indian Prosthodont Soc. 2017;17(1):35–40.
87. Perumal G, Grewal HS, Pole M, Reddy LVK, Mukherjee S, Singh H, et al. Enhanced biocorrosion resistance and cellular response of a dual-phase high entropy alloy through reduced elemental heterogeneity. ACS Appl Bio Mater. 2020;3:1233–44.
88. Cordeiro JM, Barão VAR. Is there scientific evidence favoring the substitution of commercially pure titanium with titanium alloys for the manufacture of dental implants? Mater Sci Eng C Mater Biol Appl. 2017;71:1201–15.
89. Willhite CC, Karyakina NA, Yokel RA, Yenugadhati N, Wisniewski TM, Arnold IMF, et al. Systematic review of potential health risks posed by pharmaceutical, occupational and consumer exposures to metallic and nanoscale aluminum, aluminum oxides, aluminum hydroxide and its soluble salts. Crit Rev Toxicol. 2014;44(sup4):1–80. https://doi.org/10.3109/10408444.2014.934439.
90. Aaseth J, Skaug MA, Cao Y, Andersen O. Chelation in metal intoxication – principles and paradigms. J Trace Elem Med Biol. 2015;31:260–6.
91. Huang W, Wang P, Shen T, Hu C, Han Y, Song M, et al. Aluminum trichloride inhibited osteoblastic proliferation and downregulated the Wnt/-catenin pathway. Biol Trace Elem Res. 2017;177:323–30.
92. Yang X, Huo H, Xiu C, Song M, Han Y, Li Y, et al. Inhibition of osteoblast differentiation by aluminum trichloride exposure is associated with inhibition of BMP-2/Smad pathway component expression. Food Chem Toxicol. 2016;97:120–6.

93. Xu F, Ren L, Song M, Shao B, Han Y, Cao Z, et al. Fas- and mitochondria-mediated signaling pathway involved in osteoblast apoptosis induced by AlCl3. Biol Trace Elem Res. 2018;184:173–85.
94. Yu H, Zhang J, Ji Q, Yu K, Wang P, Song M, et al. Melatonin alleviates aluminium chloride-induced immunotoxicity by inhibiting oxidative stress and apoptosis associated with the activation of Nrf2 signaling pathway. Ecotoxicol Environ Saf. 2019;173:131–41.
95. Costa BC, Tokuhara CK, Rocha LA, Oliveira RC, Lisboa-Filho PN, Costa PJ. Vanadium ionic species from degradation of Ti-6Al-4V metallic implants: in vitro cytotoxicity and speciation evaluation. Mater Sci Eng C. 2019;96:730–9.
96. Fretwurst T, Buzanich G, Nahles S, Woelber JP, Riesemeier H, Nelson K. Metal elements in tissue with dental peri-implantitis: a pilot study. Clin Oral Implants Res. 2016;27(9):1178–86.
97. Pettersson M, Kelk P, Belibasakis GN, Bylund D, Molin Thorén M, Johansson A. Titanium ions form particles that activate and execute interleukin-1β release from lipopolysaccharide-primed macrophages. J Periodontal Res. 2017;52(1):21–32.
98. Souza MEP, Lima L, Lima CRP, Zavaglia CAC, Freire CMA. Effects of pH on the electrochemical behaviour of titanium alloys for implant applications. J Mater Sci Mater Med. 2009;20(2):549–52. https://doi.org/10.1007/s10856-008-3623-y.
99. Severino VO, Napimoga MH, de Lima Pereira SA. Expression of IL-6, IL-10, IL-17 and IL-8 in the peri-implant crevicular fluid of patients with peri-implantitis. Arch Oral Biol. 2011;56(8):823–8.
100. Safioti LM, Kotsakis GA, Pozhitkov AE, Chung WO, Daubert DM. Increased levels of dissolved titanium are associated with peri-implantitis – a cross-sectional study. J Periodontol. 2017;88(5):436–42.
101. Daubert D, Pozhitkov A, McLean J, Kotsakis G. Titanium as a modifier of the peri-implant microbiome structure. Clin Implant Dent Relat Res. 2018;20(6):945–53.
102. Barão VAR, Mathew MT, Yuan JCC, Knoernschild KL, Assunção WG, Wimmer MA, et al. Influence of corrosion on lipopolysaccharide affinity for two different titanium materials. J Prosthet Dent. 2013;110(6):462–70.
103. de Lima-Souza RA, Vallarelli AFA, Viviane Mariano F, Cintra ML. Multiple cutaneous fistula after titanium dental implant: a case report. Clin Implant Dent Relat Res. 2021;23(2):270–4.
104. Shah R, Penmetsa DSL, Thomas R, Mehta DS. Titanium corrosion: implications for dental implants. Eur J Prosthodont Restor Dent. 2016;24(4):171–80.
105. Daubert DM, Pozhitkov AE, Safioti LM, Kotsakis GA. Association of global DNA methylation to titanium and peri-implantitis: a case-control study. JDR Clin Trans Res. 2019;4(3):284–91.
106. Zhang X, Song Y, Gong H, Wu C, Wang B, Chen W, et al. Neurotoxicity of titanium dioxide nanoparticles: a comprehensive review. Int J Nanomedicine. 2023;18:7183–204.
107. Shelly S, Liraz Zaltsman S, Ben-Gal O, Dayan A, Ganmore I, Shemesh C, et al. Potential neurotoxicity of titanium implants: prospective, in vivo and in vitro study. Biomaterials. 2021;276:121039.
108. Czajka M, Sawicki K, Sikorska K, Popek S, Kruszewski M, Kapka-Skrzypczak L. Toxicity of titanium dioxide nanoparticles in central nervous system. Toxicol In Vitro. 2015;29(5):1042–52.
109. Ferraro SA, Domingo MG, Etcheverrito A, Olmedo DG, Tasat DR. Neurotoxicity mediated by oxidative stress caused by titanium dioxide nanoparticles in human neuroblastoma (SH-SY5Y) cells. J Trace Elem Med Biol. 2020;57:126413.
110. Song B, Zhang Y, Liu J, Feng X, Zhou T, Shao L. Unraveling the neurotoxicity of titanium dioxide nanoparticles: focusing on molecular mechanisms. Beilstein J Nanotechnol. 2016;7:645–54.
111. Disdier C, Chalansonnet M, Gagnaire F, Gaté L, Cosnier F, Devoy J, et al. Brain inflammation, blood-brain barrier dysfunction and neuronal synaptophysin decrease after inhalation exposure to titanium dioxide nano-aerosol in aging rats. Sci Rep. 2017;7(1):12196.

112. Beger B, Goetz H, Morlock M, Schiegnitz E, Al-Nawas B. In vitro surface characteristics and impurity analysis of five different commercially available dental zirconia implants. Int J Implant Dent. 2018;4(1):13.
113. Hallab NJ, Mikecz K, Vermes C, Skipor A, Jacobs JJ. Orthopaedic implant-related metal toxicity in terms of human lymphocyte reactivity to metal-protein complexes produced from cobalt-base and titanium-base implant alloy degradation. Mol Cell Biochem. 2001;222:127–36.
114. Puskar T, Jevremovic D, Williams RJ, Eggbeer D, Vukelic D, Budak I. A comparative analysis of the corrosive effect of artificial saliva of variable pH on DMLS and cast Co-Cr-Mo dental alloy. Materials (Basel). 2014;6:6486–501.
115. Saha S, Roy S. Metallic dental implants wear mechanisms, materials, and manufacturing processes: a literature review. Materials (Basel). 2022;16(1):161.
116. Karimi S, Alfantazi AM. Ion release and surface oxide composition of AISI 316L, Co-28Cr-6Mo, and Ti-6Al-4V alloys immersed in human serum albumin solutions. Mater Sci Eng C. 2014;40:435–44.
117. Thakur L, Arora N. An investigation on the development and wear performance of chromium-MWCNTs transformed HVOF sprayed nano-WC-CoCr coatings. Surf Coat Technol. 2020;388:125610.
118. Takemoto S, Hattori M, Yoshinari M, Kawada E, Asami K, Oda Y. Corrosion mechanism of TiCr alloys in solution containing fluoride. Dent Mater. 2009;25:467–72.
119. Mellado-Valero A, Muñoz AI, Pina VG, Sola-Ruiz MF. Electrochemical behaviour and galvanic effects of titanium implants coupled to metallic suprastructures in artificial saliva. Materials (Basel). 2018;11(1):171.
120. Reclaru L, Unger RE, Kirkpatrick CJ, Susz C, Eschler PY, Zuercher MH, et al. Ni–Cr based dental alloys; Ni release, corrosion and biological evaluation. Mater Sci Eng C. 2012;32(6):1452–60.
121. Szuhanek CA, Watz CG, Avram S, Moacă EA, Mihali CV, Popa A, et al. Comparative toxicological in vitro and in ovo screening of different orthodontic implants currently used in dentistry. Materials (Basel). 2020;13:5690.
122. Saini M. Implant biomaterials: a comprehensive review. World J Clin Cases. 2015;3:52.
123. Kerosuo H, Moe G, Kleven E. In vitro release of nickel and chromium from different types of simulated orthodontic appliances. Angle Orthod. 1995;65:111–6.
124. Wang K, Wang S, Yin J, Yang Q, Yu Y, Chen L. Long-term application of silver nanoparticles in dental restoration materials: potential toxic injury to the CNS. J Mater Sci Mater Med. 2023;34(11):52. https://doi.org/10.1007/s10856-023-06753-z.
125. Murphy A, Casey A, Byrne G, Chambers G, Howe O. Silver nanoparticles induce pro-inflammatory gene expression and inflammasome activation in human monocytes. J Appl Toxicol. 2016;36(10):1311–20.
126. Hashimoto M, Imazato S. Cytotoxic and genotoxic characterization of aluminum and silicon oxide nanoparticles in macrophages. Dent Mater. 2015;31(5):556–64. https://doi.org/10.1016/j.dental.2015.02.009.
127. Di Virgilio AL, Reigosa M, de Mele MFL. Response of UMR 106 cells exposed to titanium oxide and aluminum oxide nanoparticles. J Biomed Mater Res A. 2010;92A(1):80–6.
128. Qin W, Xing T, Tang B, Chen W. Mechanical properties and osteogenesis of CFR-PEEK composite with interface strengthening by graphene oxide for implant application. J Mech Behav Biomed Mater. 2023;148:106222.
129. Li Y, Wang D, Qin W, Jia H, Wu Y, Ma J, et al. Mechanical properties, hemocompatibility, cytotoxicity and systemic toxicity of carbon fibers/poly(ether-ether-ketone) composites with different fiber lengths as orthopedic implants. J Biomater Sci Polym Ed. 2019;30(18):1709–24.
130. Masuki H, Isobe K, Kawabata H, Tsujino T, Yamaguchi S, Watanabe T, Kawase T. Acute cytotoxic effects of silica microparticles used for coating of plastic blood-collection tubes on human periosteal cells. Odontology. 2020;108(4):545–52.

131. Chen F, Li G, Zhao ER, Li J, Hableel G, Lemaster JE, et al. Cellular toxicity of silicon carbide nanomaterials as a function of morphology. Biomaterials. 2018;179:60–70.
132. Marquardt C, Fritsch-Decker S, Al-Rawi M, Diabaté S, Weiss C. Autophagy induced by silica nanoparticles protects RAW264.7 macrophages from cell death. Toxicology. 2017;379:40–7.
133. Poier N, Hochstöger J, Hackenberg S, Scherzad A, Bregenzer M, Schopper D, et al. Effects of zinc oxide nanoparticles in HUVEC: cyto- and genotoxicity and functional impairment after long-term and repetitive exposure in vitro. Int J Nanomedicine. 2020;15:4441–52.
134. Vaz R, Xavier P, Brito S, Dantas J, Duque S, Consciência JG, et al. Metallosis: a new form of autoimmune/autoinflammatory syndrome induced by adjuvants syndrome (ASIA)? Eur J Case Rep Intern Med. 2019;6(3):001034.
135. Chang X, Li J, Niu S, Xue Y, Tang M. Neurotoxicity of metal-containing nanoparticles and implications in glial cells. J Appl Toxicol. 2020;41:65–81.
136. Moretti B, Pesce V, Maccagnano G, Vicenti G, Lovreglio P, Soleo L, et al. Peripheral neuropathy after hip replacement failure: is vanadium the culprit? Lancet. 2012;379(9826):1676.
137. Oliveira CA, Candelária IS, Oliveira PB, Figueiredo A, Caseiro-Alves F. Metallosis: a diagnosis not only in patients with metal-on-metal prostheses. Eur J Radiol Open. 2015;2:3–6.
138. Igbokwe IO, Igwenagu E, Igbokwe NA. Aluminium toxicosis: a review of toxic actions and effects. Interdiscip Toxicol. 2019;12:45–70.
139. Mirza A, King A, Troakes C, Exley C. Aluminium in brain tissue in familial Alzheimer's disease. J Trace Elem Med Biol. 2017;40:30–6.
140. Mold M, Cottle J, Exley C. Aluminium in brain tissue in epilepsy: a case report from Camelford. Int J Environ Res Public Health. 2019;16:2129.
141. Savory J, Ghribi O. Can studies of aluminium toxicity in vivo and in vitro provide relevant information on the pathogenesis and aetiology of Alzheimer's disease? J Alzheimer's Dis. 2007;11:429–30.
142. Gopi G, Shanmugasundaram S, Krishnakumar Raja VB, Afradh KM. Evaluation of serum metal ion levels in dental implant patients: a prospective study. Ann Maxillofac Surg. 2021;11:261–5.
143. Daroit N, Visioli F, Magnusson A, Vieira GR, Rados P. Cell phone radiation effects on cytogenetic abnormalities of oral mucosal cells. Braz Oral Res. 2015;29:1–8.
144. Mishra S, Chowdhary R, Kumari S, Rao S. Effect of cell phone radiations on orofacial structures: a systematic review. J Clin Diagn Res. 2017;11(5):01–5.
145. Kundi M, Nersesyan A, Schmid G, Hutter HP, Eibensteiner F, Mišík M, et al. Mobile phone specific radiation disturbs cytokinesis and causes cell death but not acute chromosomal damage in buccal cells: results of a controlled human intervention study. Environ Res. 2024;251:118634.
146. Jovanovic DB, Krasic D, Cvetkovic NN, Vuckovic D, Stanković VB. Electric field and SAR distribution in the vicinity of dental implants exposed to the cell phone electromagnetic radiation. COMPEL. 2023;42(5):1052–67.
147. Siqueira EC, de Souza FTA, Ferreira E, Souza RP, Macedo SC, Friedman E, et al. Cell phone use is associated with an inflammatory cytokine profile of parotid gland saliva. J Oral Pathol Med. 2016;45(9):682–6.
148. Aisha A. Effect of mobile phone use with and without earphones on salivary nickel ion release from fixed orthodontic appliances: a cross-over trial. En [Internet]. 2018 [cited 2025 Jan 23]. Available from: https://www.semanticscholar.org/paper/Effect-of-mobile-phone-use-with-and-without-on-ion-Aisha/cbff4ac22f992a8827d64d12d3a4e7a1d7d44a59
149. Mortazavi SM, Daiee E, Yazdi A, Khiabani K, Kavousi A, Vazirinejad R, et al. Mercury release from dental amalgam restoration after magnetic resonance imaging and following mobile phone use. Pak J Biol Sci. 2008;11(8):1142–6.
150. Kavyashree M, Harish PV, Mishra SK, Chowdhary R. Cell phone radiation effect on bone-to-implant osseointegration: a preliminary histologic evaluation in rabbits. Int J Oral Maxillofac Implants. 2019;34(3):643–50.

151. Jing D, Zhai M, Tong S, Xu F, Cai J, Shen G, et al. Pulsed electromagnetic fields promote osteogenesis and osseointegration of porous titanium implants in bone defect repair through a Wnt/β-catenin signaling-associated mechanism. Sci Rep. 2016;6:32045.
152. Wessapan T, Rattanadecho P. Thermal effects of metal implants embedded in different layers of human tissues exposed to electromagnetic fields. Case Stud Therm Eng. 2024;53:103771.
153. Shojaee M, Seyed Majidi M, Jenabian N, Ebrahimi M, Yazdi M, Asgharpour F, et al. Assessment of cell phone effect on dental socket healing in rats. Minerva Dent Oral Sci. 2022;71(5):255–61.
154. Nayak RS, Shafiuddin B, Pasha A, Vinay K, Narayan A, Shetty SV. Comparison of galvanic currents generated between different combinations of orthodontic brackets and archwires using potentiostat: an in vitro study. J Int Oral Health. 2015;7(7):29–35.
155. Mathew MT, Abbey S, Hallab NJ, Hall DJ, Sukotjo C, Wimmer MA. Influence of pH on the tribocorrosion behavior of CpTi in the oral environment: synergistic interactions of wear and corrosion. J Biomed Mater Res B Appl Biomater. 2012;100B:1662–71.
156. Escalante E. Amalgam: a controversial mixture [Internet]. 2010 [cited 2025 Jan 20]. Available from: https://terapianeural.com/articulos/29-odontologia-neurofocal/216-amalgama-una-mezcla-controversial
157. Osorio Díaz Y, Fajardo MF. Bioelectronic measurements: a new diagnostic resource in dentistry. Rev Fed Odontol Colomb. 1997;54(191):36–41.
158. Nuñez-Lucio E. Electrogalvanism in neurofocal dentistry [Internet]. [date unknown] [cited 2025 Feb 10]. Available from: https://odontologosecuador.com/espanol/artodontologos/odontologia_neurofocal.htm.
159. Osorio-Diaz Y. Neurofocal dentistry: another rationality [Internet]. 2003 [cited 2020 Oct 13]. Available from: http://www.terapianeural.com/publicaciones/14-articulos-y-publicaciones/del-concepto/148-odontologia-neurofocal-qotra-racionalidadq.
160. Rost A. Dental foci: sanitation and therapy [Internet]. 2006 [cited 2025 Jan 20]. Available from: https://terapianeural.com/publicaciones/29-articulos-y-publicaciones/odontologia-neurofocal/134-focos-odontologicos-saneamiento-y-terapia
161. Cartagena-Montalvo SL. Oral rehabilitation in a patient with post-surgical sequelae from a tumor at the base of the skull from the perspective of neurofocal dentistry [Internet] [thesis]. Quito: Universidad Internacional del Ecuador; 2013 [cited 2025 Jan 10]. Available from: https://repositorio.uide.edu.ec/handle/37000/366
162. Delov V. Physiology of the muscles and nerves. In: Bykov KM, editor. Text-book of physiology. Moscow: Foreign Languages Publishing House; 1960. p. 516–670.
163. Bykov K, Konradi G. Fundamental concepts of physiology. In: Bykov KM, editor. Text-book of physiology. Moscow: Foreign Languages Publishing House; 1960. p. 15–45.
164. Speransky AD. A basis for the theory of medicine. New York: International Publishers; 1943.
165. Zueva EY, Zuev KB. The concept of dominance by A.A. Ukhtomsky and anticipation. In: Nadin M, editor. Anticipation: learning from the past: the Russian/soviet contributions to the science of anticipation. Cham: Springer International Publishing; 2015. p. 13–35. https://doi.org/10.1007/978-3-319-19446-2_2.

Chapter 45
Veterinary Neural Therapy

Rosane Aparecida Piloto Lopes Colares

1 Introduction

A few years ago, the author of this chapter received a call to schedule the care of a dog that had been found on the street, unable to walk. There was no history about the animal: it was not known if she had belonged to anyone, if she had been run over, or if there was some other factor that explained her immobility. The only relevant clinical data were that she could not move her legs or urinate on her own, and her bladder had to be compressed several times a day to empty it.

Andrea was the person who took care of the dog and brought her to the doctor's office, where she was treated with neural therapy (NT). The same night the dog was able to urinate on her own without the need for bladder compression, which brought great relief to all those who accompanied the animal's state of suffering. For the next 3 days, the dog maintained the ability to urinate unassisted; however, her legs remained immobilized. Andrea even provided a wheelchair to help the dog move, but to everyone's surprise, 4 days after the first visit, the dog started walking. It was a surprising recovery and hard to believe. The euphoria, however, was short-lived. The same day she walked again, the dog stopped urinating on her own, relying again on the compression of her bladder to eliminate urine. The situation persisted for two more days, which generated some frustration.

On the sixth day after initial care, without any therapeutic intervention having occurred beyond the start of treatment (first day), and to everyone's surprise, the dog

Supplementary Information The online version contains supplementary material available at https://doi.org/10.1007/978-3-032-03257-7_45.

R. A. Piloto Lopes Colares (✉)
Universidade Federal Fluminense, Niterói, Rio de Janeiro, Brazil
e-mail: rosluc@yahoo.com.br

L. B. Pinilla Bonilla et al. (eds.), *Neuraltherapeutic Medicine*,
https://doi.org/10.1007/978-3-032-03257-7_45

urinated again on her own and thus regained her autonomy, being able to walk and urinate without assistance.

The dog in question was named “Guria” and Andréa became her guardian. Guria became one of the great “teachers” of the neural therapy for this author, by demonstrating how the nervous system (NS) works in mysterious ways, “deciding” its priorities and capabilities, all in its own time. Guria taught the author that the human will, often guided by the linearity of logic, which guides veterinary medical treatment, is often not the determining factor in the recovery from a pathological process. The organism seems to possess an “intelligence of its own” and, through the nervous system, “chooses” its priorities by determining which circuits should be activated in response to new realities and stimuli (treatment).

It is not without reason that this brief story has been chosen to begin the chapter on veterinary neural therapy. The objective here was to draw attention to one of the theoretical bases that sustain NT, that is, the process of body self-regulation, which will be provided by a “stimulus” aimed at reducing an irritation existing in the body. This dynamic will be better explained throughout the text that will be developed.

For this chapter, the dog will be the animal of choice in the description of physiological processes and clinical reports. The choice is guided by a few reasons. First, due to the fact that this author, as a veterinarian, has a greater casuistry of canine care in relation to any other animal. This is a personal reason. Far more important than this personal reason, however, is the fact that dogs were the first animals domesticated by man, which is central to the understanding of their behavior. For veterinary NT, any analysis of a disease begins with the analysis of animal behavior. Similarly, dogs were the animals used by Pavlov in his studies of the conditioned reflex (classical conditioning) (see Chap. 13) [1–3]. Since Pavlov, there has been a clear understanding that both the behaviors and physiological dynamics of organisms have a reflex character and that pathological processes, according to Speransky, are the consequence of neurodystrophic processes[1] [4]. Understanding the relationship between reflex, behavior, and neurodystrophic processes is fundamental to the understanding of veterinary NT, as will be seen below [5].

2 Autonomic Nervous System

Sensory stimulation of any animal leads to a cascade of physiological events. A dog, for example, develops the following sequence of physiological reactions to a life-threatening situation: it will be alert, its body position will show that it is attentive.

[1] According to Toscano and Pinilla, “Neural therapy considers any pathological process as a dystrophy (from the Latin dys meaning bad and trophē, food-nutrition). This concept is taken from nervism; because the nervous system is the guide in all morbid processes, Speransky uses the term neurodystrophy to designate pathological processes. When a neurodystrophy occurs in the body, it is not the same again since it reorganizes itself to adapt by keeping a memory of its new condition, even generating cyclical phenomena, which are characteristic of chronic diseases [4]

In case the stimulus comes from another bigger dog invading his territorial limits, he must be prepared to make a decision that will be to "stay and fight" or "flee in retreat" [6].

For these reactions to occur, the dog relies on the Sympathetic Autonomic Nervous System (Sympathetic ANS) which provides behavioral responses that prepare the dog for what may happen. The dog's ears will stand erect to capture the source of the sound, the dog's pupils will dilate for greater visual acuity, and the dog will have piloerection to appear larger. Secretions from the adrenal gland will allow the muscles and heart to prepare for what is to come. The pain threshold increases, and the release of red blood cells through the spleen helps prevent injury. In order for the dog to have more energy, substrates are mobilized by stimulating lipolysis and glycogenolysis. All of these reactions occur involuntarily [6].

The NS, according to analytical physiology, has a division dedicated to involuntary processes called the Autonomic Nervous System (ANS) and the reactions described in the previous paragraph are an example of its action in the body. The ANS works as a specialization of the NS for events that require the maintenance of physiological functions in the face of constant variations in the environment, the so-called homeokinesis[2] [7].

In order for the ANS to perform homeokinesis, it has a sympathetic component and a parasympathetic component, which work in a complementary and antagonistic manner to modulate the body's actions and responses. This modulation uses feedback mechanisms to be able to measure the response of one and activate the other in a constant and uninterrupted involuntary system, that is, independent of the will or consciousness of the being [7].

The knowledge of the ANS for the veterinary neuraltherapist (VNT) is important because the behavior that the dog assumes when faced with a stimulus is the consequence of a whole machinery that involves afferent systems, coding systems, memorization systems, and effector systems. This entire process is aimed at the survival of the species [7, 8]. If any part of the entire machinery begins to "fail," some function will not be performed as expected. The "malfunction"of the organism will generate a neurodystrophic process that will be reflected in the animal's behavior.

For this reason, it is emphasized that the veterinarian who intends to study and use NT medicine must be familiar with the expected behavior of the species with which he will work, as well as knowing the physiology and anatomy of the ANS in question. Knowing these characteristics, the VNT will be able to identify changes in the ANS and this is fundamental for the detection of a possible future pathology, thus being able to act preventively. However, if the disease is already set in, he can map the pathway where there was the "failure in the information process" (irritation or neurodystrophic process for NT) and act with the aim of reestablishing homeokinesis.

---

[2] Homeokinesis: A term that encompasses homeostasis and more accurately reflects the process by showing that balance is achieved dynamically, not statically. The term encompasses many dynamic processes whose equilibrium is so highly controlled that, under abnormal circumstances, they appear static.

3 Organs of the Senses

Dog's sense organs are essential for their interaction with the environment, for their postural perception, and for communication, both with other dogs and with humans. Understanding basic aspects of the anatomy and physiology of these senses is essential to delineate how they determine the dog's behavior. As it is a patient who does not directly communicate what he is feeling (symptoms), analyzing the dog's behavior is essential to understanding the changes that may be caused by dystrophic processes of any nature.

The sensory organs play a crucial role in measuring stimuli to the nervous system (NS), allowing the latter to send information to the central nervous system (CNS) and the latter to make decisions about what behavior to adopt in different situations. The animals' CNS, as well as their sensory organs, evolved over time to meet adaptation and survival needs. In different species, some senses develop more than others, depending on environmental and behavioral demands [9]. As an example, some species have a keener sense of smell, while others have more developed hearing. This phylogenetic development is also reflected in brain organization, with specific areas of the brain, such as the olfactory cortex, occupying a greater or lesser proportion, depending on the species [1, 8].

Sensory organs are fundamental as communication channels between the environment and the NS, providing essential data for the brain to make appropriate decisions [8, 9] and similarly to the ANS's need for knowledge, the VNT can use information about the perceptions generated by the dogs' senses to identify where and how to act during consultation. An example of this need for knowledge can be identified by clinical experience. Dogs whose tails have been docked for aesthetic purposes often present excessive sensitivity in that area. The scar there can generate an increase in tactile sensitivity, indicating the origin of certain behaviors (aggression to touch, excessive fear, leakage of urine, submissive posture, scape to palpation, etc.). The kowledge nowledge of the sensory origin of these atypical behaviors is of utmost importance for identifying the type of treatment to which the patient will be subjected. In NT, the places where neurodystrophic phenomena occur (scarring, for example) usually include a wide spectrum of factors that will guide the map of possible application sites for NT techniques.

3.1 Vestibular System

The vestibular system is a specialized proprioception system that maintains the animal's orientation in relation to gravity and its natural position, whether in linear, rotational acceleration or head tilt. It plays a crucial role in coordinating the movements of the eyes, trunk, and limbs in response to the position and movement of the head [2, 5, 10].

The neurons involved in the vestibular system are located in the vestibular nucleus in the brainstem and are connected to receptors in the inner ear via cranial nerve VIII. The main receptors responsible for balance are located in the semicircular canals. To maintain proper posture and coordination of eye movements, vestibular stimuli are transmitted from the vestibular nucleus to the cerebellum by means of the medial longitudinal fasciculus which projects to the nuclei of cranial nerves III, IV, and VI [6].

In addition, the motor fibers of the vestibular nucleus project to all levels of the spinal cord through the vestibulo-spinal tracts, synapsing with interneurons in the ventral gray matter. The final effect of these projections is the facilitation of the ipsilateral extensor muscles, which is essential for the maintenance of extensor tone and the functioning of the stretch reflex. Both are fundamental components of the animal's anti-gravity system [6].

3.2 Vision

Vision is one of the most important senses for dogs, especially in relation to intra- and interspecies communication and learning behaviors. Through their body postures, dogs can express themselves, and vision plays an important role in this process. Dogs are able to visually perceive the intentions of certain postures and this is significantly reflected in their learning of behaviors, both with respect to the species itself and with respect to humans [8].

Canine vision is also essential for the protection of the animal, as it allows it to perceive threats in the environment, such as branches that can hurt it. In anatomical terms, vision is a highly developed sense, with a large number of receptors in the eye and a significant representation in the cerebral cortex [8].

The eyelid reflex protects the dog's eyes, being aided by the vibriso-palpebral reflex, which causes the animal to blink when its vibrissae (whiskers) are touched. This reflex is present even when puppies are born with their eyes closed, and light perception already begins early in development [8, 9].

Compared to humans, dogs' binocular vision spans a field of 60 to 116 degrees, while in humans it is 140 to 160 degrees. Each canine eye has an additional monocular field of 86 to 90 degrees, resulting in a total visual field of 240 to 290 degrees (see Fig. 45.1). This gives the dog a visual ability superior to that of humans, which is an evolutionary adaptation related to hunting. Blindness can alter a dog's behavior, especially when it comes to its interaction with the environment and communication with its guardians [7–9].

It is important for VNT to understand canine postures, as these postures are intimately linked to the dog's visual perception and can provide information about the animal's emotional state (see Fig. 45.2). During a veterinary consultation, observing these postures can provide crucial information about the animal's health, as well as indicating how to approach it during service to avoid unnecessary stress.

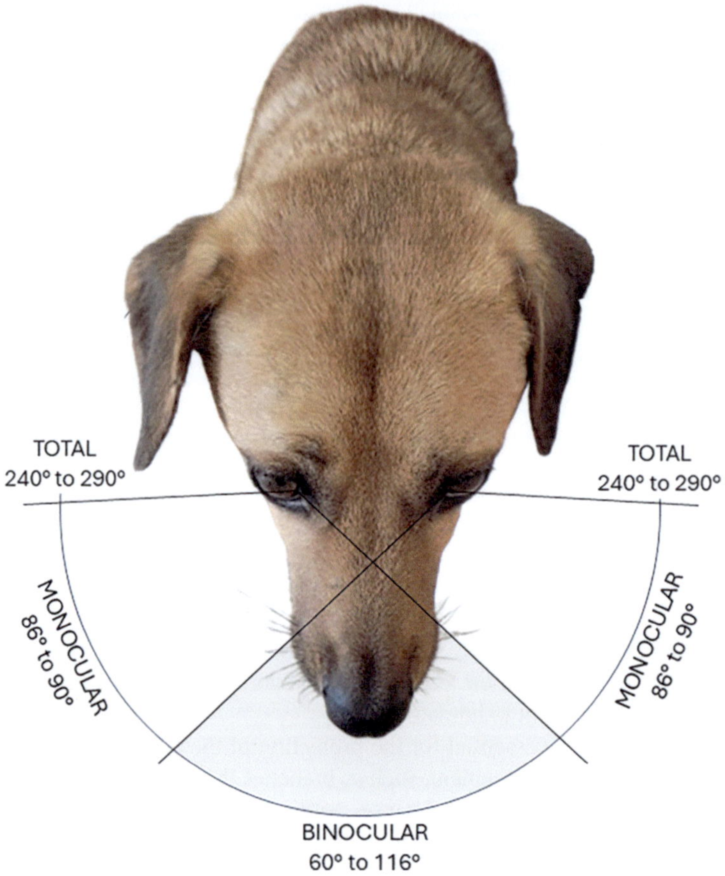

Fig. 45.1 Binocular vision of the dog. (Source: Own elaboration)

This author's clinical experience suggests that many irritative memories arise from traumas associated with vision imaging. A typical example is that of dogs that, upon seeing someone in a white coat, withdraw, flee, or become paralyzed, as they associate this image with medical-veterinary care that generated pain or discomfort. A dog that sees a veterinarian in a white coat may, for example, immediately associate it with the pain of an injection for the application of a vaccine. The knowledge that an irritative memory may have originated by sensory perception of vision is important for VNT. The observation of this aspect, associated with the life history (LH) (based on the anamnesis) and complemented by physical examinations, will lead the VNT to use the appropriate TN technique for each case.

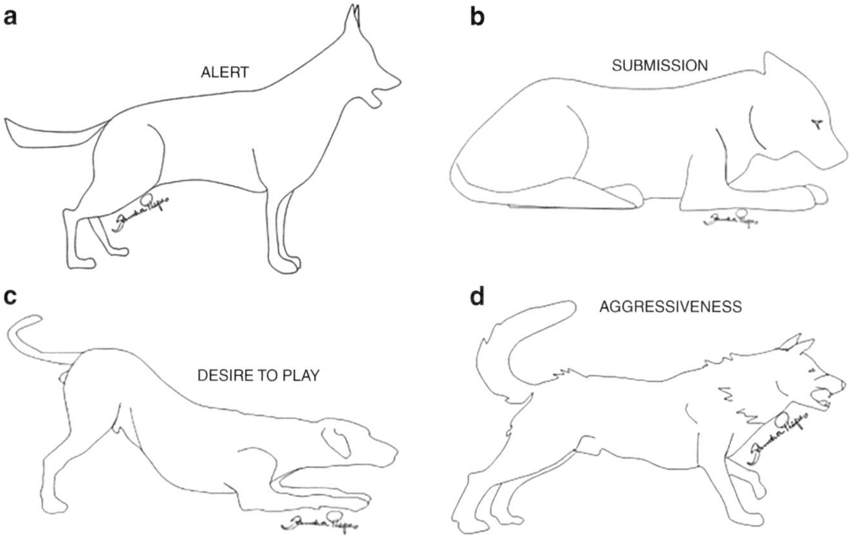

Fig. 45.2 Dog postures. (**a**) Posture of the dog on alert. (**b**) Posture of the dog in submission. (**c**) Dog pose inviting play. (**d**) Dog's posture showing aggression. (Source: Own elaboration)

3.3 Hearing

Canine hearing is also highly developed and plays a fundamental role in the animal's communication and behavior. Dogs can locate the source of sounds due to their ability to move their ears, which allows them to detect differences in the timing and intensity of sounds reaching each ear. This behavior is often observed when the dog tilts its head to better direct its ear [9].

Dogs have a hearing capacity ranging from 200 Hz to 15,000 Hz, being more sensitive to higher frequencies compared to humans, who have an auditory range of 20 Hz to 20,000 Hz. In addition, dogs' hearing sensitivity is better at frequencies above 8000 Hz [8, 9]. These data are relevant to the evaluation of the animal's hearing, as it allows VNT to better understand the dog's hearing ability and identify potential disorders.

The erection reflex in the ears, which occurs in response to a sound, is an important indicator of canine hearing. However, this reflex can be inconsistent at frequencies below 8000 Hz, which should be taken into account when performing behavioral tests to assess the dog's hearing [8, 9]. In addition, hearing also contributes to the animal's balance, aiding the limbic system and vestibular system in spatial perception and postural control [6, 7].

In terms of clinical experience, this author considers it important to highlight that many traumas and irritative memories in dogs end up occurring by virtue of their extreme auditory sensitivity, such as traumas derived from storms or fireworks. Collecting this important information in the anamnesis to detail LH well is essential for understanding the set of factors that lead to the development of fear behavior, for example.

3.4 Smell

Canine smell is notoriously superior to humans, being one of the main tools for perceiving the environment and communication. Dogs have between 220 million olfactory receptors, compared to 5 million in humans. The olfactory mucosa of dogs occupies an area of 75–150 cm^2, while in humans the area is only 5 cm^2 [9, 10].

That sense of smell allows dogs to detect smells associated with emotions and events, such as fear, and form olfactory memories linked to emotional experiences. The neural pathway that smells travels through the canine brain passes through areas such as the olfactory cortex, hippocampus, amygdala, and limbic system, which are intimately related to memory formation and emotional response [9, 11].

Smell is also related to behavior and learning, and it is possible to observe that exposure to odors associated with fearful situations can alter the animal's behavior, making it difficult to train and form bonds. This phenomenon is related to the intense connection between the olfactory system and the limbic system, which controls emotions [11].

This author's clinical experience corroborates the idea that, through smell, numerous emotional "triggers" can be activated, which can be reflected in atypical (unexpected) behaviors in dogs, which makes smell essential for the systemic analysis required for NT. Clinically, smell also seems to be associated with the formation of numerous memory registers, both positive and negative, which proves to be very important in the analysis of the association of certain olfactory experiences with trauma. As an example, this author has treated numerous dogs that, upon sniffing the scent of a feline patient in the author's white coat, bristled their hair and began to bark aggressively, evidencing that only the smell of an "unfriendly" species was enough to trigger fighting behavior, even without the visualization of another animal.

3.5 Taste

Although canine taste is less developed than smell, it also plays an important role in the perception of taste and in protecting the animal against the ingestion of potentially harmful substances. Canine taste is closely linked to smell, as both work together to determine the acceptability of a food or substance [7, 8].

3.6 Touch

Touch is a vital sense for the animal, being important not only for the perception of the environment but also for communication and social interaction, as is the case of piloerection, which can be a way of showing itself, particularly among members of a herd as well as for enemies. Touch begins to develop from birth and is essential for the animal body's perception [8].

Importantly, sensory perception is not limited to the sense organs alone. Other elements, such as dermatomes, fascia, and teeth, also play important roles in sensory inputs and can directly influence the way the body records, learns, and uses information from the environment. The process of memorization and learning from sensory stimuli is essential for the adaptation of the organism and for the formation of memories that will guide its future reactions and behaviors [1, 3, 8]. Important considerations regarding these elements will be made in the following paragraphs.

4 Dermatomes

Dermatomes are regions of the skin innervated by afferent fibers from a single spinal nerve. These regions form continuous fields and are arranged overlapping along the body, from the cranial region to the caudal region (see Fig. 45.3) [6, 12].

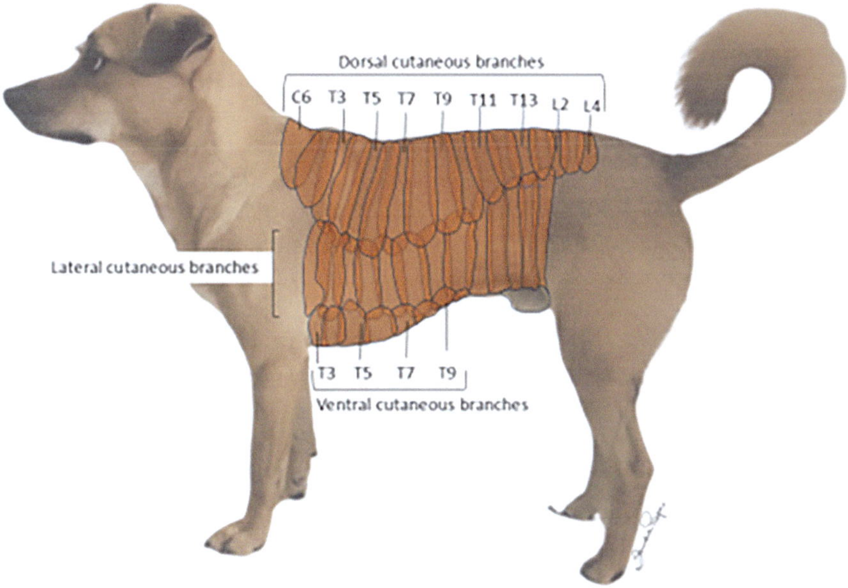

Fig. 45.3 Schematic illustration of the dog's dermatomes (thorax and part of the lumbar region). (Source: Own elaboration)

Knowledge of dermatomes is of great importance to VNT because it allows the therapist to examine and evaluate the sensory responses of the animal from a subtle pinch and roll or fold test of the skin along the entire segment of the spine [13]. This examination can help locate changes in innervation, changes in the fascia segment, as well as provide valuable information for diagnosis and treatment [13].

Observation of this author's clinical experience suggests that, during the animal's growth period, areas of possible injury or irritation of a dermatome may be modified due to expansion or displacement of body structures, which may alter the location of the original lesion. Therefore, it is critical that the VNT be attentive to these changes, tailoring assessment and treatment as needed.

5 Fasciae

The author's interest in the study of fascia arose from her clinical experience when caring for a turtle (*Trachemys dorbigni*) that had suffered a fall, resulting in a scar on its shell. The hardness of the shell restricted the choice of site for direct application of procaine (diluted local anesthetic). The inability to apply procaine directly to the site of injury led to the search for an alternative. In a fairly summarized way, it can be said that fasciae connect all parts of the body and can serve as channels for the transmission of information different from traditional synapses.

The fascination is part of Pischinger's basic system (see Chap. 11), or extracellular matrix, which also acts as a communication system, transmitting information to the body not only through synapses but in a broader and more ubiquitous way. This system facilitates the coordination and response of the body to stimuli of various natures [14, 15].

Each anatomical region of the dog has the participation of the fascia, which are commonly divided into superficial and deep. The superficial fascia is defined as an enveloping layer, located directly under the skin. It divides the hypodermis into superficial and deep compartments, the first being related to exteroception and the second to interoception. The deep fascia is a fibrous membrane that forms an intricate network, wrapping around and separating muscles, forming sheaths for nerves and vessels, strengthening the ligaments around the joints, and binding all of these structures together into a compact, firm mass [15]. Studies have shown that this complex three-dimensional network of fascia is involved in the perception and coordination of movement, as well as facilitating the transmission of muscle force and the functional connection between the body and the extremities (see Fig. 45.4). The presence of nociceptive fibers in fascial tissue has recently been discovered, which can contribute to the perception of pain and other sensations in the body [14, 15].

The clinical experience of this author suggests that knowledge about fasciae in animals helps in the diagnosis and treatment of areas affected by irritative memories, contributing to a greater understanding of the functioning of the NS of each being. It can often be an alternative to deep NT applications, as the fasciae connect

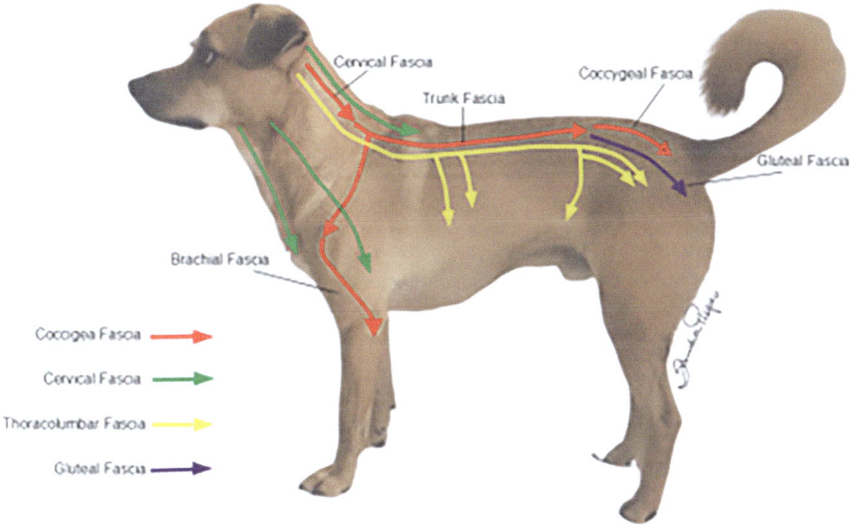

Fig. 45.4 Schematic illustration of the superficial fasciae of the dog. (Source: Own elaboration)

to deeper structures, and in veterinary medicine, the animals do not always remain immobile long enough for the deep application to be carried out safely. In this context, the application on fasciae becomes a viable option to consider.

In summary, the study of fasciae can be a viable strategy when it is not possible to make deep applications due to anatomical or behavioral limitations of the animals.

6 Teeth

Teeth play a critical role in the health and well-being of dogs, although they are often neglected. Generally, they are observed only to identify the age of the animal or detect possible dental problems without association with other health problems [16]. In the best of cases, the veterinary medical literature has linked the appearance of tartar with bacterial myocarditis [17]. However, it is important to highlight the relevance of teeth, especially in practices such as VNT [13]. Studies on teeth and their importance for NT tend to focus on human medicine, being rare or nonexistent in veterinary medicine. For this reason, it is important to clarify that the following paragraphs are based on the author's clinical experience.

Although the term neurofocal dentistry (NFD) is not used in VNT, teeth represent a significant part of therapeutic care for several reasons. From an embryonic point of view, tooth formation can be affected by circumstances such as the distemper virus, which can result in teeth without enamel [17]. This aspect can serve as an indication of the appearance of diseases during embryologic development, and, throughout the animal's life, these marks are recorded both in the formation and in

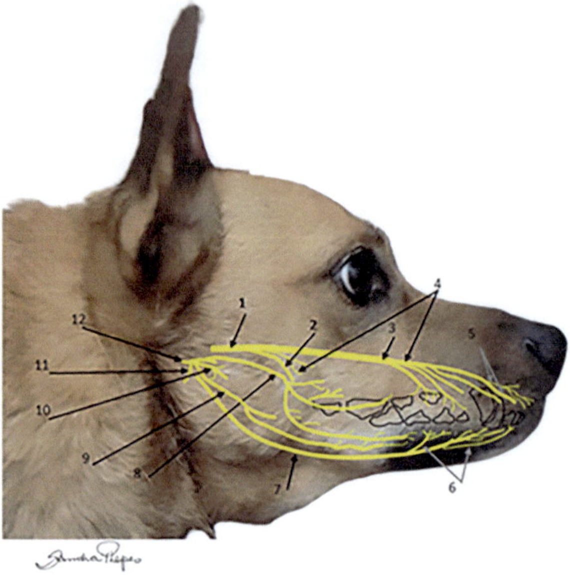

Fig. 45.5 Schematic innervation of the dog's teeth. Trigeminal nerve and branches (**a**). Ophthalmic: not illustrated; (**b**). Maxillary branches: 1, 2, 3, 4, 5; (**c**). Mandibular branches: 12, 11, 10, 9, 8, 7, 6. (1). Maxillary nerve; (2). Pterygopalatine nerve; (3). Infra-orbital nerve zygomatic nerve; (4). Upper alveolar branches; (5). Nasal and labial; (6). Mental nerves; (7). Inferior alveolar nerve; (8). Nerve buccalis; (9). Lingual nerve; (10). Maseteric nerve; (11). Auriculotemporal nerve; (12). Mandibular nerve. (Source: Own elaboration)

the change of teeth and can become an irritative memory or interfering field (IF) [13, 18].

In addition, the teeth and their innervations account for a large part of the innervation of the dog's muzzle (see Fig. 45.5) [12, 16], a highly sensitive region. The dog's mouth, for example, is capable of carrying its puppies without hurting them and, at the same time, can be used to kill or subjugate prey or foe, playing a vital role in the animal's defense and communication. In this way, the teeth also influence the dog's hierarchical position within its social group [8].

Dogs use their teeth as part of their communication [8], as they are directly connected to facial mimicry. The general condition of the teeth can, therefore, provide important information about the animal's NS, reflecting its emotional state and overall health.

Although it is not possible to state with certainty that there is an exact percentage of IF in the teeth, as discussed by Adler in his book, it is possible to state that the teeth play a significant role as IF [13]. For this reason, the VNT must always examine the condition of the animal's teeth, evaluating, for example, possible fractures of canines, which are usually common in dogs.

Another important point to consider is changing teeth in dogs. This process occurs at a critical period in the animal's life, when important events such as the animal's socialization occur [8]. In this same period, vaccines are applied. It is a period in which changes in feeding, castration, application of microchips for identification, first grooming, change of environment and training usually occur. Changing teeth, therefore, can save memories of important experiences lived by the dog, and this can have a significant impact on its behavior and development.

In addition, the condition of the gums also deserves attention since their lubrication is a direct reflection of the ANS, where the acting parasympathetic allows greater saliva production [12]. The absence of saliva production can be interpreted as a sign of stress.

Therefore, teeth are important in the afferent pathways of the ANS and, consequently, in the behavior of the animal, constituting important places of records of dystrophic phenomena.

7 Behavior, Learning Process of Dogs, and Other Interactions Related to Dystrophic Processes

The dog's behavior results from a coordinated action of the nervous system (NS), which responds to stimuli from the environment (external stimuli) and from its own body (internal stimuli) [8]. Thus, hormonal changes would be examples of internal stimuli, and the smell of a food would be the example of an external stimulus. These stimuli, in turn, always act together. The pathways by which this information (internal and external) reaches the CNS vary, depending on the type and location of the stimulus. These variations are evolutionary adaptations that the dog developed for its survival [2, 19].

The response provided by the CNS, which culminates in a behavior, depends on the coding and storage of information, in addition to the evaluation of the energy expenditure involved. That is, the CNS assesses the importance of the stimulus and coordinates the response efficiently to ensure that the behavior is as economical as possible. The multiplicity of behaviors that the dog can exhibit is influenced by several factors, including the degree of maturation of the NS itself, the development of the sense organs, and motor ability [8].

Once the basic physiological mechanism of the origin of behavior is understood, one can better understand how the relationship between man and dog is processed. The relationships between man and dog, since the process of domestication of the latter, imply the establishment of a learned behavior, then initiated by an external stimulus. This learned behavior, which was generated by an external stimulus, triggers physiological responses. These responses, in turn, can lead to the triggering of a pathology. According to Speransky, the repetition of an external stimulus, invariably and repeatedly, can trigger dystrophic phenomena (temporary or permanent) that will be reflected in any part of the body, affecting afferent or any information route to the cerebral cortex. Consequently, external stimuli, when applied invariably and repeatedly, may be related to the origin of a pathological focus [5].

What determines the organism to develop a pathological picture or not will depend on the "initial state of the cerebral cortex, the subcortical centers, the reticular formation, the vegetative nervous system, the isolated nerves and the peripheral components." This pathology may be the result of a "protective inhibition"of the NS or its "increased sensitivity" [5].

By way of conclusion, it is valid to assume that the interactions between man and dog constitute possible sources of stimuli to trigger neurodystrophic phenomena, depending on the type of external stimulus involved in the learning processes and the initial state of the system (neurophysiological conditions of the organism). Therefore, for the VNT, in addition to the clinical examination, it becomes essential to analyze the conditions that involve the learning environment of the behaviors of a given dog, which will be obtained in a good anamnesis and in the detailed description of its LH.

In the same way that an external stimulus that is mismanaged (invariably and repeatedly) in the dog's learning process can generate a neurodystrophic phenomenon, other factors can also be involved in similar irritant processes. Repeated and persistent emotions, viral or infectious diseases, or a simple castration (scar), provided that they have occurred in a weakened organism (initial stage), follow the same process of formation of pathological foci and also deserve the attention of the VNT on the occasion of medical care.

8 Local Anesthetic

The use of procaine in dogs and horses for therapeutic purposes was first proposed by I. Ya. Tijoinin under the supervision of A. V. Vishnevsky and L. S. Sapózhnikov *apud* [5] taking into account the action of procaine in the mediations of the nerve branches. Knowledge of the functioning of the ANS in animals and the conditions capable of altering it were the basis for the use of procaine in weak dilutions 0.25–0.5% as a treatment [5].

A.V. Vishnevski *apud* [5] argued and discovered that the healing effect of procaine on the somatic and vegetative nervous systems replaced a strong stimulus in the NS with a weak one; therefore, the inflammatory reaction decreases, leading to a predominance of the regenerative component.

Recent studies show that procaine is able to relieve neuropathic pain in rats [20]. Other studies have found that procaine is capable of acting on the limbic system by modifying the excitability threshold. Consequently, modifying the perception of fear in rats [21]. Other studies demonstrate decreased sinoaortic reflex under procaine action in cats [22].

However, not all mechanisms of action of procaine in animals are known, but the use of procaine in veterinary NT does not differ from NT and NFD used in humans. Scientific thinking and scientific bases are the same. The needles are the same in terms of caliber as those used in human NT and NFD. What may differ from human NT or NFD is the volume to be used at some application sites due to the anatomical differences of dog breeds and other animals compared to humans and the total dose with respect to the maximum dose of procaine in each species [23] (see Table 45.1).

The choice of diluted local anesthetic (procaine hydrochloride or lidocaine) depends on the practitioner's decision. The acquisition of the anesthetic and the current legislation on the use of local anesthetics in the country where the veterinarian

Table 45.1 Anesthetic dose and maximum dose of LA used in veterinary TN

Local anesthetic	Directions	Dose	Species
Procaine chloridrate	Nerve blocks	2–4 mg/kg	Dogs
Procaine chloridrate	Nerve blocks	Maximum dose 3–5 mg/kg	Cats
Procaine chloridrate	Nerve blocks	Maximum dose 6–10 mg/kg	Dogs
Lidocaine	Nerve block	4 mg/kg (2% solution)	Dogs and cats
Lidocaine	Nerve block	Maximum dose 5–6 mg/kg 2–3 mg/kg	Dogs, horses, cats

Source: Own elaboration

operates may vary, which may facilitate or hinder access to the drug. Another aspect that may influence the choice of LA is its metabolization pathway, where lidocaine is metabolized in the liver and procaine is metabolized by acetylcholinesterase [24, 25, 26].

The concentrations of procaine used in veterinary TN range from 0.25% to 1% [21, 24]. It should be noted that the use of procaine hydrochloride in competition horses is considered doping by sports legislation. Its metabolites are detected in the urine and bloodstream for up to 48 hours after application when used in the anesthetic dose [24, 27].

The author of this chapter has clinically observed that, invariably, the dog exhibits the behavior of licking the lips and swallowing immediately after the application of procaine 0.5%. In humans, there are reports of a metallic taste arising in the mouth after a few applications of procaine. Nothing has been found in the scientific literature about the metallic taste perceived by dogs after administration of procaine.

Current studies on the use of procaine in animals use anesthetic doses and are mostly conducted in rats. However, it is what is available as knowledge. Further research with dilute doses of procaine is still needed to confirm all mechanisms of action.

9 Consultation

The consultation at the veterinary TN follows a similar approach to the veterinary consultation. In the face of the main complaint of the guardian, the veterinarian adds the patient's identification information, history, and LH added to physical examination. Ancillary diagnostic tests can complement the consultation. Generally speaking, clinical consultation of NT does not differ significantly from consultation of NT or NFD in humans. The main difference is that, in the case of the animal, the guardian assumes the role of interlocutor, providing information about the events for which the patient was subjected.

A question about the veterinary service is: how to proceed when there is no interlocutor to tell the LH, when the animal was found at that time, or when it is a wild animal from the wild, without a guardian. Such a situation is quite common and, as the consultation, it is built on some fundamental pillars such as: observation of the animal, evaluation of behavior at the time of consultation, physical examination, and complementation with what is known about the individual identification of the patient, such as breed, sex, and general condition. Each of these elements complements the others, and in the absence of LH data, the veterinarian can use the available information, such as species, breed, coat, sex, approximate age, and general condition, so that it is possible to draw a mental map of what may be happening with the animal. The physical examination will be definitive in guiding the veterinarian through the body's responses and behavior and guiding the veterinarian where to apply the procaine.

9.1 Life History

The life history (LH) of the veterinary patient is elaborated by asking questions about all relevant aspects of the animal's life, in order of appearance, as chronologically as possible. It is an account of the events and complications that marked the patient's life, including the arrival of the animal in the lives of the guardians. It is important to inquire about: surgical events, prophylactic events, recurrent diseases, hospitalizations, and emotional and behavioral aspects of the animal. The bond between the animal and another being should be part of the list of questions.

As a guide, the following questions are suggested:

1. Daily habits: Ask about the animal's daily habits, such as food, physical exercises, and general behaviors.
2. Health history: Investigate the life complications of dogs, including frequent illnesses and episodes of parasitism (such as ticks, fleas, internal parasites, or hemoparasitism). If the animal is currently using or has previously used any medication. If she has already become pregnant in the case of females and if she has copulated in the case of males.
3. Surgical procedures: Report any surgery the animal has undergone, including the reason for the surgery, the procedure performed, and recovery. Ask if the animal is neutered or has undergone a cesarean section. Cosmetic or traumatic surgeries: Include questions about cosmetic surgeries, such as ear cutting, tail, removal of fingers or hernias, and placement of prostheses.
4. Vaccinations: Identify the vaccines applied, the place of application, and the behavior of the animal after vaccinations.
5. Oral health: Ask about tooth changes, the presence of deciduous teeth, tooth loss, fractures, or dental prophylaxis procedures.

6. Hospitalizations: Check if the animal has been hospitalized for surgeries or other health conditions.
7. Identification: Ask if the animal was microchipped or tattooed.
8. Complementary tests: If there is any imaging test or hematological or biochemical analysis.
9. Behavioral habits: Explore the animal's behavior in relation to its feeding, exercises, walks, socialization with other animals and people, as well as its general temperament.
10. Sleeping and elimination habits: Ask about the sleeping and waking habits where the animal usually sleeps, as well as its defecation and urination habits.
11. Living environment: Ask if the animal lives in a house or apartment, and if it has free access to the street. If you are afraid of thunder and rain or a phobia.
12. Link with the guardians and purpose of the animal: The veterinarian must also inquire about the arrival of the animal in the life of the guardians, the bond created between them and other members of the residence, in addition to clarifying the purpose of the animal (as a companion or working animal).

The questions asked during the consultation aim to assess the animal's general condition, how its NS reacts or processes possible irritative records throughout life, chronologically, in an attempt to establish where such irritative records occurred.

It should be noted that, even with the guardian's story, it is not always possible to obtain information about the animal's first experiences, such as birth, lactation, learning, and socialization.

Finally, complementing the LH and anamnesis, the veterinarian proceeds to the physical examination, with the aim of collecting additional data for diagnosis and treatment.

9.2 Physical Examination

The examination of the animal begins just before we put our hands on it. The observation of the animal's behavior in the face of the veterinarian's approach is already part of the examination.

The veterinarian must remain calm and approach the dog gently. Speak little and in a low tone, touching the animal gently. The veterinarian is fully attentive to any animal response during the test.

The clinical examination is extremely important not only because it provides additional information in the diagnosis and guides treatment, but it is often the only source of information that the animal provides to the veterinarian when there is no LH in cases where the animal is found and brought to the veterinary office without a tutor.

All parts of the body should be examined. In Video 45.1, there is a suggested sequence of physical examinations that the author follows with her patients.

Here follows a sequence that summarizes the canine clinical examination: (A) Head Assessment: palpation of the head gently, covering the innervations of the supraorbital, infraorbital; ears, temporomandibular joint, parotid glands, thyroid and an evaluation of the teeth and gums by placing the finger in the gingival sulcus of the teeth and gums by placing the finger in the gingival sulcus of the teeth of the mandible and maxilla. Observe the dog's behavior at the time of the examination. Areas of the head with differences in temperature of the skin, scars, absence of fur, discomfort, and/or pain should be recorded as possible areas of irritation. Include in your observation occlusion, saliva production, teeth condition, pupil reflex, and eyelids. (B) Palpation of the entire spinal column: The skin of the spine should be examined with the tips of the fingers performing a gentle impingement called "rolling clamping"to detect areas with greater or lesser sensitivity, adhesions, or normal areas that reflect the state of the dorsal nerve roots of the medulla [13]. The veterinarian may assess the dog from the nape of the neck to the base of the tail. Include the whole tail in the examination. Observe the animal's behavior at the time of the examination. Areas of the spine with subcutaneous adhesions, temperature differences, scars, absence of fur, discomfort, and/or pain should be recorded as possible areas of irritation. (C) Palpation of the ventral region of the dog: from the manubrium to the pubis, gently, checking for areas of adhesions, tumors, changes of skin color, sensitivity, discomfort, and/or pain. Observe the dog's reaction to the exam. Areas of the ventral segment with subcutaneous adhesions, temperature differences, scars, absence of fur, discomfort, and/or pain should be recorded as possible areas of irritation.

Observe the gait and positioning of the dog's body in station and in movement. Include inspection of the limbs and their joints, posture, symmetry of the dog's hole body, observe the wear of the nails, areas of the joints with painful sensitivity, pressure sores, decreased range of motion, increased volume or temperature changes, and scars, as well as the muscle mass abnormalities and painful sensitivity, should be considered at the time of the clinical evaluation of veterinary NT.

The physical examination helps to create a "mental map" of the places where there has been a reaction of the animal that, together with the LH, contributes to deciding the place of application of procaine.

Before starting the application of procaine in the animal, the guardian must be informed about the procedure, signing a free and informed consent, and authorizing the application since it is still an experimental procedure in some countries.

10 Final Considerations

The practice of NT applied to veterinary medicine is rather recent, the latter lacking works aimed at the dissemination of the specialty (NT) and the analysis of basic clinical aspects that involve the subject.

In this sense, this chapter sought to reconcile the description of the fundamentals of NT with the most relevant physiological aspects of the dog, aspects observed in the course of clinical practice during the author's career.

The description of the functioning of the sensory organs aimed to demonstrate the relationship of each of them with the NS, highlighting that these organs act systemically, which explains that a neurodystrophic process can impact any part of the body, with possible behavioral changes. The veterinarian, in his daily clinical practice, must always be attentive to changes in behavior, which constitute the first manifestations of dystrophism.

In addition to the sensory organs, other aspects relevant to NT involving the dog's physiology were appreciated. The analysis of the dermatomes shows the clinician the location, in the skin, of a neurodystrophic process originating in the dorsal root of the spine. Fascia, in turn, demonstrates that bodily connections go far beyond neural connections. Teeth, often neglected by the literature of veterinary medicine, have proven fundamental for the understanding of neurodystrophic processes by reflecting, among others, how the dog behaves and relates to the environment.

Finally, the therapeutic potencial of procaine, extending beyond its anesthetic hole, highlights the importance of proper administration by the veterinarian. A thorough understandingof its effects on de ANS is essencial for promoting funcional recovery and restoring physiological balance.

The practical guide to the physical examination and the correct obtaining of the patient's LH was a personal contribution of an empirical (practical) nature in order to facilitate and elucidate clinical aspects, which are rarely dealt with in the veterinary medical literature and, in particular, in the literature of veterinary TN. Its reading should not be dogmatic and should not be taken as the adoption of definitive and obligatory procedures, but only taken as a guide, a direction, an example.

To conclude, this author emphasizes the importance of the continuous study of anatomy, the improvement of application techniques, and the constant updating of scientific discoveries that should complement the daily life of the VNT. However, it is essential that the patient is his or her greatest teacher, where in each consultation the veterinarian has the opportunity to understand its complexities and act effectively.

References

1. Dethier VG, Stellar E. Animal behavior. São Paulo: Edgard Blusher/Edusp; 1973.
2. Bykov KM. Text-book of physiology. Moscow: Foreign Languages Publishing House; 1960. p. 767.
3. Bear MF, Connors BW, Paradiso MA. Neurosciences: unraveling the nervous system. Porto Alegre: Artmed Editora; 2017.
4. Toscano de la Torre F, Pinilla Bonilla LB. The principles of neural therapy from the fundamentals of nervism to current neuroscience. Salud UIS. 2012;44(2):57–65.
5. Plajotin MV. Manual of veterinary surgery. Moscu: Imported pub; 1983.
6. Lorenz MD, Kornegay JN. Veterinary neurology. Ciudad de México: unknown Publisher. 2006:323–44.

7. Dukes HH, Swenson MJ, Reece WO. Dukes' physiology of domestic animals. Rio de Janeiro: Editora Guanabara Koogan; 1996.
8. Manteca Vilanova X. Veterinary ethology. Barcelona: Editorial Multimedica S/A; 2009. p. 261.
9. Beaver BV. Canine behavior: a guide for veterinarians. São Paulo: Roca; 2001.
10. Melvin J, Reece WO. Dukes – physiology of domestic animals. In: Dukes HH, editor. Dukes: physiology of domestic animals. Rio de Janeiro: Editorial Guanabara Koogan S/A; 1996.
11. Nagasawa M, et al. Oxytocin-gaze positive loop and the coevolution of human-dog bonds. Science. 2015;348(6232):333–6.
12. Evans HE, Lahunta A. Miller's anatomy of the dog. 4th ed. St. Louis: Elsevier Health Sciences; 2012.
13. Draehmpaehl D, Zohmann A. Acupuncture in dogs and cats: scientific foundations and practice. Stuttgart: Georg Thieme Verlag; 1998.
14. Bordoni B, Mahabadi N, Varacallo M. Anatomy, fascia. [Internet]. 2018 [cited 2025 Jan 7]. Available from: https://www.ncbi.nlm.nih.gov/books/NBK538338/
15. Longo F, Mastrangelo G. Manual of integrated fascial technique in dogs, horses, and cats. Milano: NOI Edizioni s.r.l; 2021.
16. Román FS. Atlas of dentistry for small animals. São Paulo: Editora Manole Ltda; 1999. p. 115–9.
17. Ettinger SJ, Feldman EC. Treatise on veterinary internal medicine, vol. 1. 5th ed. St. ed. Louis: Elsevier; 2010.
18. Kidd RF. Neural therapy: applied neurophysiology and other topics. Ohnario: GeneralStore PublishingHouse; 2005.
19. Noden DN, et al. Embryology of domestic animals: developmental mechanisms and malformations. 1990.
20. Li D, et al. Procaine attenuates pain behaviors of neuropathic pain model rats possibly via inhibiting JAK2/STAT3. Biomol Ther. 2016;24(5):489–95.
21. Matulewicz P, et al. Hippocampal theta rhythm after local administration of procaine or amphetamine into the ventral tegmental area in fear conditioned rats. Neurosci Lett. 2015;589:132–7.
22. Tanikawa M. Inhibitory action of procaine upon the reflex bradycardia caused by barium, calcium, digitalis, and adrenaline. J Pharmacol. 1954;3(2):118–28.
23. Tranquilli WJ, Thurmon JC, Grimm KA, editors. Lumb and Jones' veterinary anesthesia and analgesia. 5th ed. Hoboken: Wiley; 2013.
24. Booth NH, McDonald LE. Pharmacology and therapeutics in veterinary medicine. Rio de Janeiro: ED; 1992. p. 323–5.
25. Hernández E. Manual of neural therapy in veterinary medicine: a complementary therapy for clinical practice in dogs. Mexico City: Unknown Publisher; 2006.
26. Castro RA. Bases for neural therapy in canines and felines. Buenos Aires: Dunken; 2011. p. 304.
27. Spinosa HS, Górniak SL, Bernardi MM. Pharmacology applied to veterinary medicine. Rio de Janeiro: Editora Guanabara Koogan S/A; 2006.

Chapter 46
Social Contributions to the Complex Conception of Neuraltherapeutic Medicine

Esperanza Cerón-Villaquirán, Mauricio Torres-Tovar, and Francisco Javier Echandía Bocanegra

The doctor who only knows medicine, no medicine knows

Dr. Josep de Letamendi (1828–1897)

1 Introduction

The purpose of this text is to reflect on the moment in which Neuraltherapeutic Medicine (NTM), community medicine, Primary Health Care (PHC), and Participatory Action Research (PAR) met in a concrete experience at the "La Nueva Esperanza" Health Center (NEHC), in the Department of Cauca, Colombia. This experience became a gateway through which one can continue walking and building a vision and practice from the integral complexity of health. An experience that contributed to the development of what is now known as the Julio Cesar Payán de la Roche School of Thought[1] and that allowed Dr. Payán to round off an epistemic and

[1] Dr. Julio Cesar Payán de la Roche, Physician and Surgeon, Specialist in Gynecology and Obstetrics at the University of Cauca. He joined the Faculty of Health Sciences where he was Professor of the Medicine program, Head of the Department of Gynecology and Obstetrics and Dean of this Academic Unit. Doctor of the Los Robles School of Neural Therapy, president of the CIMA Center for Research in Alternative Medicines, member of the Board of Directors and Director of the Foundation for Popular Communication, FUNCOP. Councilor of the city of Popayán, teacher of Neural Therapy in his office, at the "La Nueva Esperanza" Health Center in Popayán and in several Ibero-American countries.

E. Cerón-Villaquirán (✉) · F. J. Echandía Bocanegra
Master in Alternative Medicine, Neural Therapy Area, Faculty of Medicine,
Universidad Nacional de Colombia, Bogotá, Colombia
e-mail: fechandia@unal.edu.co; esperania@gmail.com

M. Torres-Tovar
Faculty of Medicine. Department of Public Health, Facultad de Medicina,
Universidad Nacional de Colombia, Bogotá, Colombia
e-mail: mhtorrest@unal.edu.co

L. B. Pinilla Bonilla et al. (eds.), *Neuraltherapeutic Medicine*,
https://doi.org/10.1007/978-3-032-03257-7_46

pedagogical corpus, which earned him the nickname of "philosopher of neural therapy,"as he was known in Europe.

The text is structured in three segments. The first presents some general elements of both Neuraltherapeutic Medicine and Primary Health Care, Participatory Action Research, and Community Medicine, as they together shared general bases of thought that allowed them to resonate with each other. These three approaches start with a critique of the mechanistic vision of science and the biomedical model, weaving in the discourse and practice within the pedagogical and epistemic framework of the School of Neuraltherapeutic Thought.

The second segment presents the way in which these currents were rooted in a particular way in a concrete experience of community health, through the NEHC. And in the last one, some conclusions are proposed that are expected to give rise to the continuation of this necessary dialogue of knowledge that enriches a new look at public health.

2 Approaches and Practices That Converged in the Experience

2.1 *Neuraltherapeutic Medicine*

Neuraltherapeutic medicine (NTM) arrived in Colombia by the hand of Dr. Germán Duque Mejía,[2] who studied medicine and specialized in internal medicine and gynecology in Germany [1]. A detailed story that can be read in Chap. 3 of this same book.

It arrived in the early 70 s as a therapy called Neural Therapy, which soon took root in a group of doctors who for two decades taught and practiced it in the Hacienda and therapeutic center "Los Robles" on the outskirts of Popayán, in the Department of Cauca in Colombia (see Fig. 46.1). It achieved so much success that brought patients from the most diverse corners of the country and Latin America [2, 3].

One of the reasons for the massive presence of local patients that arose, in addition to the effectiveness, was the warmth and very low costs of care. It had to do with the cultural context of the Department of Cauca, whose population was more than 80% rural, possessing a diversity of knowledge and practices of its own in health, which the anthropologist Hugo Portela calls different "cultures of health"[4]. The fact that, for centuries, isolated populations had addressed their problems with their own ancestral knowledge allowed a resonance with a medicine that explored the body a lot, listened very carefully, and did not despise the knowledge of

[2] Dr. Germán Duque Mejía, an obstetrician-gynecologist and internist trained in Germany. He studied Neural Therapy with Dr. Peter Dosh among other German pioneers. He founded in the 70s the Los Robles School-Clinic on the outskirts of Popayán, where for more than a decade, he treated and trained more than 1700 doctors from all over Latin America. As a result of the earthquake that destroyed the city of Popayán, he moved to Arbeláez, Cundinamarca, where he founded the Kirpalamar Clinic and continued his teaching work.

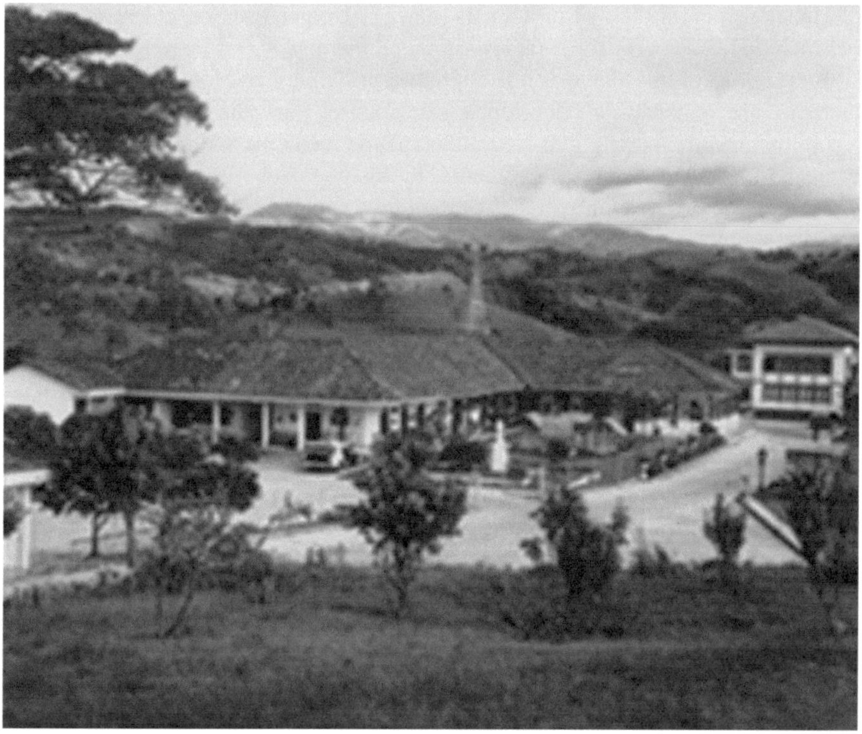

Fig. 46.1 Hacienda Los Robles, Popayán-Cauca. 1990s. (Source: Photo from personal archive of Dr. Germán Duque Mejía)

indigenous, Afro-Colombian, Roma, and peasant communities, and even less neglected the stories and explanations of the patients.

The therapeutic center "Los Robles" was a kind of Tower of Babel, where all those local and even foreign health cultures felt included and respected. It is likely that this process was also influenced by the meetings that Dr. Duque had witnessed at that time and for decades in Baden-Baden.[3]

The consultants who came to Los Robles by the dozens a day were treated with neural therapy and diet therapy, and little by little, other approaches were added. Dr. Germán Duque received frequent visits from other German doctors, namely: Dr. Reinhold Voll—father of electroacupuncture that bears his name; Dr. Franz Hopfer, Austrian physician and dentist of neural therapy; Dr. Helmut Regelsberger, neural therapist and expert in cell therapy; Dr. Ernesto Adler, father of neurofocal dentistry (NFD), Dr. Hans Haensler and Dr. Renate Haensler-Viebahn pioneers in the development of ozone therapy equipment; veterinarian Heinrich Rahn, pioneer of the use

[3] Baden-Baden, a German city that, for more than 50 years, has held meetings on alternative medicines and what they call natural medicine.

of Huneke's neural therapy in animals; and Dr. Holger Huneke, eldest son of Dr. Ferdinand Huneke, one of the fathers of neural therapy.

In Chap. 18 of this textbook, the approach, principles, and foundations of neural therapy are extensively developed. It focuses on the transformation of Neuraltherapeutic therapy into Neuraltherapeutic medicine and its gradual qualification in Latin America from Colombia. In this approach, the classic mechanistic view of biomedicine is transcended, propelling a paradigm shift from the anthropocentric to a biocentric, integral, and holistic one. This could be applied to the very concept of health-disease-well-being, and in the exercise and methods of individual, collective, and environmental health management.

Later, the NTM, incorporating elements of bio-cybernetics and quantum physics, Russian nervism, and German and English physiology, among other scientific knowledge, was organized at the National University of Colombia as a complex medical system [5–8]. Meanwhile, Dr. Payán's current movement in the southern region of Colombia was advancing philosophically and epistemologically in the area of complex and critical systemic thinking. The social and cultural fact was linked with praxis in processes of health determination, consolidating several milestones that represent significant epistemological, ontological, and hermeneutical turns for alternative medicine in the country. This brought an integrative and non-segmented vision of the living, the active and participatory listening of the patient, the reflexive dialogue of knowledge and ignorance with recognition of non-biomedical cultural and popular knowledge. Also, disease and the phenomena of society, the environment, and life were understood as a dynamic and adaptive learning process with new emerging realities with non-hierarchical relationships in health processes, among others, which frame the biocentric vision of NTM [3]. This approach is based on the individual's own potentiality to self-manage its different biological systems coordinated and integrated by the nervous system (Russian Nervism). In a similar way, the social field would correspond to the communities themselves in their different contexts and territories to manage and self-eco-organize in their health and development.

For MNT, in the health/illness/well-being process, illness and its symptoms arise "as an emerging dynamic process of life, with a self-eco-organized totalizing meaning for the individual" [9]. They become a possibility for the system to recover its vital dynamics in interaction with its environment. This conceptual basis, both doctrinal and physiological, gives rise to the deployment of a diagnostic system based on the patient's life history. Additionally, it paves the way for a therapeutic approach that employs "nonspecific procaine impulses in specific sites, through local, segmental, regional, remote (interfering fields), or systemic infiltrations, for new individual complex biological emergencies" [9–12]. While these approaches differ from those of biomedicine, they can sometimes complement each other, depending on the individual's state of dysfunction or dystrophy.

The doctrine of NTM, as conceived, inherently correlates with the social and ecological environment that encompasses human life and history [9]. In the same vein, the NTM's experience has been centered on its management in the social and community sphere, demonstrating a greater affinity for proposals such as Franco's social medicine [13]. This perspective is oriented towards the search for "good living," and to what Laurel proposes about the study and management of the health-disease of the community as an expression of social processes and not only as biological phenomena of individuals [14].

In this neuraltherapeutic vision of health, the concept of "ground"is considered, on which the processes of self-organization of complex systems are unleashed. In the context of an individual, it is referred to a sort of basic tone of the organism on which the dysfunction or dystrophism (that we call disease) develops. This "ground" is decisive for the result of both reactive care interventions and for promotion and prevention actions, in terms of the generation of comprehensive healthy lifestyle habits (food, physical activity, hydration, sleep, habitat, emotions, family relationships, socioeconomic and political conditions, environmental ecology, among others) [9, 15]. This concept is comparable to that of healthy territory when is referring to community and environmental management, which are in close and indissoluble correlation with life, and as Cerón enunciates, "there is no human health if there is no environmental health" (see Chap. 28) [16].

In the context of Los Robles, it is worth highlighting the tremendous dialogue of knowledge and ignorance aroused between doctors who, from different shores, sought answers in new scientific paradigms. This was due to the fact that the biological and mechanistic vision of the sciences did not satisfy them, and for which Los Robles constituted a propitious scenario. The more than 1700 doctors from all latitudes of Latin America who came to be trained, the dozens of medical students who came regularly to learn and, above all, the growing number of satisfied consultants account for the richness of the process.

Although Los Robles did not project itself massively towards the community in a public health experience, it did open its doors to unconventional knowledge[4] that developed community health experiences in its territories, including what was later the NEHC in Popayán.

2.2 *NTM in Dialogue with Comprehensive Health Care by and for All*

> … Humanity is not sick of fields of interference but of fields of indifference... then it needs another type of needle... which can even be the neuraltherapeutic thinking [17].
>
> Julio Cesar Payán de La Roche (1942–2020)

Primary Health Care (PHC) was born from the clamor and experiences of countries, then considered peripheral, as an example to follow in the world. This was in a context where United Nations agencies were already a space that was beginning

---

[4] In addition to homeopaths, iridologists, dowsers, magnetotherapists, shamans, "Te′Walas", masseurs, spiritists, "jaibanás", African medicines, etc., as well as spiritual healers from India, most of them arrived spontaneously, as if sensing a space of recognition.

to be questioned by the block of non-aligned countries and where it was dreamed of providing health for all in 2000. At the meeting that gave rise to the Declaration of the World Health Organization, among other experiences, those of barefoot doctors in China, Ayurveda in India, and experiences in Tanzania or Peruvian Puno were valued [18].

The concept of PHC was mistranslated, according to Dr. David Tejada de Rivero,[5] who coordinated the entire conference from WHO in 1978. It should be called "comprehensive health care for all and by everyone." This was, in fact, the spirit and the intentionality of Alma-Ata when proposing this strategy for the management of the health of the people, inspired by a broad and today, one could say, complex meaning of health.

In various interviews at the end of his life, Dr. Tejada de Rivero recounted the behind-the-scenes of the change of name to the well-known PHC by the official translators of the United Nations, who refused to give it the initial meaning despite his express request. Furthermore, he mentioned how just after the conference, UNICEF, co-convener of Alma-Ata (and financed more by private companies since then), contributed to limiting the meaning and the goals set. This opens the doors for a distorted implementation between the administrative and the technical, later characterized as selective according to the government's policies of the health systems in the countries [19]. Then, in 2008, the Pan American Health Organization (PAHO) refocused it with more comprehensive models with social participation and the definition of Social Determinants of Health, known as PHC Renewed [20, 21].

In 2017, the Environmental Determinants of Health and the 2030 framework objectives were incorporated [21, 22]. In 2018, with the Declaration of Astana in Kazakhstan, Universal Health Coverage (UHC) and the Sustainable Development Goals (SDGs) were incorporated into the 2030 agenda of "Good Health and Well-being for All" [22]. Despite these modifications, PHC has not been able to respond to the complex social processes that it intended and that implies health understood integrally and as a human right. On the contrary, it appears to be more aligned with the purposes of achieving UHC under insurance models in a framework of generating economic gains from private investment [23], which shapes the health industry crudely described by Waitzkin [24]. This deviation from the fundamental purpose of PHC was evidenced by the First International Conference on Health Promotion in Canada in 1986 and expressed its position in the so-called Ottawa Charter [25]. This charter was oriented towards the social determination of health, based on the recognition of health as a fundamental right for all inhabitants of a territory, and in a participatory way, in the management of the social and environmental determinants of health.

This is how almost all of the world's health systems have abandoned health in its complexity as a fundamental human right. They became aligned with commodification, pharmacologization, and medicalization within the framework of a hegemonic

[5] Dr. Tejada Rivero, a Peruvian physician, was deputy director of the WHO and general coordinator of the International Conference on Primary Health Care in 1978.

model of development that has managed to position itself in an exclusive and preponderant way. This model has become normalized in the imagination of all the actors involved in the health of most public health models.

Care, different from the concept of *attention*, has been assimilated to active providers for passive recipients of services. The concept of *primary* replaced the word *integral* and was translated into an elementary and cheap service for the poor. This service, then, became selective and oriented to programs to control certain risks when the Declaration of Alma-Ata spoke of essential and fundamental.

Health, despite the adjustments in the definitions that have been made by the officiality, has been oriented to the disease. Consequently, PHC, mainly in distant territories, is executed as a peripheral level of auxiliaries who carry out minimal activities of a care type, little preventive and little promotional health, and integral well-being.

From Neuraltherapeutic Medicine, it is intended to contribute to the recovery and development of the original conception of "comprehensive health care by and for all," established in the original spirit of the Declaration of Alma-Ata. This must be understood as an organic participant and participatory strategy to address health as a complex process that leads to the following:

- Realize health as a fundamental human and planetary right.
- Seek to reduce inequities.
- Promote effective solidarity and humanized health service.
- Confront injustices.
- Encompass all so-called levels of care.
- Understand it at all times as a social and political process that includes the determination and social and environmental management of health.
- Adjust it to the realities and social, cultural, environmental, economic, and political differences of each territory.
- Operate in a decentralized manner.
- Move it away from medicalization, pharmacologization, and apparatus in health.
- Understand human and ecosystem health as a tool to promote other possible worlds away from anthropocentrism.
- Recognize and enter into dialogue from the health sciences with other ways of understanding and treating bodies, minds, people, communities, and territories.
- Carry out joint actions with consultants and communities to find solutions to collective health problems and their environmental and social determinants, where health workers can enjoy decent working conditions.

It is in the missionary spirit of Neuraltherapeutic medicine and PHC to work for the highest level of human and environmental health, regardless of the scenario where the profession is practiced, which implies both individual and collective responsibility, conceiving that our work is part of the heart in the framework of the care of life.

The community operational exercise that guided and accompanied the NEHC process used two strategies. These were called by FUNCOP[6] framework events (Fig. 46.2):

> The first was called the Environmental Management and Citizenship event, which sought the promotion of health and social well-being as a vital habitat, with 3 components: public space, healthy environment, and democratic participation. The second event, known as The Health Event, encompassed two key components: health access and medical education. Access to health care was provided through the NEHC, with alternative medicines, especially neural therapy, changes in eating habits, and using methods of popular and participatory health education promoting the recovery of traditional medicines. The management of medical education was provided through the training of alternative doctors from all over the world, both in neural therapy techniques and in alternative thinking under a medical-social conception of health that explored new paradigms [9, 26].

Public health management has become a catalyst for change within the population, and the impact that health personnel have on it is significantly influenced by

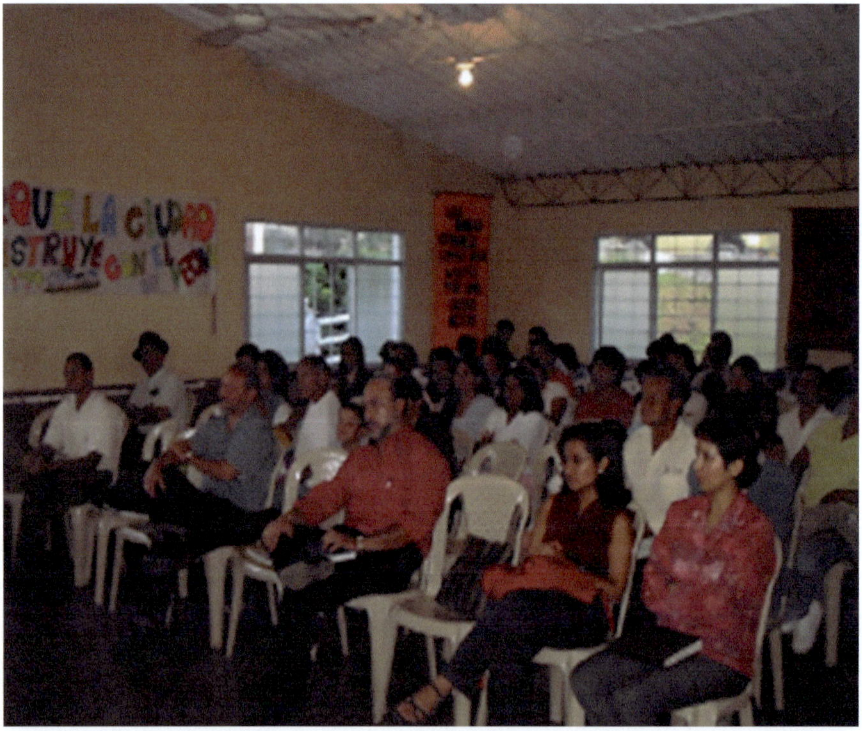

Fig. 46.2 "La Nueva Esperanza" Health Center (NEHC). Dialogues of knowledge. Popayán-Cauca. 1990s. (Source: FUNCOP—Bella M. Calucé [9])

[6] FUNCOP, Foundation for Popular Communication, created informally in the earthquake and formally registered in 1986, an NGO that played an important role in energizing health, education, organic agriculture, and community processes of women throughout the Department of Cauca between 1983 and 2023. She was co-founder of the Viva la Ciudadanía Campaign.

their "health awareness"[27] which is either acquired through their academic training or through their professional experience [9]. In this sense, the comprehensive training processes carried out by Payán in Cauca were especially important. In 2005, included more than 500 health professionals from around the world, 20 national and international events, including the Colloquia and the Eighth International Congress of Neural Therapy and Neurofocal Dentistry [9, 26]. He always had as a basis to sow the seeds of this health awareness, with a critical look at his relationship with public health, which can be seen in the colloquiums he led in Cauca [4, 28]. Here are excerpts from one of his lectures:

> ...it must have a principle of political awareness, when it intends that graduated professionals are linked to the work of the public sphere, where they acquire a critical sense to launch renewed and disruptive proposals of the orthodox, overcoming the reductionist paradigm.—That they link the living as an expression of a universal network.—That they accept that every medical act entails a political stance.—That, beyond fields of interference, they also intervene in fields of social indifference, where inserting a needle also plants a seed of self-recognition and hope. -That they see the doctor-patient relationship as a communal and participatory dialogue, accepting that there are no fixed models, only approaches that allow for flow. -That they embrace an ethics of responsibility and service beyond the barriers of the consultation room. -That they promote health and prevention in a non-imposing and respectful manner. -That they accept chaos and disorder as possible frameworks for biological and social constructs. -That they expose the paradigmatic blindness of anthropocentrism, patriarchy, positivism, mechanistic thinking, reductionist analysis, and above all, consumerism. -That they trust in life, its times, and its rhythms. -That they foster interactions and encounters… [17]

After the WHO included traditional medicines and alternative and complementary therapies within the strategies to improve the health of nations [29, 30], some countries have made progress in its implementation, including regulatory and technical measures [31]. In countries such as Colombia, NTM and other alternative disciplines managed to enter the public and private care systems, mainly in the capitals. Nevertheless, they are restricted to a primarily instrumental utilization of care, which is contingent upon the policies and programs of the government in power or the interests of the entities that provide the health insurance model. Consequently, it is imperative to establish specific state public policies with a broader scope [9].

2.3 The NTM in Dialogue with the Participatory Action Research

Orlando Fals Borda,[7] creator of the Participatory Action Research (PAR) method in its socio-anthropological foundation, remained studying in the USA between 1947 and 1953, when a sector of the academic world questioned the limits of technology

[7] Orlando Fals Borda completed undergraduate studies in English Literature and History at the University of Dubuque, (1947), a master's degree in Sociology from the University of Minnesota in 1953, and a Ph.D. degree in Latin American Sociology from the University of Florida in 1955.

given the impact of the two atomic bombs. At the same time, questioning ideas of a new biology[8] and quantum physics challenged the mechanistic paradigm in knowledge. Upon his return to the country, he brought this body of knowledge and an obsessive question: "How to investigate reality to transform it? Not to leave it printed on a shelf." With such a question on his back, between the 60 s and 70 s, immersed on the back of a mule in the depths of the Caribbean coast, he amassed a transformative sociological and methodological proposal that he called Participatory Action Research, denoting with this fist word a sense of growing continuity to the participation of the actors involved [32].

Paraphrasing Orlando Fals, PAR is a method of study and action that goes hand in hand with an altruistic philosophy of life aimed at obtaining useful and reliable results in the improvement of collective situations. It is multidisciplinary, spanning from the micro to the macro, and develops with a commitment to transform a specific reality. "Participatory-investigative work is both discovery and creation, and it takes place in an epigenetic space. His style is historical and anthropological. It seeks not only to explain but also to improve or reform situations (as is the case with clinical medicine). Therefore, in his holistic epistemology, what is can be defined in the context of the must be" [33].

PAR is a political and scientific instrument that, through a communicative interaction, creates an emergency/action through a dialogue of knowledge and ignorance[9] between actors involved in a given social process (also in the clinic), where everyone learns from each other [34, 35]. In PAR, there is no dichotomy between the subject and the object of research, but rather a situation of omnisubjectivity. That is, it is a relational field where observer-observed (health professional-consultant) are inextricably interaffected. This notion invalidates anthropocentrism in any type of research as much as it challenges the scientific method as the only valid path. The quantum experiment of the double slit has been teaching us that the observer always affects what is observed [36]. This relationship, which involves the observer being observed and the observed observing their observer, results in an action that aims to transform a specific reality. This action or set of actions is the result of this participation in omnisubjectivity.

He was a consultant to the Organization of American States (OAS) in Brazil and director general of the Ministry of Agriculture in Colombia, between 1959 and 1961. Co-founder of the Faculty of Sociology of the National University of Colombia, creator of Participatory Action Research method.

[8] Orlando Fals Borda maintained a friendly relationship with biologist Ernst Mayr, who attended his invitation to the PAR Convergence Congress in Cartagena in 1997.

[9] "The dialogue of knowledge constitutes a pedagogical action that seeks to promote the social construction of knowledge through the exchange of meanings and feelings, which is why it can be presumed that it is an ideal methodology. However, in human and social complexity, it is never possible to know everything about something, which is why it is proposed to introduce the dialogue of ignorance. Ignorance has been stigmatized as something negative when in reality it refers to the recognition of what we do not know, which complements and allows for a true exchange of democratic meanings. For more information, see: http://www.sustentabilidades.usach.cl/sites/sustentable/files/paginas/04-03.pdf

A fundamental tool for this dialogue to take place implies that the intervening actors seek to get to know each other in an authentic way. Also, it implies developing relationships of trust, for which an important step is to carry out a critical recovery of history. This means to review the contexts and epigenetics (a term that Fals Borda already used) [33], which has brought a community (or patient) to the present situation. Fals Borda introduced the concept of "feel-think" in this dialogue as a result of his investigative verification of the significance of permanently connecting, in this bidirectional relationship observer-observed, not only the feeling (such as the patient's arrival, body language, and semiology), but also the mutual thinking in each phase of the consultation and afterwards.

Everything that has touched on vital feel-think throughout individual and community history is important because it frames its own and particular phenomenological meaning. As with the life story of a consultant in a consultation room, the story does not usually end in the first interview. That is to say, history is not a successive static story as we were taught in the classroom.

In order for it to become a critical recovery of history, we must allow the memory of people and individuals to emerge as dialogue-action deepens. It is about understanding the contexts that have left traces and have led individuals and communities to certain situations that need to be transformed (Fig. 46.3). The complexity of life and the multiple factors involved in the evolution of communities and people make it difficult to do a detailed review of the different components of their stories while they are living them. Added to this aspect are the culture, ideologies, media, etc., that have contributed to or influenced them. This critical review in a joint dialogue helps to better understand such situations and, therefore, to direct solutions and accumulate learning. PAR is based on the understanding that societies are constituted in complex systems and are not simple linear phenomena of cause and effect, as is not the case with health. As Orlando Fals explained:

> This broad interdisciplinary position is shared in terms of a 'new philosophy of science' by scientists such as biologist Ernst Mayr [37], by advocating for greater recognition of stochastic processes, the pluralism of causes and effects, the emergence of unanticipated properties, and the internal cohesion of complex systems. For Mayr[10] [37], biological systems are open with homeostatic mechanisms, which leads only to probabilistic prediction, without the classical criteria of validity adopted by purists.

That is, biological knowledge will always be relative and circumstantial.

Both the PAR and the NTM simultaneously ran and continue to run a path of positive feedback. Each one, at a crossroads, encountered complex thinking, quantum physics, and new biology. Each one on its own reached points of confluence, which today we could place in that space that is developing as biocentrism. As expected from a new paradigm, PAR came to put life at the center of its concerns in all environmental, social, economic, political, and cultural dimensions [38, 39]. For the NTM, each moment and individual or collective interaction is a scenario and an opportunity for research and learning to understand the lives of all its actors.

---

[10] Op. cit. [37]. pp. 14, 19.

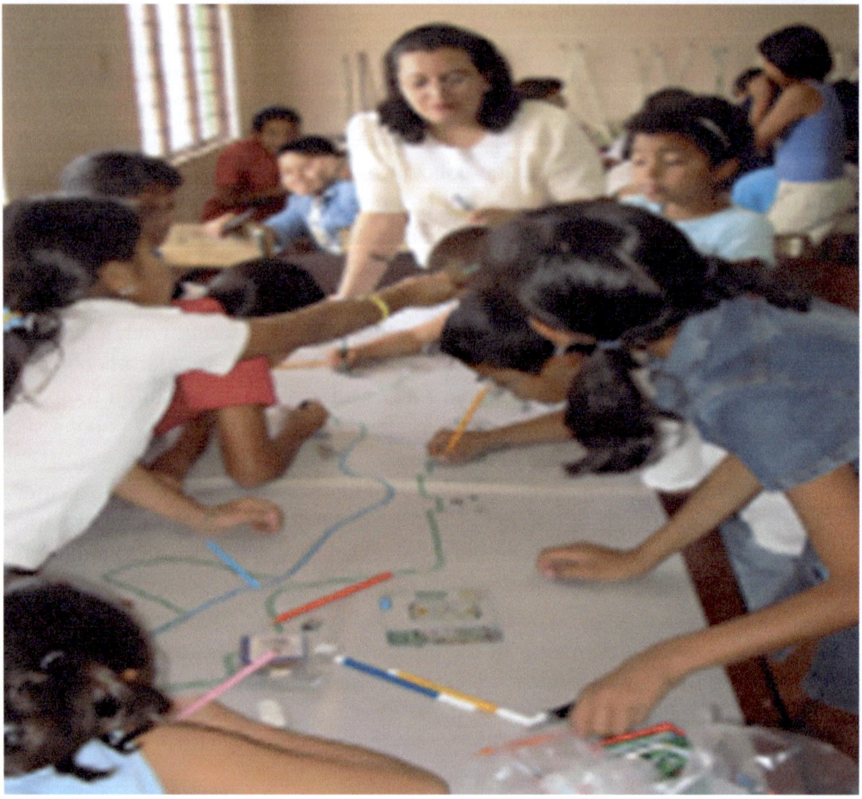

Fig. 46.3 PAR activity—social cartography at the "La Nueva Esperanza" Health Center (NEHC). Popayán-Cauca. 1990s. (Source: FUNCOP—Bella M. Calucé [9])

3 The Experience of the "La Nueva Esperanza" Health Center: Scenario of Construction of the Social Fabric

In March 1983, an earthquake semidestroyed the city of Popayán, capital of the Department of Cauca in southwestern Colombia. It left hundreds of thousands of families homeless, most of them rural migrants who lived in conditions that were already precarious. These families, in the face of the continuity of the earthquakes, occupied several nearby lands in even more disadvantageous conditions, living under plastics and without public services of any nature [9, 26].

From the very day of the earthquake, students from several faculties of the University of Cauca who had worked with Orlando Fals in an experience in northern Cauca turned to support these populations.

With regard to health, health committees were set up, made up of women who had been spontaneously trying to find daily solutions to the social and health crisis generated. Until 1985, under the leadership of these women, care was provided in 7 communities of invasion, with neural therapy, activities developed for prevention, garbage management, searching for water sources, care for infants, and prevention of gender violence. This resulted in an unusual growth of women's organizations in number and empowerment of their rights.

In 1985, in the "Colombia II Stage" neighborhood, an external organization of cooperation built a health center that was closed and not formally handed over to the health system. The women of the neighborhood realized that this center was available and unused. Therefore, they ask FUNCOP for help, an organization recently formed by the aforementioned group of students. In conjunction with the women's association, FUNCOP requests permission from the Departmental Directorate of Health to transfer the experience of care that has been taking place literally "in the open air," to that center. The health system at that time accepted the request. This was the beginning of the formal work of care that this center provided for over two decades, which was not limited to the Municipality of Popayán but also extended to the neighboring Departments of Nariño, Putumayo, Huila, and Caquetá (see Fig. 46.4) [9, 26].

NEHC was the first center to develop a community health experience attended only with NTM. Concurrently, it served as the setting for the School of Thought, which was directed by Dr. Julio Cesar Payán de la Roche, who was a member of the Center for Research in Alternative Medicines—CIMA and the Board of FUNCOP. Payán assumed the scientific coordination of the center, and all the students who came from other parts of the country and Latin America to train in neural

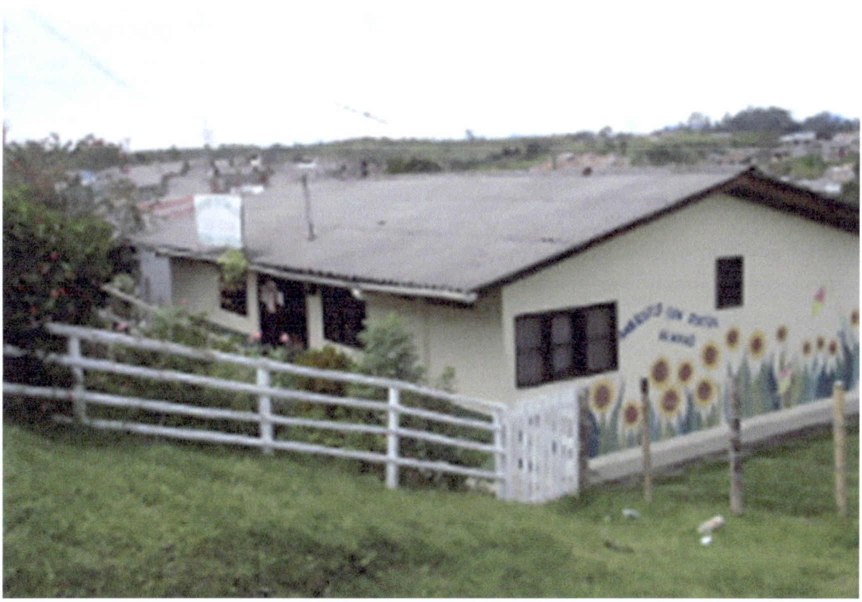

Fig. 46.4 "La Nueva Esperanza" Health Center (NEHC)—gardens and medicinal orchards. Popayán-Cauca. 1990s. (Source: FUNCOP—Bella M. Calucé [9])

therapy in his office passed through the center. Payán consolidated from there an experience of an "educating city"where the epicenter of his proposal and action was both human and environmental health. This proposal came to impact the municipal public policy of the time, ended up strengthening women's organizations, and positioned public health with a holistic approach like nowhere else in the country at the time [9, 26].

Throughout its process, it has had an impact on people and families in the benefited communities. It has also impacted the work teams themselves, in their health, their talents, and their skills in the different roles of society, which could be considered a social neuraltherapeutic impulse [9].

The NEHC was also the setting where PAR, the approach to comprehensive health care by and for all, was embodied, and the foundations of community medicine were revisited. This was an experience promoted by FUNCOP but led in daily life by the Association of Women of the Colombia II Stage Neighborhood. Without this experiential and community-based interweaving, the NTM would not have been enriched by the Latin American contribution of the social determination of health.

The NEHC, in coordination with FUNCOP's community management, developed a community-based urban process that advanced in the building of a civic culture of well-being and life. This had four main perspectives, based on the model of social determination of health under the perspective of social and community medicine in health promotion: (i) *Health*: Alternative medical care and education with critical thinking; (ii) *Environmental*: Public space and healthy environment; (iii) *Local, citizen, and social management*: formation of citizenship, social fabric, and democracy. (iv) *Equity*: Women and gender. In these perspectives, they identify with the postulates of the 1986 Ottawa Charter: peace, shelter, education, food, economic income, a stable ecosystem, sustainable resources, social justice, and equity [9].

From a health perspective, therapeutic assistance was provided through the use of benevolent, efficient, and effective neural therapy, which was characterized by its high resolving power and its support of herbalism. The promotion and prevention programs that were designed to promote the well-being and development of individuals and communities considered relational categories, including life strategies, human rights, sustainable development, socio-historical space, social class, community needs, gender and vulnerable populations, empowerment of public space, and leadership. The following elements were also taken into account in the strengthening of the ground at the individual level, as well as the territory at the collective and environmental levels: healthy eating, healthy agro-ecology, and healthy and responsible habits in the physical, mental, emotional, spiritual, and environmental spheres, among others. PAR interacted directly with community organizational forms and community structures (community action board, women's association, local leaders, schools, and colleges) [9].

In a conjunctural effort during the post-earthquake stage, the NEHC and the local health administration attempted to integrate the NEHC with the PHC in Popayán. Such an endeavor was not possible given the significant differences in approach between the anthropocentrism of the hegemonic official biomedical system and the biocentrism of the NEHC. However, it managed to remain active as a private institution, interacting with the public system to a large extent. This feat was possible because of the acceptance and leadership of the community and the social management of FUNCOP. It was also facilitated by the commitment and persistence of the School of Neural Therapists in southern Colombia, led by Dr. Payán, forming health teams with health awareness and collective management [9].

Finally, the NEHC ends up closing definitively around 2018. This happened after several attempts to survive by resisting the demands of the official health system and its quality assurance system, which never understood the alternative proposal and its contributions to the public health of the territory.

The participation of alternative and complementary medicine, and in particular NTM in public health is necessary, feasible, and accepted by several countries, in some of which it is precisely the prevalent one. In times of crisis, its necessity becomes increasingly apparent, as evidenced by Snowden's analysis prior to the Covid-19 pandemic [40]. He found that it would be more economical and probably more efficient to complement the public health care orientation with the social and community perspective of a promotion and prevention approach. This aspect coincides with what was considered in the foundation of NTM in its systemic-complex approach [9, 15].

The PHC proposal developed at the NEHC was based on the focus on processes of generating comprehensive well-being and not only on the care of the disease. They are described in the Colloquiums of Alternative Medicines and Society, promoted by Payán and Cárdenas with FUNCOP in Popayán in 1991 [4, 26, 41, 42].

The NEHC in the Colombian Cauca territory adopted collective, community, and social medicine approaches, in contrast to the so-called traditional public health developed by the biomedical model [43, 44]. It challenged public health and its main strategies, including PHC, since they fail to develop the original mission objectives, although they have included the social and environmental determinants of the health and well-being of the people.

The NTM, from the foundation and praxis, provides some elements for reflection on public health policies, as follows:

- In addition to guaranteeing coverage and access, it must be asked: What type of medicine is being made available to the community? It should be less drug-dependent medicine and more preventive and comprehensive. It should not deteriorate the "base ground of the individual," nor harm the environment in the territory [45]. It should go beyond the search for statistical compliance of UHC through selective PHC by exposure and probability programs to the risk of the insurance model [23].
- Regarding policies, to guarantee comprehensive health and well-being as a fundamental right, the greatest allocation of public resources should be focused mainly on the promotion of the integral health of communities and the prevention of disease. Such efforts should not ignore the progress and possibilities of technological developments for health care for the sick and injured.

- Health integrality requires involving the community as an active participant in the determination of their health, in the management of the social determinants of health [46].
- It is the right of the entire community to have their alternative knowledge studied and recognized, including the ancestral knowledge and cultural practices in the context of the territories. This approach is referred to as therapeutic pluralism, and it is centered on individuals rather than diseases [47]. It is a practical application of the principle of interculturality, which is based on the exchange of knowledge in order to promote the management of healthy individual, collective, and environmental lands.
- The ideal health human resources to cover a country in collective health promotion management in the territories is generally insufficient, including alternative and complementary medicines, so it is required that the academic training of human resources in health also contemplates, from the undergraduate levels, tools for community and social management of a participatory type such as PAR.
- Comprehensive health policies should not only be developed in hospitals, clinics, and health centers, so they must consider, starting with academic training, other possibilities for health and wellness services in addition to the classic intramural models. Even the home and women with their leadership have become a kind of real first level of care, self-care, and self-medication [48].
- The health management proposed by the NTM, related to health as a right and not as a business as is the case under insurance models, contemplates humanistic mission principles, which must be incorporated into the training of health personnel by developing critical political awareness of the public [17, 26, 27, 41, 42] and avoiding the wise arrogance with which epistemic violence is exercised [16].
- The possibilities of a good practice of alternative medicines in health systems must respect their epistemological foundations as complex medical systems, even adapting the regulations, to avoid their merely instrumental use, as often happens in public and private health institutions, and ultimately be part of market and business models that do not meet the mission objective of public health.

4 Conclusions

In southwestern Colombia, this rich and beautiful experience facilitated the integration of epistemic, practical, social, and political aspects into a single whole, thereby revealing the richness of a network of professionals and communities, as well as of MNT, community health, PHC, and IAP.

As part of the conclusions and lessons that can be derived from this experience, some can be mentioned, as follows:

- The intelligence and commitment of Julio Cesar Payán made it possible to collect and incorporate several elements from these experiences and approaches.

The NTM was enriched and interwoven with these elements, which were derived from the PAR, PHC in its original form, and Latin American social and community medicine.

- The NTM, in its process of advancing in consolidating itself as a complex medical system, which goes beyond the application of an effective medical technique, finds in social and community medicine how to put into practice its missionary principles of service with a biocentric orientation. This approach transcends the constraints of anthropocentrism and positivist frameworks, emphasizing holistic health and well-being through promotion and prevention, aligning with the primary objective of public health. In this case, it could be through the management of the social and environmental determinants of health, with participatory methodologies such as PAR to agree with the community in its own context, and allowing the articulation of environmental protection and the defense and protection of life [49].
- In terms of the care component that accompanies public health for the care of the disease, NTM has a resource with a very efficient and resolute comprehensive approach, with few side effects and low cost. Contrary to the drug dependence and the costly technologies employed by biomedicine, which, while facilitating significant advancements in the treatment of particular diseases, have failed to achieve substantial progress in addressing the multifactorial conditions contributing to the decline in population health.
- Public health management requires the deployment of strategies that, such as PHC, guarantee its implementation and full coverage of the population, processes in which the NTM has elements to contribute. The experience of more than 20 years that the NEHC provided as a practical exercise of the social and community component of this complex medical system showed that it is necessary to allow a deployment with autonomy and respect for the principles and epistemological foundations of its approach. It would allow a free interaction with the hegemonic system, including the elaboration and implementation of a public policy of traditional medicine and alternative and complementary therapies. This policy would facilitate the dialogue of knowledge and the approach with the territorial entities in a permanent intersectoral and transdisciplinary exercise [9].
- The public health systems of nations could improve their impact on the social management of health with greater coverage, participation, and better cost-efficiency. This would be feasible if they expanded their perspective to include other integrative health management systems and organizations, such as NTM, herbalism, traditional, and ancestral medicine, as well as other alternative and complementary therapies, alongside conventional intramural and pharmacological models.
- The incorporation of alternative health services into the public health system, beyond their merely instrumental use, requires expanding the training base of suitable human talent with social and community management skills. This proposal challenges universities and academic institutions, seeking to open up scenarios for scientific research in this field that contribute to society.

- The social and community management of NTM shows the need to develop clear and coherent public policies, not to be imposed but empowered by the community. It was very important that the community itself developed its own mechanisms for participation, organization and agency, such as community boards, groups and associations, institutions, and sectoral associations of a public, private, or mixed nature [45].
- From this experience, the political sense of the NTM was ratified, as Payan called it in his first book, "a committed medicine." The NTM is committed to the idea that health is both individual and collective, which is why it proposes to seek self-eco-socio-organization in practice [49].

References

1. Solorzano LL. The art in body and soul [Internet]. May 2008. Available from: https://www.elespectador.com/entretenimiento/gente/el-arte-en-cuerpo-y-alma-14125/
2. Sarmiento LD. History and institutionalization of neural therapy in Colombia [Master thesis] [Internet]. Universidad Nacional de Colombia. Universidad Nacional de Colombia; 2014. Available from: http://www.bdigital.unal.edu.co/43119/1/52145193.2014.pdf
3. Garzón Fuentes EC. Neuraltherapeutic medicine in Colombia [Internet] [Master Thesis]. Bogotá: Universidad Nacional de Colombia; 2024 [cited 2025 Feb 6]. Available from: https://repositorio.unal.edu.co/handle/unal/87341
4. FUNCOP-CIMA (1991–2005). Proceedings of the Colloquia on Alternative Medicine and Society. Some contents available: Unedited. Popayán, Cauca, Colombia. Retrieved September 2023.
5. Beltrán EH. Neuraltherapeutic medicine: an approach from complex medical systems. Bogotá: Universidad Nacional de Colombia; 2013.
6. Urrego D. Approach to alternative medicine as a complex medical system at the National University of Colombia. Rev Fac Med Univ Nac Colomb. 2010;58(2):155–6.
7. Luz M. Contemporary culture and alternative medicines: new health paradigms at the end of the 20th century. Rev Saude Coletiva. 1997;7(1):13–43.
8. Toscano de La Torre F, Pinilla Bonilla LB. The principles of neural therapy from the fundamentals of Nervism to current neuroscience. Salud UIS J [Internet]. 2012;44(2):57–65. Available from: http://www.scielo.org.co/scielo.php?script=sci_arttext&pid=S0121-08072012000200008
9. Echandía Bocanegra FJ. Analysis of the integration of neuraltherapeutic medicine with primary health care at the Nueva Esperanza alternative health center in Popayán, Cauca from 1987 to 2005. Case Study. [Internet] [Master's Thesis]. Bogotá: Universidad Nacional de Colombia; 2024 [cited 2025 Feb 6]. Available from: https://repositorio.unal.edu.co/handle/unal/85949
10. Fisher L. Neural therapy according to Huneke; neurophysiology, therapeutic injection techniques. 3rd ed. Niño Ibarra MC, editor. Vol. 1. Mexico: Unknown Publisher; 2012. p. 1–261.
11. Payán JC. Vital disobedience. Buenos Aires: Salbe Ediciones; 2005.
12. Oettmeier R, Pinilla L. The procaine-base-infusion: 20 years of experience of an alternative use with several therapeutic effects. HSOA J Altern Complement Integr Med. 2019; https://doi.org/10.24966/ACIM-7562/100061. Available from: https://www.heraldopenaccess.us/article_pdf/9/the-procaine-base-infusion-20-years-of-experi
13. Franco S. For social health. Medellín: Ediciones Aurora; 2017.
14. Laurell AC. The social study of the health-disease process in Latin America. 19th ed. Mexico: Cuadernos Sociales; 1982.

15. ACOLTEN-NTM, CONETSO-JCP. Neural therapy/neuraltherapeutic medicine (NTM) in the context of the pandemic. June 1, 2020. Available from: https://acolten.com.co/wp-content/uploads/2020/07/LA-TERAPIA-NEURAL-MEDICINA-NEURALTERAPEUTICA-NTM-EN-CONTEXTO-DE-PANDEMIA_compressed.pdf
16. Ceron Villaquirán E. From vital disobedience to epistemic disobedience. Bogotá: EAE Publishing; 2017. Available from: https://www.eae-publishing.com/catalog/details//store/es/
17. Payán JC. Public health and neural therapy. 2004. Available from: https://www.youtube.com/watch?v=xnRDsHmkMxQ
18. Tejada de Rivero DA. The history of the Alma-Ata conference. Rev Peru Ginecol Obstet. 2018;64(3):361–6. https://doi.org/10.31403/rpgo.v64i209.
19. Vega R, Acosta N, Mosquera P, Restrepo O. Comprehensive primary health care: a strategy for health system transformation and achieving health equity. Bogotá: Alcaldía Mayor de Bogotá, Universidad Javeriana; 2009.
20. World Health Organization. The renewal of primary health care in the Americas. Position Paper by the Pan American Health Organization/World Health Organization (PAHO/WHO); 2007. Available from: https://www.paho.org/hq/dmdocuments/2010/Renovacion_Atencion_Primaria_Salud_Americas-OPS.pdf
21. PAHO/WHO. Social determinants of health. n.d. Available from: https://www.paho.org/es/temas/determinantes-sociales-salud
22. WHO. Global conference on primary health care. 2018. Available from: https://www.who.int/teams/primary-health-care/conference
23. Latin American Association of Social Medicine – ALAMES. ALAMES declaration on the attempt to absorb PHC into the much-questioned Universal Health Coverage (UHC). Saúde Debate. 2018;42(Special Issue 1):431–3. https://doi.org/10.1590/0103-11042018S129.
24. Waitzkin H. Medicine and public health at the end of empire. 1st ed. New York: Taylor & Francis; 2011. Available from: https://www.taylorfrancis.com/books/edit/10.4324/9781315633473/medicine-public-health-end-empire-howard-waitzkin
25. Canadian Public Health Association. First international conference on health promotion. Ottawa Charter: Canadian Public Health Association; 1986.
26. González Bermúdez N, Jaramillo Molina JA. Popayán, a social process for sustainability. Popayán: FUNCOP-CAUCA, Fondo para la Acción Ambiental, Ecofondo; 2005.
27. Arouca S. The Preventivist Dilemma. Contributions to Understanding and Critique of Preventive Medicine. Región y sociedad. 2008;2. Available from: https://www.scielo.org.mx/pdf/regsoc/v2
28. Payán JC. History and current state of neural therapy in Colombia. 2004. Available from: https://www.terapianeural.com/index2.php?option=com_content&task=emailform&id=95
29. WHO. WHO strategy on traditional medicine 2002-2005. Geneva: WHO; 2002. Available from: https://apps.who.int/iris/bitstream/handle/10665/67314/WHO_EDM_TRM_2002.1_spa.pdf?sequence=1&isAllowed=y.
30. WHO. Strategy on traditional medicine 2014-2024. 2014. Available from: https://apps.who.int/iris/bitstream/handle/10665/95008/9789243506098_spa.pdf
31. Barajas YAJ. Technical guidelines for the integration of alternative and complementary medicines and therapies within the framework of the general system of social security in health. Bogotá: Ministry of Health and Social Protection; 2018. Available from: https://www.minsalud.gov.co/sites/rid/Lists/BibliotecaDigital/RIDE/VS/TH/lineamientos-mtac-sgsss.pdf
32. Fals Borda O. Double history of the coast. Bogotá: Universidad Nacional de Colombia, Banco de la República, El Áncora; 2002.
33. Orlando F. A feel/thinking sociology for Latin America. Bogotá: Siglo del Hombre Editores, CLACSO; 2009. p. 312.
34. Borda F. Participatory research and rural Praxis. Bogotá: Punta de Lanza; 1979.
35. Fals Borda O. How to investigate reality to transform it. 1979. Available from: http://biblioteca.clacso.edu.ar/clacso/se/20160308051848/09como.pdf
36. Penrose R. The emperor's new mind. Barcelona: Grijalbo Mondadori; 1991.

37. Mayr E. Toward a new philosophy of biology. Cambridge: Harvard University Press; 1988. p. 21.
38. Ortiz MB. Participatory action research: Fals Borda's contribution to popular education. Espacio Abierto. 1992;17(4):615–27.
39. Wikipedia contributors. Participatory action research [Internet]. Wikipedia. 2025. Available from: https://en.wikipedia.org/wiki/Participatory_action_research
40. Snowden F. Epidemics and society: from the black death to the present. Yale University Press; 2019. Available from: https://history.yale.edu/publications/epidemics-and-society-black-death-p.
41. FUNCOP. Medicine, ecology, and society: critical foundations for alternative thinking. Popayán: FUNCOP Editions; 1991.
42. Cárdenas JJ. Public health for all. Neural therapy course booklet. Popayán: FUNCOP; 2004. Available from: https://acolten.com.co/wp-content/uploads/2025/02/COLOQUIO-Dr.-Payan.pdf
43. Morales M. Collective health and public health: are they talking about the same thing? 18 Doctoral Course Notebooks. 1st ed. 2016;16–30. Available from: https://medicina.bogota.unal.edu.co/facultad/consejo-de-facultad/actas-cf/category/46-adelantos-editoriales?download=869:investigacion-en-salud-colectiva-entre-ciencias-sociales-y-ciencias-de-la-salud
44. Hernández LJ, Ocampo J. The WHO model as a guide in public health based on social determinants. Rev Salud Pública. 2017;19(3):393–5. Available from: http://www.scielo.org.co/scielo.php?script=sci_arttext&pid=S0124-00642017000300393&lng=en. https://doi.org/10.15446/rsap.v19n3.68470.
45. FUNCOP. Inclusive health video: a contribution of neural therapy for building healthy public policies. Popayán: FUNCOP; 2003. Available from: https://drive.google.com/file/d/13JBJKCPPqqbIOg9re5AdpaBoM6J8eGCL/view
46. Sánchez LV. Social determination vs social determinants: reflections from the perspective of critical epidemiology. [cited 2024 Feb 25];38–51. Available from: https://revistainclusiones.org/index.php/inclu/article/view/2047
47. Carvalho IMS. Experiences and reflections on traditional, complementary, and integrative medicines in health systems of the Americas. 2021. Available from: https://docs.bvsalud.org/biblioref/2021/03/1151530/mtci-america-observapics-rede-mtci.pdf
48. Menéndez E. Care models for ailments: theoretical exclusions and practical integrations. Ciênc Saúde Coletiva [Internet]. 2003;8(1):185–207. https://doi.org/10.1590/S1413-81232003000100014
49. Declaration of Colombia 2022. Bogotá D.C.: ACOLTEN; 2022. Available from: https://acolten.com.co/declaration-of-colombia-2022/

Declaration of Colombia 2022[1]

In the 19 years since the Declaration of Colombia emerged from the First World Meeting of Neural Therapy and Neurofocal Dentistry, held in Bogotá, several conceptual, scientific, and academic transformations in the fields of medicine and dentistry have also emerged. This Third International Congress of Neuraltherapeutic Medicine and Neurofocal Dentistry was conceived to reflect these changes in our profession.

From Neural Therapy to Neuraltherapeutic Medicine

Colombia is the birthplace of the "Complex Systemic School." Through the academic framework developed in the Master's Program at the National University of Colombia, Neural Therapy has experienced a transformation important enough to warrant the proposal of a new designation for our discipline: Neuraltherapeutic Medicine. This name has been accepted by the Ministry of Health. The conception of this medical system transcends the idea that Neural Therapy is simply a system of procaine injections. It represents a new epistemological approach, a biocentric cosmology that is consistent with the ideas of Dr. Julio Cesar Payán.

This approach, which also follows the principles of the Russian and British Nervism schools, conceives of the nervous system as the coordinator of all pathophysiological states in the organism. It suggests that health and disease are

[1] Asociación Colombiana de Terapia Neural/Medicina Neuralterapéutica (ACOLTEN), Asociación Colombiana de Terapia neural Julio César Payán de la Roche (CONETSO), Asociación de Odontólogos neurofocales de Colombia (ODNF). Third International Congress of Neuraltherapeutic Medicine and Neurofocal Dentistry, Bogotá, October 6–8, 2022. Bogotá: ACOLTEN, 2022. Available from: https://acolten.com.co/declaration-of-colombia-2022/

L. B. Pinilla Bonilla et al. (eds.), *Neuraltherapeutic Medicine*,
https://doi.org/10.1007/978-3-032-03257-7

cybernetic, dynamic, nonlinear, and self-organizing processes. It also involves an integrative conception of the body in which the health of the oral cavity is relevant to the whole.

Its teachings include an interpersonal and intercultural perspective, with an understanding that the health of an individual, or that of a community, is dependent on nonhierarchical relationships with regard to cultural orientation and gender.

Additionally, it assumes a critical and proactive perspective within the field of public health which promotes the autonomy of individuals and communities, respecting a diversity of cultures and beliefs. This new understanding of the contextual process of health and disease suggests a need for reassessment of public policies.

This pedagogic guidance has been built from respectful dialogues designed to overcome relationships based on hierarchical authority. It recognizes collaborative learning processes, and the development of knowledge through critical and creative thinking.

Neuraltherapeutic Medicine and the New Paradigms

Neuraltherapeutic Medicine is built upon a particular academic, social, and scientific approach. The biocentric nature of this approach implies that it supports the preservation of life. It assumes the union of body and mind, objective and subjective, without divisions. It conceives of the complexity of life and its emergent properties as an open, thermodynamic, autopoietic process that highlights the self-organizing, nonhierarchical interdependencies of all living beings in nature and the cosmos.

This approach recognizes that health and disease are not opposites, but integral parts of life itself. As Hippocrates said, "there are no diseases, but people who are ill." The state of health of any individual, or any community, is unique.

Neuraltherapeutic Medicine recognizes that individuals became human through relationships with others. Our social lives are inherent to our humanity. The strong coupling of humans to others, and to the environment suggests the phrase, "I am because we are." The ethics which guide Neuraltherapeutic Medicine reflect the "inter-self," which represents inclusion, recognition, respect, and social and cultural visibility. It seeks to retain an ecology of knowledge, with open dialogue between cultures. Neuraltherapeutic Medicine comes from a place of love, from heart–mind, and from human dignity.

Global Perspectives: Public and Environmental Health

There is no human health without environmental health. Climate scientists for the United Nations insist that the situation facing human and environmental health is increasing in seriousness, threatening an extinction of all life. Due to globalization, health care access has become an example of the politics of inequality, and our current systems are unprepared for our future challenges. Neuraltherapeutic Medicine recognizes the interdependence of humans with the health of the planetary biomass. That is why we repeat, privately and publicly, the assertion that human health is a fundamental right.

Health is a dialectic process encompassing biology, sociology, the individual, and the universe. As Julio Cesar Payán said, health is "an adaptive process within a society, (encompassing its) cultural, political, economic, environmental, vital, and historic processes." From this perspective, Neuraltherapeutic Medicine has emerged as a response to the societal need for health, understanding that the individual represents a node in the network of social relationships, influence, and feedback.

In this context, Neuraltherapeutic Medicine supports the claim from the 1978 Alma Ata WHO Conference that future decision-making in primary health care will require increased participation of individuals and their communities as the needs for healthy food, climate change mitigation, and protection of soils and biomass, accelerate. Hence, the recognition of health as a fundamental human right is an unwavering commitment. The neuraltherapeutic approach should be loving, caring, and ethical for the individual, for the planet, and, as Dr. Payán used to say, for Andromeda.

About the Training in Neuraltherapeutic Medicine

Education in neuraltherapeutic medicine originated in the informal, warm settings of rural states, private offices, and conferences that allowed for such a complex doctrine to emerge. Since the 1970s, these schools of thought were developed in Colombia and Latin America under the leadership of Dr. Julio Cesar Payán. Several of the aforementioned paradigmatic and scientific concepts were integrated into his teaching, including the recognition of neurofocal dentistry, thanks to the collaborative work of both the medical doctors and dentists in the field of neural therapy.

Nowadays, at the fundamental core of neural therapy's identity is a complex medical system that is concerned with the deeper dimensions of social and political health in addition to those of clinical investigation. So, this is an invitation to the guild of neuraltherapeutic practitioners to continue teaching from this reflexive, self-critical, and collaborative perspective. As Julio Cesar often repeated, a loving, ethical, academic path that accepts both our knowledge and our ignorance gives us hope for the future of life.

Index

L. B. Pinilla Bonilla et al. (eds.), *Neuraltherapeutic Medicine*,
https://doi.org/10.1007/978-3-032-03257-7

D

E

O

P

W